PHYSIOLOGY
Prep Manual for Undergraduates

PHYSIOLOGY
Prep Manual for Undergraduates

FIFTH EDITION

Vijaya D Joshi, MD
Ex Professor and Head
Department of Physiology
Dr DY Patil Medical College
Nerul, Navi Mumbai, India
Formerly, Professor of Physiology
Seth GS Medical College, Parel, Mumbai

Sadhana Joshi-Mendhurwar, MD
Professor
Department of Physiology
Dr DY Patil Medical College
Nerul, Navi Mumbai, India

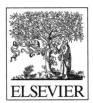

ELSEVIER
A division of
Reed Elsevier India Private Limited

Physiology: Prep Manual for Undergraduates, 5e
Joshi & Joshi-Mendhurwar

©2014 Reed Elsevier India Private Limited

First Edition 1995
Second Edition 2001
Third Edition 2005
Fourth Edition 2010
Fifth Edition 2014

ISBN: 978-81-312-3629-1
e-book ISBN: 978-81-312-3873-8

Notices

Knowledge and best practice in this field are constantly changing. As new research and experience broaden our understanding, changes in research methods, professional practices, or medical treatment may become necessary.

Practitioners and researchers must always rely on their own experience and knowledge in evaluating and using any information, methods, compounds, or experiments described herein. In using such information or methods they should be mindful of their own safety and the safety of others, including parties for whom they have a professional responsibility.

With respect to any drug or pharmaceutical products identified, readers are advised to check the most current information provided (i) on procedures featured or (ii) by the manufacturer of each product to be administered, to verify the recommended dose or formula, the method and duration of administration, and contraindications. It is the responsibility of practitioners, relying on their own experience and knowledge of their patients, to make diagnoses, to determine dosages and the best treatment for each individual patient, and to take all appropriate safety precautions.

To the fullest extent of the law, neither the Publisher nor the authors, contributors, or editors, assume any liability for any injury and/or damage to persons or property as a matter of products liability, negligence or otherwise, or from any use or operation of any methods, products, instructions, or ideas contained in the material herein.

Please consult full prescribing information before issuing prescription for any product mentioned in this publication.

The Publisher

Published by Reed Elsevier India Private Limited
Registered Office: 305, Rohit House, 3 Tolstoy Marg, New Delhi-110 001
Corporate Office: 14th Floor, Building No. 10B, DLF Cyber City, Phase II, Gurgaon-122 002, Haryana, India

Senior Project Manager-Education Solutions: Shabina Nasim
Content Strategist: Renu Rawat
Project Coordinator: Goldy Bhatnagar
Sr Operations Manager: Sunil Kumar
Production Manager: NC Pant
Sr Production Executive: Ravinder Sharma
Sr Graphic Designer: Milind Majgaonkar

Typeset by GW India

Printed and bound in India at EIH Ltd – Unit Printing Press (Manesar, Haryana)

Dedicated
to
Dr DV Joshi

Foreword

It gives me great pleasure in writing the foreword for this book. Physiology is one of the basic medical sciences which needs to be thoroughly studied by medical students for proper understanding of the clinical subjects, particularly pathology, pharmacology and medicine. This subject is so vast that students often find it difficult to revise it adequately from large textbooks before examinations. There has been a long felt need for a book which is concise and covers the subject in a format that provides quick revision and easy comprehension.

It is my belief that Dr Vijaya Joshi's book in the present form should meet the requirements of the students fully, both for theory and viva-voce examinations. All the topics are comprehensively covered in a simplified way. The author has made an attempt to systematically analyse and present the relevant data in question and answer form. Another strength of the book is the large number of excellent line drawings that should assist in comprehending the subject with ease. The students will therefore find it very helpful in revising the subject quickly and facing the examinations with confidence.

This book will also be useful for dental, paramedical, physiotherapy, homeopathy and ayurvedic students.

A lot of meticulous work seems to have gone into preparing this book for which Dr Vijaya Joshi deserves all praise.

I wish this book all success.

Dr PB Patil
President, Terna Charitable Trust
Formerly, Minister of Energy and Irrigation
Government of Maharashtra

Preface to the Fifth Edition

We are pleased to write the Fifth Edition of this book. In addition to our recommended updates, this revision incorporates feedback, suggestions and requests from faculty, students and readers. Accordingly, appropriate modifications have been incorporated to make this edition crisper and more focused towards students preparing for their examinations. Some of these modifications include:

1. To improve understandability and aid memorization, key contents have been tabulated and suitably referenced.
2. To help students achieve the most in least time, extraneous and unimportant matter has been pruned. However, in some chapters, e.g. Central Nervous System, many new questions are included.
3. Prioritization of overall content, in line with typical assessment expectations. Chapter Nutrition is completely omitted.

We hope students will appreciate the changes, and find this edition beneficial. Any suggestions from the readers will be highly appreciated.

Vijaya D Joshi
Sadhana Joshi-Mendhurwar

Preface to the First Edition

The curriculum of physiology for the medical students is very vast and the time available for its study is comparatively short. Students have to prepare for theory as well as viva-voce examinations. In viva examination, the students have to answer several questions within a short time and the answers must be precise and correct to secure good marks. With my experience as an examiner over the years, I have noticed that many students find it difficult to answer the theory paper properly and complete it within the stipulated time. All this has prompted me to write this manual in concise form to facilitate preparation of the students both for viva and theory examinations. I would, however, like to emphasize that it is not intended as a textbook on physiology but a supplement for revision purposes.

The book is divided into fourteen chapters and covers all important topics. The important points in each topic are reviewed. Each topic is described in the form of questions and answers. The book is written in a simple and easy to understand language. Wherever possible the information is given in the form of tables and flowcharts. It is well illustrated.

I feel that, at the time of examination, the students will be able to revise the subject quickly with the help of this manual. It would also be useful for post-graduate entrance examinations.

I do hope the students will appreciate this book as a resource for securing good marks in the examination. Any suggestions, comments from the readers will be highly appreciated.

I am very much thankful to Dr PB Patil (President, Terna Public Charitable Trust) and Dr (Smt) CP Patil for giving me permission to write this book. I wish to express my sincere gratitude to (Smt) Sushma R Apte and Mr RP Apte for their valuable help in preparing the manuscript.

I am grateful to B.I. Churchill Livingstone for their valuable suggestions, supplying the line drawings and publishing this book in a professional manner.

Vijaya D Joshi

Contents

CHAPTER 1
The Cell and General Physiology

CELL AND CELL ORGANELLES

What is a cell?

Cell is a basic living unit of the body. Each cell is enveloped by a cell membrane. Fluid inside the cell is termed cytoplasm. Cytoplasm contains minute and large dispersed particles and organelles. The clear fluid portion of cytoplasm in which organelles are suspended is termed 'cytosol'.

What is protoplasm?

The different substances that make up the cell are collectively called protoplasm. Protoplasm is mainly composed of water, electrolytes, proteins, lipids and carbohydrates.

Describe the structure of cell membrane.

The cell membrane measures 75 nm in thickness. It is composed mainly of lipids, proteins and carbohydrates.

1. *Lipids.* Basic structure of a membrane is a lipid bilayer (2 molecules thick), which is continuous over the entire cell surface. This lipid bilayer is composed of phospholipid and cholesterol. Each lipid molecule has one hydrophilic part which is soluble in water and other hydrophobic part which is soluble in lipid. In phospholipid molecule phosphate part is hydrophilic and fatty acid radicals are hydrophobic. In cholesterol molecule hydroxyl radical is hydrophilic and steroid nucleus is hydrophobic.

Because hydrophobic portions of both these molecules are repelled by water, they have a natural tendency to line up, occupying the centre of the membrane. Hydrophilic portions project to two surfaces (inside and outside of the cell).

The membrane lipid bilayer is the major barrier to usual water soluble substances (e.g. urea, glucose, ions). Fat soluble substances such as alcohol, CO_2, O_2 can easily penetrate through lipid bilayer.

2. *Proteins.* Proteins of the membrane are of two types:
   - Integral proteins
   - Peripheral proteins

Integral proteins. At intervals, lipid bilayer is replaced by globular proteins known as integral proteins. They act as channels (pores) for passage of water soluble substances.

Integral proteins have selective properties causing preferential diffusion of certain substances more than others. Some integral proteins act as carriers allowing active transport of certain substances. Some integral proteins act as enzymes.

Peripheral proteins. They are present mostly on the inside surface of the membrane, attached to integral proteins. They act as enzymes.

   3. **Carbohydrates.** Carbohydrates are mainly present in combination with lipid (as glycolipids) or in combination with proteins (as glycoproteins). Some integral proteins are glycoproteins and about one-tenth lipid molecules are glycolipids.

Other important carbohydrate compounds are proteoglycans which are mainly carbohydrate substances bound together by small protein cores. They form a loose carbohydrate coat which covers the entire surface of the cell. This coat is termed glycocalyx.

The functions of carbohydrate moieties are as follows:

- Because of their negative charges they give cell an overall negative surface that repels other negative objects.
- Glycocalyx causes attachment of cells to each other.
- Many carbohydrates act as receptor substances for binding hormones like insulin.
- Some carbohydrates enter into immune reactions.

What are the functions of cell membrane?

1. Acts as a selective barrier allowing some molecules to cross, excluding others. Thus it regulates the passage of substances in and out of the cell and hence separates two aqueous compartments of dissimilar compositions.
2. Plays important role in receiving chemical signals from other cells by detecting the chemical messenger arriving at the cell surface.
3. Links adjacent cells together.
4. Provides sites for attachment of protein filaments associated with generation and transmission of force to the cell surface.

Name the different cytoplasmic organelles and enumerate their functions.

For details see Table 1.1.

CELL DIVISION

What are the types of cell division?

Cell division is of two types:

  (a) Mitosis
  (b) Meiotic

In mitosis number of chromosomes in two daughter cells remains the same as that of a parent cell (i.e. diploid cells are formed).

In meiotic division, number chromosomes is halved (becomes half) and haploid cells are formed.

Table 1.1 Cytoplasmic Organelles and Their Functions	
Name (Figure 1.1)	**Functions**
Nucleus with nuclear membrane	1. The nucleus is the main control centre of the cell. It controls the rate of different chemical reactions occurring in the cell. 2. Responsible for transmission and expression of genetic information. 3. Chromatin is a network of threads present in the nucleus. It is composed of DNA and proteins. 4. Chromosomes are fine thread-like structures formed from chromatin at the time of cell division. They store genetic information and pass it over from cell to cell each time when a cell divides. There are 46 (23 pairs) chromosomes in the cell. Out of these 44 (22 pairs) are somatic chromosomes and 2 (1 pair) sex chromosomes.
Centrioles	Initiates the process of cell division.
Granular (with ribosomes) and smooth (without ribosomes) endoplasmic reticulum	• Transports substances from one part of the cell to the other. Granular • Granular endoplasmic reticulum (with ribosomes) is involved in packaging of proteins that are secreted by the cell. Ribosomes are small granular structures attached to endoplasmic reticulum. They are composed of ribonucleic acid (RNA) and proteins. They do the function of protein synthesis. Smooth • Smooth endoplasmic reticulum (without ribosomes) is the site of lipid synthesis. • Smooth endoplasmic reticulum contains enzymes controlling glycogen breakdown. • Smooth endoplasmic reticulum also contains enzymes capable of detoxifying substances that are damaging to the cell.

Continued

Table 1.1	Cytoplasmic Organelles and Their Functions—cont'd
Name (Figure 1.1)	**Functions**
Mitochondria	Mitochondria are 'power houses' of the cell. Almost all oxidative reactions occur inside the mitochondria and energy that is released is used to form high energy compound termed ATP (adenosine triphosphate). This ATP is stored in the mitochondria and is made available for supplying energy for different functions of the cell.
Golgi apparatus	1. Site for concentration of proteins and polysaccharides. 2. Sorts out the different types of proteins received from endoplasmic reticulum into vesicles which are delivered to the various parts of the cell. Vesicles delivered to plasma membrane release their protein contents outside the cell. They are known as secretory vesicles. 3. Site for completion of synthesis of carbohydrate moiety of glycoproteins which are major components of ground substance in the interstitial spaces.
Lysosomes	Lysosomes are a highly specialized intracellular digestive system. They contain about 50 different hydrolytic enzymes. They breakdown bacteria and debris from dead tissue cells that have been taken into the cell. They play important role in various specialized cells that make up defence system of the body.
Peroxisomes	Peroxisomes contain oxidases. They destroy certain products formed from oxygen, notably hydrogen peroxide that can be toxic to the cell.
Filament and tubular structures of cell, e.g. cilium, flagellum	The fibrillar proteins of the cell are organized into filaments or tubules. These originate as precursor protein molecules synthesized by ribosomes in cytoplasm. The precursor molecules then polymerize to form filaments.
Microtubules	Main function of microtubules is to act as a cytoskeleton to provide rigid physical structures for some parts of cells. A specific type of shift filament composed of polymerized tubulin molecules is used to construct strong tubular structures called microtubules.

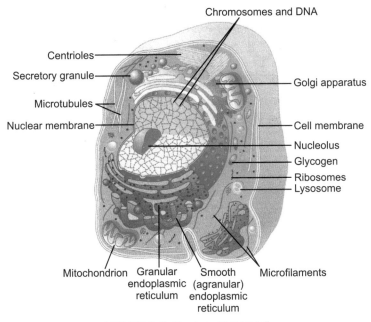

FIGURE 1.1 Structure of typical cell.

CELL DEATH

What is apoptosis?

It is a process of programmed cell death in which body cells die and get phagocytosed (absorbed) under genetic control.

SIGNIFICANCE

- It is responsible for removal of inappropriate clones of immune cells.
- Important in degeneration and regeneration of neurons within central nervous system and for formation of synapse.
- Is responsible for cyclical shedding of endometrium at the time of menstruation.

Abnormal apoptosis is seen in cancers, autoimmune diseases, etc.

What is a tissue?

Collection of cells having same structure and function is termed tissue.

HOMEOSTASIS

What is 'milieu interieur'?

Cells live in the environment of extracellular fluid and this extracellular fluid is called 'milieu interieur'.

Define homeostasis.

Homeostasis means maintenance of static or constant conditions in the internal environment of cells.

Explain the role of various systems of the body in homeostasis.

Homeostasis, i.e. maintenance of constant conditions in the internal environment (extracellular fluid) is very essential for normal functioning of various cells.

The following factors must be maintained for homeostasis:

- pH
- Temperature
- Electrolyte concentrations
- Supply of nutrients
- Supply of O_2
- Hormone levels
- Metabolic end products
- Water content

Almost all systems of the body are involved in maintenance of internal environment.

1. *Circulatory system.* Nutrients and O_2 from extracellular fluid are constantly utilized by the cells. Waste products from the cell constantly diffuse from cells to the extracellular fluid. This changes the composition of extracellular fluid. For maintaining constancy in this fluid, the body has circulatory system which causes constant flow of blood to various tissues. In tissues, blood passes through capillaries which are thin walled and can cause exchange of materials very easily. There is diffusion of nutrients and O_2 from blood to interstitial fluid and the waste products in the opposite direction. Also there is a constant exchange of fluid from blood and extracellular fluid. Small amount of protein-free plasma comes out of capillaries at the arterial end and almost equal quantity is absorbed at the venous end. Thus circulatory system causes circulation of blood to different tissues and allows constant exchange of materials between blood and the interstitial fluid.

2. *Respiratory system.* Blood is also circulated to lungs. It picks up O_2 in the alveoli needed for the cell. CO_2 from blood diffuses out in alveoli of lungs for excretion.

3. *Gastrointestinal tract.* Large amount of blood is pumped by the heart to the wall of gastrointestinal tract. Here different digested materials such as amino acids, fatty acids, glucose, etc. are absorbed from lumens of the gastrointestinal tract into the blood. Thus nutrients required for cells are obtained. All the substances which are absorbed may not be utilized by the cells. The absorbed substances first pass to the liver which changes the chemical compositions of some of them and make them utilizable by the tissue cells. Liver can also store the excess materials for future use.

4. *Musculoskeletal system.* This allows the person to move to appropriate places either for obtaining food, water or for protection against adverse surroundings.

5. *Kidneys.* Water and water soluble waste products are selected from the blood and are excreted by kidneys in urine. Kidneys assist in the maintenance of water balance, electrolyte balance with the help of endocrine system. Kidneys also help in regulation of pH of the extracellular fluid.

6. *Hormonal system (Endocrine glands).* Each endocrine gland secretes hormone or hormones, which are transported to all the parts of the body in the extracellular fluid. Hormones regulate metabolic functions of different body cells, e.g. insulin controls glucose metabolism. Adrenocortical hormones control levels of different ions and protein metabolism. Parathyroid hormone controls calcium level of extracellular fluid and also the bone metabolism.

7. *Nervous system.* It is composed of the sensory portion, the central nervous system (CNS) which is the integrator, and the motor portion.

Sensory portion receives information from the surroundings, e.g. eyes give visual image of the surrounding area, ears hear the sounds.

Brain and spinal cord form the CNS which collects and stores the information received from sensory portion, can generate thoughts, determines the plan of action in response to sensory stimulation.

Motor system receives information from brain and spinal cord about its plan of action and the actions are actually executed by the motor system (which mainly supplies skeletal muscles and causes movements as desired by the person).

8. *Reproductive system.* It helps to maintain static conditions by generating new beings to take the place of ones that are dying.

Different systems involved in homeostasis operate through two feedback mechanisms, viz. (a) negative and (b) positive.

(a) *Negative feedback mechanism.* Most of the control systems of the body act by this mechanism.

If there is any change in the output of the systems, the effects of the change are made to known (feedback) to the sensor which initiates the sequence of events. In negative feedback system, increase in output of a system results in a decrease in the input leading to stability of the system. If some factors become excessive or too little, control system initiates a feedback which tends to push the factors in the direction opposite (negative) to the direction of original change, e.g. a decrease in body temperature leads to responses which tend to increase body temperature, i.e. return it to original value. Negative feedback is the most common homeostatic mechanism in the body as it is capable of causing stability of an internal environment variable (factor). Homeostatic control mechanisms cannot maintain complete constancy of any given factor of internal environment. Therefore, any regulatory factor (variable) will have a narrow range of normal values.

Gain of a control system. The degree of effectiveness with which the control system maintains constant conditions is expressed by a gain of the negative feedback control system.

$$\text{Gain} = \frac{\text{Correction}}{\text{Error}}$$

For example, baroreceptor system controls arterial blood pressure. Normal level of arterial blood pressure is 100 mmHg. If any factor changes it to 175 mmHg, baroreceptor system starts functioning and causes correction so that blood pressure falls to 125 mmHg (instead of 100 mmHg which is normal). Thus, feedback control system has caused the correction of -50 mmHg (from 175 to 125 mmHg) but error of 25 mm of Hg still remains. Therefore, gain of this system becomes -50 mmHg/25 mmHg $= -2$. This means if any extraneous factor tends to change arterial blood pressure can do so only one third as much as would occur if this control system were not present.

(b) *Positive feedback mechanism.* In this the initial disturbance in the system sets off a train of events that increases the disturbance even further. Thus positive feedback does not favour stability and often displaces a steady state away from its steady state operating point. Positive feedback is therefore also known as 'vicious cycle'. A mild degree of positive feedback can be overcome by negative feedback control mechanisms of the body and thus a vicious cycle fails to develop.

Example of a positive feedback is the release of oxytocin hormone on stretching of cervix of uterus at the time of labour. This positive feedback occurs as follows:

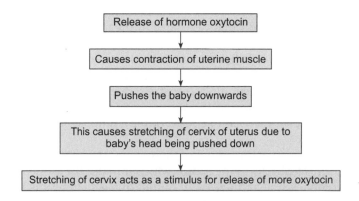

This positive feedback leads to a vicious cycle which causes greater and greater oxytocin secretion leading to greater and greater contraction of uterine muscle, ultimately leading to delivery of the baby.

Another example is the blood clotting mechanism which is a very useful positive feedback. When a blood vessel is ruptured, multiple enzymes called clotting factors are activated. Some of these enzymes act on other yet inactivated enzymes of the immediately adjacent blood, activating them and causing still more clot. This process continues until the hole in the vessel is plugged by the clot and bleeding no longer occurs.

TRANSPORT ACROSS THE CELL MEMBRANE

Enumerate the different transport mechanisms which transport substances through the cell membrane.

Different transport mechanisms (Fig. 1.2) are classified as follows:

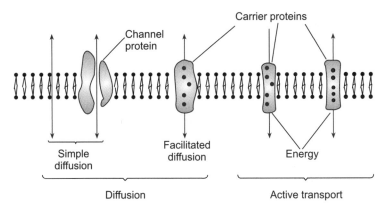

FIGURE 1.2 Transport pathways through the cell membrane.

Enumerate the different transport mechanisms (Chart 1.1).

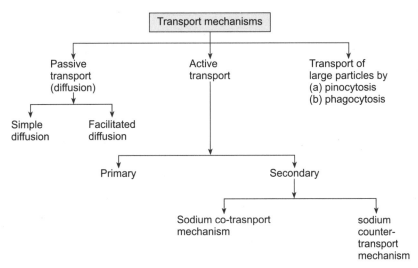

CHART 1.1 Different transport mechanisms.

What is passive transport or diffusion?

Passive transport is the transport of a substance along the electrochemical gradient. It occurs by diffusion of molecules and does not require energy.

What is active transport?

Active transport is the transport of a substance against electrochemical gradient. It requires energy as it has to transport the substance uphill (against the gradient).

SIMPLE DIFFUSION

What is simple diffusion?

The random thermal motion of the molecules in a liquid (or a gas) that tends to re-distribute them uniformly throughout the liquid is called simple diffusion. Simple diffusion of a substance through cell membrane occurs from higher to lower concentration simply due to thermal motion of molecules. It does not require a carrier.

Enumerate the substances which pass through the cell membrane by simple diffusion.

Substances passing through the lipid bilayer of the cell membrane by simple diffusion are:

- All lipid soluble substances.
- Lipid soluble gases mainly CO_2, O_2 and N_2.
- Though water is not lipid soluble still it passes quickly through lipid bilayer because of its small molecular size and high kinetic energy. Water molecules pass like a bullet through the lipid bilayer before hydrophobic character of lipid can stop them.

Substances passing through the protein channels of the cell membrane by simple diffusion are:

- Ions mainly Na^+, K^+ and Ca^{++}.
- Water molecules.

Why ions, though of smaller size, cannot diffuse through lipid bilayer?

Ions cannot diffuse through lipid bilayer because of the presence of electric charge. Electric charge impedes the passage in two ways:

1. Electric charge of ion causes multiple water molecules to become bonded with the ion to form hydrated ion. This increases the size of the ion.
2. Each half of lipid bilayer is formed of polar lipids having either negative or positive charges. By these, both negatively as well as positively charged ions are repelled.

What are the characteristics of protein channels?

1. Selective permeability (e.g. channels through which mainly sodium ions can pass are called sodium channels).
2. Many channels are opened or closed by gates.

How is opening or closing of gates of protein channels controlled?

There are two mechanisms controlling opening or closing of protein channels (Fig. 1.3).

1. *Voltage gating.* Opening or closing of gates depends on the voltage across the cell membrane.

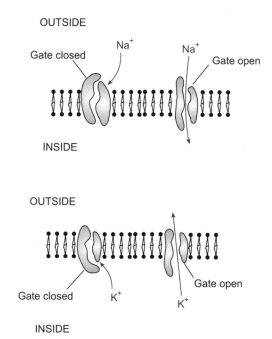

FIGURE 1.3 Transport of Na$^+$ and K$^+$ ions through ion channels.

2. *Ligand gating.* Binding of membrane protein with another molecule called ligand, which controls opening or closing of protein channels.

How is current flow through single channel recorded?

Current flow through single channel can be recorded by 'patch-clamp' technique.

FACILITATED DIFFUSION

What is facilitated diffusion?

It is diffusion of a substance which is mediated by a carrier.

Describe the mechanism of facilitated diffusion.

Facilitated diffusion is a carrier-mediated diffusion. The specific carrier facilitates the diffusion of a substance to the other side.

Carrier protein causing facilitated diffusion has a receptor site for binding with a specific substance. Protein also has a channel which is large enough to transport a specific molecule only halfway but not all the way through the membrane. Facilitated diffusion of a molecule of specific substance occurs as follows:

- Molecule of a specific substance binds with the receptor site.
- Then within a fraction of a second conformational change occurs in a carrier protein and this causes channel to open on the opposite side of the

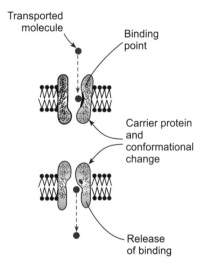

Transported
molecule

Binding
point

Carrier protein
and
conformational
change

Release
of binding

FIGURE 1.4 Process of facilitated diffusion.

membrane (to close on the side which was open before filling of the receptor site).

- Because of the weak binding force between the molecule and the receptor site, molecule breaks away from the site and diffuses to the opposite site.
- After the detachment of a molecule from the receptor site, another conformational change occurs in a carrier molecule and it gets the shape as before so that the channel now is open only half way. Another molecule of a substance to be transported gets attached to receptor site and the entire cycle repeats to cause diffusion of this molecule to opposite side (Fig. 1.4).

The mechanism allows the transported molecule to diffuse in either direction through the membrane (diffusion occurs along the electrochemical gradient).

The rate of transport by facilitated diffusion depends on two factors:

- Number of carrier molecules available in the cell membrane.
- Rate at which carrier molecule can undergo conformational change back and forth between its two states.

Most important substances which are transported by facilitated diffusion are glucose and many of the amino acids.

Describe the characteristics of facilitated diffusion.

Facilitated diffusion is carrier mediated and therefore has following characteristics:

1. V_{max}. Facilitated diffusion has a maximum rate of absorption (V_{max}) beyond which the rate cannot be increased. In case of simple diffusion if one goes on increasing the concentration of a substance on one side, there is proportionate increase in the rate of diffusion. However, in case of facilitated diffusion, this increase in rate of diffusion occurs only to a certain limit, i.e. at some concentration it

reaches the maximum (V_{max}), beyond which it cannot be increased even if concentration increases further. This is because as concentration of a substance rises more and more number of carrier molecules get involved in diffusing the substance. Once all the carrier molecules (there is a limited number of carrier molecules in the cell membrane) become involved in diffusion of a substance, the rate becomes maximum. This difference between simple diffusion and facilitated diffusion is illustrated in Fig. 1.5.

2. *Specificity.* A carrier is specific only for a substance or group of substances of a similar kind, e.g. the carrier molecule for glucose is a protein of molecular weight of 45,000 and it can also transport several other monosaccharides that have structures similar to glucose, e.g. mannose, galactose, xylose.

3. *Competitive inhibition.* If the carrier is common for two or more substances, e.g. glucose and galactose have a common carrier, these substances compete for the carrier receptor site, inhibit the rate of transport of the other substance. If only glucose is to be transported, rate of transport is more than when glucose and galactose both are present for getting transported.

4. *Non-competitive inhibition.* In this type of inhibition two substances A and B can get attached to the receptor site of the carrier. Substance A is transported across the membrane whereas substance B is not transported but only blocks the receptor site of the carrier. As a result the rate of transport of substance A is reduced when substance B is also present. Substance B does not compete for getting transported and therefore it is termed non-competitive inhibition.

Note. Active transport mechanisms have all the above characteristics as they are also carrier mediated. In addition they require energy because the substance is to be transported against the electrochemical gradient. This energy is obtained from ATP of the cell.

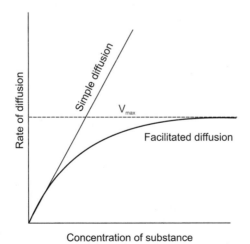

FIGURE 1.5 Effect of concentration of a substance on the rate of diffusion.

Enumerate the factors affecting the rate of diffusion through the cell membrane.

The factors affecting rate of diffusion are:

1. Permeability of membrane. It is the rate of diffusion per unit area of membrane per unit concentration difference. It depends on:
   - thickness of the membrane.
   - lipid solubility of substance which is passing through lipid bilayer.
   - number of protein channels per unit area for substances passing through protein channels.
   - temperature.
   - molecular weight of a substance.
2. Concentration difference across the membrane.
3. Electrical gradient across the membrane (for ions).
4. Pressure difference across the membrane.

ACTIVE TRANSPORT

How does primary active transport mechanism differ from secondary active transport mechanism?

In primary active transport mechanism, carrier protein molecule possesses ATPase activity. It splits ATP molecule and obtains energy for uphill transport (Fig. 1.6).

In case of secondary active transport mechanism, carrier protein molecule does not have ATPase activity. Energy for active transport of a substance is obtained from sodium gradient, and the sodium gradient is maintained because of Na^+-K^+ pump activity.

PRIMARY ACTIVE TRANSPORT

Describe the mechanism of primary active transport.

In primary active transport, the substance is transported against the electrochemical gradient and the energy required is obtained directly by breakdown of adenosine triphosphate (ATP) or some other high-energy phosphate bond.

Sodium, potassium, calcium, hydrogen, chloride ions are transported by this mechanism. The mechanism of primary active transport which is studied in greatest detail is the Na^+-K^+ pump which is present in membranes of all the body cells.

Na^+-K^+ pump. Carrier protein of this pump is made up of two globular proteins. One of them has a molecular weight of 100,000, and the other 55,000. The function of the smaller protein is not known.

The larger protein molecule of the carrier has the following features:

- Three receptor sites for binding Na^+ ions on the portion of protein protruding to the interior of the cell.
- Two receptor sites for K^+ ions on the outside surface.
- Inside portion of protein near the sites for Na^+ ions has ATPase activity.

OUTSIDE

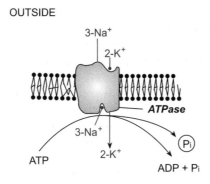

FIGURE 1.6 Mechanism of the Na$^+$-K$^+$ pump.

MECHANISM OF PUMP (Fig. 1.6)

- Three Na$^+$ ions bind on the inside surface of protein (at the receptor sites).
- Two K$^+$ ions bind on the outside surface of protein (at their receptor sites).
- ATPase function of protein is activated.
- ATP splits into ADP and high-energy phosphate bond. Thus energy is liberated.
- The energy liberated causes conformational change in protein carrier molecule which pumps Na$^+$ ions outward and K$^+$ ions inwards. Precise mechanism of the conformational change is yet unknown.

What are the functions of Na$^+$-K$^+$ pump?

1. The pump helps in maintaining the concentrations of Na$^+$ and K$^+$ ions inside and outside the cell constant. Normally concentration of Na$^+$ ions in extracellular fluid is greater than that of intracellular fluid. Concentration of K$^+$ ions is greater in intracellular fluid than that in extracellular fluid. Na$^+$ ions therefore tend to diffuse inward and K$^+$ ions tend to diffuse outward through leak channels. This is likely to change their concentrations in extracellular and intracellular fluid. In case of excitable tissues like nerve and muscle, the passage of impulse results into diffusion of Na$^+$ ions inwards and diffusion of K$^+$ ions outwards. Hence after passage of many impulses, the concentrations of Na$^+$ and K$^+$ ions are likely to change in extracellular and intracellular fluid. However, because of Na$^+$-K$^+$ pump, these concentrations are maintained constant. As soon as concentration of Na$^+$ ion inside the cell rises to a certain concentration, the Na$^+$-K$^+$ pump is activated and pumps Na$^+$ ions outward and K$^+$ ions inward and thereby brings their concentration in extracellular and intracellular fluid, back to normal levels.

2. It helps in maintaining the cell volume constant. This occurs as follows. Inside the cell there are large number of proteins and other organic compounds that cannot come out of the cell. Most of these are negatively charged, and

therefore collect around them a large number of positive ions as well. As a result this causes total number of molecules to be present in slightly more number inside the cell as compared to outside. This causes osmotic pressure of intracellular fluid to be slightly higher than that of extracellular fluid which tends to cause osmosis of water to the interior of the cell. Unless this is checked, the cell will swell and will burst open. However, this is prevented by Na^+-K^+ pump. As soon as cell size increases, Na^+-K^+ pump is activated causing pumping of three Na^+ ions outward and two K^+ ions inward with each cycle. Thus there is a net loss of one ion in each cycle. This increases the total number of molecules in extracellular fluid leading to osmosis of water from inside of the cell to outside. This brings the size of the cell back to normal. Thus activity of the pump tries to maintain the cell volume constant.

3. It acts as electrogenic pump. It pumps two K^+ ions inside the cell and three Na^+ions outside the cell with each cycle. So there is a net loss of one positive charge outwards with each cycle. This creates positivity outside the cell and thus creates a membrane potential across the cell membrane.

SECONDARY ACTIVE TRANSPORT

Describe the types of secondary active transport mechanisms.

There are two types of secondary active transport mechanisms:

1. Sodium co-transport mechanism.
2. Sodium counter-transport mechanism.

In sodium co-transport mechanism, both sodium and the substance to be transported move in the same direction, whereas in sodium counter-transport mechanism, sodium is transported in one direction and the substance is transported in the opposite direction.

MECHANISM OF CO-TRANSPORT

- Normally there is a large concentration gradient of Na^+ across the membrane. Concentration of sodium is very high outside the cell and is very low inside. This gradient represents a storehouse of energy, because excess sodium outside the cell membrane is always attempting to diffuse to the interior. This diffusion of sodium can literally pull the other substance along with it under appropriate conditions and hence the substance is transported against the electrochemical gradient (though sodium ion diffuses along the gradient). Thus gradient energy is used for transporting the substance against the electrochemical gradient. In this mechanism because the substance is transported along with the sodium in the same direction, it is called sodium co-transport mechanism.
- There is a carrier protein in the cell membrane, with a receptor site for Na^+ as well as for the molecule of a substance which is transported along with on the outside surface. When both the receptor sites are filled, conformational changes occur in a carrier protein. The energy gradient of the sodium ion causes both sodium and other substance to be transported together to the interior of the cell.

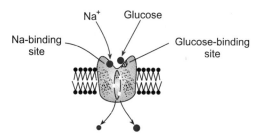

FIGURE 1.7 Process of sodium co-transport of glucose.

- Glucose and many amino acids are transported by this mechanism into the cells especially into the small intestinal epithelial cell against the gradient (Fig. 1.7). Energy is required for maintaining low concentration of Na^+ inside the cell. It is achieved by activity of Na^+-K^+ pump.

MECHANISM OF COUNTER-TRANSPORT

This mechanism is absolutely the same as Na^+ co-transport mechanism except that here Na^+ and the substance to be transported move in the opposite direction. Na^+ ions move to the interior of the cell and the other substance or ion moves to the exterior against the electrochemical gradient. In this mechanism carrier protein contains the receptor sites for Na^+ and the other ion but site for Na^+ ion is present on the outside surface of the cell and that for the other ion is present on the inside surface. Conformational change occurs in a carrier protein molecule when both the sites are filled. This change causes Na^+ ions to diffuse inwards along the concentration gradient and the other ion is transported outward against the gradient. The Na^+ gradient energy is used for the transport. Na^+ gradient is maintained by activity of the Na^+-K^+ pump. Examples of Na^+ counter-transport are: (a) Na^+-calcium counter-transport occurs in almost all the cells, (b) Na^+-H^+ counter-transport especially occurs in proximal tubular cells of kidneys.

PINOCYTOSIS AND PHAGOCYTOSIS

Describe the mechanism of pinocytosis and phagocytosis.

Entry of large particles into the cell is termed endocytosis. It occurs in two principal forms, pinocytosis and phagocytosis. In pinocytosis small vesicles are ingested whereas in phagocytosis large particles such as bacteria, cells or parts of degenerating tissues are ingested.

Pinocytosis. It occurs in all the cells but specially occurs very rapidly in some cells, e.g. macrophages. Pinocytosis is the only means by which very large macromolecule such as protein molecules can enter the cell.

Pinocytosis occurs as follows (Fig. 1.8):

- Molecules of protein attach to the cell membrane. These molecules usually get attached to specific receptors present on the surface of cell membrane. The receptors are concentrated in small pits in the cell membrane called coated pits. Beneath coated pits there is a lattice work of fibrillar

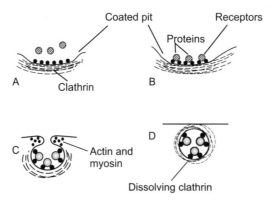

FIGURE 1.8 Mechanism of pinocytosis.

protein, clathrin. Contractile filaments of actin and myosin are also present here.

- Binding of protein molecules at the receptor site changes the surface properties of the membrane leading to invagination of the entire pit inward.
- Contractile proteins cause the closing of borders of the invaginated part. Ultimately borders close over the attached protein. The invaginated portion of membrane breaks away from the surface forming pinocytic vesicle. The usual diameter of pinocytic vesicle is from 100 to 200 nanometers (nm). This vesicle contains protein molecules with some extracellular fluid. Contraction of actin and myosin and breaking away of invaginated membrane portion requires presence of calcium ions in the extracellular fluid. The energy required is obtained by ATP of the cell.
- One or more lysosomes get attached to the pinocytic vesicle and empty their enzymes in it, forming a digestive vesicle. Enzymes hydrolyze proteins, glycogen, nucleic acid, mucopolysaccharides and other materials present in the vesicle. Products of digestion (amino acids, glucose, etc.) diffuse through the membrane of the vesicle and enter in the cell cytoplasm. What is left in digestive vesicle is only an undigested material and the vesicle is now termed residual body.
- Residual body is excreted out through cell membrane by mechanism of exocytosis which is essentially opposite to endocytosis.

Phagocytosis. It occurs in much the same way as pinocytosis but has the following differences:

- Phagocytosis involves large particles rather than molecules.
- Phagocytosis occurs only in certain cells such as macrophages and some of the white blood cells.
- In case of phagocytosis of bacteria, bacteria usually get attached to specific antibodies and then to the receptor. This intermediation of antibodies is called opsonization and is necessary before phagocytosis of bacteria can occur.
- Phagocytic vesicle is larger than a pinocytic vesicle.

OSMOSIS AND OSMOTIC PRESSURE*

What is osmosis?

The most abundant substance that diffuses across the cell membrane is water. This movement of water occurs because of concentration difference of water and is termed osmosis. When solutes are concentrated more on one side of the membrane (side 1) than the other side (side 2), it means that water concentration is more in side 2 as compared to side 1. This causes diffusion of water from side 2 to side 1, i.e. along the concentration gradient for water. This is termed osmosis.

What is osmotic pressure?

Amount of pressure required to stop osmosis of water is termed osmotic pressure. It depends on number of osmotically active solute particles per unit volume of fluid and not by mass of particles. This factor that determines osmotic pressure is concentration of solution in terms of number of particles.

To express the concentration of solution in terms of number of particles, a unit called osmole is used in place of grams.

One osmole is 1 gram molecular weight of osmotically active solute; thus for undissociating solutes like glucose, 180 grams of glucose is equal to 1 gram molecular weight of glucose which is equal to one osmole. For solute which dissociates into two ions, one gram molecular weight of solute becomes two osmoles.

When 1 osmole of solute is dissolved in each kilogram of water the osmolality of that solution is 1 osmole/kg. 1/1000th of osmole is miliosmole.

At body temperature of 37°C, concentration of one osmole per litre causes 19300 mmHg osmotic pressure in solution. Therefore, one milliosmole per litre solution has osmotic pressure of 19.3 mmHg. Concentration of solutes in body fluids is 300 milliosmoles per litre; therefore, total osmotic pressure of body fluids is

$$19.3 \times 300 = 5790 \text{ mmHg}$$

(Observed value of osmotic pressure of body fluids is 5500 mmHg. This is because many ions in the body fluid are attracted towards each other and therefore do not remain in dissociated form.)

RESTING MEMBRANE POTENTIAL

What is a resting membrane potential? How is it recorded?

Electrical potential existing across the cell membrane under resting state is called resting membrane potential.

One microelectrode is placed into the interior of the cell and another is placed outside the cell in interstitial fluid. These electrodes are connected to appropriate

---

*For details refer Vaz M, Kurpad A, Raj T, editors. *Guyton & Hall Textbook of Medical Physiology*. Elsevier: New Delhi, 2013, p. 40.

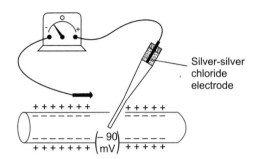

FIGURE 1.9 Measurement of the membrane potential of the nerve fibre using a microelectrode.

voltmeter for recording resting membrane potential (Fig. 1.9). It varies from -65 to -90 mV (with negativity inside the cell) in different cells.

What is the basic cause of production of resting membrane potential?

The resting membrane potential is due to diffusion potential caused by diffusion of diffusible ions across the membrane. Diffusion of these ions occurs because of their unequal distribution across the membrane. This unequal distribution occurs due to the presence of negatively charged ions (proteins, organic phosphates) inside the cells and the cell membrane is not permeable to ions. The presence of these non-diffusible ions inside the cell has the following effects at equilibrium which is called Gibbs–Donnan's equilibrium:

1. Solutions on either side of the membrane (intra- and extracellular fluids) are electrically neutral, i.e. the total charges on cations are equal to those of anions.
2. The product of diffusible ions on one side of membrane is equal to the product of diffusible ions on the other side.

Diffusible anions $\times$ Diffusible cations = Diffusible anions $\times$ Diffusible cations
(inside the cell)   (outside the cell)

At equilibrium, concentration of diffusible cations is greater than the concentration of diffusible anions inside the cell (i.e. side of the membrane containing non-diffusible anions). Opposite is true for anions, i.e. their concentration is greater outside the cell.

3. Because of unequal distribution of diffusible ions, ions tend to diffuse along their concentration gradient and this causes development of electrical potential across the membrane. For understanding this one has to imagine the hypothetical experiment where the membrane separates two solutions: 0.15 molar NaCl on side 1 and 0.15 KCl on side 2. Side 1 represents extracellular fluid and side 2 represents intracellular fluid. The membrane is only permeable to K^+ ions. There are concentration gradients for Na^+ ions and K^+ ions across the membrane but no gradient for Cl^- ions. As membrane is only permeable to K^+ ions, they diffuse from side 2 to side 1, due to the concentration force. This diffusion creates positivity in compartment one. This positivity opposes the diffusion of positively charged potassium ions. Thus electrical force is developed across the membrane due to diffusion of

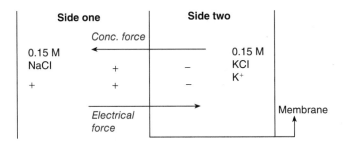

K$^+$ ions. It is termed diffusion potential. As more and more number of K$^+$ ions diffuse due to concentration force, more and more electrical force will develop and will oppose the diffusion potential. When concentration force tending to cause diffusion of K$^+$ ions from side 2 to side 1 becomes equal to electrical force which opposes the diffusion, the stage of equilibrium will be reached. At this stage, the force developed will be exactly equal but opposite to concentration force and there will be no net diffusion of potassium ions. Membrane potential that develops at this equilibrium is termed Nernst potential for K$^+$ ions. Thus Nernst potential for any ion is the equilibrium potential at which there is no net diffusion of ion in any direction, when membrane is permeable only to that ion.

In the above example, the membrane was permeable only to K$^+$ ions but Nernst potential for Na$^+$ ions and Cl$^-$ ions can also be calculated in a similar manner.

Nernst potential for different ions can be calculated by Nernst equation.

Nernst equation for positively charged ions is as follows:

$$EMF \ (mV) \ = \ -61 \log \frac{\text{concentration of ion inside the cell}}{\text{concentration of ion outside the cell}}$$

Nernst potential for negatively charged ions is calculated as:

$$EMF \ (mV) \ = \ -61 \log \frac{\text{concentration of ion outside the cell}}{\text{concentration of ion inside the cell}}$$

OR

$$EMF \ (mV) \ = \ +61 \log \frac{\text{concentration of ion inside the cell}}{\text{concentration of ion outside the cell}}$$

Cell membrane is differentiately permeable to different ions. Diffusion potential of different ions contributes towards the development of resting membrane potential. Goldmann has prepared an equation for finding out resting membrane potential by considering:

(i) Polarity of ion
(ii) Concentration gradient for ion across the cell membrane
(iii) Permeability of the cell membrane for the ion

Goldmann's equation is as follows:

$$\text{EMF (millivolts)} = -16 \log \frac{C_{Na^+i} + P_{Na^+} + C_{K^+i} \, P_{K^+} + C_{Cl^-o} \, P_{Cl}}{C_{Na^+o} + P_{Na^+} + C_{K^+o} \, P_{K^+} + C_{Cl^-i} \, P_{Cl}}$$

where,

C	=	Concentration,
(i)	=	Inside the cell,
(o)	=	Outside the cell,
P_{Na^+}	=	Permeability of membrane for sodium,
P_{K^+}	=	Permeability of membrane for potassium and
P_{Cl^-}	=	Permeability of membrane for chloride.

Under the resting state, cell membrane is most permeable to K^+ ions and hence the resting membrane potential is mainly caused due to diffusion potential for K^+ ions. The resting membrane potential of the cell is therefore nearer to Nernst's potential for K^+ ions.

Thus diffusion potential caused by diffusion of diffusible ions (mainly K^+ ions) is the main cause of development of resting membrane potential.

Another cause of development of resting membrane potential is the Na^+-K^+ pump. This pumps out three Na^+ ions outward and two K^+ ions inwards with each cycle. Thus there is a net loss of one positive charge with each cycle. Thus pump is responsible for creating potential gradient across the membrane.

Calculate Nernst potentials for K^+ and Na^+ ions.

Nernst potential for K^+ ions
Concentration of K^+ ions inside the cell = 140 mEq/L
Concentration of K^+ ions outside the cell = 4 mEq/L

$$\text{EMF (mV)} = - 61 \log \frac{140}{4}$$
$$= - 61 \log 35$$
$$= - 94 \text{ mV}$$

Thus, Nernst potential for K^+ ions is − 94 mV.
Nernst potential for Na^+ ions
Concentration of Na^+ ions inside the cell = 14 mEq/L
Concentration of Na^+ ions outside the cell = 142 mEq/L
∴ According to Nernst equation

$$\text{EMF (mV)} = - 61 \log \frac{14}{142}$$
$$= - 61 \log - 1$$
$$= + 61 \text{ mV}$$

Thus, Nernst potential for Na^+ ions is + 61 mV.

CHAPTER 2
Blood

BODY FLUIDS

Classify body fluid compartments.

Water constitutes about 45 to 75% of body weight. Total body water is distributed in two major compartments (Fig. 2.1):

1. *Intracellular fluid*: 55%
2. *Extracellular fluid*: 45%

Extracellular fluid is further subdivided into smaller compartments as follows:

- Plasma of blood (7.5% of total body water).
- Interstitial fluid (20% of total body water). It includes fluid between cells and lymph.

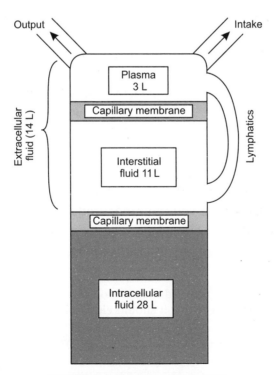

FIGURE 2.1 Distribution of body water.

- Fluid in dense connective tissue, such as cartilage (constitutes 7.5% of total body water).
- Transcellular fluid: Fluid present in different compartments and as fluid in GI tract, biliary and urinary tracts, intraocular fluid, cerebrospinal fluid, fluids present in serous spaces such as pleural, peritoneal, pericardial cavities, etc. It constitutes 2.5% of total body water.
- Inaccessible bone water (7.5% of total body water).

Which is the major cation of extracellular and intracellular fluids?

Major cation of extracellular fluid is sodium and that of intracellular fluid is potassium.

Which are the major anions of extracellular and intracellular fluids?

Major anion of extracellular fluid is chloride whereas those of intracellular fluid are phosphates, proteins and organic metabolic intermediates.

How do you account for difference in composition of extracellular and intracellular fluids?

Differences in extracellular and intracellular fluids are brought about by transport mechanisms of the cell membrane.

MEASUREMENTS OF VOLUMES OF DIFFERENT FLUIDS

Mention the principle used in determining volume of any fluid compartment.

Dilution principle is used in determining the volume of fluid compartment:

$$\text{Volume of compartment (in ml)} = \frac{\text{Quantity of test substance instilled}}{\text{Concentration of substance per ml after dispersement in the fluid}}$$

How is extracellular fluid volume measured?*
How is intracellular fluid volume measured?*
How is plasma volume measured?

The substances to be used for determination of plasma volume should have the following criteria:

- Substance should be retained in the blood vessels, i.e. it should not pass out through capillaries. For this it should either bind to plasma proteins or to red blood cells.
- Substance itself should not change the blood volume.

---

*For details refer Vaz M, Kurpad A, Raj T, editors. *Guyton & Hall Textbook of Medical Physiology*. Elsevier: New Delhi, 2013, p. 49.

- Substance should get evenly distributed in plasma.
- Substance should be non-toxic.
- The plasma volume is 2.8 to 3.0 litres.

The substances used for measuring plasma volume are:

- Dye Evans' blue.
- ^{131}I labelled albumin.

How is blood volume measured?

Blood volume can be measured by various methods.

1. A sample of blood is removed from a superficial vein. It is placed in a graduated tube (Wintrobe's tube) and is centrifuged for about 30 minutes. The red blood cells sediment and packed cell volume is read on the tube. Normally it is 45 (in 100 ml blood there are 45 ml cells and 55 ml plasma). The total blood volume is then calculated as follows:

$$\text{Total blood volume} = \frac{\text{Plasma volume}}{100 - \text{Haematocrit}} \times 100$$

$$= \frac{\text{Plasma volume}}{100 - 45} \times 100$$

2. Radioactively labelled (with ^{51}Cr) blood cells are injected into the circulation (RBCs are labelled with radioactive chromium *in vitro*). After they have mixed in circulation, a sample of blood is collected and its radioactivity is measured. Total blood volume is calculated by determining the degree of dilution of radioactivity (as in plasma volume).

What is oedema? What are its causes?

Oedema means presence of excess fluid in the tissues of the body mainly in the extracellular fluid compartment. It is due to:

1. Abnormal leakage of fluid from the capillaries. This in turn is due to:
   - Increased capillary pressure.
   - Decreased plasma proteins.
   - Increased capillary permeability.
2. Failure of lymphatic system to return the fluid from extracellular compartment back to circulation.
3. Retention of water and salt by the kidneys.

AETIOLOGY

1. Cardiac oedema.
2. Mechanical obstruction to veins.
3. Renal disease.
4. Inflammatory area (increased capillary permeability).

5. Malnutrition (lack of proteins).
6. Toxic substances (increased capillary permeability).

What are the safety factors which normally prevent oedema?

There are three major safety factors preventing oedema:

1. *Low compliance of interstitium.* Normally interstitial fluid hydrostatic pressure is −3 mmHg. Small increase in interstitial fluid volume causes relatively large increase in interstitial fluid pressure which opposes further filtration of fluid into the tissue (thus preventing oedema). Once interstitial fluid pressure rises above zero mmHg. Compliance of tissues rises markedly, allowing large amount of fluid to accumulate in tissues (oedema) with relatively small additional increase in interstitial fluid hydrostatic pressure.
2. *Ability of lymph flow to increase ten to fiftyfold.* Lymphatics act as safety factor against oedema because lymph flow can increase ten to fiftyfold when fluid begins to accumulate in tissues. This allows lymphatics to carry away large amount of fluid and proteins in response to increased capillary filtration, preventing interstitial fluid pressure from rising into positive range.
3. *Wash down of interstitial fluid protein concentration.* In most of the tissues protein concentration of interstitium decreases as lymph flow is increased. Due to this large amount of protein is carried away than can be filtered out of capillaries. This in turn causes lowering of concentration of protein in interstitial fluid which lowers net filtration force across capillaries and tends to prevent further accumulation of fluid.

What is effusion?

When oedema occurs in subcutaneous tissues, oedema fluid also collects in potential spaces. Collection of fluid in potential spaces is termed effusion. Potential spaces include pleural cavity, pericardial cavity, synovial cavity, etc.

Excess fluid collected in pleural cavity is termed pleural effusion.

Enumerate the forces concerned with dynamics of fluid exchange at capillary level.

At the arterial end of capillaries different forces cause movement of fluid out through capillary membrane. The low pressure at the venous end of capillaries leads to movement of fluid into the capillaries.

1. FACTORS CAUSING FILTRATION OF FLUID AT THE ARTERIAL END OF CAPILLARIES

(a) Forces tending to move fluid outward   30 mmHg
- Capillary pressure   3 mmHg
- Negative interstitial free fluid pressure   8 mmHg
- Interstitial fluid colloid osmotic pressure   41 mmHg
Total outward force

(b) Forces tending to move fluid inward
  - Plasma colloid osmotic pressure   28 mmHg
    Total inward force   28 mmHg

SUMMATION OF FORCES

(a) Outward   41 mmHg
(b) Inward   28 mmHg
Net outward force   13 mmHg

Thus at the arterial end of capillaries there is a net filtration force of 13 mmHg which causes movement of fluid outward from the capillaries.

2. FACTORS CAUSING REABSORPTION OF FLUID AT THE VENOUS END OF CAPILLARIES

(a) Forces tending to move fluid inward
  - Plasma colloid osmotic pressure   28 mmHg
    Total inward force   28 mmHg
(b) Forces tending to move fluid outward
  - Capillary pressure   10 mmHg
  - Negative interstitial fluid pressure   3 mmHg
  - Interstitial fluid colloid osmotic pressure   8 mmHg
    Total outward force   21 mmHg

SUMMATION OF FORCES

  - Inward   28 mmHg
  - Outward   21 mmHg
    Net inward force   7 mmHg

Net reabsorption pressure at venous ends of capillaries is 7 mmHg which causes reabsorption. The reabsorption pressure at venous end is less than the filtration pressure at the arterial ends of capillaries but venous capillaries are more numerous and more permeable than the arterial capillaries, so less pressure is required to cause inward movement. About nine-tenth of filtered fluid is absorbed at the venous end.

What is Starling's equilibrium?

EH Starling pointed out that under normal condition a state of near equilibrium exists at capillary membrane. The amount of fluid filtering out from capillaries equals almost exactly the quantity of fluid that is returned to the circulation by absorption. The slight disequilibrium that occurs accounts for small amount of fluid that is eventually returned by way of the lymphatics.

Chart showing principles of Starling's equilibrium (pressures at arterial and venous ends of capillaries are averaged to calculate mean capillary pressure).

MEAN FORCES TENDING TO MOVE FLUID OUTWARD

  - Mean capillary pressure   17.3 mmHg
  - Negative interstitial free fluid pressure   3.0 mmHg
  - Interstitial fluid colloid osmotic pressure   8.0 mmHg
    Total outward force   28.3 mmHg

MEAN FORCE TENDING TO MOVE FLUID INWARD

▪ Plasma colloid osmotic pressure	28.0 mmHg
Total inward force	28.0 mmHg

SUMMATION OF FORCES

▪ Outward	28.3 mmHg
▪ Inward	28.0 mmHg
Net outward force	0.3 mmHg

Thus for total capillary circulation one finds a near-equilibrium between total outward and inward forces.

What is isotonic fluid?

A fluid in which normal body cells can be placed without causing either swelling or shrinkage of the cells is said to be isotonic with the cells. 0.9% sodium chloride and 0.5% glucose solutions are isotonic for human cells.

What is hypertonic fluid?

A fluid in which body cells 'shrink' when suspended is called hypertonic fluid. Sodium chloride of greater than 0.9% concentration is hypertonic.

What is hypotonic fluid?

A fluid in which body cells 'swell' is called hypotonic fluid. Sodium chloride solution with less than 0.9% concentration is hypotonic.

BLOOD

What is blood?

Blood is a fluid connective tissue in which cells are suspended in plasma.

Give the composition of blood.

Blood is composed of:

1. **Plasma.** Plasma contains the following constituents:
   - Water: 93%.
   - Electrolytes: Mainly sodium, potassium, calcium, magnesium.
   - Proteins: Albumin, globulin, fibrinogen and others.
   - Gases: CO_2, O_2 and N_2.
   - Various nutrients: Glucose, amino acids, trace elements, vitamins, lipids, cholesterols, etc.
   - Waste products: Urea, creatinine, uric acid, bilirubin, etc.
   - Different hormones.

2. **Cells**. Mainly three types of cells are present which are also called formed elements of blood. They are as follows:
   - Red blood cells (RBCs).
   - White blood cells (WBCs).
   - Platelets.

Enumerate the functions of blood.

- Picking up of O_2 from the lungs and delivering it to the various tissues. Most important is uninterrupted delivery of O_2 to heart and brain.
- Delivery of glucose to various tissues.
- Carries amino acids, fatty acids and other nutrient substances to the tissues.
- Transports various hormones from different endocrine glands to the target tissues to modulate metabolic processes.
- Helps in maintenance of pH of body fluids.
- Transports various waste products to excretory organs (such as CO_2 to lungs, urea, uric acid to kidneys and bilirubin to liver).
- Transports heat from deep organs to the skin and lungs for dissipation, thus helping in maintaining of temperature of the body.
- White blood cells combat against different microorganisms entering the body.
- White blood cells also initiate immune responses.

BLOOD VOLUME

What is normal blood volume?

Normal blood volume varies from 5 to 5.5 litres in adult person (75 to 80 ml/kg). Normal plasma volume is about 3 litres and cell volume is 2 litres.

What is the relative volume of plasma and cells or corpuscles?

Plasma volume is 55% whereas cell volume is 45%.

What is haematocrit or packed cell volume (PCV)? How is it determined?

Haematocrit or PCV is the volume of red blood cells expressed as percentage of the total volume of blood.

It is determined by Wintrobe's method. Oxalated blood is filled in Wintrobe's tube up to '0' mark and the tube is centrifuged for half an hour. The cells settle down. Reading of haematocrit is noted. The Wintrobe's tube is again centrifuged for 5 minutes and reading of PCV is noted. Procedure is repeated till the successive readings for PCV are the same. This is done to ensure that all the cells have settled down.

What is observed haematocrit?

It is the value of haematocrit obtained by the above experiment.

What is true haematocrit?

Even if the red cells are fully packed, about 2% of the plasma is trapped in between the cells. Therefore, true haematocrit is calculated by multiplying observed haematocrit by 0.97 to 0.99.

What is body haematocrit? How is it calculated?

Body haematocrit is average of haematocrit values of blood present in large and small vessels. It is calculated by multiplying observed haematocrit by 0.87.

This correction is required because red blood cells (RBCs) mass is unevenly distributed in the circulating blood. Usually, venous blood is collected for determining haematocrit. Haematocrit of the venous blood is higher than the whole blood haematocrit. In capillaries, haematocrit is lower than that of the venous blood. In vessels with larger diameter, haematocrit is greater than in smaller vessels (capillaries) because of axial streaming of RBCs. Average of haematocrit in both the large and the small vessels is called body haematocrit.

What is the normal specific gravity of blood?

Normal specific gravity of blood varies from 1.055 to 1.062. Specific gravity of RBCs is greater (1.090) than that of plasma (1.030).

Name the mechanisms of blood volume regulation.

Mechanisms of regulation of blood volume are as follows:

1. **Capillary fluid shift mechanism.** If there is increase in blood volume, there is increased capillary pressure leading to increased leakage of fluid from capillary to interstitial fluid which decreases the blood volume back to normal. If there is decreased blood volume, exactly reverse events occur.

2. **Reflex mechanisms (Baroreceptor reflex).** When blood volume increases, baroreceptors are stretched and are stimulated. There is reflex inhibition of sympathetic nervous system leading to dilatation of renal arteries allowing excess urinary output.

3. **Hormonal mechanism.**
   - *Atrial natriuretic factor (ANF).* Excess blood volume causes release of atrial natriuretic factor (from atria of heart). This ANF increases sodium and water excretion through kidneys.
   - *Aldosterone.* Decrease in blood volume stimulates aldosterone secretion from adrenal cortex. It increases absorption of sodium and water from kidney tubules.
   - *Angiotensin.* It is released when blood volume is decreased. It causes retention of water and salt.
   - *ADH (Anti-diuretic hormone).* Increased blood volume decreases release of ADH and allows water loss through kidneys and vice versa.

4. **Thirst mechanism.** When blood volume is decreased, thirst mechanism is stimulated.

5. **Renal mechanism.** It controls blood volume by changing urinary output as follows:

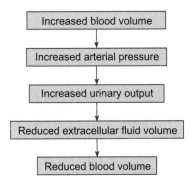

When blood volume falls below normal, exactly reverse events occur.

Name the conditions leading to increased blood volume.

PHYSIOLOGICAL CONDITIONS

- *Age.* In infants, blood volume is more when compared to body weight and less when compared to surface area. It is 80 ml/kg in infants and 70 ml/kg in adults.
- *Sex.* Blood volume is greater in males than in females because of more erythropoietin activity, more body weight and greater surface area.
- Exposure to warm environment increases the blood volume.
- *Pregnancy.* Blood volume is increased by 20 to 30% in pregnancy.
- *Exercise.* Increases blood volume due to contraction of spleen and release of stored blood in circulation.
- *High altitude.* Due to hypoxia there is increased erythropoietin secretion at high altitude. This in turn increases the production of red blood cells which leads to increased blood volume.
- *Emotional disturbance.* Sympathetic stimulation causes contraction of spleen which releases stored blood in circulation.

PATHOLOGICAL CONDITIONS

- *Congestive cardiac failure.* Blood volume increases due to retention of sodium and water.
- *Hyperthyroidism.* Blood volume increases because thyroxine increases red cell production rate.
- *Hyperaldosteronism.* Increased aldosterone causes greater absorption of sodium and therefore water by the kidneys. This increases extracellular fluid volume and blood volume.
- *Cirrhosis of liver.* This condition is associated with secondary aldosteronism because the damaged liver cannot metabolize the hormone. Excess aldosterone causes greater absorption of sodium and water by kidneys.
- *Polycythaemia vera.* Mainly red blood cells increase.

Name the conditions which reduce blood volume.
PHYSIOLOGICAL CONDITIONS
- Acute exposure to cold.
- *Posture.* Blood volume is low in erect position than in recumbent state. This is because the pooling of blood in lower limbs during erect posture increases the hydrostatic pressure and passage of fluid from blood vessels into the tissue spaces.
- *Obesity.* Blood volume per kilogram of body weight in an obese person is lower but it is normal when considered in relation to the body surface.

PATHOLOGICAL CONDITIONS
- *Haemorrhage or blood loss.* Acute external or internal haemorrhage occurs in accidents. It occurs in females from uterus during menstruation or various abnormalities. It occurs from bleeding peptic ulcer.
- *Fluid loss.* It occurs in burns, vomiting, diarrhoea, excessive sweating and polyuria in diabetes mellitus or diabetes insipidus.
- *Reduction in red blood cells.* In anaemia or excessive destruction of red cells by various haemolytic agents causes reduction in blood volume. But sometimes in anaemia blood volume may be maintained by entry of fluid into the blood vessels causing haemodilution.
- *Myxoedema.*

BLOOD pH

What is pH? What is the normal blood pH?
pH is negative logarithm of H^+ ion concentration to the base 10. Normal blood pH is 7.4 (range 7.38 to 7.42).

What is acidosis?
It is a condition when pH of blood falls below 7.38.

What is alkalosis?
It is a condition when pH of blood is more than 7.42.

What is buffer?
A buffer is a substance that has the ability to bind or release H^+ ions in solution, thus keeping pH of the fluid relatively constant despite addition of considerable quantities of base or acid.

What are the buffer systems?
Buffer systems of body are weak acids that exist as a mixture of a pronated form and an unpronated form in the physiological pH range. Buffer systems are most immediate defences against pH changes.

What are the buffer systems present in blood?

- Haemoglobin: Very effective and major protein buffer.
- Plasma proteins.
- Phosphate buffer: Mainly acts as a buffer in intracellular fluid because its concentration in extracellular fluid is less.
- Bicarbonate buffer.

PLASMA PROTEINS

Name the plasma proteins. Where are they synthesized?

Important plasma proteins are:

1. *Albumin.*
2. *Globulins.* Globulin fraction is further divided into:
   - Alpha 1
   - Alpha 2
   - Beta
   - Gamma globulin
3. *Fibrinogen.*

Albumin and majority of globulins (except immunoglobulins) are synthesized in the liver. Immunoglobulins (gamma globulin) are synthesized by B-lymphocyte. Fibrinogen is also synthesized in the liver.

In addition, there are other plasma proteins like alpha-one protease inhibitor, alpha-two macroglobulin and carrier proteins like haptoglobin, transferrin and two major lipoproteins.

What is the normal plasma protein level?

Total plasma protein in blood is 7.4 g/100 ml (normal range is 6.4 to 8.3 g%) out of which albumin level is 3.5 to 5.0 g/100 ml, globulin level is 1.5 to 2.5 g/100 ml and fibrinogen level is 150 to 300 mg/100 ml of blood.

What is the normal albumin–globulin ratio? When does it get changed?

Normal albumin–globulin ratio is 1.8:1 to 2:1. Synthesis of albumin exclusively occurs in liver but many globulins (immunoglobulins) are synthesized by B-lymphocyte. Therefore, ratio changes in liver diseases because only albumin synthesis is reduced.

Enumerate the methods used for separation of plasma proteins.

1. *Precipitation by salting out.*
   (a) *Ammonium sulphate solution.*
   (b) *Sodium sulphate solution.*
2. *Cohn's fractionation method.*
3. *Electrophoresis.*
4. *Immunoelectrophoresis.*
5. *Sedimentation with ultracentrifugation.*

Describe the functions of plasma proteins.

Plasma proteins have the following functions.

1. **Colloid osmotic pressure.** Proteins of blood exert colloid osmotic pressure which is normally 25 to 30 mmHg. Albumin contributes 70 to 80% of osmotic pressure. Colloid osmotic pressure plays important role in exchange of water between tissue fluid and blood. At the arterial end of capillary, hydrostatic pressure exerted is greater than colloid osmotic pressure. This causes filtration of fluid out from vessels to tissue spaces. At the venous end colloid osmotic pressure of blood is greater than hydrostatic pressure. This causes absorption of fluid from tissue spaces into the vessels.

2. **Viscosity.** Owing to the presence of plasma proteins blood is a viscous fluid. Fibrinogen and globulins, mainly because of their asymmetrical shape, account for the viscosity. The viscosity of blood provides resistance to flow of blood in blood vessels, to maintain blood pressure in the normal range.

3. **Buffering action.** Serum proteins like other proteins are amphoteric and thus can combine with acids and bases. In acidic pH, NH_2 group acts as base and can accept proton and is converted to NH_4. In alkaline pH, COOH group acts as acid and can donate a proton and thus become COO^-. At normal pH of blood, proteins act as acids and combine with cations (mainly sodium). Plasma proteins are responsible for about 15% of buffering capacity of blood.

4. **Binding and transport function.** CO_2 is transported by plasma proteins in the form of carbamino compound.

Several hormones are transported in blood in association with plasma proteins, e.g. thyroxin is transported in association with an alpha-globulin called thyroxine binding protein (TBP). Cortisol is transported by a mucoprotein called transcortin.

Many drugs and dyes are transported in plasma in combination with albumin. Half of calcium of plasma is bound to protein for transport. Beta one globulin transports iron in plasma (transferrin).

Lipids and fat soluble vitamins (A, D and E) are transported by high and low density lipoproteins (HDL and LDL).

Bilirubin is associated with albumin and also with fractions of the alpha globulins.

Ceruloplasmin (alpha$_2$ globulin) binds with copper. Transcobalamine binds with vitamin B_{12}. Haptoglobin binds with free haemoglobin in the vessels and carries it to reticuloendothelial system.

5. **Immunity.** Gamma globulins in plasma are antibodies and they protect body against bacterial infections.

6. **Clotting of blood.** Whenever there is injury to the blood vessel fibrinogen is converted to fibrin which forms blood clot. This clot seals the hole in the vessel and therefore prevents blood loss.

7. **Reserve proteins.** Amino acids from plasma proteins can be taken up by tissues and used for building up new tissue proteins and vice versa.

8. **Nutritive value.** Albumin is largely involved in the nutritive functions of plasma proteins owing to its high concentration. It is effective as a source of protein in hypoproteinaemic states.

9. **Fibrinolysis.** Intravascular clot (thrombus) is digested by the enzymes of fibrinolytic system present in plasma, which saves from disastrous effects of thrombosis.

Which plasma protein can pass through capillary endothelium?

Normally capillary endothelium is almost impermeable to all plasma proteins. In diseases with increased capillary permeability, albumin because of its lower molecular weight (68,000) is the first protein that would pass through the capillary membrane.

Which is the principal plasma protein influencing erythrocyte sedimentation rate?

Erythrocyte sedimentation rate is mostly influenced by fibrinogen.

Which plasma protein has got the highest molecular weight?

Fibrinogen has got the highest molecular weight, i.e. 450,000.

What is crystalloid osmotic pressure? Does it play any role in tissue fluid formation?

Osmotic pressure exerted by crystalloids is known as crystalloid osmotic pressure. Crystalloids can pass back and forth across the capillary wall with great ease. Therefore, they do not contribute to the effective osmotic pressure and hence do not play any role in tissue fluid formation.

What is plasmapheresis? What are the conclusions drawn from the experiment?

Plasmapheresis is the experimental procedure first performed by Whipple in dog to demonstrate the importance of plasma proteins.

Conclusions drawn from the experiment:

- Plasma proteins are normally formed from food proteins.
- Efficacy of food proteins depends upon degree of its chemical resemblance in amino acid pattern to the plasma protein which it is going to form.
- Plasma proteins can be satisfactorily synthesized if essential amino acids are present in the diet.
- Some proteins (those from muscle and viscera) favour albumin formation.
- Some proteins (plant and grain proteins) favour globulin formation.
- Presence of infection depresses protein regeneration.
- Regeneration of plasma proteins occurs within 14 days. Rate of regeneration is very fast within first 24 hours.

What is isoelectric pH?

Proteins can ionize either as acids or bases owing to the fact that their constituent amino acids contain both amino groups (NH_2) and carboxyl groups (COOH). In alkaline solution, proteins ionize as acids and free protein anions (negatively charged) are formed. In acid solution, proteins (amino groups) act as bases taking up H^+ ions and the proteins carry positive charges.

At an intermediate pH (specific for each protein) the protein molecule carries equal number of positive and negative charges and hence has a net zero charge. This pH value at which the molecule shows electrical neutrality is known as iso-electric pH.

NON-PROTEIN NITROGENOUS SUBSTANCES

What are the important NPN (non-protein nitrogenous) substances in plasma?

- Urea
- Uric acid
- Creatinine

BLOOD CELLS
HAEMOPOIESIS—FORMATION OF BLOOD CELLS

What are the sites of haemopoiesis?

In early embryonic life, blood cells are produced in the liver and to a lesser extent in the spleen. At 20th week of intrauterine life, haemopoiesis begins in the bone marrow. During later months, haemopoiesis increases in the bone marrow and decreases in the liver and spleen.

After birth, all blood cells except lymphocytes are formed in the bone marrow. In young children, active haemopoietic marrow is found in both axial skeleton and bones of extremities. In adults, haemopoietic bone marrow is confined to axial skeleton (cranium, ribs, sternum, vertebrae and pelvis) and proximal ends of femur and humerus.

RED BLOOD CELLS

What is erythropoiesis?

Erythropoiesis is the process of formation of RBCs.

Enumerate the stages of erythropoiesis.

There are pluripotent haemopoietic stem cells in the bone marrow from which all the cells of circulating blood can be derived. Some cells are converted to committed cells. Committed stem cell which gives rise to erythrocyte is called colony-forming unit erythrocyte.

Stages of erythropoiesis are depicted in Figure 2.2.

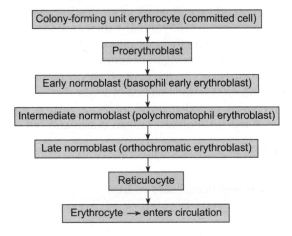

Describe the various changes occurring in RBC during erythropoiesis?

1. **Size.** Size of the cell goes on decreasing with subsequent stages.

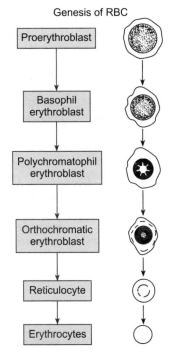

FIGURE 2.2 Stages of erythropoiesis.

2. **Nucleus.** Nucleus first condenses and then becomes pyknotic. Final remnant of nucleus is thrown out of cell and nucleus finally disappears.

3. **Haemoglobin synthesis.** Haemoglobin first appears at intermediate normoblast stage and then its content gradually increases.

4. **Staining property.** Before the appearance of haemoglobin, cell is basophilic (stained by basic dye). When haemoglobin appears, cell is stained by both acidic and basic dye (polychromatophilic). In the stage of late normoblast when haemoglobin synthesis is completed, cytoplasm is stained by acidic dye.

5. **Mitosis.** Seen only in earlier stages up to the stage of intermediate normoblast. At the stage of late normoblast, mitosis ceases and cell only matures.

For details see Table 2.1.

Table 2.1	Different Precursors of RBC				
Name of the cell	Size (in microns)	Nucleus	Cytoplasm	Percentage of haemoglobin	Mitosis
1. Haemocytoblast	18 to 23	Large	Small amount; therefore, thin rim of deep basophilic cytoplasm	Not present	Present
2. Proerythroblast	14 to 19	Large with distinct nucleoli and reticulum of fine chromatin threads	Basophilic and scanty	Not present	Present
3. Early normoblast (basophil erythroblast)	11 to 17	Nucleus and chromatin more dense. Nucleoli are absent or rudimentary	Basophilic and Scanty	Not present	Present
4. Intermediate normoblast (polychromatophil erythrocyte)	10 to 14	More condensed often eccentric. No nucleoli	Becomes polychromatic because of appearance of haemoglobin	Appears	Present
5. Late normoblast (orthochromatic erythrocyte)	7 to 10	Nucleus very dense and takes a deep stain (pyknotic)	Polychromatic	Increases in amount	No
6. Reticulocyte (stained by vital stain such as cresyl blue)	7 to 7.5 (almost same as mature erythrocyte)	Disappears	Net-like structure (reticulum) in cytoplasm	Same quantity as in mature erythrocyte	No
7. Erythrocyte (mature RBC)→ Released in blood					

What is reticulocyte? Why is it so called?

Reticulocyte is the last stage in the formation of erythrocyte, i.e. the young red cell. It is so called because on vital staining with cresyl blue a network of reticulum is apparent in the cytoplasm of the cell.

Do reticulocytes appear in circulation?

Reticulocytes enter the peripheral circulation but the number entering is very small. It is only 0.5 to 1% of circulating erythrocytes in adults.

What is reticulocytosis?

Increase in circulating reticulocytes up to 25 to 35% is called reticulocytosis. This is seen when the rate of erythropoiesis is very high, e.g. injection of haemolytic poisons, after treatment of pernicious anaemia with vitamin B_{12}.

How is erythropoiesis regulated?

Erythropoiesis is regulated by erythropoietin. The main function of red blood cells is to supply oxygen to the tissues (which is carried by haemoglobin present in the red blood cells). Therefore, whenever there is hypoxia (decreased oxygen supply to the tissues), there is a release of renal erythropoietic factor from juxtaglomerular cells of kidney. Renal erythropoietic factor acts on plasma alpha globulin (erythropoietinogen) to form erythropoietin. Erythropoietin acts on the bone marrow and stimulates erythropoiesis. Levels of erythropoietin vary with degree of hypoxia or number of circulating red blood cells. If number of red blood cells is less in circulation, greater erythropoietin is formed. This increases the rate of erythropoiesis and brings red blood cells number to normal. If number of red blood cells in circulation is more, erythropoietin level is lowered.

Negative feedback mechanism regulating RBC count

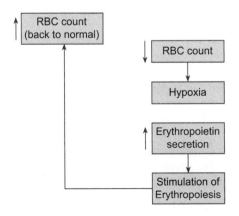

If RBC count increases, exactly opposite events occur

Discuss the factors necessary for erythropoiesis.

For development and maturation of erythrocytes the following factors are necessary: (1) General factors, (2) Maturation factors, (3) Factors necessary for haemoglobin formation.

1. GENERAL FACTORS

Erythropoietin stimulates erythropoiesis and for this it promotes the following processes:

- Production of proerythroblast from the stem cell in CFU-E of bone marrow.
- Maturation of proerythroblasts into matured red cells through various normoblastic stages. It also promotes haem synthesis.
- Release of matured erythrocytes in circulation through the capillary membrane of bone marrow. Even some reticulocytes are released along with the matured red blood cells.

Hypoxia is the fundamental stimulus for erythropoiesis. Other factors that stimulate erythropoietin secretion are:

- Products of red cell destruction enhance the production of erythropoietin and hence increase the rate of erythropoiesis. This would be a physiological feedback process for maintenance of red blood cell count constant.
- *Hormones.* Androgen stimulates erythropoietin secretion. This leads to higher haemoglobin and red cell count in males.

ACTH and adrenocortical steroids increase erythropoietin secretion and hence the rate of erythropoiesis.

Thyroxine, TSH, growth hormone, prolactin stimulates secretion of erythropoietin.

(b) *Growth inducers.* Some growth inducers (e.g. interleukin-3) stimulate the growth of stem cells for red blood cells.

(c) *Vitamins.* Vitamin B_{12}, C and D are required for erythropoiesis and their deficiency causes anaemia along with pellagra, scurvy and rickets respectively.

2. MATURATION FACTORS

They are the factors required for maturation of red cells.

(a) *Vitamin B_{12}.* It is present in the diet and is also synthesized by bacterial flora of colon. It is stored in large amounts in liver and when necessary is transported to bone marrow. Vitamin B_{12} is essential for the synthesis of DNA and its deficiency leads to failure in maturation of nucleus, and of cell and reduction in cell division; also cells are larger and are more fragile. Vitamin B_{12} is not absorbed readily in absence of intrinsic factor (produced by oxyntic cells of gastric glands). Therefore, severe gastritis, ulcers and gastrectomy lead to pernicious anaemia (vitamin B_{12} deficiency causes pernicious anaemia).

(b) *Folic acid.* It is also necessary for synthesis of DNA and therefore maturation. Its deficiency causes anaemia with cells of larger size. This anaemia is termed megaloblastic anaemia.

3. FACTORS NECESSARY FOR HAEMOGLOBIN PRODUCTION

(a) *First class proteins* provide amino acids required for synthesis of globin part of haemoglobin, stroma proteins and nucleoproteins of red cells.

(b) *Iron* is necessary for formation of haem part of haemoglobin. Deficiency of iron leads to microcytic hypochromic (small size and decreased haemoglobin) type of anaemia. Iron is supplied in the diet. In addition when old red blood cells are destroyed iron portion can be reutilized for production of red cells.

(c) *Copper* is required for absorption of iron from gastrointestinal tract.

(d) *Cobalt and nickel.* Cobalt is a part of vitamin B_{12}. These metals act as catalytic agents for incorporation of iron in haemoglobin.

(e) *Vitamins.* Vitamin C, riboflavin, nicotinic acid, pyridoxine are essential for the formation of haemoglobin.

(f) *Calcium* helps indirectly for conserving iron and its subsequent utilization.

(g) *Bile salts.* Presence of bile salts in the intestine is necessary for proper absorption of metals (copper, nickel, etc.) which are important factors in synthesis of haemoglobin.

What is the physiological stimulus for erythropoiesis?

Basal levels of erythropoietin in the blood are the normal physiological stimulus for erythropoiesis.

What is the shape of red blood cells? What are the advantages of the shape?

Red blood cells have circular biconcave shape (diameter 7.2 microns).

ADVANTAGES OF BICONCAVE SHAPE

1. Due to greater surface area as compared to volume, it can take in some quantity of fluid before getting haemolyzed. That means it can resist haemolysis to certain extent when placed in hypotonic solution.

2. It exhibits remarkable deformability because of its typical shape. This is especially important while the cells are passing through the small capillaries.

3. O_2 and CO_2 exchange occurs easily because of greater surface area.

Name the different variations that occur in the shape of red blood cells.

Abnormal shapes of the RBCs are given below. Some abnormalities in shape occur in certain types of anaemia.

1. **Shrinkage or crenation.** It occurs when red blood cells are suspended in hypertonic solutions. The water from the red cell diffuses outward giving rise to crenation.

2. **Spherocyte.** The globular shape of RBCs is seen in a hereditary disease called spherocytosis. Such cells cannot be compressed and therefore rupture more easily than the normal red blood cells.

3. **Elliptocyte.** The elliptical shape occurs in certain anaemias.

4. **Sickle cell.** The cell is crescentic in shape and is seen in sickle cell anaemia because of presence of abnormal haemoglobin (haemoglobin S).

5. **Poikilocytes.** This unusual shape of RBCs is due to deformed cell membrane. The shape may be like flask, hammer or any other abnormal shape.

What is normal RBC count?

In adult male, it varies from 5 to 6.5 million/mm^3 of blood.
In adult female, it varies from 4 to 4.5 million/mm^3 of blood.

HAEMOGLOBIN

What is haemoglobin?

Haemoglobin is a protein containing haem, which is iron containing porphyrin known as iron porphyrin IX. Porphyrin nucleus is formed by four pyrrole rings joined by methine bridges. Protein globin combines with haem to form haemoglobin (Fig. 2.3).

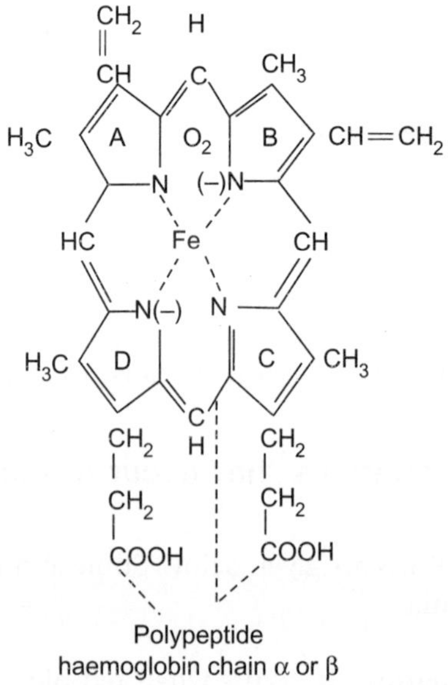

Polypeptide
haemoglobin chain α or β

FIGURE 2.3 Structure of haemoglobin.

How is haemoglobin synthesized?

- Haemoglobin is synthesized mainly from acetic acid and glycine. Most of the synthesis occurs in mitochondria. Acetic acid is converted to succinyl CoA.
  (a) 2 Succinyl CoA + 2 Glycine → Pyrrole
  (b) 4 Pyrrole → Protoporphyrin IX
  (c) Protoporphyrin IX + Iron → Haem Molecule
  (d) Haem + Globin (4 chains) → Haemoglobin
- Globin has four different types of protein chains called alpha, beta, gamma and delta. Normal adult haemoglobin contains two alpha chains and two beta chains.

Enumerate the nutrients required for haemoglobin synthesis.

1. Proteins.
2. Vitamins (vitamin B_{12}, folic acid, pyridoxine, ascorbic acid).
3. Minerals (iron, copper, cobalt).

What are the physiological varieties of haemoglobin?

Different varieties of haemoglobin are due to variations in the composition of peptides of globin fraction; haem moiety is same in all types.
   There are following physiological varieties of haemoglobin in human:

1. Adult haemoglobin is of two types:
   (a) Haemoglobin A (globin contains two alpha and two beta chains).
   (b) Haemoglobin A_2 (globin contains two alpha and two delta chains). It is a minor component of adult haemoglobin.
2. Foetal haemoglobin is called haemoglobin F (globin contains two alpha and two gamma chains).

State the important haemoglobinopathies.

Haemoglobinopathies occur due to disorders of globin synthesis (haem synthesis is normal).

   There are two types of disorders of globin synthesis:

   1. Abnormal polypeptide chains formed due to substitution of an abnormal amino acid in the chain of HbA, e.g. haemoglobin S in which there is substitution of valine for glutamic acid at position 'six' in the beta chain of HbA. HbS gives rise to change in the shape of the red cell called sickling when HbS is reduced.

   2. The synthesis of polypeptide chain of globin is repressed, e.g. in thalassaemia there is impaired synthesis of one or more of the polypeptide chains of globin.

   Beta thalassaemia in which β-globin chains are depressed is common. Red cells get rapidly haemolyzed in thalassaemia.

Name the different derivatives of haemoglobin.

1. **Compounds:**
   - Oxyhaemoglobin: Compound of Hb with O_2.
   - Methaemoglobin: Compound of Hb with O_2 after treating blood with potassium ferricyanide.
   - Carbaminohaemoglobin: Compound of Hb with CO_2.
   - Carboxyhaemoglobin: Compound of Hb with CO.
   - Sulphaemoglobin: Formed by combination of Hb with H_2S.
2. **Derived products:**
   - *Iron containing:*
     - (i) Haematin: acid or alkali haematin, by action of acid or alkali with Hb.
     - (ii) Haemochromogen: obtained by reduction of alkali haematin.
     - (iii) Cathaemoglobin: compound of Hb containing ferric iron with denatured globin.
     - (iv) Haem.
   - *Iron free:*
     - (i) Haematoporphyrin.
     - (ii) Haemopyrrole.
     - (iii) Haematoidin.
     - (iv) Bilirubin.

METABOLISM OF B_{12}

What is the daily requirement of vitamin B_{12}?

1–2 micrograms (μg) in adults.

What are extrinsic and intrinsic factors?

Extrinsic factor is vitamin B_{12}. Intrinsic factor is the factor released by gastric mucosa which combines with vitamin B_{12} and increases its absorption. Intrinsic factor is also known as Castle's intrinsic factor.

What is the role of vitamin B_{12} and folic acid in erythropoiesis?

Vitamin B_{12} and folic acid are required for DNA synthesis during the formation of red blood cells. Therefore, deficiency of these two factors prevents maturation of red blood cells giving rise to megaloblastic type of anaemia.

How is megaloblastic anaemia treated?

Megaloblastic anaemia is treated by giving folic acid orally and vitamin B_{12} intramuscularly because usually deficiency of vitamin B_{12} occurs due to lack of absorption caused by lack of intrinsic factor synthesis.

Vitamin B_{12} also corrects the neurological symptoms caused due to subacute combined degeneration of the spinal cord which occurs during megaloblastic or pernicious anaemia.

METABOLISM OF IRON

What is the daily requirement of iron?

From the iron taken in the food, only 10% is absorbed. Therefore, daily amount of iron required in the food is as follows:
   Adult males: 5 to 10 mg/day.
   Adult females: 20 mg/day to compensate the menstrual loss.

Name the factors influencing absorption of iron.

About 10% of the dietary iron is absorbed and is used for haemoglobin synthesis. Absorption mainly occurs in duodenum and upper jejunum. Factors affecting iron absorption are:

   1. State of iron. Ferrous (Fe^{++}) iron is better absorbed than ferric (Fe^{+++}) iron. Therefore, reducing substances such as vitamin C (ascorbic acid) enhance iron absorption by converting Fe^{+++} to Fe^{++} state.
   2. Presence of phosphates or phytates in foods (cereals) reduces iron absorption by forming insoluble iron salts.
   3. Haem is absorbed directly without splitting off of iron.
   4. Decrease in iron stores of the body enhances iron absorption (e.g. iron deficiency anaemia, increased erythropoiesis). Increased iron stores decrease the rate of absorption of iron.

How is iron transported in blood?

Iron absorbed from the intestine combines with a beta globulin, apotransferrin, to form transferrin. Iron loosely combines with globulin molecule and can be released to any of the tissue cells at any point in the body.

How is iron stored in the body?

Iron can be stored in all the cells of the body, but is especially stored in reticulo-endothelial (RE) cells and liver hepatocytes. In these cells iron mainly combines with protein apoferritin to form ferritin. Ferritin is thus the storage form of iron. Some amount of iron is also stored as a compound haemosiderin in reticuloen-dothelial cells when the intake of iron in the diet is in extremely large quantities.

What is the mechanism of absorption of iron?

Iron is absorbed from all parts of small intestine by the following mechanism:
   The liver secretes moderate amount of apotransferrin into bile which flows through bile duct into duodenum.
   In small intestine apotransferrin binds with free iron and iron compounds (Hb, myoglobin). This combination is called transferrin. Transferrin is then attracted to and binds with receptors of membranes of intestinal epithelial cells.

Then by pinocytosis transferrin molecule carrying with it its iron store is absorbed into epithelial cells and later is released into blood capillaries beneath these cells in the form of plasma transferrin.

How is iron absorption regulated?

There are two mechanisms for regulating iron absorption:

1. When essentially all apoferritin in the body is saturated with iron, it becomes difficult for transferrin to release its iron to the tissue cells. Transferrin also becomes fully saturated with iron (normally only one-third transferrin is saturated with iron) and therefore it does not accept any iron from intestinal mucosal cells. Iron thus builds up in mucosal cells, which depresses iron absorption.

2. When body has excess stores of iron, there is decreased rate of synthesis of apo-ferritin in liver, and thus less iron is absorbed from the intestinal cells.

ANAEMIA

What is the normal haemoglobin content?

Normal haemoglobin content of blood in males varies from 14 to 18 g/100 ml whereas in females it varies from 12 to 14 g/100 ml of blood.

What is anaemia?

Anaemia is defined as decreased oxygen carrying capacity of blood. One gram of haemoglobin carries 1.34 ml of O_2.

Give the classification of anaemia.

Anaemia can be classified on the basis of its cause, size of RBCs or amount of haemoglobin per red blood cell.

A. CLASSIFICATION ON THE BASIS OF CAUSE

1. *Anaemias caused by blood loss or increased blood destruction:*

   (a) Posthaemorrhagic anaemia. The haemorrhage may be acute (e.g. in accident), or chronic (as a result of peptic ulcer, piles, ancylostomiasis, purpura, etc.). In chronic blood loss there is loss of iron leading to iron deficiency anaemia.

   (b) *Haemolytic anaemia* due to greater red cell destruction as a result of:
   - Chemical haemolytic poisons such as lead, coal tar, arseniuretted hydrogen.
   - Infections like malaria, septicaemia.
   - Abnormal structure of red cells which renders them more susceptible to disintegration in blood stream or to phagocytosis, e.g. chronic congenital haemolytic anaemia (Cooley's anaemia). Sickle cell anaemia is due to abnormal haemoglobin (HbS).

- Anaemia due to endogenous haemolysins of unknown nature, e.g. chronic congenital haemolytic jaundice.
- Anti-Rh and occasionally anti-A and anti-B agglutinins causing haemolytic disease of newborn.

In haemolytic anaemia there is rise in concentration of bile pigment in the plasma (this gives indirect Van den Bergh's reaction). There is associated jaundice.

2. *Anaemia due to defective formation of blood.* They are of following types:
   (a) *Nutritional anaemias*
   - Iron deficiency may be due to excessive loss of iron from the body as in chronic haemorrhage or due to inadequate quantity of iron in the diet (common in infants, adolescents, pregnancy where iron requirement is increased).
   - Protein deficiency is less common.
   - Lack of folic acid, vitamin C, pyridoxine, riboflavin, nicotinic or pantothenic acids in the diet.
   - Macrocytic anaemia of sprue is atrophy of intestinal mucous membrane leading to failure of absorption especially of vitamin B_{12}.

   (b) *Lack of failure in absorption or utilization of any of the antianaemic factor* especially cyanocobalamin (vitamin B_{12}).

   (c) *Aplasia of bone marrow.* It means failure of bone marrow to function. The resulting anaemia is termed aplastic anaemia. Aplasia may result due to following:
   - Primary failure of bone marrow to function.
   - Enormous exposure to X-rays or gamma rays.
   - Cancer in bone morrow.
   - Poisoning from aromatic organic chemicals or some toxins, e.g. benzol, gold, salts, radium, syphilitic toxins or bacterial toxins.
   - Kidney disease.

   Aplastic anaemia is normocytic normochromic.

   (d) *Infections.* Anaemia accompanying infection is usually a mild, normocytic normochromic type.

B. CLASSIFICATION ON THE BASIS OF SIZE OF THE CELL

The size of the cell is judged by calculating MCV (mean corpuscular volume). Normal MCV is 82 to 92 cubic microns. The types of anaemia based on MCV are:

- Microcytic (size of the cell smaller than normal).
- Normocytic (size of the cell normal).
- Macrocytic or megaloblastic (size of the cell is larger than normal).

C. CLASSIFICATION BASED ON AMOUNT OF HAEMOGLOBIN PRESENT PER RED BLOOD CELL

Amount of haemoglobin per RBC is determined by calculating MCH (mean corpuscular haemoglobin). Normally MCH varies from 28 to 32 micro-micrograms.

The types of anaemia based on MCH are:

- Hypochromic (MCH is lesser than normal).
- Normochromic (MCH is normal).
- Hyperchromic (MCH is more than normal).

What are the symptoms and signs of anaemia?

- Colour of skin, buccal and pharyngeal mucous membrane, conjunctiva, lips, tongue, palm, nail bed become pale.
- Increase in heart rate and velocity of blood flow.
- Increase in rate and force of respiration.
- Common symptoms of gastrointestinal tract like nausea, vomiting, constipation.
- Disturbance in menstrual cycle in females.
- Common symptoms like headache, loss of concentration, irritability, drowsiness, fainting.

What are the effects of anaemia on circulatory system?

Effects of anaemia on circulatory system:

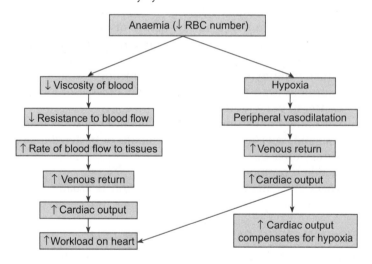

How do you determine type of anaemia?

Type of anaemia is determined by determining blood indices mainly:

- MCV (82 to 92 cubic microns).
- MCH (28 to 32 micro-micrograms).
- MCHC (mean corpuscular haemoglobin concentration). 32 to 38%.

What is colour index?

Ratio of percentage of haemoglobin to percentage of red blood cells is called colour index.

Haemoglobin concentration of 14.5 g/100 ml is considered as 100% and RBC count of 5 million/mm^3 is considered as 100%.

Colour index (CI) normally varies from 0.85 to 1.1. Usually both haemoglobin and cells percentage increase or decrease in the same proportion and thus colour index remains normal. Therefore, colour index is not very useful index for determining the type of anaemia.

POLYCYTHAEMIA

What is polycythaemia?

Increase in red blood cells above the normal range is known as polycythaemia.

What is secondary polycythaemia?

When tissues become hypoxic, the larger number of red blood cells are produced resulting in polycythaemia. This is called secondary polycythaemia. It occurs due to following reasons:

1. At high altitudes due to decreased PO$_2$ in atmosphere, hypoxic hypoxia results which causes polycythaemia, which is also called physiological polycythaemia.

2. Hypoxia caused due to cardiac failure.

What is polycythaemia vera?

Polycythaemia vera is the condition where red blood cell count increases as high as 7 to 8 million/mm^3. It is due to tumourous condition of the organs that produce red blood cells.

LIFE SPAN AND FATE OF RBC

What is haemolysis?

Disruption of red blood cells with release of haemoglobin is known as haemolysis.

What is the normal life span of red blood cell?

120 days.

Enumerate the methods for determination of life span of red blood cells.

1. *Differential agglutination method*
2. *Radioactive chromium method*

What are the causes of reduction in the life span of red blood cells?

Causes of reduction in the life span of red blood cells are as follows:

1. *Defects in red blood cells (corpuscular defects)*
   - *Spherocytosis.* It is the hereditary disease in which red blood cells are spherical rather than biconcave and are smaller in size. These cells cannot be compressed; therefore they get easily ruptured while passing through pulp of the spleen or by slight compression. This decreases the life span of red blood cells.
   - *Sickle cell anaemia.* This is the condition in which red blood cells contain abnormal haemoglobin called haemoglobin S. When this haemoglobin is exposed to low concentration of O_2 (in tissues), it precipitates as long crystals giving sickle-shaped appearance to red blood cells. This precipitation also damages the cell membrane and makes red blood cell more fragile. Cell gets easily haemolyzed and thus its life span is reduced.
2. *Extracorpuscular defects*
   - Transfusion of mismatched blood.
   - Reactions to drugs, malaria.
   - Hypersplenism.

What is the fate of red blood cells?

Cell remains in circulation for about 120 days. Its membrane becomes very fragile and cell ruptures while passing through some tight spots in circulation (many red cells fragment in spleen). Haemoglobin released after haemolysis is taken up by macrophages present in different tissues, but especially into those of liver, spleen and bone marrow. Macrophages break the haemoglobin molecule into haem and globin. Iron released from it enters into the circulation and is carried to bone marrow for utilization or to other tissues for storage in the form of ferritin.

Porphyrin portion of haem is converted to bile pigment bilirubin which is released into the blood. Bilirubin entered in circulation is taken up by the liver where it is made soluble by binding it with glucuronic acid or sulphate and is excreted in bile. In the intestine it is converted into urobilinogen by the intestinal bacteria. Most of the part of urobilinogen is excreted in faeces. It is oxidized to urobilin on exposure to air, or in faeces it is altered and oxidized to form stercobilin. Some part of urobilinogen is absorbed in blood and is excreted in urine.

Which is the principal cation in red blood cells?

The principal cation in red blood cells is potassium.

FRAGILITY

Define fragility.

Fragility is the index of resistance of the red blood cell to haemolyze in hypotonic solution (osmotic fragility).

Haemolysis of red blood cells commences at 0.46 to 0.38% of sodium chloride solution.

Why are venous red blood cells more fragile?

- Due to entry of CO_2 in red blood cells in tissues, chloride ions from plasma enter into the cells and ions of cells diffuse out into the plasma (chloride shift). This shift increases osmotic pressure of the cell causing entry of water from plasma into the cell (osmosis).
- Thus in venous blood, red cells have imbibed some quantity of water and therefore when placed in hypotonic solution, they can now take in smaller quantity of water as compared to arterial red blood cells, i.e. they become more fragile (get easily haemolyzed).

ESR

What is ESR?

Erythrocyte sedimentation rate (ESR) is the rate at which red blood cells settle down when blood containing an anticoagulant is allowed to stand in a vertically placed tube. It is expressed in millimeter at the end of one hour.

Name the methods used to determine ESR.

- Westergren's method.
- Wintrobe's method.

Which is the method preferred for ESR? Why?

Westergren's method is preferred for determination of ESR. Westergren's tube is longer and therefore chance of error in measurement of ESR is lesser than that in Wintrobe's method.

What is the clinical significance of ESR?

Erythrocyte sedimentation rate is not a diagnostic test, because it increases in large number of pathological conditions. But it is used as prognostic test, i.e. to judge the progress of the disease in patients under treatment. It is especially used in diseases like tuberculosis and rheumatic fever.

As ESR is increased in various diseases, it is also used as a routine investigation to rule out any organic disease.

Enumerate the main factors affecting ESR.

1. **Rate of rouleaux formation.** The red cells sediment because their density is greater than that of plasma, this is particularly so when the cells aggregate to form a rouleaux (i.e. the cells are piled on top of each other). Fibrinogen favours

rouleaux formation and causes increase in ESR. Protein which enters the plasma in inflammatory (globulins) and neoplastic diseases also favours rouleaux formation and hence increases ESR. Rate of rouleaux formation also depends on cell size and shape. Ratio of surface area to mass is an important factor. Therefore, increase in MCV or decrease in MCH retards rouleaux formation and hence decreases ESR.

2. **Number of red blood cells.** When the number of red cells is more, ESR is decreased and vice versa.
3. **Viscosity of blood.** ESR is reduced when the viscosity is more.

State various physiological variations in ESR.

- **Age.** In infants, ESR is low. It gradually increases up to puberty and then decreases until old age.
- **Sex.** ESR is greater in females.
- **Pregnancy.** ESR begins to increase at about third month of pregnancy and returns to normal 3 to 4 weeks after the delivery.
- **High altitudes.** ESR is less because of polycythaemia.

State various pathological variations in ESR.

1. Pathological increase in ESR occurs in following conditions:
   - All acute infections.
   - Acute episodes of chronic infections.
   - Bone diseases like rheumatoid arthritis, tuberculosis and osteomyelitis.
   - Tuberculosis of lung.
   - Malignant diseases.
   - Collagen diseases.
   - Anaemia.
2. Pathological decrease in ESR occurs in following conditions:
   - Polycythaemia due to any cause (various heart and lung diseases).
   - Decreased fibrinogen level.

JAUNDICE

What is jaundice? Name the different types of jaundice. How do you differentiate them?

Jaundice is a yellow discolouration of skin and mucous membrane due to presence of an excess of bilirubin in plasma and tissue fluids. Normal bilirubin level varies from 0.3 to 1 mg per 100 ml. An excess bilirubin can result from:

- Excessive breakdown of red blood cells—haemolytic jaundice (prehepatic jaundice).
- Infective or toxic damage to the liver cells—hepatic jaundice or hepatocellular jaundice.
- Obstruction to bile ducts—obstructive or posthepatic jaundice.

Bilirubin formed in RE cells is lipophilic, non-water soluble and exists in plasma as a protein conjugate. It is therefore not excreted in urine; hence in haemolytic jaundice urine does not show bilirubin. Bilirubin from plasma is conjugated to glucuronic acid. In liver cells bilirubin glucuronides (mono and di) are formed which are soluble in water and are excreted in urine. These conjugates are also regurgitated back into the blood stream and escape in urine when bilirubin glucuronide level rises above 2 mg per 100 ml. Bile salts also escape in blood stream and are excreted in urine in hepatic and posthepatic jaundice but not in prehepatic jaundice. In hepatic and posthepatic jaundice due to decreased secretion of bile salts into the intestine, fat digestion is affected. Fat content of stool rises. Haemolytic jaundice is not associated with any abnormalities of fat digestion.

Van den Bergh test. This test is done to differentiate different types of jaundice. In this test diazo agent (mixture of sulphanilic acid, hydrochloric acid and sodium nitrite) is added to serum. If serum contains increased bilirubin glucuronide (soluble bilirubin) reddish-violet colour results, the maximum colour intensity is reached within 30 seconds. This is the so-called *direct reaction.*

Sometimes there is delayed direct reaction where reddish colour appears (when diazo reagent is added to serum) which gradually becomes violet in 5 to 15 minutes.

Sometimes there is a biphasic reaction. A reddish colour appears promptly after addition of diazo reagent to serum and after much longer time becomes violet.

In hepatic jaundice (which is also called toxic or infective jaundice) Van den Bergh test is direct or biphasic.

When diazo reagent is mixed with a serum containing insoluble bilirubin (bilirubin protein complex) no colour develops. By adding alcohol, reddish-violet colour develops and then test is said to be *indirect positive.*

In haemolytic jaundice plasma gives an indirect Van den Bergh reaction, whereas in hepatic and posthepatic (obstructive) jaundice plasma will give direct Van den Bergh reaction.

WHITE BLOOD CELLS

What is the normal leucocyte (WBC) count?

Normal leucocyte count varies from 4000 to 11,000/mm^3 of blood.

Classify leucocytes.

Leucocytes are broadly classified on the basis of presence or absence of granules in the cytoplasm into:

- *Granulocytes*
- *Agranulocytes*

Granulocytes are of three types:

- *Neutrophils:* They contain granules which take both acidic and basic stain (Fig. 2.4).

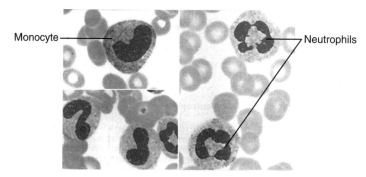

FIGURE 2.4 Neutrophils.

- *Eosinophils:* They contain granules which take acidic stain (Fig. 2.5).
- *Basophils:* They contain granules which take basic stain (Fig. 2.5).

Agranulocytes are of two types:

- *Lymphocytes* (Fig. 2.6).
- *Monocytes* (Fig. 2.7).

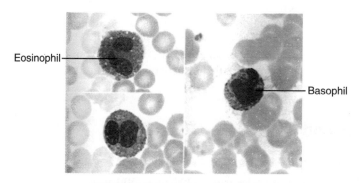

FIGURE 2.5 Eosinophils and basophils.

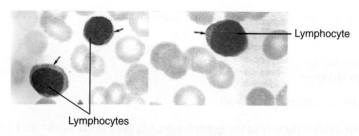

FIGURE 2.6 Lymphocytes.

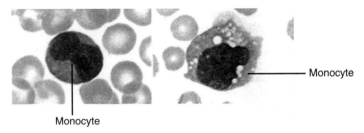

Monocyte

Monocyte

FIGURE 2.7 Monocytes.

Describe the functions of white blood cells (WBCs).

1. **Defence mechanism.** WBCs, mainly neutrophils and monocytes, constitute the second line of defence against the microorganisms, viruses and other injurious agents that enter the body; macrophages already present locally in the tissues act as first line of defence. These cells engulf foreign particles or bacteria and digest them. This process is called phagocytosis. These cells are the free cells and wander freely through the tissues. When bacteria invade the body these cells are attracted to the site by means of chemo-taxis. After reaching the area neutrophils and monocytes can pass out of blood vessels. They can move from place to place by diapedesis and with the help of pseudopodial processes they engulf the bacteria or foreign material.

Neutrophils entering the tissues are already mature cells that can immediately begin phagocytosis. On approaching a particle to be phagocytosed, neutrophil first attaches to the particle, then project pseudopodia in all directions around the particle. Pseudopodia meet each other on the opposite side and fuse. This creates an enclosed chamber with phagocytosed material. It breaks away from membrane forming a phagocytic vesicle. Neutrophil can usually phagocytose 5 to 20 bacteria before it itself becomes inactive or dead.

Monocytes after entering in the tissue get converted to macrophages. These are more powerful phagocytes than neutrophils and are capable of phagocytosing as many as 100 bacteria. They also have ability to engulf larger particles such as red blood cells, malarial parasites. Neutrophils are not capable of phagocytosing particles much larger than bacteria.

Once the phagocytic vesicle is formed in neutrophil or monocyte, lysosomes immediately come in contact with the vesicle and pour their enzymes into the vesicle. There are large number of proteolytic enzymes especially geared for digesting bacteria in lysosomes of neutrophils and macrophages. In addition lysosomes of macrophages also contain lipases which can digest the thick lipid membranes possessed by certain bacteria.

In addition neutrophils and macrophages also contain bactericidal agents which can kill most of the bacteria even when lysosomal enzymes fail to digest them. This is important because some bacteria have a protective coat which prevents their destruction by digestive enzymes. Much killing effect results from oxidizing agents (superoxide, H_2O_2, etc.) formed by enzymes in membrane of the phagosome or by organelle called peroxisome.

Some bacteria like tubercle bacterium have coats which are resistant to lysosomal digestion and even secrete some substances that resist killing effects of neutrophils and macrophages. Such types of bacteria are responsible for causing chronic diseases.

Eosinophils are not very motile and are weak phagocytes but still play important role in defence mechanism. Eosinophils increase in number in parasitic infections. Parasites are too large to be phagocytosed but eosinophils attach to juvenile form of parasites and kill them by:

- releasing hydrolytic enzymes.
- releasing highly reactive forms of oxygen that are lethal.
- releasing highly larvicidal polypeptide called major basic protein.

2. **Role in allergic reaction.** Eosinophils also increase in number in allergic conditions like bronchial asthma, hay fever. They are capable of detoxifying inflammation inducing substances released by mast cells and basophils. They phagocytose and destroy antigen-antibody complexes.

Basophils and similar cells located immediately outside the capillaries called mast cells release histamine, bradykinin, serotonin, heparin, slow reacting substances of anaphylaxis and large number of lysosomal enzymes. These substances in turn cause local vascular and tissue reactions that cause many allergic manifestations. Basophils and mast cells also release eosinophil chemotactic factor that causes eosinophils to migrate toward the inflammed allergic tissue. Eosinophils then phagocytose and destroy antigen-antibody complexes and prevent spread of local inflammatory process.

3. **Role in parasitic infection.** In parasitic infections, eosinophils are produced in large numbers into tissues which are diseased by parasites. Eosinophils attach themselves by way of special surface molecules to parasites and release substances which kill many of the parasites, e.g. releasing hydrolytic enzymes, releasing highly larvicidal polypeptide called major basic protein, releasing reactive form of oxygen which is lethal.

4. **Immunity.** Immunity is the capacity of human body to resist all types of microorganisms and their toxins that tend to damage the tissue or organ. Lymphocytes play important role in immunity. They are classified as B-lymphocytes and T-lymphocytes. B-lymphocytes are responsible for humoral immunity. Humoral immunity is by the antibodies which are circulating in the blood. These antibodies are gamma globulins produced by B-lymphocytes. They fight against the invading organisms. Humoral immunity is the major mechanism of defence against the bacterial infections. Macrophages play important role in the development of humoral immunity. Antibodies protect body against invading organisms by direct action and making organism inactive by agglutination, precipitation, neutralization or lysis.

Antibodies can also act through complement system (a system of plasma enzymes C_1 to C_9 and 3 subunits of C_1). These enzymes are activated by classical or alternative pathway (details are given in Chapter 3 on Immunity).

T-lymphocytes are responsible for cell-mediated immunity. It is a major defense against infections due to viruses and few bacteria. It also helps to defend against tumours (details are given in Chapter 3 on Immunity).

5. **Release of heparin.** Basophils release heparin into the blood. Heparin prevents clotting of blood.

What are macrophage and neutrophil responses during inflammation?

- Tissue macrophage is first line of defence against infection.
- Neutrophil invasion of inflamed area is second line of defence.
- A second macrophage invasion (monocytes) into the inflamed tissues is third line of defence.
- Increased production of granulocytes and monocytes by bone marrow is fourth line of defence.

Describe the feedback control of macrophage and neutrophil responses.

Various factors are involved in control of macrophage response to inflammation. These factors are formed by activated macrophages and T cells in inflamed tissues and other inflamed tissue cells.

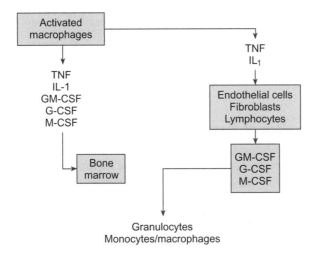

Which is the largest WBC in peripheral blood?

Monocyte.

Which is the more matured cell—large lymphocyte or small lymphocyte?

Small lymphocyte.

What is the clinical significance of doing differential WBC count?

Differential count (DC) is done to find out which type of WBCs are increased or decreased. In different diseases, different types of WBCs increase, e.g. in acute infections there is increase in the number of neutrophils.

In allergic conditions, there is increase in number of eosinophils.

What is absolute count? What is its importance?

Absolute count is the number of particular type of WBC/cumm of blood. If DC shows increase in number of any type of WBC, it may be a relative increase and not an absolute increase, e.g. increase in one type of cell may be due to relative decrease in other types of WBCs. Therefore, to know actual decrease or increase in the number of particular type of WBC, absolute count is necessary.

FORMATION OF WBCs

What is the life span of WBCs?

Granulocytes released from the bone marrow remain in circulating blood for 6 to 8 hours and then they enter the tissues where they live for 4 to 5 days. In cases of severe infection, life span may become as short as few hours.

Monocytes have short time in circulation (10 to 20 h), but in tissues they get converted to macrophages and can live for a few months or even for a year unless destroyed while doing phagocytic functions.

Lymphocytes remain in circulation for a few hours, then pass to the tissues and re-enter the blood through lymph. They have life span of months or a year depending upon body's need for these cells.

What are the sites of formation of leucocytes?

Granulocytes and monocytes are formed in the red bone marrow. Lymphocytes are produced in various lymphogenous organs including lymph glands, spleen, thymus, tonsils, lymphoid tissue in the bone marrow and GI tract.

Give the process of formation of WBCs.

There is differentiation of the pluripotential haemopoietic stem cells into different type of committed cells (Fig. 2.8).

Granulopoiesis occurs in bone marrow. Monocytes are also formed in the bone marrow.

Granulocytes and monocytes are formed from colony-forming unit GM (CFU-GM) as shown in the Figure 2.8.

Stem cells of lymphocytes are present in the bone marrow. The pluripotent stem cell gives origin to lymphoid stem cells (LSC) in addition to colony-forming units. Lymphoid stem cell forms lymphoblast which develops into lymphocytes (lymphocytes are produced mainly in the various lymphogenous organs including lymph glands, spleen, thymus, tonsils, bone marrow, Peyer's patches present underneath epithelium of gut wall).

Then some lymphocytes enter thymus (just before and after birth) and are processed there. They come out as T-lymphocytes. Some lymphocytes are processed in liver (in foetal life) and bone marrow (after birth). They are converted to B-lymphocytes.

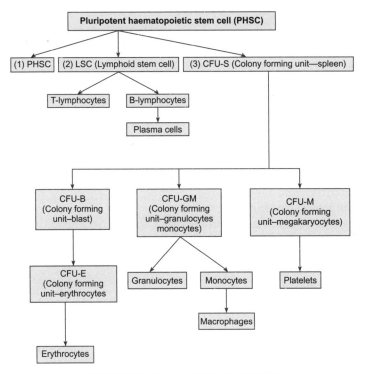

FIGURE 2.8 Process of formation of WBCs.

Granulocytes are formed in the bone marrow and are stored in the bone marrow. When need arises they are released in circulation. Normally about three times as many granulocytes are stored in the marrow as circulate in the entire blood.

How is leucopoiesis regulated?

1. Colony stimulating factors (CSF):
   (a) G-CSF (granulocyte CSF).
   (b) M-CSF (monocyte CSF).
   (c) GM-CSF (granulocyte-monocyte CSF).
2. Interleukins. They are cytokines which stimulate lymphocyte production.

ABNORMALITIES

What is leucocytosis?

Increase in total WBC count above 11,000/mm^3 is called leucocytosis.

State the physiological conditions causing leucocytosis.

- Newborn babies up to the age of one year. At birth WBC count is about 18,000/mm^3 but it drops gradually to adult level.

- After muscular exercise.
- After food intake.
- Mental stress—in severe pain, emotional states, etc.
- Exposure to very low temperature.
- Pregnancy—at full term, total WBC count is 12,000 to 15,000/mm³.
- Parturition.

Enumerate the pathological conditions causing leucocytosis.

- Acute bacterial infections especially by pyogenic organisms. Infection may be localized (e.g. boil, abscess) or generalized (pneumonia, bronchitis).
- Haemorrhage and burns.
- Malignant diseases cause leucocytosis if there is secondary infection.
- Post-operative.

What is leucopenia?

Decrease in total WBC count below 4000/mm³ is called leucopenia.

Enumerate the pathological conditions causing leucopenia.

- Infections by non-pyogenic bacteria, e.g. typhoid fever, paratyphoid fever, malaria, viral infections such as influenza, smallpox, mumps, etc.
- Drugs such as chloromycetin, cytotoxic drugs used in malignant diseases cause leucopenia.
- Repeated exposure to X-ray or radium.
- Aplasia of bone marrow.
- Chemical poisons like arsenic, dinitrophenol, antimony cause depression of bone marrow.
- Malnutrition.

What is leukaemia?

Leukaemia is a malignant disease in which there is abnormal increase in WBC count with presence of immature WBCs in the peripheral blood. Total WBC count may be as high as 100,000 to 300,000/mm³.

What are the types of leukaemia?

Types of leukaemia:

- Lymphocytic
- Myelogenous

Lymphocytic leukaemia is caused due to cancerous production by lymphoid cells usually beginning in lymph nodes or other lymphocytic tissues and spreading to other areas of the body.

In myelogenous leukaemia there occurs cancerous production of young myelogenous cells in bone marrow and then spreads throughout the body so that white blood cells are produced in extramedullary organs especially lymph nodes, spleen and liver.

What is neutrophilia? When does it occur?

Increase in circulating neutrophils (increase in neutrophil counts) is known as neutrophilia. It is the commonest cause of leucocytosis.

CAUSES OF NEUTROPHILIA

Physiological causes	Pathological causes
▪ Newborn babies.	▪ Acute bacterial infections, especially by cocci (streptococci, staphylococci, pneumococci or meningococci), acute *E. coli* and *Shigella* infections, plague, etc.
▪ After meals.	
▪ Muscular exercise.	
▪ Pregnancy.	
▪ Parturition.	▪ Certain acute viral infections, e.g. smallpox, chickenpox, poliomyelitis.
▪ Emotional stress.	▪ Non-infective inflammatory conditions like gout, acute rheumatic fever, burn, after surgical operations, etc.
	▪ Intoxication—uraemia, diabetic ketoacidosis.
	▪ Acute haemorrhage.
	▪ Myeloproliferative disorders like polycythaemia vera.

What is neutropenia? When does it occur?

Decrease in neutrophil count is known as neutropenia. It occurs in following conditions:

- Typhoid, paratyphoid fever.
- Malaria.
- Aplastic anaemia due to depression of bone marrow.
- Drugs depressing bone marrow, e.g. chloramphenicol.
- Radiation.

What is basophilia? When does it occur?

Increase in basophil count is known as basophilia. It occurs in chronic myeloid leukaemia (CML).

What is Arneth's count? What is the information obtained from it?

Counting number of neutrophils with different nuclear lobes and expressing the count as percentage of cells with different number of nuclear lobes is called Arneth's count.

What is agranulocytosis?

Absence of granulocytes in the blood is known as agranulocytosis.

What is lymphocytosis? When does it occur?

Increase in the lymphocyte count is known as lymphocytosis.

Physiological causes

- Young infants.
- During menstruation.

Pathological causes

- Chronic infections like tuberculosis, whooping cough.
- Virus infections inducing rash.
- Autoimmune diseases.
- Infectious mononucleosis.
- Lymphatic leukaemia.

What is lymphopenia? When does it occur?

Lymphopenia is decrease in lymphocyte count. It occurs in patients on steroid therapy.

What is eosinophilia? When does it occur?

Increase in eosinophil count is known as eosinophilia. It occurs in following conditions:

- Various allergic conditions like bronchial asthma, hay fever, tropical eosinophilia.
- Scarlet fever.
- Worm infestations.
- Skin diseases.

What is eosinopenia? When does it occur?

Decrease in eosinophil count is known as eosinopenia. It occurs in patients on steroid therapy, in stressful conditions and in acute pyogenic infections.

What is monocytosis? When does it occur?

Increase in monocyte count is known as monocytosis. It occurs in following conditions:

- Infectious mononucleosis.
- Malaria.
- Kala-azar.
- Collagen diseases.
- Subacute bacterial endocarditis.
- Protozoal infections.

PLATELETS

What is normal platelet count?

It varies from 150,000 to 450,000/mm^3.

Describe the structure of platelet.

Platelet is an oval disc, 2 to 4 micrometre in diameter. It does not have nucleus and therefore cannot reproduce. In its cytoplasm it has following active factors:

1. **Actin and myosin molecules and thrombosthenin.** Actin and myosin molecules are similar to those of contractile proteins of muscle. In addition there is thrombosthenin. These proteins can cause the platelet to contract.

2. **Residual endoplasmic reticulum and Golgi's apparatus.** These structures synthesize various enzymes and store large quantities of calcium.

3. **Mitochondria.** These are capable of forming ATP adenosine triphosphate) and ADP (adenosine diphosphate).

4. **Enzymes for synthesis of prostaglandins.** Prostaglandins act as local hormones and have local vascular and tissue reactions.

5. **Fibrin stabilizing factor.** It is an important protein having role in blood coagulation.

6. **Growth factor.** This causes growth of vascular endothelial cells, vascular smooth muscle cells and fibroblasts, and helps in repair of damaged vessel wall.

7. **von Willebrand factor.** It is responsible for adherence of platelets.

Cell membrane of platelet has a coat of glycoproteins on its surface which causes it to avoid adherence to normal endothelium and yet to adhere to injured areas. Membrane of platelet contains phospholipids containing platelet factor III which plays activating role at several points in blood clotting process.

Describe the functions of platelets.

Platelets do the following functions.

1. **Haemostasis.** It means prevention of blood loss. Platelets do the function of haemostasis in two ways:

(a) Platelets secrete 5-HT which causes constriction of blood vessel when blood vessel is injured or ruptured.

(b) Plug formation. Platelets repair the vascular openings by formation of plug. When platelets come in contact with a damaged vascular surface such as collagen fibres in the vascular wall or damaged endothelial cells, they change their characteristics. They begin to swell and assume irregular forms with large number of pseudopodia protruding from the surface. Their contractile proteins contract forcefully and cause release of granules that contain multiple factors. They become sticky and therefore stick to the collagen fibres of the vessel. They secrete large quantities of ADP and their enzymes form thromboxane A$_2$ which is also secreted into the blood. ADP and thromboxane act on nearby platelets and cause their activation. Stickiness of these additional platelets causes them to adhere to originally activated platelets. Thus at the site of any rent in a vessel a vicious cycle is initiated which causes successive activation of more and more number of platelets thus forming a platelet plug. At first it is a fairly loose plug but is successful in blocking the blood loss if vascular opening is small (during subsequent process blood clot is formed at the site forming tight and unyielding seal).

Platelet plug mechanism is important in closing the minute ruptures in very small blood vessels that occur hundreds of time daily. Multiple holes in endothelial cells are closed by platelets.

2. **Clot formation.** Platelets are responsible for forming intrinsic prothrombin activator. It is initiated by trauma to blood itself or exposure of blood to collagen in a traumatized blood vessel. This causes activation of factor XII and release of platelet phospholipid which contains the lipoprotein called platelet factor III. This plays an important role in subsequent reaction which leads to formation of prothrombin activator which is responsible for onset of blood clotting.

3. **Clot retraction.** Within few minutes after clot formation, it begins to contract and usually expresses most of the fluid called serum (plasma without fibrinogen and other clotting factors) within 20 to 30 minutes. Platelets are necessary for clot retraction.

Platelets are attached to fibrin fibres of the clot in such a way that they actually bond different fibres together. Platelets entrapped in the clot continue to release procoagulant substances like fibrin stabilizing factor which causes more and more cross linking bonds between different fibrin fibres. Platelet thrombosthenin, actin and myosin (the contractile proteins of platelets) cause strong contraction of platelet spicules attached to fibrin fibres. This helps to compress the fibrin meshwork into a smaller mass. Contraction is activated by thrombin and calcium ions present in the mitochondria, endoplasmic reticulum and Golgi apparatus of platelets.

4. When platelets disintegrate, 5-hydroxytryptamine (5-HT) and histamine are liberated. 5-HT has vasoconstrictor effect and helps in haemostatic mechanism.

How are platelets formed?

Platelets are formed in the bone marrow. Pluripotent stem cell gives rise to CFU-M (colony-forming unit macrophage). This develops into megakaryocyte, the largest cell in the bone marrow. The cytoplasm of megakaryocyte forms pseudopodia. A portion of pseudopodium is detached to form platelet which enters circulation.

What is the life span of platelets?

From 7 to 10 days.

Enumerate the physiological variations in platelet count.

Physiological variations in platelet count are uncommon. Platelet count may increase after severe muscular exercise and at high altitudes. Sometimes platelet count decreases during menstruation.

Enumerate the pathological variations in platelet count.

Pathological variations in platelet count are as follows:

1. *Thrombocytopenia* (decrease in platelet count) occurs in:
   - Idiopathic thrombocytopenic purpura.
   - Bone marrow depression due to cytotoxic drugs.
   - Leukaemia or secondary deposits of malignancy in the bone marrow.
   - Acute septic fever.
   - Toxaemia—septicaemia, uraemia, etc.
2. *Thrombocytosis* (increase in the platelet count) occurs after removal of spleen.

What is the normal bleeding time?

It varies from 1 to 6 minutes.

What is purpura?

Purpura is a condition in which bleeding time is prolonged while clotting time remains normal.

How is purpura classified?

Purpura is classified into:

1. Primary idiopathic purpura which is probably an autoimmune disease.
2. Symptomatic idiopathic purpura due to allergy, cancer, drugs and irradiation.

CLOTTING OF BLOOD

What is coagulation or clotting of blood?

Transformation of blood into a solid gel is termed blood coagulation or clotting.

What is thrombus?

Clot that is developed in a vessel is known as thrombus.

What is normal clotting time?

Normal clotting time is about 6 to 10 minutes.

Mention the steps in coagulation.

There are three steps in coagulation:

1. **Formation of prothrombin activator.** Prothrombin activator is a complex substance formed in response to rupture of the vessel or damage to the blood itself.

2. **Conversion of prothrombin to thrombin.** Prothrombin activator which is formed catalyzes conversion of prothrombin (protein present in blood) to thrombin.

3. **Conversion of fibrinogen to fibrin.** Thrombin acts as an enzyme converting soluble fibrinogen (protein present in the blood) to insoluble fibrin threads. These fibrin threads form the meshwork in which blood cells are entangled.

Enumerate the different clotting factors present in the blood.

Clotting factor		Synonym
Fibrinogen	...	Factor I
Prothrombin	...	Factor II
Tissue thromboplastin	...	Factor III, tissue factor
Calcium	...	Factor IV
Labile factor proaccelerin AC—globulin (AC-G)	...	Factor V
Stable factor—Serum prothrombin conversion accelerator (SPCA)	...	Factor VII
Antihaemophilic factor (AHF)	...	Factor VIII
Antihaemophilic globulin (AHG) (Christmas factor)	...	Factor IX
Stuart factor	...	Factor X
Plasma thromboplastin antecedent (PTA)	...	Factor XI
Hageman factor	...	Factor XII
Fibrin-stabilizing factor	...	Factor XIII
Fletcher factor	...	Prekallikrein
Fitzgerald factor	...	High-molecular-weight kininogen platelets

How is the clot formation initiated?

Clot formation is initiated either due to trauma to the vascular wall and adjacent tissues, trauma to blood or contact of blood with damaged endothelial cells or collagen or other tissue elements outside the vessel. Clot is initiated by formation of prothrombin activator. Prothrombin activator can be formed in two basic ways:

- Extrinsic pathway
- Intrinsic pathway

Describe the extrinsic mechanism of initiation of clotting.

Extrinsic mechanism of initiation of clotting begins with trauma to vessel wall or extravascular tissues. It occurs in three basic steps as follows:

- **Release of tissue thromboplastin.** Traumatized tissue releases complex of several factors called tissue thromboplastin. This includes phospholipids of membranes of the tissues and lipoprotein complex containing glycoprotein which acts as an enzyme.

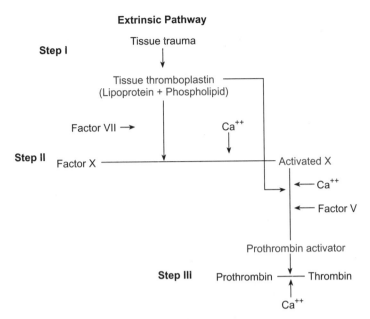

Extrinsic Pathway

FIGURE 2.9 Extrinsic mechanism of clot formation.

- **Activation of factor X to form activated factor X.** Lipoprotein complex of tissue thromboplastin complexes with factor VII in presence of tissue phospholipids, and calcium ions act enzymatically on factor X to convert it into activated factor X.
- **Effects of activated factor X to form prothrombin activator.** Activated factor X complexes with tissue phospholipid (as a part of tissue phospholipid or released from platelets) and also with factor V to form a complex called prothrombin activator. The extrinsic pathway is illustrated in Figure 2.9.

Describe the intrinsic mechanism of initiation of clot formation.

Intrinsic mechanism of clot formation is initiated due to trauma to blood itself or exposure of blood to collagen in a traumatized vascular wall. It is formed of series of cascading reactions illustrated in Figure 2.10.

What is the role of calcium in intrinsic and extrinsic pathway?

Except for the first two steps in intrinsic pathway, calcium ions are required for promotion of all reactions. Therefore, in absence of calcium, blood clotting will not occur.

When does only intrinsic mechanism initiate coagulation?

When blood is removed from the body and held in a test tube, intrinsic pathway alone initiates clotting. This usually results due to contact of factor XII and platelets with the wall of test tube which activates both of them to initiate intrinsic mechanism.

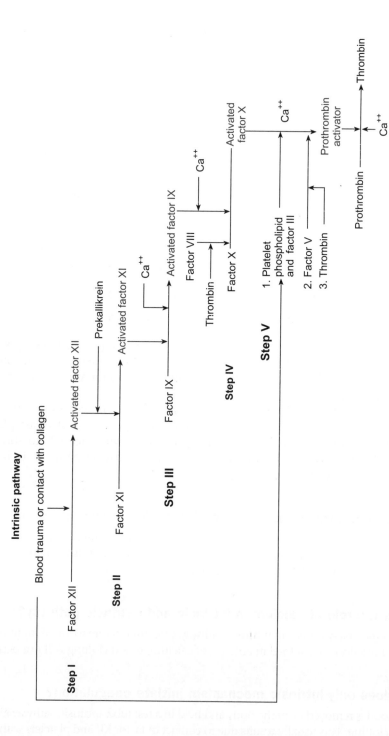

FIGURE 2.10 Intrinsic mechanism of clot formation.

When blood vessel is ruptured, how is clotting initiated?

When blood vessel is ruptured, clotting is initiated by both intrinsic and extrinsic pathways simultaneously. Tissue thromboplastin initiates extrinsic pathway and contact of factor XII and the platelets with collagen in the vascular wall initiates the intrinsic pathway.

What is the difference between extrinsic and intrinsic mechanism for initiation of clotting?

Extrinsic pathway can be explosive in nature. Once initiated its speed of occurrence is only limited by amount of tissue thromboplastin and factors X, VII and V in the blood. Clotting occurs as quickly as within 15 seconds if there is severe tissue damage.

Intrinsic pathway is much slower and it takes 1–6 minutes to cause clotting.

How is clotting of blood inside the vascular system prevented?

There are several factors which prevent intravascular clotting as follows:

1. **Endothelial surface factors.**
   - Smoothness of endothelial lining prevents initiation of intrinsic mechanism.
   - A layer of glycocalyx (mucopolysaccharide) adsorbed to the inner surface repels clotting factors and platelets.
   - A protein bound with endothelial membrane called thrombomodulin binds thrombin. This slows the clotting process by removal of thrombin. In addition, combined thrombomodulin-thrombin complex also activates plasma protein (protein C) which acts as anticoagulant by inactivating factors V and VIII.
2. **Fibrin and antithrombin III actin.** Alpha globulin called antithrombin III and fibrin threads are powerful anticoagulants in the blood because they remove thrombin from blood.
3. **Heparin.** Heparin is another powerful anticoagulant present in the blood. But its concentration in the blood is so less that under physiological conditions it has very little anticoagulant effect.
4. **Alpha-2 macroglobulin.** This is a very large globulin molecule present in the blood. It acts as a binding agent for several coagulation factors and prevents their proteolytic actions until they can be destroyed in various ways. Thus it plays an important role in preventing blood clotting.

Describe the mechanism by which heparin acts as anticoagulant.

Heparin by itself does not have anticoagulant property. It acts in following ways:

- It combines with antithrombin III and increases its effectiveness in removing thrombin.
- Complex of heparin with antithrombin III also removes several other activated coagulation factors such as factors XII, XI, IX and X.

Where are clotting factors synthesized?

With few exceptions, almost all the clotting factors are synthesized in liver.

Name the vitamin K dependent clotting factors.

Vitamin K is required for formation of four most important clotting factors:

1. Prothrombin.
2. Factor VII.
3. Factor IX.
4. Factor X.

What is haemophilia?

Haemophilia is a disorder in which clotting time is prolonged. It is a hereditary coagulation disorder and is of two types:

1. *Classical haemophilia (haemophilia A)* is due to deficiency of clotting factor VIII. In 85% of haemophilia cases there is deficiency of factor VIII.
2. *Christmas disease (haemophilia B)* is due to deficiency of factor IX. In 15% of haemophilia cases, factor IX is deficient.

Why is haemophilia uncommon in females?

Haemophilia occurs due to deficiency of clotting factor VIII or IX. Both these factors are transmitted genetically by way of female chromosome as a recessive trait. Therefore, female does not suffer from haemophilia if at least one of the two female chromosomes will have appropriate genes. If one of the X-chromosomes is deficient, she will be a haemophilic carrier.

What happens to bleeding time in haemophilia?

Bleeding time is normal in a haemophilic person, only clotting time is prolonged.

What are physiological variations in clotting time?

Physiologically clotting time is reduced during menstruation and before and during parturition.

Give the pathological variations in clotting time.

Clotting time is prolonged in:

- Haemophilia (due to lack of factor VIII).
  - Liver disease.
  - Afibrinogenaemia.
  - Christmas disease (due to lack of factor IX).
  - Vitamin K deficiency.
  - Disseminated intravascular coagulation (DIC).

ANTICOAGULANTS

What are anticoagulants?

Anticoagulants are the substances which prevent clotting of blood.

Name anticoagulants used in vitro.

Anticoagulants used *in vitro* are:

- Sodium citrate 3.8%
- Potassium ammonium oxalate
- Sodium edetate (ethylenediaminetetraacetic acid—EDTA)
- Heparin

They act by sequestering calcium.

Name anticoagulants used in vivo.

Anticoagulants used *in vivo* are:

1. **Heparin.** It can be used *in vitro* as well as *in vivo*. It can be injected in patients to prevent the development or spread of venous thrombosis. Its action begins within a few minutes and lasts for hours. Heparin can also be given intravenously.

2. **Dicoumarol.** This is a coumarin derivative. Because of its chemical resemblance with vitamin K, it acts as antivitamin K by the process of substrate competition. In liver it replaces vitamin K but does not carry out physiological function of vitamin K. So vitamin K deficiency develops leading to decreased synthesis of prothrombin, factors VII, IX and X. Thus dicoumarol acts as anticoagulant only *in vivo*. It is given orally, the effect of one lasting for several days. It is used in venous and coronary thrombosis.

3. **Other anticoagulants acting as vitamin K antagonists** are phenindione, warfarin, nicoumalone. Their speed of onset and duration of action are different from dicoumarol.

4. **Sodium citrate (3.8%)** chelates calcium and thereby acts as anticoagulant. It is added to the blood collected for transfusion.

What is the antidote for heparin?

Protamine is the antidote for heparin. It reverts clotting mechanism to normal when heparin is injected in excess and leads to the serious bleeding crisis.

Enumerate the factors which hasten and retard coagulation.

Factors hastening coagulation:

- Exposure of blood *in vitro* to a negatively charged surface such as glass surface. It allows contact activation of platelets and factor XII to initiate intrinsic mechanism of clot formation.
- Increase in temperature.

Factors delaying clotting time:

- When siliconized containers are used for collecting blood, blood does not clot for a long time (an hour or more).
- Lowering the temperature of blood.
- Dilution of the blood.

DISEASES

What is disseminated intravascular coagulation?

When clotting mechanism becomes activated in widespread areas of the circulation condition, disseminated intravascular coagulation (DIC) is produced. It is mostly due to large amounts of traumatized or dying tissue in the body which releases thromboplastin into the blood (e.g. septicaemic shock). In this condition there is plugging of small vessels with clots resulting in decreased O_2 and nutrients supply to the tissues. In this condition a person begins to bleed because of removal of clotting factors by widespread clotting and very few precoagulants present in the remaining blood.

Name the conditions which cause excessive bleeding in human being.

- Deficiency of vitamin K.
- Haemophilia.
- Thrombocytopenia (deficiency of platelets).
- Diseases of liver such as hepatitis, acute yellow atrophy (because most of the clotting factors are formed in liver).

METHODS FOR DETERMINATION OF DEFECTS IN BLOOD CLOTTING

What are the methods for determination of clotting time?

Clotting time is determined by two methods:

- **Capillary method.** Using glass capillary.
- **Lee and White method.** Ideal method.

Name the important tests for determination of defects in blood clotting.

- Clotting time.
- Prothrombin time.
- Thromboplastin generation test.

What is prothrombin time? What is the significance of doing this test?

From the citrated blood, plasma is separated. To this plasma, large excess of calcium and tissue thromboplastin is added and time required for coagulation is measured. This is prothrombin time. In this test, calcium nullifies the effect of oxalate and tissue thromboplastin acts as prothrombin activator, i.e. it initiates extrinsic pathway.

This test gives indication of total quantity of prothrombin in the blood. Normal prothrombin time is 10 to 12 seconds. Similar test can also be designed for other clotting factors.

CLOT LYSIS

What is clot lysis? How does it occur?

Clot lysis is a process of liquefaction of clot. Plasma protein euglobulin contains enzyme plasminogen (profibrinolysin) which when activated to plasmin or fibrinolysin causes cleavage of fibrin threads, breaking fibrin into successively smaller soluble fragments called fibrin degradation products.

Normally plasmin is present in blood in inactive form called plasminogen. Large amount of plasminogen is trapped in the clot. Injurious tissue and vascular endothelium release a powerful plasminogen activator.

What is plasmin inhibitor? What is its role?

Plasmin not only destroys fibrin but it also digests fibrinogen and number of other clotting factors. Therefore, a small amount of plasmin in circulation would seriously impede the activation of clotting system, if there is no plasmin inhibitor. α_2 antiplasmin acts as plasmin inhibitor. This binds with plasmin and inhibits it.

What is the significance of plasmin system?

Plasmin system causes lysis of blood clots allowing slow clearing of extraneous blood clots in the tissue. It also allows reopening of clotted vessels. Especially it removes minute clots which are formed in millions of tiny peripheral vessels which would eventually occlude if there is no plasmin system.

BLOOD GROUPS

What are the different blood group systems?

Different blood group systems are: ABO, Rhesus, MNSs, P, E, Kell, Duffy, Lutheran, Lewis, etc.

How are the blood groups under 'ABO' type classified?

ABO groups are classified as A, B, AB and O according to the type of agglutinogen present in the red blood cells of the person.

Persons having 'A' agglutinogen are called A group persons.
Persons having 'B' agglutinogen are called B group persons.
Persons having 'A and B' agglutinogens are called AB group persons.
Persons having no agglutinogen are called O group persons.

State Landsteiner's law.

Landsteiner's law states that if an agglutinogen is present in the red cells of the blood, the corresponding agglutinin must be absent from the plasma; if the agglutinogen is absent, corresponding agglutinin must be present in the plasma.

What are the agglutinins present in ABO group system?

Person having 'A' group has anti B or beta agglutinins in plasma.
  Person having 'B' group has anti A or alpha agglutinins in plasma.
  Person having 'AB' group does not have any agglutinins in his plasma.
  Person having 'O' group has both anti A and anti B agglutinins in his plasma.

Describe the inheritance of ABO group system.

1. Agglutinogens (antigens) A and B are inherited as Mendelian dominant and first appear in six week of foetal life. Their concentration is low at birth but, progressively rises up to puberty. Blood group antigens are present on the RBC membrane. They are also present in many other tissues like salivary glands, pancreas, kidneys, liver, lungs, testes and body fluids (saliva semen amniotic fluid).
2. Specific agglutinins (antibodies) are present in the plasma and appear at 10th day after birth and rise peak level at 10 years of age.

Phenotype and possible genotypes are given in the following table:

Phenotype	Genotype
Group A	AA, AO
Group B	BB, BO
Group AB	AB
Group O	OO

The above four blood groups depend on 3 genes—A, B and O. Genes A and B can be demonstrated by use of anti A and anti B. Presence of 'O' gene is not easily demonstrated. Antiserum cells react alive with AA and AO genotype and therefore, serologically, both are group A (phenotype).

If the mother has B group and father has A group offspring will have following blood group.

	Father	Mother
Phenotype	A	B
Genotype	AA, AO	BB, BO
Inherited gene	A A A O	B B B O
	I II III IV	1 2 3 4

Offspring have the following combinations and blood groups:

		1	2	3	4
I	Genotype	AB	AB	AB	AO
	Phenotype	AB	AB	AB	A
II	Genotype	AB	AB	AB	AO
	Phenotype	AB	AB	AB	A
III	Genotype	AB	AB	AB	AO
	Phenotype	AB	AB	AB	A
IV	Genotype	BO	BO	BO	OO
	Phenotype	B	B	B	O

BLOOD TRANSFUSION

What is a donor and is a recipient?

Person who donates the blood is a donor and person who receives blood is a recipient.

What is universal donor? Is this term used correctly?

'O' group person is called universal donor because he does not contain any agglutinogen and he can donate blood to any person. But this term is no longer valid as it ignores the complications produced by existence of Rh factors and other blood group systems (especially Rh group also must be considered).

What is universal recipient? Is this term true?

Person having 'AB' group is called universal recipient because he does not contain any agglutinins. So he can receive blood from group A, group B as well as group O or group AB person. But this term is not valid because it ignores the complications produced by the existence of the Rh factors and other blood group systems.

How is the blood stored?

Blood is collected with complete aseptic precautions. It is stored in a sterile container. To each 480 ml of blood 120 ml of ACD (acid citrate dextrose) mixture is added. Blood is stored at 4°C. It can be used up to 21 days if stored under above precautions.

ACD mixture contains:

- Acid citric (monohydrous)   0.48 g
- Trisodium citrate   1.32 g
- Dextrose   1.47 g
- Distilled water   100 ml

What is the purpose of addition of glucose to ACD mixture?

Red blood cells in the blood tend to swell and haemolyze unless sodium-potassium pump remains active. Pump activity maintains the size of the cell. This pump requires energy. When blood is taken out of the body, this energy is provided by glucose added to ACD mixture. If glucose is not added, rate of haemolysis of RBCs would be very high.

What precautions are taken while selecting the donor?

- He should be healthy.
- He should not suffer from diseases like malaria, AIDS, etc. which are spread through blood.
- Haemoglobin and PCV should be within normal range. This is grossly determined by measuring specific gravity of fresh capillary blood.
- Cross matching of blood should be done.

What is cross-matching of blood?

Blood is collected from donor as well as recipient. Plasma and red blood cells are separated in each. Then donor's cells are mixed with recipient's plasma (major cross) and recipient's cells are mixed with donor's plasma (minor cross). This is called cross-matching. If there is no agglutination in either of the cases described above, recipient can safely receive donor's blood.

Why is matching of donor's cells with recipient plasma called major cross-matching?

When mismatched blood is transfused in a recipient, the donor's cells get agglutinated because against their agglutinogen, there is a high agglutinin concentration in the recipient's plasma. Because of high concentration of agglutinins, reaction between donor's cells and recipient's plasma can easily take place and therefore matching of donor's cells with recipient's plasma is called major cross-matching.

Why is matching of recipient's cells with donor's plasma called minor cross-matching?

Reaction of donor's plasma and recipient's cells is not very important and usually does not occur on giving mismatched blood transfusion. Normally amount of donor's blood given is 500 ml. Half of it is plasma (about 250 ml). This donor's plasma when enters recipient's circulation, gets diluted with recipient's blood. Therefore, concentration of donor's agglutinins in the recipient's blood is very low, not sufficient to cause agglutination of recipient's cells. Therefore, matching between donor's plasma and recipient's cells is called minor cross-matching.

What precautions should be taken during blood transfusion?

- Transfusion should be done only if it is absolutely indicated.
- Donor's and recipient's blood groups (ABO as well as Rh) should be checked and cross-matching should be done to exclude mismatching of blood groups other than ABO and Rh.
- Rh-positive blood should never be transfused to Rh-negative person.
- Before starting the blood transfusion, label on the blood bottle should be checked for the name and the blood group.
- Transfusion should be given at a slow rate (not more than 20 drops/min). If it is given fast, citrate present in stored blood may cause chelation of calcium leading to decreased serum calcium level and tetany.
- Proper aseptic precautions must be taken during transfusion.

What are the indications of blood transfusion?

Blood transfusion is indicated in following conditions:

- Major operations.
- Cases where there is severe blood loss.
- Haemophilia.
- Aplastic anaemia.
- Agranulocytosis.

What are the hazards of mismatched blood transfusion?

- Agglutination of donor's red blood cells in the recipient's circulation.
- Agglutinated cells may block certain vessels leading to tissue ischaemia.
- Agglutinated red cells get haemolyzed leading to greater breakdown of haemoglobin and greater formation of bile pigments, causing haemolytic type of jaundice.
- Acute renal shut down (anuria). It occurs within a few minutes to a few hours after transfusion of mismatched blood, and continues until the person dies of renal failure. It results from three causes:
  1. Release of toxic substances from the haemolyzing blood cause powerful renal vasoconstriction.
  2. Loss of circulating red cells and toxic substances both cause circulatory shock leading to fall in arterial blood pressure and decreased renal blood flow.
  3. Haemolysis of red cells causes haemoglobinaemia, i.e. increased circulating haemoglobin. Total free haemoglobin becomes more than that can bind with haptoglobin (plasma protein binding haemoglobin). Free haemoglobin leaks through glomerular membrane and enters in renal tubules. If this amount is high it precipitates and blocks the renal tubules (especially if urine is acidic).
- Anuria leads to uraemia, shock and unconsciousness. This may be lethal if untreated.

Rh BLOOD GROUP SYSTEM

What is Rh factor? Who discovered it? Why is it so named?

Rh factor is an agglutinogen found in red blood cells of some human beings (called Rh-positive persons). It was discovered by Landsteiner and Wiener in 1940. It is so named because it was found first in Rhesus monkeys.

What are the various Rh agglutinogens in Rh system?

There are six important agglutinogens as C, c, D, d, E, e. Out of these Rh 'D' is of clinical importance.

Describe the inheritance of Rh Group

Three types of Rh antigens C, D and E are recognized. But, 'D' antigen is commonest and produces transfusion reactions. Therefore, for all practical purposes Rh antigen is referred to as 'D' antigen. Person possessing 'D' antigen is Rh positive and not possessing 'D' antigen is Rh negative.

Antigen 'D' is inherited as dominant gene. When 'D' is absent from chromosome, its place is taken by 'd'.

Phenotype	Genotype
Rh +ve (85%)	DD 35%, Dd (50%)
Rh −ve (15%)	dd

What is the clinical importance of Rh group?

In Rh group system, natural antibodies against Rh agglutinogens are not present, i.e. Rh-negative person does not have agglutinins against Rh antigen. Therefore, if by chance a Rh-negative person receives Rh-positive blood for the first time, Rh antigen causes sensitization, i.e. stimulation of immune system. Large number of antibodies (agglutinins) is formed against Rh antigen. Thus when that person is given Rh-positive blood next time, he gets severe reaction.

Similarly, in Rh-negative woman bearing Rh-positive child for the first time sensitization occurs. At the time of delivery foetal cells enter maternal circulation. Mother is sensitized and agglutinins against Rh antigen are formed. If next time also the woman bears Rh-positive child, it is likely to suffer because of agglutinins passing from mother to foetus through placenta. These agglutinins cause agglutination of foetal red blood cells leading to disease called erythroblastosis fetalis.

How can erythroblastosis fetalis be prevented?

Erythroblastosis fetalis can be prevented by desensitizing the pregnant Rh-negative mother (bearing Rh-positive foetus) by injecting antibodies IgH (anti-D agglutinins).

What is the clinical picture of erythroblastosis fetalis?

Baby suffering from erythroblastosis fetalis if anaemic at birth, has jaundice. Haemopoietic tissue of baby attempts to replace the haemolyzed red blood cells. Because of rapid production of red blood cells, earlier forms (erythroblasts) appear in peripheral blood. Hence, the name of the disease is erythroblastosis fetalis. Liver and spleen are also enlarged. Because of haemolysin and excess bilirubin production, there is damage to motor areas of brain due to precipitation of bilirubin in neurons causing their destruction. This condition is known as kernicterus.

What is the treatment for erythroblastosis fetalis?

Treatment for erythroblastosis fetalis is replacement of newborn baby's blood with Rh-negative blood. Baby's own Rh-positive blood is removed slowly and about 400 ml of Rh-negative blood is infused over a period of 1.5 hours or more. This is called exchange transfusion.

What is the importance of MN blood group?

MN blood group is important in medicolegal cases of paternity dispute.

LYMPHATIC SYSTEM

What is lymph?

Lymph is the tissue fluid (interstitial fluid) that enters the lymphatic vessels. It drains into the blood via thoracic and right lymphatic ducts.

What is the protein content of lymph?

Lymph is derived from interstitial fluid and therefore it has almost the same composition as that of interstitial fluid of the tissue. In most of the tissues, protein concentration of interstitial fluid is 2 g/100 ml, so lymph also has same content of protein. However, lymph from the liver has protein concentration of 6 g/100 ml whereas lymph from intestine has protein concentration of 3–4 g/100 ml. About two-third of the lymph is derived from liver and intestine; therefore, thoracic duct lymph (mixture of lymph from different areas) has usually a protein concentration of 3–5 g/100 ml.

What is the rate of lymph flow?

Rate of lymph flow is 100 ml/h through thoracic duct and about 20 ml/h through other channels. So, every hour 120 ml of lymph flows back to circulation.

Enumerate the factors determining lymph flow.

1. **Interstitial fluid pressure.** Increase in interstitial fluid pressure increases lymph flow up to a certain limit.

2. **Lymphatic pump.** Valves exist in all lymph channels. In large lymphatics, valves exist every few millimetres. In smaller lymphatics they are much closer than this.

3. **Intrinsic pumping by lymph vessels.** When lymph vessels become stretched with fluid, smooth muscle of the vessel automatically contracts.

4. **Pumping by external compression of the lymphatics.** This occurs due to contraction of muscles, movements of different body parts, arterial pulsations and compression of tissue by objects outside the body.

5. **Lymphatic capillary pump.** Lymphatic capillary is also able to pump the lymph in addition to lymphatic pump in larger vessels.

6. **Capillary surface area.** Increase in capillary surface area by capillary distension (due to increased capillary pressure, increase in local temperature and infusion of fluid) increases the flow.

7. **Capillary permeability.** Increase in temperature, capillary toxins and decreased O_2 leads to increased permeability of capillary membrane which in turn increases the lymph flow.

8. **Increased functional activity of the tissue** increases lymph flow.

Enumerate the functions of lymphatic system.

1. Returns proteins, water and electrolytes from tissue spaces to the blood and thus controls concentration of proteins in interstitial fluid, volume of interstitial fluid and interstitial tissue fluid pressure.

2. Absorption of nutrients especially fats from the gastrointestinal tract.

3. Acts as a transport mechanism to remove red blood cells that have lost into the tissues as a result of haemorrhage.

4. Lymph nodes act as efficient filters. They have sinuses lined with phagocytic cells that engulf bacteria, red blood cells and other particulate matter (bacteria or toxins are carried to them through lymph).

5. **Nutritive.** It supplies nutrition and O_2 to those parts where blood cannot reach.

Describe the spleen and its functions.

Spleen is a lymphoid and highly vascular organ. It has outer serous coat and inner fibromuscular coat. From the capsule, trabeculae and trabecular network arise. The substance of spleen lying between the trabeculae is red pulp and white pulp. Red pulp consists of venous sinus and cords of structures like blood cells, macrophages and mesenchymal cells. White pulp has a central artery surrounded by splenic or Malpighian corpuscles which are formed by the lymphatic sheath containing lymphocytes and macrophages.

Spleen has the following functions:

1. **Formation of blood.** In the embryo spleen functions as haemopoietic organ. During second half of foetal life, spleen forms red blood cells. Spleen contains lymphoid tissue which like that elsewhere forms lymphocytes and plasma cells.

In certain pathological conditions like leukaemia normal cells of splenic pulp are replaced by lymphoid cells in lymphatic leukaemia, and myeloblasts and myelocytes in myeloid leukaemia.

2. **Destruction of blood cells.** The old red cells, white cells and platelets are destroyed by the spleen. Thus spleen acts as a filter which removes old useless cells and allows only young active cells to pass in circulation.

When red blood cells become older the cell membrane becomes more and more fragile. Diameter of capillaries is equal to or less than that of a red cell. When, therefore, these old red cells try to squeeze through the capillaries, they are destroyed. The destruction occurs mostly in the capillaries of spleen because splenic capillaries have a thin lumen. After breakdown of red cells, haemoglobin released is broken down and bilirubin (bile pigment) is formed from it in the spleen. Iron from haemoglobin is stored in splenic pulp and is gradually transferred to liver for storage.

3. **Reservoir of blood.** Spleen acts as a reservoir of blood. In animals it stores much larger amount of blood than in human beings. Spleen when contracts may release about 150 ml of blood (mainly erythrocytes) in circulation. In certain emergency conditions like haemorrhage, asphyxia, severe muscular exercise, high altitude, spleen contracts and releases the stored blood (mainly red blood cells), which is used for carrying oxygen.

4. **Defence function.** The lymphoid tissue and reticuloendothelial cells (macrophages) like those of tissues elsewhere, participate in defence reactions against toxins (diphtheria, tetanus), bacteria and larger parasites by formation of antibodies or phagocytosis.

Describe the reticuloendothelial system and its functions.*

Reticuloendothelial system is a system of primitive cells which play an important role in the defence mechanism of the body. Reticuloendothelial cells form:

- Endothelial lining of vascular and lymph channels.
- Reticular cells of connective tissue and some organs such as spleen, liver, lungs, lymph nodes, bone marrow form macrophage system. There are two types of RE cells. Macrophage is a large cell having a property of phagocytosis.

FUNCTIONS OF RETICULOENDOTHELIAL SYSTEM

1. Reticuloendothelial cells play important role mainly in defence mechanism of the body. Blood monocytes are immature cells and migrate to the site of injury or infection where they come out from circulation in the tissue and get converted to macrophages. They are more powerful phagocytes than neutrophils. Their lysosomes contain large number of proteolytic enzymes geared for digesting bacteria and other foreign matter. Macrophages also contain bactericidal agents that kill bacteria when enzymes fail to digest them. Some bacteria

*For details refer Vaz M, Kurpad A, Raj T, editors. *Guyton & Hall Textbook of Medical Physiology*. Elsevier: New Delhi, 2013, p. 127.

have protective coats, which are digested by peroxidase and other oxidizing enzymes present is peroxisomes of macrophages.

2. Macrophages in lymph nodes trap foreign particles in the meshwork of sinuses (lined by tissue macrophages).

3. In each tissue local macrophages phagocytose invading bacteria and kill them, e.g. bacteria may enter the body through respiratory tract, where alveolar macrophages phagocytose and digest them. Bacteria entering through GI tract reach liver through portal circulation. Kupffer cells (macrophages of liver) phago-cytose and digest them very quickly. Invading organisms are thus not allowed to succeed in entering general circulation. If they do succeed macrophages of spleen and bone marrow phagocytose them.

4. Macrophages after engulfing the bacteria by phagocytosis liberate antigenic products of the organism. These antigens activate B-lymphocytes and helper T-lymphocytes.

5. Macrophages also engulf inorganic particles like carbon dust and silicon when injected into the body.

6. Macrophages secrete hormonal substance like interleukin-1 which activates the maturation and proliferation of specific B-lymphocytes and T-lymphocytes.

7. RE cells of spleen destroy senile red blood cells and release haemoglobin.

8. RE cells convert haemoglobin to bile pigments—bilirubin and biliverdin.

CHAPTER 3
Immunity

INTRODUCTION

Define immunology.

Immunology is the study of physiological responses by which the body destroys or neutralizes the foreign matter (living or non-living) as well as cells of its own that have become altered.

What is immunity?

Capacity of human body to resist all types of microorganisms and their products (toxins) that tend to damage tissues or organs is called immunity.

CLASSIFICATION

How do you classify immunity?

There are two categories of immunity:

1. *Non-specific immunity.* This protects against foreign substances or cells non-selectively, i.e. without recognizing their specific identities. This is also called innate immunity.
2. *Specific immunity.* This protects against foreign substances or cells after recognition of substance or cell to be attacked. This is also termed acquired immunity.

Name the cell-mediated immune response.

Cell-mediated immune responses are:

Leucocytes. Neutrophils, eosinophils, monocytes and lymphocytes (B cells and T cells of various types).

Plasma cells. They differentiate from B-lymphocytes and are present in peripheral lymphoid tissues.

Macrophages. They differentiate from monocytes and are present in almost all the organs and tissues.

Mast cells. They differentiate from basophils and are also present in all the tissues and organs.

NON-SPECIFIC IMMUNITY

What are the factors responsible for non-specific immunity?

External barriers

- Barrier for invasion of microorganisms, e.g. skin.
- All secretions (sweat, lacrimal, sebaceous) secrete antibacterial chemicals.
- Mucus secreted by respiratory tract lining and gastrointestinal lining is sticky. Particles get adhered to it and thus are prevented from entering the blood. Then these particles are either swept by ciliary action or engulfed by microphages, present in the linings.
- Specialized surface barriers are hair in nose, acid secretions in the stomach, cough reflex, sneeze reflex, etc.

Local response to infection or injury called inflammation

This response causes the following effects locally:

- Vasodilatation.
- Increased permeability of capillary membrane for proteins.
- Exit of neutrophils and monocytes out of the capillaries. They cause phagocytosis of the invaded bacteria.
- Tissue repair.

What is diapedesis?

It is the process by which monocytes and neutrophils squeeze out through the pores of blood vessels.

What is chemotaxis?

Many chemical substances in the tissues cause neutrophils and monocytes to move towards them. This phenomenon is called chemotaxis. This is the mechanism by which these cells are collected in inflamed tissue.

What is phagocytosis? Which cells do this function?

Engulfing of foreign living and non-living particles is known as phagocytosis. Neutrophils and monocytes do this function.

What is the difference in phagocytosis caused by neutrophils and monocytes?

1. Neutrophil can usually phagocytose 5 to 20 bacteria before its death; whereas, monocyte can phagocytose about 100 bacteria before death.
2. Monocytes have ability to engulf larger particles as compared to neutrophils. They can engulf the whole red blood cell or malarial parasite. Neutrophils cannot phagocytose particles much larger than bacteria.
3. Monocytes lysosomes contain enzymes known as lipases which can digest thick lipid membrane possessed by some bacteria.

SPECIFIC IMMUNITY

How do you classify specific immune responses?

Specific immune responses are classified as follows:

1. *Antibody-mediated or humoral response*. This response is mediated by anti-bodies secreted by plasma cells (which arise from activated B-lymphocytes). They mainly cause protection against bacteria and viruses.

2. *Cell-mediated response*. This response is mediated by cytotoxic T-lymphocytes and natural killer cells. This constitutes major defence against intracellular viruses and cancer cells. Both the above mechanisms are facilitated by helper T-lymphocytes and are inhibited by suppressor T-lymphocytes.

What are antigens?

Any foreign molecule that can trigger immune response is termed antigen. Most of the antigens are either proteins or very large polysaccharides.

What is antibody?

Antibody is a protein called immunoglobulin. It has four polypeptide chains, two long chains called heavy chains and two small ones called light chains.

Antibody consists of one Fc (stem) chain and two prongs. Each prong contains single antigen-bearing site. Two heavy chains make Fc chain forming a constant portion.

Two light chains form the two prongs which form variable portion, different for each antibody. Thus antibody is highly specific.

What are the different types of lymphocytes?

There are three types of lymphocytes:

1. *B-lymphocytes*. These cells mature in the bone marrow and are carried through blood to peripheral lymphoid organs. All generations arising from these cells by mitosis in peripheral lymphoid tissue are identical to parent cell, i.e. B-lymphocyte.

2. *T-lymphocytes*. These cells leave bone marrow in immature state during foetal or early neonatal life. They are carried to thymus where they mature and then carried to peripheral lymphoid organs (production of T cells is completed in early life by thymus).

In peripheral lymphoid tissue these cells undergo mitosis to produce identical T cells. But during maturation process in thymus, there exist four types of T cells: (a) cytotoxic T cells, (b) helper T cells, (c) suppressor T cells and (d) memory T cells.

3. *Natural killer cells*. They are also called third population of lymphocytes. Their origin is still unknown (also called non-B, non-T-lymphocyte). They kill cells which have undergone malignant transformation, and act as first line of defence against viral infection.

HUMORAL IMMUNITY

Classify immunoglobulins (Igs). Where are they produced?

Immunoglobulins (antibodies) are divided on the basis of differences in amino acid sequences in the heavy chains into five major classes:

1. *IgM (μ chain)*. Large share of antibodies formed during primary response are of this type. They have 10 binding sites which make them highly effective in protecting the body.
2. *IgG (gamma chain)*. These are most common and are also called gamma globulins.
3. *IgA (alpha chain)*. These are secreted by linings of gastrointestinal tract, respiratory tract, etc. Generally they act locally and do not enter into the circulation.
4. *IgD (delta chain)*. Functions are not yet clear.
5. *IgE (epsilon chain)*. They mediate allergic responses and participate in defence against multicellular parasites.

Depending on serological and physicochemical differences in their class specific heavy chains, immunoglobulins are further subclassified as follows:

- IgM is of two types: μ_1 and μ_2.
- IgA is of two types: Alpha 1 and Alpha 2.
- IgG has four types: Gamma 1, Gamma 2, Gamma 3 and Gamma 4.

B-lymphocytes get converted into plasma cells which synthesize immunoglobulins.

What is antigen processing?

An antigen is processed in the body before lymphocytes can interact with it. Macrophages do this function and link between non-specific and specific immune response. Macrophages phagocytose microbe or non-cellular antigen (non-specific response). Phagocytosed material is broken down into fragments capable of reaction with receptors on the surface of lymphocyte.

Describe the stages of specific immune response.

Typical specific immune response is divided into three stages:

1. *Recognition of antigen by lymphocytes*. Lymphocyte recognizes the specific antigen which it encounters. Antigen gets bound to specific receptor on the surface of lymphocyte. (This binding is physicochemical meaning of the word 'recognize'). Differentiation of one antigen from other is determined by nature of receptors lymphocytes have.
2. *Lymphocyte activation*. Lymphocyte that has combined with antigen undergoes cycles of mitotic divisions. This process is termed lymphocyte activation and usually occurs at the site of recognition, i.e. mostly in peripheral lymphoid tissue.
3. *Attack*. Activated cells attack against the antigen of the kind that has initiated the immune response. Nature of attack varies with the type of lymphocyte. It may be antibody-mediated (humoral) or cell-mediated. B-lymphocytes are responsible for humoral type of attack; whereas, T-lymphocytes and natural killer cells (NK cells) are responsible for cell-mediated response.

Describe the antibody-mediated response.

Antibodies are proteins present in the plasma membrane of B-lymphocytes. These B cells get differentiated into plasma cells which secrete these antibodies and through lymph these antibodies enter the circulation.

Antibodies combine with antigen and then direct an attack that eliminates antigen or cell bearing the antigens. Elimination is done either by phagocytosis or by complement.

What is the mechanism of action of antibody?

Antibodies act on the invading agent in two ways:

1. *By direct attack on the invading agents.* Because of bivalent nature of antibody and multiple antigen sites on most invading agents, antibodies inactivate the invading agent in the following ways:
   - *Agglutination.* Large number of particles (bacteria or red cells) with antigens on their surfaces are bound together to form a clump.
   - *Precipitation.* Antibody-antigen complex is formed which is large and insoluble, therefore, it precipitates.
   - *Neutralization.* Antibodies cover the toxic sites of antigen.
   - *Lysis.* Antibodies attack the membranes of cellular agents thereby causing rupture of cell.

2. *Complement system.** Complement is the term used to describe different proteins which mostly act as enzyme precursors. The main proteins are 11 in number which are named as, C_1, C_2, C_3, C_4, C_5, C_6, C_7, C_8, C_9, B and D. All these are present in plasma as well as in tissue fluid. This system acts in two ways as follows:

   (a) *Classical pathway.* This is activated by antigen-antibody reaction. When antibody binds with antigen, a specific reactive site on the constant portion of the antibody becomes uncovered and binds directly with protein C_1 itself. This produces a cascade of sequential reactions which causes activation of successive proteins leading to multiple products causing the following effects:
   - Opsonization. Activation of neutrophils and macrophages to engulf the bacteria.
   - Lysis. Destruction of bacteria by rupturing the cell membrane.
   - Chemotaxis. Attraction of leucocytes to the site of antigen-antibody reaction.
   - Agglutination. By causing of clumping of foreign bodies like red blood cells.
   - Neutralization. Covering the toxic sites of antigenic products.
   - Activation of mast cells and basophils. This causes liberation of histamine. Histamine causes dilatation of blood vessels and increases capillary permeability; therefore, plasma proteins from blood enter the tissues and antigenic products are inactivated.

   (b) *Alternate pathway.* The compliment system can also be activated sometimes without antigen-antibody reaction. A protein in circulation called factor I

---

*For details refer Vaz M, Kurpad A, Raj T, editors. *Guyton & Hall Textbook of Medical Physiology.* Elsevier: New Delhi, 2013, p. 136–137.

binds with polysaccharide present in the cell membrane of the invading organism. This binding activates C_3 and C_5 which ultimately attack the antigenic products of the invading organism. Because this pathway does not involve antigen-antibody reaction, it is one of the first lines of defence against invading organism. This pathway especially occurs in response to large polysaccharide molecule in the cell membrane of invading organism.

What is the effect of transformation of B-lymphocyte into plasma cell?

When B-lymphocyte is converted to plasma cell, its cytoplasm expands. It is filled with granular endoplasmic reticulum. Therefore, plasma cell now produces thousands of antibody molecules per second (before they die in a day or so). Antibodies thus secreted enter the extracellular fluid or into blood through peripheral lymphoid organs. At the site of infection they leave the blood and combine with antigen.

What is active immunity? How is it produced?

Resistance built-up (antibody formation) as a result of the body's contact with microorganisms and their toxins or other antigenic components is known as active immunity. Active immunity, therefore, can be developed by suffering from an infection or by injection of microbial derivatives (vaccines).

What is passive immunity?

Direct transfer of actively formed antibodies from one person (or animal) to another, causes recipient to receive preformed antibodies. This is called passive immunity.

Such transfers normally occur between mother and foetus, through breast milk. In adult, pooled gamma globulin can be injected for protecting the person against infection. But the protection offered is short-lived as compared to that offered by vaccine.

Name the varieties of T-lymphocytes and their functions.

Varieties of T-lymphocytes:

- Helper or inducer T cells.
- Suppressor T cells.
- Cytotoxic T cells (effector or killer T cells).
- Memory T cells.

Functions
Helper T cells and suppressor T cells are involved in the regulation of antibody formation by B-lymphocytes. Helper T cells secrete protein messengers that act on B cells and cytotoxic T cells. Suppressor T cells inhibit the function of both B cells and cytotoxic T cells. Cytotoxic T cells destroy transplanted and other foreign cells. Memory T cells do not make an initial response but are readily converted to effector cells by a later encounter with the same antigen. They remain in the body without dividing for months or years.

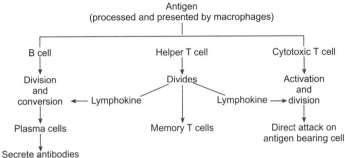

Role of B, helper T and cytotoxic T cells

What is the role of humoral immunity?

Humoral immunity is due to circulating antibodies and is a major defence against bacterial infections.

CELL-MEDIATED IMMUNITY

Write a note on cell-mediated immunity.

The term cell-mediated immunity refers to the specific immune responses that do not involve antibodies. T-lymphocytes are responsible for cell-mediated immunity.

ACTIVATION OF LYMPHOCYTES

The macrophages are present along with lymphocytes in almost all lymphoid tissues. When bacteria, viruses, foreign protein or toxins enter the body, macrophages ingest them by phagocytosis. The antigenic products of these organisms are then liberated by macrophages. These antigenic products activate T- and B-lymphocytes. On exposure to antigen, T-lymphocytes of specific lymphoid tissue clone proliferate and release large number of activated T cells. Activation of B-lymphocytes causes release of antibodies. The principal difference is that instead of releasing antibodies, whole activated T cells are formed and released into the lymph and then enter into circulation through which they are distributed throughout the body. They also pass out through capillary walls and enter in tissue fluid present in tissue spaces from where they enter back into the lymph, then to lymphoid tissue and once again in blood. Thus, T-lymphocytes circulate again and again throughout the body, sometimes lasting for months or years.

T-lymphocyte memory cells are also formed. When a clone of T-lymphocytes is activated, many of the newly formed lymphocytes are preserved in lymphoid tissue to become additional T-lymphocytes of that specific clone. These are memory cells spread throughout the lymphoid tissues of the entire body. Therefore, on subsequent exposure to the same antigen, release of T cells occurs far more rapidly and much more powerfully than in the first response.

Antigenic products from macrophage also cause activation of helper T cells, which in turn stimulate activation of T and B cells, by secreting interleukins 2, 3, 4, 5 and 6, granulocyte-monocyte colony stimulating factor and interferon 4.

These secretions are proteins called lymphokines. These activate formation of cytotoxic cells and suppressor T cells (especially interleukin 2). Suppressor T cells suppress the activity of cytotoxic T cells and play an important role in preventing cytotoxic T cells from destroying body's own tissues along with invader organisms.

ACTION OF CYTOTOXIC T CELLS

1. The outer membrane of cytotoxic T cells contains some receptor proteins. These bind the antigens or organisms tightly with cytotoxic T cells. Then these T cells enlarge and release cytotoxic substances like the lysosomal enzymes. These substances destroy the antigen or invaded organisms. Like this, each cytotoxic cell can destroy large number of organisms one after another.

2. At times T cells also destroy body's own cells containing the antigen. Therefore, they are also called killer cells. The receptor proteins on the surfaces of cytotoxic cells cause them to bind tightly with the cells that contain their binding specific antigen. After binding, the cytotoxic cell secretes hole-forming proteins called perforins. These proteins literally punch round holes in the membrane of the attacked cell. Then fluid rapidly flows into the cell from interstitial space. In addition, cytotoxic cells also release cytotoxic substances directly into the attacked cell. Almost immediately the attacked cell becomes greatly swollen and usually dissolves shortly thereafter. Cytotoxic killer cells can pull away from the victim cells after they have punched holes, and then move on to kill many more such cells. After destruction of invaders these killer cells persist in the tissue for months.

Some T cells are especially lethal to body tissue cells that have been invaded by viruses (many virus particles become entrapped in the membrane of these cells). The antigen of viruses attracts the T cells. The cytotoxic T cells then kill the affected cells along with viruses.

3. Cytotoxic or killer T cells also destroy cancer cells, transplanted heart or kidney cells or other types of cells that are foreign to the person's own body.

What are the major histocompatibility complex (MHC) proteins?

The major histocompatibility complex (MHC) proteins are the group of proteins coded in the gene known as major MHC located in short arm of human chromosome 6. No two persons except identical twins can have same MHC proteins on plasma membranes of their cells.

There are two subclasses—class I and class II. Class I MHC proteins are found on surface of virtually all the cells of the body excluding erythrocytes. Class II proteins are only found in macrophages, B-lymphocytes and some other cells.

What are lymphokines? What are their functions?

Lymphokines are the protein mediators secreted by helper T cells. They are named as:

- Lymphocyte transforming factor.
- Macrophage activating factor.

- Macrophage migration inhibition factor.
- Chemotactic factor.
- Interleukin-2.
- Interleukin-3.
- Interleukin-4.
- Interleukin-5.
- Interleukin-6.
- Granulocyte-monocyte colony stimulating factor.

FUNCTIONS
1. Stimulate growth and proliferation of cytotoxic T cells and suppressor T cells.
2. Activate macrophage system to cause far more efficient phagocytosis.
3. They have feedback stimulatory effect on the helper cells themselves.

What is clone of cells?

When any antigen enters in the body, it is processed by antigen binding cell to the appropriate lymphocyte. These cells are stimulated to divide, forming large number of cells which respond to this antigen. Thus, a group of cells responding to a single specific antigen forms clone of cells.

What is primary and secondary response?

Primary response is response for forming antibodies that occurs on first exposure to a specific antigen and secondary response is one which occurs on second exposure to the same antigen.

Primary response shows delay in appearance, and it has weak potency and short life. In contrast, secondary response begins rapidly after exposure to antigen (within hours), is far more potent and forms antibodies for many months rather than few weeks.

What are memory cells?

Few lymphoblasts formed by activation of clone of B-lymphocytes do not go on to form plasma cells but instead form moderate number of new B-lymphocytes similar to those of original clone. They also circulate throughout the body to populate all of the lymphoid tissue. Immunologically they remain dormant until activated once again by new quantity of the same antigen. These lymphocytes are called 'memory cells'. They are responsible for secondary response.

Why is transplanted tissue rejected?

Transplanted tissue is rejected because the recipient develops an immune response to the transplanted tissue (cell-mediated immune system driven by T-lymphocytes is mainly responsible). Only transplants which are not rejected are those from an identical twin. Except in identical twin, class I MHC proteins on the cells of the graft are different than those of the recipient, so also class II MHC molecules on macrophages. Both these are therefore recognized as foreign.

How can graft rejection be prevented?

Graft rejection can be reduced by giving radiation and drugs that kill actively dividing lymphocytes and thereby decrease T cell population. Drug cyclosporin which does not kill lymphocytes, but alters their function has proved effective in reducing rejection. It blocks production of lymphokines by helper T cells and thus eliminates critical signal for proliferation of cytotoxic T cells. In addition, injection of antilymphocyte serum will lead to decrease in 'T' cell population.

FACTORS AFFECTING RESISTANCE TO INFECTION

Name the factors that alter body's resistance to infection.

1. *Nutritional state.* Protein calorie malnutrition is the single greatest contributor for decreased resistance to infection.
2. *Previous disease.* Either infectious or non-infectious disease can predispose body to infection, e.g. diabetes.
3. *Person's state of mind.* Physiological link between state of mind and resistance to infection is not yet determined, but lymphoid tissue becomes inert. The cell-mediated immunity possesses receptors for many neurotransmitters and hormones. Therefore, it seems likely that nervous system and endocrine glands interact with immune system in important ways, e.g. production of antibodies can be altered by psychological conditioning.
4. *Development of basic resistance mechanism.* If basic resistance mechanism itself is deficient (e.g. congenital deficiency of plasma gamma globulins), it leads to frequent, life-threatening infections. It is prevented by giving regular injections of gamma globulins.
5. *Decreased production of leucocytes.* This may be the effect of certain drugs.
6. *Age.* At birth, thymus weighs 10–72 gm and cell-mediated immunity is well developed. Development of peripheral lymphoid tissue (lymph nodes and spleen) is very minimal and immunoglobulins secretion is small. IgG is present in serum in high concentration in the neonatal plasma (IgG from mother diffuses through placenta). After birth IgG concentration falls for 2–3 months when child's own IgG production takes over. IgG rises gradually in years with advancing age. Many people become susceptible to infections and malignancy because T cells become less responsive to antigens. This is due to age-related atrophy of thymus or decreased production of thymic hormones. Beta cells also become less responsive and therefore antibody levels do not increase rapidly, leading to greater susceptibility to infections.
7. *Sex.*

ALLERGY

What is allergy?

In certain people exposure to dust, pollens and food constituents (which are almost harmless antigens) elicits a specific immune response that produces distressing symptoms and causes body damage. This phenomenon is known as allergy or hypersensitivity and is due to inappropriate immune response to the stimulus.

What is anaphylactic shock?

Mostly allergic symptoms are localized at the site of entry of antigen. But rarely, large amount of chemicals released by mast cells enter circulation resulting in systemic symptoms which cause severe hypotension and bronchiolar constriction. This sequence of events is called anaphylactic shock. It can cause death due to circulatory and respiratory failure.

What is autoimmune disease?

Normally, lymphocytes recognize body's own proteins and therefore, antibodies are not developed against them. But sometimes body suffers from antibody-mediated or cell-mediated attack against its own tissues, causing damage of normal cells and their function leading to autoimmune disease.

AIDS

What is acquired immunodeficiency syndrome?

Acquired immunodeficiency syndrome (AIDS) is the disease which is an example of lack of basic resistance mechanism. It is caused by human immunodeficiency virus (HIV). HIV belongs to retrovirus family. Its nucleic acid core is RNA rather than DNA. The virus possesses an enzyme called reverse transcriptase that once inside the host cell transcribes the virus RNA into DNA which is then integrated into host cell's chromosomes. The association is permanent. Every time the host cell reproduces, it also reproduces the retrovirus RNA. Virus may remain dormant inside the cell for years without symptoms, but the individual shows antibodies against HIV in their blood. When virus becomes active and undergoes rapid replication inside the cell resulting in cell death, person suffers from actual disease.

HIV preferentially enters and resides in helper T cells. Active disease causes depletion of these helper T cells. Without adequate number of helper T cells, B cells cannot make antibodies and cytotoxic T cells also cannot function fully. Thus, AIDS patient dies of infections or cancers that ordinarily are handled readily by immune system.

Transmission of HIV occurs through transfer of contaminated blood or blood products from one person to the other, e.g. during sexual intercourse with an infected partner. It is also transmitted from infected mother to a child.

CHAPTER 4

Digestion and Absorption

INTRODUCTION

What is digestion?

Conversion of complex insoluble large organic molecules (food) into soluble smaller and simpler molecules is called digestion. Simple, soluble molecules formed by digestion can be easily absorbed.

What is absorption?

Movement of digested molecules from the lumen across the epithelial layer of gastrointestinal tract to enter into blood or lymph is called absorption.

What is hunger?

Hunger is intrinsic desire for food.

What is an appetite?

Appetite is desire for particular type of food.

What is the importance of hunger and appetite?

Hunger determines the amount of food ingested by the person whereas type of food the person would preferentially take is determined by appetite.

GASTROINTESTINAL TRACT (GI TRACT)

Name the various parts of gastrointestinal system.

- Gastrointestinal tract includes mouth, pharynx, oesophagus, stomach, small intestine, large intestine, rectum and anal canal.
- Glandular organs—salivary glands, liver, gall bladder and pancreas.

What is the total length of gastrointestinal tract?

Total length of gastrointestinal tract from mouth to anus is about 15 feet in adults. It is open at both the ends.

What are the functions of gastrointestinal system?

- Transfer of food, salt and water from external environment to gastrointestinal tract.
- Digestion of foodstuffs with the help of hydrochloric acid and digestive juices containing various enzymes.
- Absorption of digested material into the blood or lymph (which in turn flows to various tissues to supply absorbed nutrients).
- Excretion of unwanted, undigested food by process known as defaecation.
- Stomach secretes intrinsic factor which is responsible for absorption of vitamin B_{12} (extrinsic factor) from food. Vitamin B_{12} is required for maturation of erythroid cells and thus is essential for erythropoiesis.

Name the different layers present in the wall of gastrointestinal tract.

- Serosa.
- Muscular layer, divided into an outer longitudinal and inner circular coats.
- Submucosa.
- Mucosa. In deeper layers of mucosa there is muscularis mucosae layer formed of smooth muscle.

What is the type of smooth muscle present in the wall of gastrointestinal tract?

Single unit type of smooth muscle is present in gastrointestinal tract. It is a syncytium, i.e. when an action potential is initiated anywhere in the mass of muscle, it generally travels in all directions in the muscle. This is because the muscle fibres are electrically connected to each other through gap junctions having very low electrical resistance.

What are the functions of secretory glands of gastrointestinal tract?

Secretory glands are located in the mucosa layer of gastrointestinal tract. They have two functions:

- Digestive enzymes are secreted by glands present in mucosa up to distal end of ileum. Enzymes cause digestion of foodstuff.
- Secrete mucus for lubrication as well as for the protection of all parts of gastrointestinal tract.

Describe the nerve supply of digestive tract.

The nerve supply to digestive tract consists of intrinsic part and extrinsic part.

1. *Intrinsic part*. It consists of nerve cells and fibres originating and located in the intestinal wall itself. Intrinsic neural structures supply the smooth musculature of GI (gastrointestinal) tract (i.e. GI muscles except upper oesophagus and external anal sphincter which are made up of striated muscles). There are two important intramural plexuses:
   - Myenteric (Auerbach) plexus present between longitudinal and circular muscle layers of the wall.

- Meissner's plexus present in submucosal layer. These plexuses are responsible for spontaneous movements of GI tract occurring after cutting the extrinsic supply.
2. *Extrinsic part*. It is represented by vagal fibres and postganglionic sympathetic fibres.

Sympathetic fibres which are branches of splanchnic nerves originate in coeliac ganglion (superior mesenteric) and supply smooth muscle and blood vessels within intestinal wall. They do not make synaptic connections with intramural plexuses.

Preganglionic parasympathetic fibres originate in medulla, come through vagus and supply stomach, small intestine and half of large intestine. They also make synaptic connection with intramural plexuses.

A few preganglionic parasympathetic fibres originate in sacral spinal cord, pass though pelvic nerves to hypogastric (pelvic) ganglion and postganglionic fibres, supply the lower half of large intestine and rectum.

External anal sphincter is supplied by somatic nerve fibres. Sympathetic stimulation causes excitation of ileocaecal and internal anal sphincters, smooth muscle of muscularis mucosa throughout (to increase number of folds) and are inhibitory to rest of the musculature. Parasympathetic stimulation causes excitation of all the musculature except the sphincters to which it inhibits.

MASTICATION

What is mastication or chewing?

Grinding of food into smaller particles with the help of teeth and jaw muscles is known as mastication.

What is chewing reflex?

Mastication or chewing though voluntary is coordinated by chewing reflex. The presence of bolus of food in mouth causes reflex inhibition of muscles of mastication which causes lower jaw to drop. Drop of lower jaw stretches the muscles of mastication and leads to their contraction through stretch reflex, thereby raising the jaw to cause closure of the mouth. This compresses bolus against the lining of mouth which inhibits jaw muscles once again allowing jaw to drop and again contract jaw muscles due to stretch reflex. This is repeated again and again to cause mastication.

What are the functions of different types of teeth?

- Incisors provide strong cutting action.
- Canines are responsible for tearing action.
- Premolar and molars have grinding action.

What is the importance of mastication?

1. Mastication breaks the undigestible cellulose membranes present around the nutrient portions of most fruits and raw vegetables.

2. Food is broken down into smaller particles. Digestive enzymes act mainly on the surfaces of food particles. Breaking of food particles into large number (by mastication) increases the surface area and hence the rate of digestion.
3. Grinding of food to very fine particles prevents damage which the food may cause to the mucosa of gastrointestinal tract.
4. Chewing causes mixing of food with saliva. This causes initiation of starch digestion by salivary amylase and lubricates bolus.
5. Due to chewing, food is brought into contact with taste receptors which generate sensation of taste. It also releases odour stimulating olfactory receptors. Stimulation of taste and smell receptors increases pleasure of eating and stimulate gastric secretion.

SALIVARY GLANDS

Name the different salivary glands.

There are three pairs of main salivary glands:

- **Parotid.** Cause serous type of secretion containing enzyme ptyalin.
- **Submandibular.**
- **Sublingual.** Both glands mainly cause mucous secretion containing mucin for lubrication purpose.

  In addition there are small buccal glands present in mucosa covering the mouth.

How much is pH of saliva?

pH of normal saliva varies from 6 to 7.4.

How much saliva is secreted per day?

Normal salivary secretion is 800 to 1500 ml/day.

Name the important constituents of saliva.

Main constituents of saliva:

- Water: 99.5%.
- Solids: 0.5%.

Solids are further divided into:

- Organic (0.3%). Organic solids are ptyalin lysozyme, small amounts of urea, uric acid, cholesterol, mucin. Enzyme kallikrein is secreted which acts on plasma alpha globulin to release bradykinin which is a vasodilator.
- Inorganic (0.2%). Inorganic solids are $NaCl$, KCl, Ca_3CO_3, potassium thiocyanate (more in smokers).

Describe the innervation of salivary glands.

Salivary glands receive both parasympathetic and sympathetic nerves. But parasympathetic innervation is more important.

Parasympathetic supply. Parasympathetic fibres for parotid gland arise from inferior salivary nucleus (dorsal nucleus of IX nerve) of medulla. Preganglionic fibres run via tympanic nerve and small superficial petrosal nerve to otic ganglion. Postganglionic fibres from the ganglion join auriculotemporal nerve to reach parotid gland where fibres are supplied along with blood vessels of the gland.

Parasympathetic fibres for submandibular and sublingual gland originate in superior salivary nucleus (dorsal nucleus of VII nerve). Preganglionic fibres run in the nervus intermedius and join the facial nerve and leave by its chorda tympanic branch to join lingual nerve. They synapse in ganglion present near the glands and postganglionic fibres from here are supplied along with blood vessels of the glands.

Sympathetic supply. Sympathetic fibres for all the three pairs of salivary glands arise from first and second thoracic segments of spinal cord, relay in superior cervical ganglion and postganglionic fibres are supplied to the glands along with their blood supply.

What are the effects of parasympathetic and sympathetic stimulation of salivary glands?

Parasympathetic stimulation of the salivary glands causes secretion of water, enzyme, kallikrein and vasodilation. Thin, watery saliva is thus produced. Sympathetic stimulation causes secretion of viscous saliva with higher solid contents and vasoconstriction.

Name ducts of different pairs of salivary glands. Where do they open in the mouth cavity?

Parotid gland on each side opens upon the inner surface of cheek opposite upper second molar tooth by single duct called Stenson's duct.

Submandibular gland opens by Wharton's duct into the floor of mouth on the side of frenulum of tongue.

Sublingual gland opens by a number of fine ducts into the floor of the mouth.

What is the mechanism of secretion of saliva?

Salivary glands have a racemose structure. They contain acini and ducts. Salivary secretion occurs in two stages. Acini secrete a primary secretion, containing ptyalin (salivary amylase), mucin and ions in concentrations almost the same as in extracellular fluid.

As primary secretion passes through ducts it gets modified. Two major active transport processes modify the ionic concentration of saliva. Sodium ions are actively reabsorbed from all salivary ducts and potassium ions are actively secreted in exchange. This greatly reduces sodium concentration and raises the potassium concentration of saliva. However, there is excess of reabsorption of sodium over potassium secretion which creates negativity of about –70 mV in the salivary ducts. This negativity causes reabsorption of chloride ions passively. Chloride concentration therefore falls to very low level (matching the decrease of sodium concentration).

Bicarbonate ions are secreted by ductal epithelium into the lumen. This bicarbonate secretion is partly active and partly passive (exchange for chloride ions).

Thus under resting conditions concentration of sodium in saliva is 15 mEq/L that of potassium is 30 mEq/L and concentration of bicarbonate ions is 50 to 70 mEq/L.

During maximal salivation, rate of formation of primary secretion by acini can increase as much as twentyfold. The primary secretion therefore flows through ducts very rapidly and lesser time is available for reabsorption and secretion of different ions. Therefore, when large quantities of saliva are secreted, sodium chloride concentration rises and potassium concentration falls.

In presence of excess aldosterone there is greatly increased reabsorption of sodium and chloride from salivary ducts. This may reduce sodium chloride concentration of saliva almost to zero and increase potassium concentration equal to or higher than that of plasma.

How is the salivary secretion controlled?

Salivary secretion is a purely reflex phenomenon and is regulated through nerves by superior and inferior salivary nuclei. They in turn are stimulated or inhibited by impulses coming from higher centres of CNS, e.g. appetite area in hypothalamus, taste, smell centres and cortex.
There are two types of reflexes involved in salivation.

1. *Conditioned reflex*. Sight and smell of food causes salivary secretion. Various conditioned stimuli can be established.
2. *Unconditioned reflex*. Presence of food in the mouth (or even non-edible material) stimulates secretion of saliva. Chewing, sensation of taste, irritation of mucosa due to food acts as sensory stimuli, which reflexly produce salivary secretion. Afferent path runs in chorda tympani, pharyngeal branches of vagus and glossopharyngeal nerves and lingual, buccal palatine branches of trigeminal nerves. Centre is salivary nucleus in medulla and efferent pathway comes through fibres of chorda tympani nerve. The secondary factor that affects secretion is blood supply because secretion requires nutrition.

Name the various phases of salivary secretion.

Phases of salivary secretion are:

1. *Cephalic phase.* Secretion before food enters mouth. Presence of sight or smell of food causes salivary secretion through conditioned reflex.
2. *Buccal phase.* Presence of food in mouth causes salivary secretion through unconditioned reflex. Appetite area of brain partially regulates these effects.
3. *Oesophageal phase.* When food passes through oesophagus, it stimulates salivary secretion to a slight degree.
4. *Gastric phase.* Presence of food in the stomach causing salivary secretion. Specifically presence of irritant food in stomach acts as a stimulus (e.g. increased salivation before vomiting).
5. *Intestinal phase.* Presence of irritant food in upper intestine causes salivary secretion.

Enumerate the functions of saliva.

1. MECHANICAL FUNCTIONS

- Assists mastication, mixes with the food forming bolus.
- Lubricates the mouth and therefore helps in swallowing.
- Continuous secretion of saliva (at a basal rate of 0.5 ml/min) keeps the mouth moist and helps in speech.

- Dilutes hot and irritant food substances thus preventing injury to mucous membrane of the mouth.
- Decreases the risk of buccal infections and dental caries and maintains oral hygiene. This is because:
  - Continuous secretion of saliva washes away food debris and pathogenic bacteria.
  - Thiocyanate ions and proteolytic enzyme lysozyme attack the bacteria and kill them.
  - Saliva contains significant amount of protein antibodies which destroy bacteria including bacteria causing dental caries.

2. DIGESTIVE FUNCTIONS

The main enzyme present in saliva is salivary amylase or ptyalin. It acts on boiled starch, glycogen and dextrin. It digests starch to maltose in the following way:

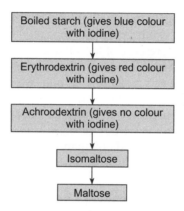

Salivary amylase is an alpha amylase and therefore acts on alpha 1 to linkage (but not on alpha 1 to 6 linkage).

3. EXCRETORY FUNCTION

Certain heavy metals and thiocyanate ions are excreted in saliva.

4. HELPS IN TEMPERATURE REGULATION

- When there is dehydration, there is reduced salivary secretion which induces thirst.
- Panting mechanism: In dogs, saliva is evaporated from the surface of tongue to cause evaporative heat loss.

5. HELPS IN TASTE SENSATION

Taste is a chemical sense and therefore unless the food is in a dissolved state, it cannot be tasted. Saliva acts as a solvent for various foodstuffs.

Why salivary amylase cannot act on unboiled starch?

Salivary amylase is not capable of breaking the cellulose covering present over the raw starch grain and therefore it can act only on boiled starch.

What is the difference between salivary amylase and pancreatic amylase?

Salivary amylase can act only on boiled starch whereas pancreatic amylase can act on boiled as well as unboiled starch and action is much more rapid.

DEGLUTITION

What is deglutition? What are the stages of deglutition?

Deglutition is swallowing of food.
Stages of deglutition are:

- **Oral stage (voluntary stage):** Bolus is rolled from mouth to pharynx.
- **Pharyngeal stage:** Food moves from pharynx to oesophagus.
- **Oesophageal stage:** Food moves from oesophagus to stomach.

Describe the oral or voluntary stage of deglutition.

When food is ready for swallowing, bolus formed is put over the dorsum of the tongue. Tongue is pressed against the palate and is moved backward, moving the bolus from mouth to pharynx.

Describe the pharyngeal stage of deglutition.

When bolus moves from mouth to the pharynx, receptors present around the opening of pharynx are stimulated (especially over tonsillar pillars). Impulses from these areas pass to the brain stem deglutition centre to initiate series of muscular contractions in the following sequence:

- Soft palate moves upwards and closes posterior nasal openings to prevent the entry of food into the nose.
- Palatopharyngeal folds on either side of the pharynx approximate to make a slit like opening for food, allowing only properly masticated food to pass through (selective action).
- Vocal cords of larynx strongly approximate. Larynx is pulled upward and anteriorly by neck muscles. Epiglottis swings backwards to close laryngeal opening. All this prevents entry of food into the trachea.
- Upward movement of larynx enlarges the opening of oesophagus (which is normally slit). Pharyngo-oesophageal sphincter relaxes.
- At the same time, entire muscular wall of the pharynx contracts from superior to inferior part, originating a fast peristaltic wave which also continues in oesophagus. This wave pushes the food from pharynx to oesophagus.

Describe the nervous control of pharyngeal phase.

Pharyngeal stage of swallowing is a reflex. It is initiated by tactile stimulation in the area of opening of pharynx (especially tonsillar pillars which are very sensitive).

Impulses are carried from these areas through 5th and 9th cranial nerves to medulla (deglutition centre). Efferent impulses from the centre pass through 5th, 9th, 10th and 12th nerves to cause different sequential events in the pharyngeal phase.

Entire pharyngeal stage of swallowing lasts for 1 to 2 second. Pharynx is a common pathway for food and air. Therefore, during pharyngeal stage airway above (nasal cavity) and below (trachea) is closed to prevent entry of food into the respiratory passage. In addition, swallowing centre inhibits respiratory centre of the medulla to halt the respiration during any time in its cycle. This momentary stoppage of respiration is known as deglutition apnoea.

Describe the oesophageal stage of deglutition.

Oesophageal stage conducts food from oesophagus to stomach by movements as follows:

1. *Primary peristalsis.* It is simply a continuation of peristaltic wave initiated in pharynx. It takes 8 to 10 seconds to carry food to the stomach. But in upright posture food passes in the stomach earlier (5 to 8 seconds) because of gravity.
2. *Secondary peristalsis.* If primary peristaltic wave fails to carry all the food to the stomach, secondary peristaltic wave is initiated in oesophagus due to distension of oesophagus with food. These waves continue till all the food entered is emptied into the stomach. These waves are produced due to intrinsic neural circuits in the wall and partly due to vagal reflex.

What type of muscles form oesophagus?

Musculature of pharynx and upper one-third of oesophagus is formed of skeletal muscles, whereas lower two-third of oesophagus is formed of smooth muscles.

What is receptive relaxation of the stomach?

Peristalsis is defined as wave of relaxation preceding the wave of contraction, therefore when peristaltic wave passes down the oesophagus, entire stomach is relaxed to accept the food. This is called receptive relaxation of the stomach.

Where is cardiac sphincter? What is its function?

At the lower end of oesophagus at about 3 to 5 cm above its junction with stomach, oesophageal circular muscle coat is thickened to form a sphincter known as lower oesophageal sphincter or gastro-oesophageal sphincter or cardiac sphincter. Its tonic contraction prevents the reflux of acid stomach contents into the oesophagus and thus protects oesophageal mucosa from damage. When peristaltic wave approaches the lower end of oesophagus, this sphincter relaxes (due to receptive relaxation) allowing passage of food from oesophagus to the stomach.

What is achalasia? What is its effect?

When lower oesophageal sphincter does not relax satisfactorily, the condition is known as achalasia. It is due to destruction of local nerve plexus. Because of this, food transmission to stomach is impeded. When it is severe, oesophagus fails to empty the swallowed food into stomach for several hours. Over months and years, oesophagus becomes enlarged and infected due to long standing stasis of food.

What is chalasia?

Chalasia is a condition in which lower oesophageal sphincter remains in a relaxed state inducing gastro-oesophageal reflux.

Is there any other factor other than cardiac sphincter which prevents reflux of food in oesophagus?

There is a valve-like mechanism of the short portion of oesophagus lying beneath the diaphragm before reaching the stomach. Increased intra-abdominal pressure caves the oesophagus inward at this point. Thus valve-like action of lower oesophagus prevents high abdominal pressure from forcing the stomach contents into the oesophagus.

ANATOMY OF STOMACH

Name the different parts of stomach.

- Fundus
- Body
- Pyloric antrum
- Pyloric canal (Fig. 4.1)

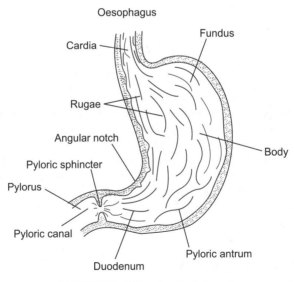

FIGURE 4.1 Different parts of stomach.

FUNCTIONS OF STOMACH

MOTOR FUNCTIONS

Enumerate the motor functions of stomach.

- Storage of food till it can be accommodated in duodenum.
- Mixing of food with gastric secretion to form semisolid chyme.
- Slow emptying of food into the small intestine.

Describe the storage function of stomach.

As food enters the stomach, it forms concentric circles in body and fundus of the stomach. Newest food therefore lies closest to oesophageal opening and oldest lying near the wall of the stomach. When food enters the stomach, stomach relaxes through a vagal reflex, so the wall of the stomach can progressively bulge outward, accommodating greater and greater quantities of food without much increase in pressure up to a certain limit (i.e. 1.5 litres).

What is chyme? How is it formed?

Chyme is a semisolid mixture of food and gastric secretion. It is obtained due to mixing of food with gastric juice mainly through mixing movements of the stomach.

What is basic electrical rhythm of stomach?

Slow electrical waves occurring spontaneously in the stomach wall are called basic electrical rhythm (BER). It is probably caused by a slow undulation of pumping activity of Na^+-K^+pump.

Describe the mixing waves of stomach.

- Peristalsis is a coordinated pattern of smooth muscle contraction and relaxation, where wave of relaxation precedes wave of contraction; peristaltic contractions are produced by periodic changes in membrane potential (BER or slow waves).
- They originate in pacemaker present in fundus (longitudinal muscle of greater curvature as constrictive ring). Initially their velocity is less, i.e. 1 cm/sec, but as the contraction wave approaches the antrum, its speed becomes 4 cm/sec. As wave proceeds towards the pylorus, it deepens.
- When it reaches terminal portion of pylorus, chyme also moves along with but wave of contraction reaches pyloric sphincter (causes its contraction) before the chyme does. When chyme reaches a sphincter it is pushed back into the body of the stomach (retropulsion). Forward and backward movement (caused by peristalsis and retropulsion) breaks the chyme into smaller pieces and mixes it with the gastric secretion. Mixing waves occur at rate of 3/min.

Describe the emptying of stomach.

Emptying of stomach depends on force of gastric peristalsis. Most of the time peristaltic waves are weak in the region of pyloric antrum and they mainly do the function of mixing of food. But about 20% of the time (while food is in the stomach), antral contractions become very intense. They begin at incisura angularis of stomach and then spread over the antrum as strong peristaltic ring-like contractions creating a pressure of 50 to 70 cm of H_2O (6 times as powerful as that produced by mixing waves). When pyloric tone is normal, each strong antral peristaltic wave forces several millilitres of chyme into the duodenum. Thus peristaltic waves provide a pumping action known as pyloric pump. Tone of pyloric sphincter keeps the pylorus open only slightly to allow the passage of water. Tone of pyloric sphincter normally prevents passage of larger food particles. So unless food is properly mixed, the semisolid chyme is not formed, it is not allowed to pass. Degree of contraction of pyloric sphincter can be changed by nervous and hormonal factors.

CONTROL OF PYLORIC SPHINCTER

During fasting, pyloric sphincter remains open. When food enters the stomach, the sphincter closes. Thus it opens at intervals. With a mixed diet opening of the sphincter depends on the following factors:

1. *Motility of stomach.* If mixing waves are strong, mixing quickly occurs forming semisolid chyme which easily passes into the duodenum.
2. *Quantity and quality of food present in stomach.* Greater the volume of food greater is the stretching of stomach walls. This excites pyloric pump through myenteric reflex and inhibits tone of pyloric sphincter. This increases rate of emptying. Presence of certain foods (e.g. meat) causes releases of gastrin which enhances the activity of the pump.
3. *Stage of digestion.* Digestion causes formation of large number of particles and rise in osmotic pressure therefore better is the digestion, quicker is the emptying.
4. *pH of contents.* High acidity on gastric side causes opening of sphincter whereas high acidity in duodenum closes it. Gastric juice contains HCl therefore as gastric juice secretion proceeds acidity in stomach rises, when it reaches a critical level, sphincter opens and gastric contents are pushed into the duodenum. Entry of acid chyme in duodenum raises acidity in duodenal contents. When it reaches a critical level pyloric sphincter closes.
5. *Pressure gradient.* When peristaltic wave of stomach becomes sufficiently strong, there is a pressure rise in stomach which causes opening of the pyloric sphincter (i.e. when mixing wave becomes stronger and gets converted into emptying wave).
6. *Presence of type of food.* Rise in level of partially digested proteins (proteoses and peptones) causes opening of the sphincter so that gastric contents are propelled to the duodenum. Once sufficient quantity is expelled, there occurs fall in level of proteoses and peptones in stomach which closes the sphincter. When after sometime concentration of proteoses and peptone rises the cycle is repeated. Similar cycle occurs with rise and fall of glucose and fatty acid concentrations in stomach.
7. *Osmotic pressure of gastric contents.* Rise of osmotic pressure in stomach causes opening of the pyloric sphincter and vice versa. As digestion proceeds, number of dissolved particles increases. This causes rise in osmotic pressure. When it rises up to a critical level, the sphincter opens and gastric contents are expelled into the duodenum thereby causing reduction in osmotic pressure in stomach. When it reduces to a critical level, the pyloric sphincter closes. As time goes and further digestion occurs the cycle is repeated.

Enumerate the factors regulating the emptying of stomach.

The operation of pyloric sphincter (i.e. opening and closing of the sphincter and factors affecting as given above) regulates gastric emptying in cooperation with antral peristalsis.

Factors affecting emptying of stomach are:

1. *Fluidity of the chyme.* Rate of emptying of solids depends upon rate at which chyme is broken down into small particles. Therefore, it depends on the intensity of mixing waves. Liquids empty much faster than solids.
2. *Gastric factors.* The gastric factors promoting emptying of stomach are:
   ▪ *Volume of food.* Greater the volume of food in the stomach, greater is the stretching of stomach wall which through local vagal and myenteric reflexes excites the activity of pyloric pump and inhibits pyloric sphincter slightly thereby increasing the rate of emptying.
   ▪ *Hormone gastrin.* Presence of certain types of food (meat) causes release of gastrin from antral mucosa. Gastrin enhances the activity of pyloric pump and therefore promotes emptying of stomach.
3. *Duodenal factors.* The duodenal factors which inhibit emptying of stomach are:
   ▪ *Enterogastric reflex.* Distension, high or low osmolarity fluid, low pH, fat and protein digestion products in duodenum, elicit enterogastric reflex which is initiated in duodenal wall. It passes to stomach through myenteric plexus and also extrinsic nerve to inhibit or even stop emptying by inhibiting antral propulsive contraction and increasing slightly the tone of pyloric sphincter.
   ▪ A variety of intestinal hormones inhibit stomach emptying. The stimulus for producing the hormones is mainly fats entering the duodenum.

On entering the duodenum fats extract several hormones from duodenal and jejunal mucosa. These hormones are carried by blood to the stomach and cause inhibition of stomach emptying. They inhibit the activity of pyloric pump and also to certain extent increase the tone of pyloric sphincter.

The most potent hormone causing such effect is CCK (cholecystokinin) which is released from mucosa of jejunum in response to fat in chyme. This hormone acts as a competitive inhibitor to block the increased stomach motility caused by gastrin.

Hormone released from duodenal mucosa in response to gastric acid contents has a general but weak effect of decreasing gastrointestinal motility.

Hormone, gastric inhibitory peptide (GIP), is released from upper small intestine in response to mainly fat in the chyme and to a lesser extent carbohydrate in the chyme. It reduces gastric motility under some conditions but in physiological concentration it probably mainly stimulates secretion of insulin from pancreas.

What is the purpose of enterogastric reflex?

A variety of stimuli cause the enterogastric reflex resulting into decreased rate of stomach emptying. It prevents flow of chyme from exceeding the ability of intestine to handle it (especially longer time is required for fat digestion). It does not allow disturbance in electrolyte balance even if hypo or hypertonic solutions are drunk.

What are hunger contractions?

When stomach is empty for a long time, intense peristaltic contractions occurring in the stomach are known as hunger contractions. When they become extremely strong, they fuse to cause tetanic contraction lasting for 2 to 3 minutes.

How are the movements of stomach studied in man?

The movements in man are studied by introducing rubber tube with a balloon attached to it. After passing the tube, balloon is inflated. Pressure changes in balloon are recorded by attaching manometer to the tube. Alternatively inner wall of the balloon can be coated with barium to make it opaque to X-ray. Then the change in shape can be directly watched under X-ray.

VOMITING

What is vomiting?

Vomiting is a forceful expulsion of food from stomach and intestine.

How is vomiting initiated?

Vomiting is activated by two ways:

1. Direct activation of vomiting centre in the medulla, e.g. due to injury or increased intracranial pressure. This causes projectile vomiting, i.e. rapid forceful vomiting not accompanied by nausea.
2. Activation of chemoreceptor trigger zone by:
   - afferent impulses from GI tract.
   - circulating emetic agents.

This type of vomiting is accompanied by nausea.

Describe the sequence of events occurring during vomiting.

- Deep inspiration with closure of glottis.
- Pressure wave originates in the intestine and propels chyme towards the stomach.
- Increase in intra-abdominal pressure forces the chyme from stomach to oesophagus and out through mouth.

SECRETORY FUNCTION

Name the types of glands present in stomach mucosa.

- **Main gastric glands (oxyntic glands)** (80%). Present in mucosa of the body and fundus.
- **Pyloric (antral) glands** (20%). Found in mucosa between the level of incisura angularis and the pylorus.
- **Cardiac tubular glands**. Near the cardiac end.

Name the types of cells present in the main gastric gland. What do they secrete?

There are three types of cells present in the main gastric gland:

- **Mucous cells** (in the neck of gland). Mainly secrete mucus but also small quantity of pepsinogen.
- **Peptic or chief cells.** Secrete large quantities of pepsinogen.
- **Parietal or oxyntic cells.** Secrete hydrochloric acid and intrinsic factor.

What is the function of pyloric glands?

Pyloric glands mainly secrete mucus rich alkaline viscid juice. Mucus is supposed to lubricate the surface over which a large volume of chyme moves back and forth during digestion. In their deeper portions, these glands contain 'G' cells which secrete hormone gastrin.

What is the function of cardiac glands?

Cardiac glands secrete mucus.

What are the important constituents of gastric juice?

The important constituents of gastric juice are:

1. *Water.* 99.45%.
2. *Solids.* 0.55%. They are further classified into:
   - *Inorganic* (0.15%): NaCl, KCl, $CaCl_2$, calcium phosphate, magnesium phosphate, bicarbonate, etc.
   - *Organic* (0.4%): Mucin, intrinsic factor, enzymes—pepsin, gastric lipase, gastric amylase, gastric gelatinase.

Gastric juice contains free HCl (0.4 to 0.5%) and is strongly acidic with pH 0.9 to 1.5.

How much is the quantity of gastric juice secreted per day?

About 500 to 1000 ml.

Describe the mechanism of secretion of hydrochloric acid.

Hydrochloric acid is secreted in the intracellular canaliculi of parietal cells. These canaliculi open into the lumen of the gastric gland (Fig. 4.2).

HCl synthesis (Fig. 4.3) occurs in three steps as follows:

1. There is active transport of chloride ions from cytoplasm of the cell into the canaliculi which as a result develops a negative potential of -40 to -70 mV. This causes passive flow of potassium ions and a small number of sodium ions from cytoplasm into the canaliculi.

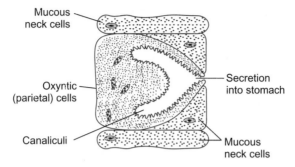

FIGURE 4.2 Anatomy of canaliculi in an oxyntic cell.

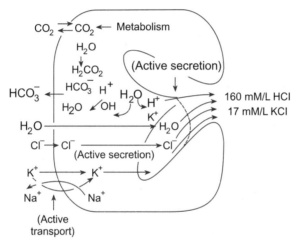

FIGURE 4.3 Mechanism of secretion of hydrochloric acid.

2. Water is dissociated into H^+ and OH^- ions in the cell cytoplasm. H^+ ions are actively secreted into the canaliculi in exchange for potassium ions by H^+-K^+ ATPase. In addition sodium ions are actively reabsorbed by separate sodium pump. Thus most of the potassium and sodium ions diffused into the canaliculi are reabsorbed and H^+ ions take their place. This results in the formation of strong solution of HCl.

3. Water enters from cell to canaliculi by osmosis and canaliculi contain final secretion of HCl of 155 mEq/L.

4. CO_2 formed due to cell metabolism or entering the cell from blood, combines with hydroxyl ions of water under the influence of enzyme carbonic anhydrase to form bicarbonate (HCO_3^-) ions. These HCO_3^- ions diffuse out of cell into extracellular fluid in exchange for chloride ions that enter the cell and later into the canaliculi.

Enumerate the functions of HCl.

- Provides optimal pH for action of pepsin.
- Prevents the growth of pathogenic bacteria.
- Causes hydrolysis of proteins, carbohydrates to certain extent.

Name the substances affecting HCl secretion.

The substances which stimulate HCl secretion are:

1. **Acetylcholine** is neurotransmitter and is released on stimulation of para-sympathetic nerves innervating parietal cell. It also stimulates mast cells to secrete histamine.
2. **Histamine** is released by mast cells present locally. It directly stimulates HCl secretion. Drugs like cimetidine which are used as ulcer treatment act as histamine antagonists.
3. **Gastrin** is the hormone released from 'G' cells of the pyloric portion of stomach. It passes via blood to parietal cells and directly increases HCl secretion as well as it stimulates secretion of histamine by mast cells.

The substance which inhibits HCl secretion is:

Somatostatin. It is neurotransmitter released by interneurons within the intrinsic nervous plexus of GI tract. It inhibits HCl secretion in two ways:

- It directly inhibits HCl secretion by parietal cells.
- It inhibits secretion of gastrin by 'G' cells.

How is HCl secretion regulated?

There are different mechanisms for regulating HCl secretion in different phases of gastric secretion:

1. During *cephalic phase,* vagus stimulation causes release of acetylcholine and inhibition of somatostatin release. Both these enhance HCl secretion.
2. During *gastric phase,* HCl secretion is stimulated by:
   - Presence of proteins in the stomach. Buffer action of proteins keeps the ideal pH for HCl secretion.
   - Certain amino acids directly stimulate parietal cells to release acid.

During this phase, secretion of HCl is inhibited by:

- Decreased pH of gastric contents (below 3) directly inhibits acid secretion. This feedback mechanism maintains pH of gastric contents.
- Lowering of pH of gastric contents causes release of somatostatin.

3. During intestinal phase, presence of products of protein digestion causes increase in HCl secretion by:
   - Release of unidentified hormone from the small intestinal mucosa.
   - Absorbed amino acids directly stimulating the HCl secretion.

During this phase, HCl secretion is inhibited as follows:

- Release of hormones from duodenal mucosa due to presence of H^+ ions, fatty acids and increased osmolarity, inhibit HCl secretion. Gastric inhibitory peptide (GIP) is the most important enterogastrone. GIP inhibits release of gastrin and stimulates the release of somatostatin.

What is the importance of feedback regulation of acid secretion?

Regulation of gastric acid secretion maintains the optimum pH of gastric contents for the action of enzyme pepsin. It does not allow pH to go below 3, and thus prevents damage to the gastric mucosa due to excessive acidity.

Describe the secretion and activation of gastric enzymes.

Several pepsinogens are secreted by peptic and mucous cells of gastric glands and all of them have almost the same function. They do not have digestive activity but are activated to form pepsin as they come in contact with hydrochloric acid and previously formed pepsin.

Other enzymes secreted in gastric juice are gastric lipase, amylase and gelatinase.

In addition a substance known as intrinsic factor, required for absorption of vitamin B_{12} secreted by parietal cells.

How is pepsinogen secretion regulated?

Pepsinogen secretion is regulated by:

- Vagus stimulation.
- HCl secretion.
- Gastrin.

Enumerate the different phases of gastric secretion.

- Cephalic phase.
- Gastric phase.
- Intestinal phase.

Describe the cephalic phase of gastric secretion.

Cephalic phase of gastric secretion occurs before the entry of food into the stomach. Sight, smell, taste or even thought of food causes gastric secretion. It results due to signals originating in cerebral cortex and appetite centres of amygdala or hypothalamus. The impulses are transmitted to dorsal vagal nuclei and from there through vagi to the stomach. Vagal fibres stimulate parietal cells as well as chief cells, therefore both HCl and pepsinogens secretion is increased.

It also stimulates mucus secretion. Rate of secretion is high about 500 ml/hour but this phase lasts for a short time and therefore accounts for about one-fifth of the total gastric secretion in a meal.

Describe the gastric phase of gastric secretion.

Gastric phase of gastric secretion occurs when food enters the stomach.

1. Distension of stomach results into local myenteric and vagovagal reflexes which stimulate the gastric secretion.

2. Distension of pyloric antrum initiates local as well as vagally mediated reflexes which result in release of gastrin from 'G' cells. Secretion of HCl lowers the pH. When pH goes below 3, gastrin secretion is inhibited.
3. Low pH causes increased pepsinogen secretion through local reflexes.

The rate of secretion of gastric juice is less (200 ml/h) as compared to that in cephalic phase but this phase remains for a long time (as long as food remains in the stomach). It accounts for about two-third of the gastric secretion per meal.

What is gastrin? From where is it secreted? What is its action?

Gastrin is a hormone secreted by 'G' cells. It is a polypeptide which occurs in two forms, viz G_{34} which is a large form having 34 amino acids and G_{17} which is a small form containing 17 amino acids. G_{17} is present in more amount.

Gastrin released is absorbed in the blood and through blood it is carried to gastric glands. It strongly stimulates parietal cells and also chief cells but to a lesser extent.

Decreased pH of gastric contents below 3 blocks the gastrin mechanism. This feedback mechanism prevents excessive acid secretion and protects gastric mucosa against high acidity and also maintains pH for enzyme action.

Describe the intestinal phase of gastric secretion.

Presence of food in upper small intestine (especially duodenum) stimulates gastric secretion. This is due to small amount of gastrin released by duodenal mucosa, on distension of duodenum by food or chemical stimuli. To a lesser extent, reflexes and several other hormones also stimulate secretion.

Describe the intestinal factors which inhibit gastric secretion during gastric phase.

Intestinal factors inhibit gastric secretion during gastric phase by the following mechanisms:

1. *Enterogastric reflex.* Distension of small intestine, presence of acid or protein breakdown products in upper intestine and irritation of mucosa initiate this reflex, which passes through intrinsic as well as extrinsic sympathetic and vagus nerves and inhibit gastric secretion.
2. *Hormonal mechanism.* Presence of acid, fat, protein breakdown products, hyper or hypotonic solutions and irritating factors in upper small intestine release several hormones such as secretin, cholecystokinin, gastric inhibitory peptide, vasoactive intestinal polypeptide and somatostatin which inhibit gastric secretion.

Enumerate the functions of gastric secretion.

1. HCl secreted provides optimal pH for enzyme action, hinders growth of bacteria and causes breakdown of proteins.

2. Digestive functions:
   - *Protein digestion.* About 10% of ingested protein is broken down completely in the stomach by pepsin in acid medium (pH 1.8 to 3.5). Pepsin facilitates later digestion of protein by breaking apart meat particles (by action on collagen).
   - *Carbohydrate digestion.* Digestion of carbohydrate by salivary amylase continues in stomach until pH of stomach contents is lowered. Gastric amylase also digests carbohydrate to certain extent.
   - *Fat digestion.* Gastric lipase is tributyrase acting on tributyrin which is a butter fat. It has almost no lipolytic activity on the other fats due to restriction of gastric lipase activity to triglycerides containing short chain (less than 10 carbons) fatty acids.
   - Pepsin and acid break fat emulsions so that fat coalesce into droplets which float and empty fast.
3. Intrinsic factor helps in absorption of vitamin B_{12}.

How are gastric lining cells protected from damage by intramural HCl?

Gastric cells are mainly protected by a thick viscous mucous layer that measures about 1 mm in thickness and is secreted by mucous cells. Turnover rate of gastric mucous cells is very high. Mild injury causes increased mucus secretion. Gastric mucosa is thus prevented from damage by HCl.

Name the substances absorbed by stomach mucosa.

Actually very little absorption of nutrients takes place in stomach. Highly lipid soluble substances (e.g. unionized triglycerides of acetic, propionic and butyric acids) are absorbed to an appreciable extent.

Ethanol (ethyl alcohol) is rapidly absorbed in proportion to its concentration. Water soluble substances like Na^+, K^+, glucose and amino acids are absorbed in insignificant amounts.

How is mechanism of gastric secretion studied in animals?

During interdigestive period, amount of gastric juice secreted is very small. After meals though amount of gastric secretion is large, it cannot be collected without contamination with the food. This offered difficulty in collecting gastric juice. To solve this problem in animals, there are two main experiments done: (1) Experiment of sham feeding, (2) Preparing pouches from the stomach.

1. Sham feeding.
2. Preparing Pavlov's pouch. Stomach is divided by an incomplete division into a larger and a smaller portion. From the pouch, juice is collected with different stimuli and can be analysed. Although gastric pouch gives information regarding a secretory activity of the portion of stomach which is excised, pouches may be prepared from different portions of stomach to study function of different parts of gastric mucosa.

How is gastric secretion studied in man?

Gastric secretion is studied in man by fractional test meal (gastric analysis).

Procedure. The person is given normal diet in the previous evening and called empty stomach the next morning. Thin flexible rubber tube—Ryle's tube (Fig. 4.4) is passed into the stomach through nose or mouth. The tube has got three markings. It is passed up to the second mark to ensure that it has entered the stomach. After passing the tube, stomach contents are collected. A test meal is then given to stimulate gastric juice. Any one of the following standard test meals can be given:

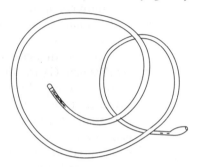

- 50 ml of 7% alcohol.
- 200 ml oatmeal gruel.
- Dry toast and a cup of tea.

FIGURE 4.4 Ryle's tube.

After 15 minutes of giving the test meal, a sample of gastric content (20 ml of fluid) is aspirated. The procedure is repeated every 15 minutes for 3 hours. Thus including the fasting sample total of 13 samples are collected. Each sample is collected in a separate container and is analysed for free acidity, combined acidity, starch and sugar, bile, total chlorides, blood, lactic acid, mucus, etc. (Fig. 4.5).

Free acidity. It is defined as amount of standard alkali required to titrate 100 ml of gastric juice up to pH 3.5 (Topfer's reagent as indicator). Normally in fasting sample it is only 10–20 ml. It increases and reaches a peak value one hour after the test meal. It remains high for half an hour. The acid level comes back to the resting level within 3 hours.

Total acidity. It is defined as amount of standard alkali required to titrate 100 ml of gastric juice to pH 8.5 (phenolphthalein is used as indicator). The curve for

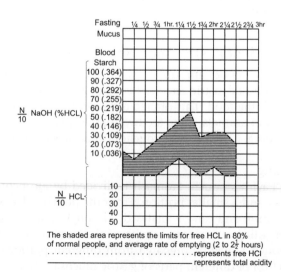

FIGURE 4.5 Fractional gastric analysis in a normal person.

total acid is parallel to that of free acidity but at higher level. The peak total acidity may be as high as 70 to 80 ml.

Combined acidity. The portion between total acidity and free acidity curves indicate combined acidity.

Blood. Blood may be normally present only in first one or two samples because of injury caused due to passage of tube. If it is present in all the samples, it indicates ulcer or cancer.

Bile. Bile comes in the sample because of regurgitation from duodenum. It therefore indicates that pyloric sphincter is open and stomach has started emptying. Generally it appears in the second hour.

Total chlorides. This includes chlorides of HCl, combined HCl and other inorganic chlorides.

Lactic acid. It is obtained by fermentation of carbohydrates. Therefore, if HCl is less, lactic acid is high.

Starch and sugar. It is present in the test meal. Its absence indicates that stomach is completely emptied.

Mucus. Excess mucus indicates irritation of stomach mucosa.

Pepsin. Presence of pepsin indicates normal secretion from chief cells.

Samples are also examined microscopically for presence of blood cells, epithelial cells, tumour cells, bacteria, etc.

What is achlorhydria?

Achlorhydria is a condition where there is no secretion of HCl.

What is hypochlorhydria?

Decreased secretion of free HCl is known as hypochlorhydria.

What is hyperchlorhydria?

Increased secretion of free HCl is known as hyperchlorhydria.

What is histamine test? When is it done?

If one finds that after fractional test meal (with standard meal) there is achlorhydria (absence of free HCl secretion), then histamine test is done to differentiate between true and false achlorhydria. Sometimes HCl is secreted but is neutralized and therefore false achlorhydria is obtained.

To differentiate it from true achlorhydria, 0.5 mg histamine is injected subcutaneously instead of giving test meal (test described earlier as fractional test meal is repeated by giving histamine). Histamine is selected because it is a very powerful stimulator of acid secretion. It stimulates parietal cells to secrete acid if the test meal has failed to do so.

Secondly, due to histamine injection, acid level increases very rapidly and therefore there is no time for neutralization of acid. If there is no free acid present in any of the samples even after histamine injection, then it is called true achlorhydria or histamine fast achlorhydria.

What is insulin test? When is it done?

Insulin test is done by giving 7 units of insulin injection and testing the gastric samples for acid level as done in gastric analysis.

Insulin causes lowering of glucose level which stimulates vagus nerve. Excitation of vagus nerve causes secretion of acid from the stomach. Acid secretion occurs after insulin injection (positive test) only if the vagus is intact. Therefore, insulin test is done after vagotomy operation (for gastric ulcer) to know whether all the fibres of nerve supplying stomach are cut or not. If vagotomy is done properly, insulin test is negative.

SMALL INTESTINE

STRUCTURE

Describe the structure of the small intestinal mucosa.

Small intestine consists of duodenum, jejunum and ileum. It is 5 m long but the total absorptive area (mucosa) is above 250 m².

Surface area of the mucosa is increased as follows:

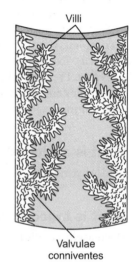

Villi

Valvulae conniventes

FIGURE 4.6 A longitudinal section of the small intestine showing the valvulae conniventes.

1. Mucosa shows many folds called valvulae conniventes (folds of Kerckring) which increase the surface area by threefold (Fig. 4.6).
2. From the surface of mucosa there are millions of small villi which project one millimetre from the surface mucosa. Villi are very densely packed and increase the surface area further by tenfold.
3. Each intestinal cell has brush border, i.e. about 600 microvilli project from each cell into the lumen. This increases the surface area further by twentyfold. Thus total increase in absorptive area is six hundredfold. This favours absorption.

Describe the structure of villus.

Villus collects the nutrients after they are absorbed for which it has an advantageous arrangement of vascular system. Each villus is supplied by an arteriole which gives rise to a capillary tuft at the tip of villus (Fig. 4.7 a,b). Capillaries coalesce into venules which drain into the portal vein. Portal vein carries the nutrients to the liver.

Branches of lymphatic also extend up to the tip of villus. There is one central lacteal. These lymphatics carry absorbed fats, which is carried by them to thoracic duct which opens into circulation.

Where are the Brunner's glands located? What is their function?

Brunner's glands are located in the mucosa of first few centimetres of duodenum (between pylorus and papilla of Vater). These glands mainly secrete mucus. They are

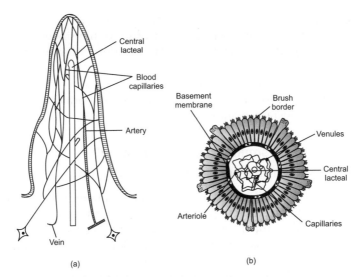

FIGURE 4.7 Functional organization of a villus.

stimulated by tactile stimuli, irritating stimuli, nervous and hormonal stimuli (especially secretin). Mucus secreted protects the duodenal wall from digestion by gastric juice. Brunner's glands are inhibited by sympathetic stimulation (one of the factors causing peptic ulcer).

SECRETION

What is the mechanism of secretion of succus entericus (intestinal secretion)?

On the entire surface of small intestine there are crypts of Lieberkuhn. Intestinal secretion is formed by epithelial cells present in the crypts. There is active secretion of chloride and bicarbonate ions into the crypts which causes electrical force leading to diffusion of sodium ions. All these ions cause osmotic movement of water. Thus there is a marked secretion of watery fluid without enzymes. Epithelial cells covering villi contain intracellular enzymes such as several peptidases, sucrase, maltase, isomaltase, lactase and intestinal lipase. Epithelial cells deep in the crypts of Lieberkuhn continuously undergo mitosis and migrate from the base towards the tip of villus and finally get shed into intestinal secretion. Thus enzymes enter the intestinal secretion. This mode of secretion of enzymes is known as holocrine mode of secretion.

Give the composition of succus entericus.

Succus entericus contains 98.5% water and 1.5% solids. The pH varies from slightly acidic to slightly alkaline.
The solids are:

1. *Inorganic (0.8%).* Sodium, potassium, calcium, magnesium with chloride, bicarbonate and phosphate.

2. *Organic (0.7%)*. The enzymes present are as follows:
   - Enterokinase (enteropeptidase): activator of trypsinogen.
   - Erepsin: proteolytic enzyme containing group of aminopeptidases and dipeptidases.
   - Nuclease, nucleotidase, nucleosidase.
   - Arginase: acts on arginine producing urea and ornithine.
   - Amylase, sucrase, maltase, lactase and isomaltase.

How is secretion of small intestine regulated?

Intestinal secretion is mainly regulated by two mechanisms:

1. *Local stimuli.* Tactile and irritative stimuli initiate local nervous reflexes which are initiated due to presence of chyme and regulate small intestinal secretion. This is the most important means of regulation.
2. *Hormonal regulation.* Secretin, cholecystokinin and other hormones extracted from small intestine stimulate intestinal secretion (mainly CCK and secretin) but this mechanism is less important in regulation.

Enumerate the functions of succus entericus.

1. There are several peptidases (erepsin) present which digest peptides into amino acids.
2. There are disaccharidase, sucrase, maltase, lactase, isomaltase which split disaccharides into monosaccharides.
3. Intestinal lipase splits triglycerides. It mainly causes hydrolysis of the primary ester linkage.

Monoglycerides are the main products of digestion. Lesser percentage of fat is converted to fatty acids and glycerol. Most of the enzymes are present near the brush border. They cause hydrolysis of foodstuff just before absorption.

4. Enterokinase activates trypsinogen to trypsin.

MOVEMENTS

Enumerate the different movements of small intestine.

There are two types of movements of small intestine:

- Segmentation movement.
- Peristaltic movement.

In addition, there are movements of villi due to contraction of muscularis mucosa. Villi alternately elongate and contract causing milking of villi resulting in free flow of lymph from central lacteal into the lymphatic system. They are initiated by local nervous reflexes in response to presence of chyme in small intestine.

Describe the segmentation movements of small intestine.

Distension of small intestine with chyme stretches the intestinal wall and initiates the segmentation movements (Fig. 4.8). There are localized concentric contractions

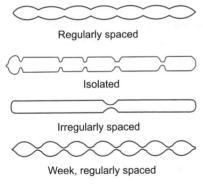

Regularly spaced

Isolated

Irregularly spaced

Week, regularly spaced

FIGURE 4.8 Segmentation movements.

(about 1 to 2 cm in length) spaced at intervals along the intestine. They divide the intestine into spaced segments. These contractions force the chyme back towards the stomach and towards the colon and last for 5 to 6 seconds. When muscle relaxes, chyme comes back to the area from which it is displaced. A new set of contractions then begins at new points between previous contractions. Segmentation movements occur at a rate of 8 to 12 minutes. Maximum frequency is present in duodenum (12/min) and proximal jejunum. In terminal ileum it is 8 to 9/min.

Segmentation contractions occur throughout the digestive period.

FUNCTIONS

1. Segmentation contractions move the food back and forth as explained above. This enables chyme to become thoroughly mixed with the digestive juices and to make proper contact with absorptive surface of the intestinal mucosa.
2. Higher frequency of segmentation in proximal intestine than in distal intestine, propels the chyme slowly towards the colon.

CONTROL

The segmentation contractions can occur only if the slow waves (basic electrical rhythm) produce action potential. Action potential appears on slow waves when the membrane potential is sufficiently depolarized. Frequency of segmentation is directly related to the frequency of slow waves and is controlled by pacemaker cells of the small intestine.

But segmentation contractions become very weak on blocking the nervous system by atropine, i.e. the contractions are not really effective without the background excitation by enteric nervous system (especially myenteric plexus) though slow waves in the smooth muscle control the segmentation contractions. Slow wave amplitude is also increased by hormones, gastrin, cholecystokinin, motilin and insulin. Secretin and glucagon reduce the slow wave amplitude.

Describe the peristaltic movements of small intestine.

Peristalsis is a wave of contraction preceded by wave of relaxation. Peristaltic wave can be initiated in any part of the small intestine. It moves analwards at a rate of 0.5 to 2 cm/min but it is weak and dies out after travelling only 3 to 5 cm, very rarely up to 10 cm. So net movement of the chyme in analward direction is slow (1 cm/min; Fig. 4.9).

FUNCTIONS

- Peristaltic waves propel the chyme in analward direction.
- As chyme enters the intestine, it spreads along the entire length of the intestine due to peristaltic waves for proper digestion and absorption.

CONTROL

Peristalsis is controlled by nervous and hormonal factors.

Nervous control. Peristalsis in the small intestine increases immediately after meals due to gastroenteric reflex. Distension of stomach due to meal initiates this reflex. Impulses pass through myenteric plexus from stomach to the small intestine along the wall of small intestine causing increase in the peristaltic activity.

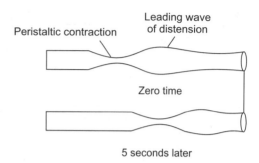

FIGURE 4.9 Peristaltic movement of small intestine.

Hormonal control. Gastrin, cholecystokinin, insulin and serotonin enhance the intestinal motility. Secretin and glucagon decrease the motility.

What is peristaltic rush?

Intense irritation of intestinal mucosa causes very powerful and rapid peristalsis called peristaltic rush. It is partly initiated by extrinsic nervous reflex and partly by myenteric reflex. Powerful peristaltic contractions travel long distances in small intestine within minutes. It sweeps the contents of intestine into the colon and relieves small intestine of either irritative chyme or excessive distension.

What is the function of ileocaecal valve?

Ileocaecal valve prevents back flow of faecal contents from colon into the small intestine. The valve usually resists pressure of 50 to 60 cm of water.

What is ileocaecal sphincter?

Immediately preceding the ileocaecal valve, the wall of ileum for several centimetres has a thickened muscular coat which is called ileocaecal sphincter. Tonic contraction of this sphincter slows emptying of meal contents into caecum. The contents stay in the ileum for a long time which facilitates absorption. Gastroileal reflex and gastrin cause relaxation of the ileocaecal sphincter. Its degree of contraction is also controlled by reflexes from caecum.

PANCREAS

Give the important constituents of pancreatic juice.

Pancreatic juice has alkaline pH.

Inorganic contents. High bicarbonate content with principal bases, sodium and potassium. Small amounts of calcium, magnesium and zinc are also present.

Organic contents. Enzymes of pancreatic juice are trypsinogen, chymotrypsinogen, procarboxypeptidase, nucleotidase (ribonuclease, deoxyribonuclease), lipase and amylase.

How much is the daily amount of pancreatic juice?
Amount of pancreatic juice secreted daily is about 500 to 1000 ml.

Name the types of cells in the pancreas with their functions.
The types of cells in pancreas are:

- *Endocrine cells.* Alpha and beta cells of islets of Langerhans. They secrete hormones, insulin, glucagon, somatostatin and pancreatic polypeptide directly into the blood.
- *Exocrine cells.* They are organized in acini. They produce four types of digestive enzymes, viz. amylases, peptidases, nucleases and lipases.
- *Ductal cells.* They secrete high quantity of bicarbonate into the pancreatic juice.

How much is the concentration of bicarbonate ions in pancreatic juice?
Bicarbonate ions in pancreatic juice can be as high as 145 mEq/L.

Describe the mechanism of secretion of pancreatic juice.
Enzyme secretion. Pancreatic alpha amylase, lipase are secreted in active forms by cells of acini. Pancreatic proteases (trypsin, chymotrypsin and carboxypeptidase) are secreted in inactive form. Trypsin inhibitor is also secreted by the same cells. It inhibits activation of proteolytic enzymes in pancreas preventing its autodigestion. Sodium and potassium concentrations are the same as in plasma.

Sodium bicarbonate secretion. Bicarbonate concentration of pancreatic juice is much higher than that of plasma. Bicarbonate is secreted into the juice by ductal cells as follows:

- CO_2 diffuses from blood to the cell and combines with water to form carbonic acid in presence of enzyme carbonic anhydrase. Carbonic acid dissociates into H^+ and HCO_3^- ions. HCO_3^- ions are actively transported from the cell to the lumen of the duct.
- H^+ ions are exchanged for sodium ions through blood border of the cell.
- Na^+ ions either diffuse or are actively transported from cell into the lumen of the duct.
- Thus there is formation of sodium bicarbonate in the duct. This creates osmotic gradient and causes water to enter the duct by osmosis. Thus bicarbonate solution is formed.

How are proteolytic enzymes of pancreas activated?
Proteolytic enzymes of pancreas are activated only when the pancreatic juice comes to the intestine. Trypsin inhibitor prevents their activation in the pancreas. Enterokinase secreted by small intestine activates trypsinogen to trypsin. Once small quantity of trypsin is formed, it can by itself activate the trypsinogen.

Trypsin also activates chymotrypsinogen and procarboxypeptidase to chymotrypsin and carboxypeptidase respectively.

State the functions of pancreatic juice.

1. Pancreatic juice causes neutralization of acidic contents of the chyme emptied into the duodenum from the stomach because of high bicarbonate content. It also provides alkaline pH for enzyme action ($HCl + NaHCO_3 \rightarrow NaCl + H_2CO_3$).
2. Pancreatic alpha amylase hydrolyzes glycogen, starch and most other complex carbohydrates except cellulose to form disaccharides.
3. Pancreatic lipases (lipase, cholesterol lipase and phospholipase) hydrolyze water soluble esters without the action of bile salts and water insoluble esters with the help of bile salts.
4. Trypsin is endopeptidase. It acts on native proteins as well as on products of protein digestion (metaprotein, proteases, peptones, polypeptides) and converts them into lower peptides (tri and dipeptides). Thus trypsin has a very wide range of action as compared to that of pepsin. Chymotrypsin is also an endopeptidase converting protein into di and tripeptides. Carboxypeptidase splits of amino acid (possessing a free carboxyl group) from protein.
5. Nucleotidases digest nucleoproteins.

Name the different phases of pancreatic secretion and their regulation.

Regulation of different phases of pancreatic secretion is described below:

1. *Cephalic phase.* Sight, smell or thought of food causes pancreatic secretion. Both acinar as well as ductal cell secretion is enhanced due to vagal stimulation. Enzyme secretion is enhanced due to stimulation of enteric neurons which release acetylcholine. Bicarbonate secretion is increased by stimulation of enteric neurons which release noradrenergic transmitter.

Very little secretion actually flows from pancreatic ducts into the duodenum during this phase because of small quantity of water and electrolyte secretion along with enzymes.

2. *Gastric phase.* When stomach is distended with food, there is increased secretion of pancreatic juice by the following mechanisms:
   - Distension of stomach with food elicits vago-vagal reflex stimulating low volume of pancreatic secretion containing HCO_3 and enzymes. Acetylcholine is the transmitter.
   - Protein breakdown products cause release of gastrin from 'G' cells of stomach. Gastrin released into the blood causes low volume, high enzyme juice secretion from pancreas.

3. *Intestinal phase.* It occurs after the chyme enters the intestine. This phase is controlled by secretin and cholecystokinin hormones released from endocrine cells of duodenal and jejunal mucosa. Cholecystokinin is released from

'I' cells of duodenal and jejunal mucosa due to presence of proteases and peptides and long chain fatty acids in upper small intestine. Cholecystokinin passes via blood to pancreas and causes effects similar to vagal stimulation but more pronounced, i.e. increased amount of enzymes are secreted which is known as ecbolic effect. Secretin is secreted by 'S' cells of duodenum and jejunum in the inactive form known as prosecretin. When chyme enters the intestine, it causes a release and activation of secretin. Acid in the chyme is the most potent stimulator for secretin release. Secretin released is absorbed in the blood and reaches pancreas. It mainly stimulates duct cells to secrete large quantities of bicarbonate and fluid. Very little secretion of enzymes occurs because secretin does not stimulate acinar cells. Release of secretin depends on pH of the intestinal content. It greatly increases when pH falls below 3. Release of secretin causes large amount of bicarbonate secretion for neutralization of acid chyme. Thus it is a protective mechanism against development of duodenal ulcer. Secondly, high bicarbonate content also maintains alkaline pH for the action of pancreatic enzymes. Effect of secretion is termed hydroelectric effect.

BILE

Give the composition of bile.

The bile contains 97.5% water and 2.5% solids.
Composition of the solids:

- Bile salts: 1.1%.
- Bilirubin: 0.04%.
- Cholesterol: 0.1%.
- Lecithin: 0.04%.
- Fatty acids: 0.12.
- Inorganic salts: 0.8%.

Explain the formation of bile.

Bile is secreted by liver epithelial cells called hepatocytes and by epithelial cells lining the bile ducts (ductal cells).
The bile secretion occurs in two stages:

- Hepatocytes secrete bile which contains large amounts of bile acids, cholesterol and other organic substances.
- When bile flows into the ducts, ductal cells secrete water, sodium and bicarbonate ions. It increases the total quantity of bile secreted by as much as additional 100%. Cholesterol and phospholipids present in bile are not soluble in water but they are solubilized by the bile salts micelles.

How much bile is secreted daily?

Daily about 500 to 1100 ml of bile is secreted.

What are bile salts? How they are synthesized?

Bile salts are sodium and potassium salts of bile acids. Bile acids are synthesized from cholesterol which is absorbed through microvilli lining the serosal border of hepatocytes. Bile acids are then conjugated with either glycine or taurine to form conjugated bile acids. Sodium and potassium salts of these acids are the bile salts. They are actively secreted into the biliary canaliculi.

What are bile pigments? How are they formed?

Bilirubin and biliverdin are the bile pigments. They are metabolites of haemoglobin. They are formed in reticuloendothelial system (liver, spleen, bone marrow). In pigmented epithelium cells, haem and globin are separated. Porphyrin ring of haem is broken, iron is removed and bilirubin is formed which is brought to the liver. In the liver it conjugates with glucuronic acid or sulphates and is made soluble. It is then excreted in bile.

On excretion, bilirubin is converted to urobilin by intestinal bacteria. Urobilin gives brown colour to the stools.

Describe the functions of bile.

Bile is required for digestion and absorption of fat and fat soluble vitamins. Bile salts present in the bile do both these functions as follows:

1. **Act as detergent**. They reduce surface tension of the fat particles, which makes them easily breakable. With agitation in the intestinal tract, fat globule is broken into multiple minute sized globules. This is called emulsification of fat. Emulsification increases the surface area of fat globule. As fat is insoluble in water, lipases which are water soluble can act only on the surface of the fat. By increasing the surface area, action of lipases is enhanced.

2. **Form minute complexes called micelles**. About 20 to 40 bile salt molecules aggregate and form micelle. Micelles are highly water soluble because of electrical charges. In formation of micelle, polar groups of bile salts project outward to cover the surface of the micelle and steroid nuclei collect in the centre to form small fat globule.

Micelles do the function of ferrying monoglycerides and fatty acids (formed during digestion) to intestinal mucosa for absorption. Digestion of triglycerides produces fatty acids and monoglycerides, but if these digested products are collected at the site, triglycerides can be reformed as it is a reversible reaction. This quickly blocks digestion. Micelles take digested products (monoglycerides and fatty acids) away from the site of digestion as rapidly as they are produced. Micelles also carry these digested products for absorption to the brush border of intestine. They are easily absorbed because of their high lipid solubility. They simply get dissolved in lipid of the membrane and diffuse through it.

3. Bile salts keep insoluble cholesterol of bile in solution due to its hydrotropic action. Ratio of cholesterol to bile salts is 1:20 to 1:30. When ratio falls to 1:13, cholesterol is precipitated and then gall stones can be formed.

Thus bile salts when present in sufficient amount prevent formation of gall stones.

4. When bile salts are absorbed from the intestine into blood (during entero-hepatic circulation) and go back to liver they act as important choleretic agent and stimulate bile secretion.

5. Bile pigments are excreted in bile.

Where is bile stored?

Bile is secreted continuously by liver cells and is normally stored in gall bladder until needed in the duodenum. Capacity of gall bladder is 20 to 60 ml.

Describe the biliary pathway.

Bile is secreted by hepatocytes into biliary canaliculi that lie between the hepatic cells in hepatic plates. Canaliculi empty into the terminal bile ducts present in interlobular septa. Then bile passes through progressively larger and larger ducts and then into the hepatic duct and common bile duct. From here, bile either enters the gall bladder through cystic duct or enters the second part of duodenum (where the common bile duct opens).

How is gall bladder filled?

At the opening of common bile duct (CBD) into the duodenum, there is a sphincter known as "sphincter of Oddi". During interdigestive period, this sphincter remains contacted and therefore opening of CBD into duodenum remains closed. As bile is secreted by liver continuously, it gets accumulated in CBD. When pressure of bile in the duct rises, it forces its way through cystic duct into the gall bladder. Thus gall bladder is filled up during the interdigestive period.

Describe the process of emptying of gall bladder.

When food reaches upper intestine and its digestion begins, gall bladder begins to empty. Basic cause of emptying is contractions of the wall of gall bladder with simultaneous relaxation of sphincter of Oddi.

CONTROL OF EMPTYING OF GALL BLADDER

1. The main stimulus for gall bladder contraction and relaxation of sphincter of Oddi is the hormone cholecystokinin. When chyme enters small intestine, fat and protein digestion products directly stimulate production of cholecystokinin from the small intestinal mucosa. It is absorbed in blood. When it reaches gall bladder, contraction of gall bladder occurs and sphincter of Oddi relaxes by three mechanisms:
   - Cholecystokinin has a relaxing effect on sphincter of Oddi.
   - Rhythmic contractions of gall bladder transmit peristaltic waves down common bile duct to sphincter of Oddi leading to receptive relaxation of sphincter.

- The intestinal peristaltic waves travel over the wall of duodenum. Relaxation phase of each wave strongly relaxes the sphincter of Oddi along with the relaxation of the muscle wall.
2. In addition to cholecystokinin, vagal stimulation also causes contraction of gall bladder and relaxation of sphincter of Oddi. Vagal stimulation occurs during the cephalic phase of digestion and indirectly during vago-vagal reflexes occurring in gastric phase of digestion.

How is the function of gall bladder studied?

Function of gall bladder is studied by cholecystography. In this test tetraiodophenolphthalein is given at night in the form of oral tablets (this substance is radioopaque and is excreted in bile). This is followed by fasting for 14 hours. During fasting period, bile secreted by liver gets collected in the gall bladder. If X-ray is taken after 14 hours, shadow of gall bladder can be seen. After this, the person is given fatty meal which promotes emptying of gall bladder. If X-ray is taken hours after the fatty meal, gall bladder is completely empty in a normal person.

Enumerate the functions of gall bladder.

- Stores the bile by absorbing water and concentrating it by 10 times.
- Equalizes the pressure within biliary passage.
- Secretes mucus which is the main source of mucin in bile.

What are the effects of cholecystectomy (removal of gall bladder)?

After removal of gall bladder, bile empties slowly but continuously in the intestine allowing digestion of fat sufficient to maintain health and nutrition. But only fat meals should be avoided.

How are gall stones formed?

Gall stones are composed chiefly of cholesterol or calcium bilirubinate.

Cholesterol and lecithin are insoluble in water but they are kept in solution because of formation of micelles of bile salts. When proportions of lecithin, cholesterol and bile salts are altered, cholesterol crystallizes leading to stone formation. Cholesterol stones are radiolucent.

When there is biliary tract infection it leads to deconjugation of conjugated bilirubin by bacteria. Unconjugated bilirubin is insoluble in water. It precipitates to begin the stone-forming process. Calcium bilirubinate crystals are radiopaque.

What is the difference between liver bile and gall bladder bile?

Gall bladder bile is 10 times more concentrated. Gall bladder absorbs salt, therefore alkalinity of gall bladder bile becomes slightly less. Gall bladder secretes mucus, therefore mucin content of the bile increases.

How is the bile secretion regulated?

Volume of biliary secretion and amount of bile salts in that secretion are regulated separately.

1. **Amount of fluid and electrolytes in bile is regulated as follows:**
The fluid is secreted by ductal cells. It has high concentration of bicarbonate ions. It is regulated by hormone secretin. Therefore, secretin causes bile-independent fraction of biliary secretion (fluid and electrolyte) and thus is called hydrocholeretic agent.

2. **Regulation of quantity of bile salts secreted:**
It is called bile-dependent fraction of biliary secretion. Bile salts secreted by hepatocytes depend on the following factors:

- Amount of bile salts secreted by hepatocytes is directly proportional to the amount absorbed by them from portal circulation.
- Increase in synthesis of bile salts: Substances that enhance the synthesis of bile salts are called choleretic agents. Bile salts and bile acids are major choleretic agents.

Synthesis of bile salts by liver is not controlled by any hormonal or nervous factor.

What are cholagogue and choleretic agents?

Cholagogue agents increase release of bile from the gall bladder.

Choleretic agents increase synthesis of bile salts from liver. Bile salts in circulation are choleretic agents. Secretin is hydrocholeretic agent and increases secretion of only water and salts in the bile.

What is enterohepatic circulation of bile salts? What is its significance?

This is recirculation of bile salts from liver to small intestine and back again.

Path of circulation. Bile salts are transported from liver to duodenum via CBD during digestion. When bile salts reach the terminal ileum, they are reabsorbed into the portal circulation. Liver cells extract them from the portal circulation and secrete them once again into the bile. About 90 to 95% of the bile salts entering the small intestine are reabsorbed in terminal ileum. Remaining bile salts are excreted in faeces.

Importance of enterohepatic circulation:

1. This circulation is necessary because of the limited pool of bile salts available. The same bile salts are utilized and reutilized because of this circulation.
Any condition that disrupts the enterohepatic circulation leads to decreased bile acid pool and malabsorption of fat and fat soluble vitamins. Clinical manifestation of such condition is steatorrhoea (undigested fat in faeces) and nutritional deficiency.
2. Absorbed bile salts present in portal circulation act as choleretic agent and stimulate their own synthesis by hepatocytes.

LARGE INTESTINE

Describe the mucosa of large intestine.

Mucosa of large intestine has crypts of Lieberkuhn but there are no villi. Epithelial cells contain no enzymes. Surface epithelium contains large number of mucous cells dispersed among the other epithelial cells.

Name the various secretions from mucosa of large intestine and their functions.

Large intestinal mucosa mainly secretes mucus and large amount of bicarbonate ions. Mucus secretion is stimulated by tactile stimuli and by local nervous reflexes. Mucus protects the wall against excoriation and provides the medium for holding faecal matter together. It also protects intestinal wall from bacterial activity that takes place inside the faeces. Bacterial activity also produces acid for which mucus acts as a barrier.

Large quantities of water and electrolytes are secreted by mucosa of large intestine only when it is intensely irritated.

Enumerate the movements of large intestine and their functions.

There are two types of movements of large intestines, namely: (1) Haustral contractions and (2) mass movement. Their functions are to:

- Increase the efficiency of colon for water and electrolytes absorption.
- Promote excretion of faecal matter.

Describe the haustral contractions.

Haustral contractions are similar to segmentation movements of small intestine.

Large circular bands of constriction occur at regular intervals. At each of these constrictive points 2.5 cm of circular muscle contracts. Longitudinal muscles (*Taenia*) also contract. This causes unstimulated portions of large intestine to bulge in a bag like sacs called haustrations. Contraction disappears within 60 seconds. After a few minutes, haustral contractions are initiated in a nearby area.

The function of this movement is to expose the faecal matter to mucosal surface for absorption. It also causes slow propulsion of faecal matter.

Describe the mass movements of large intestine.

Mass movements only occur 3 to 4 times a day. They are just like peristalsis of small intestine. Much propulsion of faecal matter in caecum and ascending colon results due to haustral contractions. From beginning of transverse colon to the sigmoid colon, mass movements cause propulsion. Mass movements are initiated after breakfast or meal due to gastrocolic or duodenocolic reflexes, initiated by distension of stomach or duodenum. First constrictive ring appears at an irritated point (usually transverse colon), then about 20 cm colon distal to it contracts as a unit forcing faecal matter in this segment down the colon. Relaxation occurs within 2–3 minutes. Then mass movement is initiated at the next point. Usually mass movements once initiated persist for about 10 to 30 minutes. Irritation of colon (ulcerative colitis) can also initiate mass movements. When mass movements force the faecal matter into the rectum, desire for defaecation is felt.

What is defaecation?
Process by which faecal material is excreted is called defaecation.

Describe the process of defaecation.
Usually the rectum is empty. Due to mass movements, faecal matter enters the rectum causing its distension. A rectosphincteric reflex relaxes the anal sphincter and generates urge to defaecate. Defaecation involves both voluntary and reflex activity. Ordinarily defaecation is initiated by defaecation reflexes as follows:

1. *Intrinsic reflex.* It is mediated by intrinsic nerve plexus. Distension of rectum with faeces initiates afferent signals which pass through myenteric plexus to descending colon to initiate a peristaltic wave. As peristaltic wave approaches lower end of rectum, it causes relaxation of internal anal sphincter (made up of smooth muscle). If external sphincter is relaxed (which is made up of skeletal muscle and is under voluntary control) defaecation occurs.

2. *Spinal cord reflex.* Intrinsic reflex is weak and is reinforced by this reflex. Distension of rectum due to faeces causes transmission of signals to sacral segments of spinal cord. Signals are transmitted from here through pelvic nerves (parasympathetic fibres) to colon to intensify the peristaltic waves and relaxation of inner anal sphincter. It converts intrinsic defaecation reflex from weak movement to powerful process of defaecation that results into emptying of large bowel from splenic flexure to anus.

In addition to defaecation reflexes, the abdominal muscles and diaphragm contract, increase the intra-abdominal pressure forcing the faeces through the anal canal.

Defaecation can be prevented by voluntarily contracting the external anal sphincter. If defaecation does not occur, internal anal sphincter closes, rectum relaxes to accommodate faecal matter within it.

In newborn babies or in person with transacted spinal cord, defaecation reflex causes automatic emptying of lower bowel without normal voluntary control on external anal sphincter.

DIGESTION AND ABSORPTION

Describe the digestion of carbohydrates.
The main carbohydrates in human diet are sucrose, lactose (milk), starch, amylose, amylopectin and cellulose. There is no enzyme in the human gastrointestinal tract for digestion of cellulose. So it is excreted unused.

Total carbohydrate intake is 200 to 800 g/day, i.e. about 50 to 60% of the diet.

Describe the absorption of water and electrolytes from the intestine.

Water and sodium in the diet and in the salivary, gastric, intestinal, biliary and pancreatic secretions are absorbed in small intestines.

1. *Water absorption.* Active reabsorption of electrolytes and nutrients creates an osmotic gradient for water. Water is absorbed passively and iso-osmotically. In duodenum, entry of chyme increases osmotic pressure causing water to flow in the intestine. In jejunum and ileum, active reabsorption of NaCl creates osmotic gradient which favours water reabsorption.

2. *Absorption of sodium and chloride.*
   - Sodium is first transported from the lumen into the intestinal cell (enterocyte) and then across the basolateral membrane into the intestinal interstitium.
   - Sodium enters the enterocyte in three ways:
     - About 30% is transported into the cell by a Na^+-glucose, Na^+-amino acid co-transport system.
     - About 30% is transported into the cell by a Na^+-Cl^- co-transport system.
     - The remainder enters the cell passively down an electrochemical gradient.
   - Once inside the enterocyte, Na^+ is transported across the basolateral membrane by a Na^+-K^+ ATPase active transport system.
   - For the most part, Cl^- flows passively through the enterocyte down the electrochemical gradient established by the active transport of Na^+.

Describe the digestion and absorption of carbohydrates, proteins and fats.

Refer Table 4.1.

Table 4.1   Digestion and Absorption of Carbohydrates, Proteins and Fats

	Carbohydrates	Proteins	Fats
		Digestion	
In Mouth	• Salivary alpha amylase acts on boiled starch and converts it into maltose.	-	-
In Stomach	-	• Pepsin of the stomach digests about 10–15% of ingested protein completely. • Pepsin breaks apart the meat particles and facilitates further digestion of proteins because of ability of pepsin to digest collagen, which is the main intercellular substance (connective tissue constituent).	• Gastric lipase acts on butter.
In Small Intestine	• Pancreatic alpha amylase is more powerful, so it acts on boiled as well as unboiled starch and varieties of other oligosaccharides.	• Proteolytic enzymes of pancreas play major role in their digestion. • All the pancreatic proteolytic enzymes are secreted in inactive form. They are converted to active form after they enter small intestine.	• Bile salts cause the emulsification of fat. The enzyme which plays major role in fat digestion is pancreatic lipase. It digests almost all the triglycerides of food to fatty acids, glycerol and monoglycerides.

Continued

Table 4.1 Digestion and Absorption of Carbohydrates, Proteins and Fats—cont'd

	Carbohydrates	Proteins	Fats
		Digestion	
	• Oligosaccharides are converted to monosaccharides by brush border enzymes of small intestine such as maltase, sucrase, lactase, isomaltase.	• Enterokinase from succus entericus activates trypsinogen to trypsin. Once small quantity of trypsin is formed, it activates trypsinogen, chymotrypsinogen as well as procarboxypeptidase. • Trypsin and chymotrypsin are endopeptidases and they break proteins and protein breakdown products into small lower peptides, mainly into tripeptides and dipeptides. Trypsin has a wider range of action as compared to that of pepsin. • Carboxypeptidase splits the amino acid possessing a free carboxyl group from protein. • Peptidases (amino polypeptidases and dipeptidases) secreted by intestinal epithelial cells convert polypeptides into lower polypeptides and amino acids. • Nucleoproteins are digested by nucleosidase, nucleotidase and nucleases secreted in pancreatic juice and succus entericus.	• Small intestinal epithelial cells contain small quantities of intestinal lipase which can also digest triglycerides. Thus end products of triglyceride digestion are free fatty acids, monoglycerides and very small quantity of diglycerides. • Cholesterol in the food is in the form of cholesterol esters (cholesterol + one molecule of fatty acid). Cholesterol esterase enzyme digests it to cholesterol and fatty acid. • Phospholipids are digested by phosphorylase A2 which separates fatty acid from phospholipid.
End Products	• Glucose, Galactose, Fructose	• Amino Acids, Dipeptides, Tripeptides	• Fatty Acids, Glycerol

Absorption of End Products

- Glucose and Galactose are absorbed by secondary active transport or Na⁺ co-transport mechanism. Fructose is absorbed by facilitated diffusion, converted to glucose and lactic acid within the intestinal cells to maintain high concentration gradient for fructose across the membrane. Monosaccharides are transported across the basolateral membrane by facilitated diffusion into the intestinal interstitium and diffused into capillaries of villus.

- Amino acids are absorbed by secondary active transport or Na⁺ co-transport mechanism similar to that for monosaccharides. But there are number of transport systems, e.g. separate transport systems are available for basic amino acids, acidic amino acids and neutral amino acids. There are also tripeptide and dipeptide transporters.

- Absorped tripeptides and dipeptides are digested to amino acids in the intestinal cells by intracellular peptidases.

- Amino are transported through basolateral surface of the intestinal cell by facilitated or simple diffusion into the interstitium and then they enter the capillaries of villus by simple diffusion.

- Sometimes whole protein is absorbed by the mechanism of pinocytosis. This is responsible for allergic reaction to food proteins.

- Products of lipid digestion get dissolved in the central fatty portion of micelle. Micelles move along the microvilli surface allowing their lipids to diffuse through the membrane of microvilli into the cell. Lipid gets dissolved in the membrane lipid of microvilli and then diffuses to the interior of the intestinal cell. Lipids, cholesterol, lipid soluble vitamins are very rapidly removed from micelles, once they make contact with microvilli. So the rate limiting step in lipid absorption is migration of micelles from intestinal chyme to microvilli surface. Once the bile salts are freed, they again go back to intestinal chyme for ferrying more fat digestion products.

Continued

Table 4.1 Digestion and Absorption of Carbohydrates, Proteins and Fats—cont'd

Carbohydrates	Proteins	Fats
Digestion		
		• Once the digested fat enters the intestinal cell, it is reconstituted as follows:
		• Monoglycerides are converted to triglycerides.
		• Lysophosphatides combine with fatty acid to form phospholipid.
		• Cholesterol is re-esterified.
		• These reformed lipids form chylomicrons which are small lipid droplets in the smooth endoplasmic reticulum of cell. The chylomicrons are covered by beta-lipoprotein (apo β-48). It is because of covering of B-apolipoprotein that exocytosis of chylomicrons is possible. After coming out from the cell they diffuse into lacteals and then into hepatic circulation.
		• Most of the absorption of fat occurs in duodenum and upper jejunum. Therefore, by the time food reaches mid-jejunum, almost all the dietary fat is absorbed. Small quantities of short chain fatty acids are absorbed directly into the portal blood.
		• Lipid malabsorption occurs when there is inadequate supply of pancreatic lipase or bile.

CHAPTER 5
Excretory System

What is excretion?

Throwing out of waste product is known as excretion.

Name the various organs through which excretion occurs.

1. *Kidneys:* Excrete water and water soluble waste products.
2. *Lungs:* Excrete carbon dioxide, water vapour and other volatile substances such as acetone.
3. *Skin:* Excretes water and salts mainly in the form of sweat.
4. *Gastrointestinal tract:* Excretes undigested food.

Enumerate the functions of kidneys.

1. Regulation of water and inorganic ion balance.
2. Removal of metabolic waste products from the blood and their excretion in urine.
3. Removal of foreign chemicals from the blood and their excretion in urine.
4. Secretion of hormones:
   - Erythropoietin, which controls erythrocyte production.
   - Renin which controls formation of angiotensin. Angiotensin influences the blood pressure and sodium balance.
   - 1, 25-dihydroxyvitamin D_3 which influences calcium balance.
5. Help in maintenance of pH of body fluids.

Name the important metabolic waste products excreted by kidneys.

Metabolic waste products excreted by kidneys are:

- Urea from protein.
- Uric acid from nucleic acid.
- Creatinine from muscle creatine.
- End products of haemoglobin breakdown.

STRUCTURE OF NEPHRON

What are nephrons? Name the different types.

Nephron is a structural and functional unit of the kidney. Each nephron is capable of forming urine. There are two types of nephrons:

   1. *Cortical nephrons.* Glomeruli are present near the surface of the kidneys. These nephrons constitute about 86% of total nephrons.
   2. *Juxtamedullary nephrons.* Glomeruli lie at the junction of cortex and medulla of the kidney. These constitute 14% of the nephrons.

What is the main function of cortical nephrons?

The main function of cortical nephrons is absorption of sodium.

What is the main function of juxtamedullary nephron?

The main role of juxtamedullary nephron is to increase concentration of medullary interstitial fluid.

What is the total number of nephrons?

Two kidneys together have two million nephrons.

Describe the parts of nephron.

Nephron consists of two major parts:

- Glomerulus.
- A long renal tubule (Fig. 5.1).
   1. *Glomerulus.* It is made up of tuft of capillaries which connect afferent arteriole with an efferent arteriole. Capillaries have single layer of endothelial cells attached to a basement membrane.

   Bowman's capsule encloses the glomerulus and is formed of two layers: inner layer which covers the glomerular capillaries is called visceral layer, and the outer layer is called parietal layer. Space between visceral and parietal layers is continued as the lumen of the tubular portion.
   2. *Renal tubule.* It is mainly formed of three parts:
      (a) Proximal convoluted tubule.
      (b) Loop of Henle consisting of:
         - Thin segment walls of descending limb and lower end of ascending limb are very thin. Therefore, they are termed thin segment.
         - Hair pin bend.
         - Thick ascending limb or segment.
      (c) Distal convoluted tubules. They open into initial arched collecting ducts called cortical collecting ducts present in renal cortex. Seven to ten such ducts form straight collecting duct which passes into medulla, thus forming medullary collecting ducts. In the inner zone of medulla

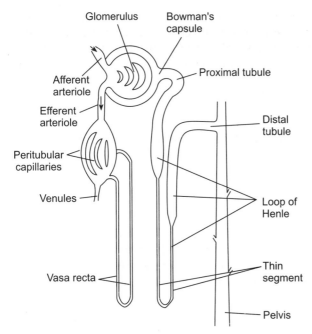

FIGURE 5.1 The functional nephron.

they form papillary ducts or ducts of Bellini. These open into papilla of minor calyces. Three or four minor calyces unite to form one major calyx. The major calyces open into pelvis of ureter. The pelvis is an expanded portion present in renal sinus and it continues as ureter.

Describe the glomerular membrane and its permeability.

Membrane of glomerular capillaries is known as glomerular membrane. It consists of 3 major layers (Fig. 5.2):

- Endothelial layer of the capillary itself.
- A basement membrane.
- A layer of epithelial surface present on the outer surface of the glomerular capillaries.

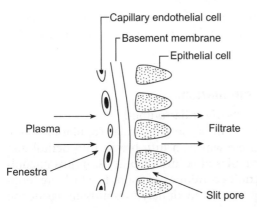

FIGURE 5.2 Functional structure of the glomerular membrane.

Glomerular membrane permeability is very high. Substances with a molecular weight of 5200 and 100% dissolved substances are filtered as easily as water but in case of protein of molecular weight of 69,000, only 0.5% of protein molecules filter (e.g. albumin is the smallest plasma protein with a molecular weight of 69,000 daltons). Glomerular membrane is almost impermeable to plasma proteins.

What are the reasons for high degree of molecular selectivity by glomerular membrane?

There are two reasons for high degree of molecular selectivity:

1. Pores of membrane are large enough to allow molecules of about 8 nanometre to pass through.
2. Basement membrane portions of glomerular pores are lined by proteoglycans which have a very strong negative electrical charge. Plasma proteins also have strong negative electrical charges, therefore they are repelled (though albumin has molecular size of 6 nanometre, it is usually not allowed to pass).

What is Bowman's space?

Bowman's capsule is a balloon-like capsule in which glomerular capillary tuft protrudes. The part of Bowman's capsule in contact with glomerular capillaries is pushed inwards but does not make contact with opposite side of the capsule. Accordingly a fluid-filled space, Bowman's space, is formed within the capsule. Blood of capillary and fluid of Bowman's space are separated by the glomerular membrane. From the Bowman's capsule, tubule of the nephron extends, the lumen of which is continuous with the Bowman's space.

BLOOD FLOW TO KIDNEYS

What is the rate of blood flowing to kidneys?

Rate of blood flow to kidneys is 1200 ml/min. This is quite high as compared to their size. It constitutes about 21% of the total cardiac output and can vary from 12 to 30%.

State the peculiarities of renal circulation.

1. Very high blood supply, about 21% of cardiac output.
2. Two sets of capillaries. One of them is the glomerular capillaries. These combine to form efferent arteriole which in turn breaks into peritubular capillary network around the tubules of cortical nephrons. In juxtamedullary nephrons, the efferent arterioles continue as vasa recta which are loop-shaped vessels. These loops dip into the medullary pyramids alongside the loops of Henle.

3. Glomerular capillary bed is a high pressure bed (i.e. hydrostatic pressure of blood in capillaries is high) because efferent arteriole is of a smaller diameter than afferent arteriole which offers considerable resistance to blood flow.
4. Peritubular capillary bed is a low pressure bed.
5. Only 1 to 2% of blood flows through vasa recta. The flow is very sluggish.
6. Renal blood flow shows remarkable constancy in face of blood pressure changes due to autoregulation.

What is the effect of sympathetic stimulation on renal blood flow?

Mild to moderate stimulation of sympathetic nerves usually has mild effects on renal blood flow because of autoregulatory mechanisms. But strong acute stimulation of sympathetic nerves constricts renal arterioles (both afferent and efferent) so greatly that renal blood flow greatly decreases (even to 10 to 30% of normal) temporarily. It recovers back to normal within 20 to 30 minutes.

What is autoregulation of renal blood flow?

There are local feedback control mechanisms in kidneys which keep the renal blood flow constant. This is called autoregulation of renal blood flow.

Which mechanism is important in regulation of renal blood flow?

Afferent arteriolar vasodilatation is the important mechanism for regulation of renal blood flow which is as follows:

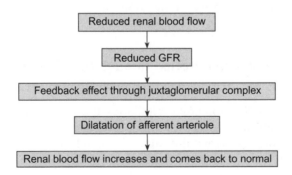

Describe the myogenic and cell separation theories for autoregulation of renal blood flow.

Autoregulation of renal blood flow is not due to influence of renal nerves because it persists even after denervation of kidney. Mainly cortical blood flow is autoregulated. The mechanism of autoregulation is explained by the following theories:

1. *Myogenic theory.* When there is a rise in perfusion pressure, there is a stretch on afferent arterioles, which results in contraction of smooth muscles of arterioles.

This reduction in calibre increases resistance to blood flow and the flow is reduced (comes back to normal).

2. *Cell separation theory.* It is claimed that with increase in perfusion pressure, the viscosity of blood in cortical region, mostly in the distal parts of interlobular arteries, is greatly increased due to higher haematocrit value. In a large blood vessel, erythrocytes remain in the axis and smaller branches get supply of blood devoid of erythrocytes and they are mainly perfused with cell free plasma. This is termed plasma skimming or cell separation. In kidneys, with increase in perfusion pressure, resistance and viscosity in interlobular arteries are increased greatly due to greater accumulation of red blood cells. This leads to decreased rate of blood flow (comes back to normal). Thus constancy of blood flow is maintained.

FORMATION OF URINE

Name the basic processes in urine formation.

Urine is formed by three basic processes:

1. Glomerular filtration.
2. Tubular absorption.
3. Tubular secretion.

GLOMERULAR FILTRATION

What is the function of glomerular capillaries?

Glomerular capillary bed is a high pressure bed and therefore does the function of filtration of fluid from plasma in the same way as the fluid filters at the arterial end of capillary.

Explain the dynamics of filtration through the glomerular membrane.

The forces which cause filtration of fluid through glomerular capillary are:

- Pressure inside the glomerular capillaries. It is 60 mmHg.
- Colloid osmotic pressure of the proteins in the Bowman's capsule. Very little protein is actually filtered. Therefore, this factor is not very significant.

The forces which oppose filtration are:

(a) Colloid osmotic pressure of plasma proteins. It varies from 28 to 36 mmHg as blood passes through capillaries (proteins get concentrated in blood as part of fluid from the blood is filtered), so average colloid osmotic pressure is about 32 mmHg.

(b) Hydrostatic pressure in the fluid of Bowman's capsule. It is about 18 mmHg. Normal filtration pressure therefore is equal to glomerular pressure minus sum of colloid osmotic pressure of blood in glomerular capillaries and capsular pressure which is equal to $60 - (32 + 18)$ mmHg = 10 mmHg.

Filtration pressure (10 mmHg) is the net pressure forcing fluid through the glomerular membrane.

What is the composition of glomerular filtrate?

Glomerular filtrate has almost the same composition as that of plasma except that it has no significant amount of proteins.

What is the normal glomerular filtration rate (GFR)?

In a normal person, quantity of glomerular filtrate formed each minute by all the nephrons of both the kidneys is 125 ml. Total quantity of glomerular filtrate formed per day is equal to 180 litres.

What is filtration fraction?

Filtration fraction is the fraction of renal plasma flow that becomes glomerular filtrate. Normal plasma flow to both the kidneys is 650 ml/min and rate of glomerular filtration is 125 ml/minute. So an average filtration fraction is approximately 1/5th or 19%.

What is filtration coefficient?

Filtration coefficient is glomerular filtration rate of both the kidneys per millimetre of mercury of filtration pressure. Normal filtration coefficient is therefore 12.5 ml/min/mmHg of filtration pressure (125 ml/10 mm where 125 ml/min is glomerular filtration rate and 10 mmHg is net filtration pressure).

It is termed K_1.

Enumerate the factors affecting glomerular filtration rate.

Glomerular filtration rate is determined by net filtration pressure and filtration coefficient K_1.

$$GFR = K_1 \times \text{net filtration pressure}$$

Various factors affect GFR in the following way:

1. *Filtration coefficient (K_1).* Increased K_1 raises GFR and decreased K_1 reduces GFR. However, changes in K_1 do not provide primary mechanism for normal day-to- day regulation of GFR. However, in some diseases K_1 is lowered due to:

(a) *Reduction in number of functioning capillaries.* This reduces the surface area for filtration which in turn reduces GFR.

(b) *Increase in thickness of capillary membrane.* In some diseases there is increase in thickness of capillary membrane and therefore GFR is reduced.

(c) *Permeability of capillary membrane.* In abnormal conditions like hypoxia, presence of toxic agents increases the permeability of renal capillary membrane. In such conditions GFR is increased because plasma proteins are also filtered to a variable degree. This causes an increase in colloid osmotic pressure of Bowman's capsular fluid (normally this is zero because proteins are not filtered) which in turn increases GFR.

2. *Hydrostatic pressure in Bowman's capsular fluid.* This pressure opposes filtration and therefore GFR is inversely related to it. Changes in this pressure normally do not serve as a primary mechanism for regulating GFR.

In certain pathological conditions associated with obstruction of urinary tract (e.g. presence of stones lodging and obstructing the tract), Bowman's capsular hydrostatic pressure increases markedly, causing serious reduction in GFR.

3. *Glomerular capillary hydrostatic pressure.* GFR is directly proportional to this pressure. Normally it is 60 mmHg. Changes in this pressure serve as a primary means for physiological regulation of GFR. Glomerular capillary hydrostatic pressure mainly depends on the following:

(a) *Arterial pressure.* Increased arterial pressure tends to raise glomerular capillary hydrostatic pressure and hence tends to raise GFR. Decreased arterial pressure has the opposite effect. However, this effect on GFR is buffered by autoregulatory mechanisms of GFR. Therefore, variation in arterial blood pressure from 60 mmHg to 180 mmHg (normal pressure is 100 mmHg) does not cause significant variation in glomerular capillary hydrostatic pressure. Thus GFR remains almost constant until arterial pressure decreases below 60 mmHg or rises above 180 mmHg.

(b) *Renal blood flow.* This is the most important factor determining GFR. GFR is directly proportional to renal blood flow. Increase in renal blood flow tends to increase glomerular capillary hydrostatic pressure and hence GFR and vice versa. However, renal blood is controlled by autoregulatory mechanisms.

(c) *Afferent arteriolar resistance.* Constriction of afferent arterioles reduces glomerular capillary hydrostatic pressure and therefore reduces GFR. Dilation of afferent arterioles increases GFR.

(d) *Efferent arteriolar resistance.* Efferent arteriolar constriction has a biphasic effect. When constriction is moderate, there is an increase in resistance to outflow from the glomerular capillaries. This raises glomerular hydrostatic pressure and increases GFR moderately (as long as efferent resistance does not reduce renal blood flow). If constriction of efferent arterioles is severe, there is stagnation of blood in glomerular capillaries causing large amount of protein free plasma to be filtered (increase in filtration fraction). This results into greater rise in colloid osmotic pressure of blood in glomerular capillaries which opposes filtration and decreases GFR.

4. *Glomerular capillary colloid osmotic pressure.* GFR is inversely proportional to colloid osmotic pressure exerted by proteins of blood. When plasma protein level is increased or there is haemoconcentration, colloid osmotic pressure rises and this decreases GFR. During hypoproteinaemia colloidal osmotic pressure is less and therefore GFR is increased.

Colloid osmotic pressure in renal capillaries also depends on filtration fraction. Normally, about one-fifth of plasma is filtered into Bowman's capsule. This causes concentration of plasma proteins (as they are not filtered) in blood to rise. If normal colloid osmotic pressure is 28 mmHg in arterial blood, by the time blood reaches efferent arteriole it becomes 36 mmHg (average is 32 mmHg). If more amount of protein free plasma is filtered (increase in filtration fraction), it causes greater concentration of plasma proteins which in turn increases colloid osmotic pressure and decreases GFR.

5. *Sympathetic stimulation.* Sympathetic nerves supply both afferent and efferent arterioles. Sympathetic stimulation causes constriction of both these arterioles. Mild to moderate sympathetic stimulation has no significant effect on renal blood flow and GFR because of their autoregulatory mechanisms.

Strong sympathetic stimulation causes severe constriction of blood vessels. The effect is more on efferent arterioles than on afferent arterioles and this causes reduction in GFR.

What do you mean by autoregulation of GFR?

There are local feedback control mechanisms in the kidneys to keep glomerular filtration rate at constant level. This is called autoregulation of GFR.

Why glomerular filtration rate should be autoregulated?

A small change in glomerular filtration rate has great effect on urinary output and therefore on loss of solutes and water, e.g. with small decrease in GFR, tubular fluid will pass through the tubules so slowly that essentially all would be absorbed and kidneys will fail to excrete the waste products (solutes and water).

What is juxtaglomerular complex (juxtaglomerular apparatus)?

Juxtaglomerular complex (juxta = near) is a specialized organ situated near the glomerulus of nephron, hence the name juxtaglomerular apparatus (Fig. 5.3). It consists of the following:

1. *Macula densa cells.* Initial part of distal tubule passes in the angle between afferent and efferent arterioles of the glomerulus. Epithelial cells of this part of distal tubule are specialized and termed macula densa cells. They are not well adapted for reabsorption and do not show the signs of secretory activity. But

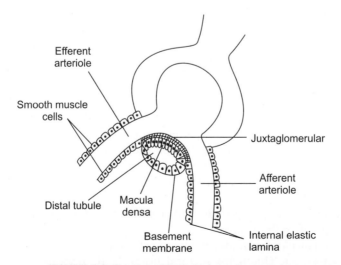

FIGURE 5.3 Structure of the juxtaglomerular apparatus.

characteristically they have their Golgi apparatus directed towards the arterioles, suggesting that these cells may be secreting a substance toward the arterioles.

2. *Juxtaglomerular cells.* Modified muscle cells in the walls of afferent and efferent arterioles are termed juxtaglomerular cells. They have well developed Golgi apparatus and endoplasmic reticulum, abundant mitochondria and ribosomes. They contain secretory granules and therefore also called granular cells. The granulation increases when there is sustained hypotension in afferent arteriole, e.g. in sodium deficiency. The granules contain renin.

Describe the functions of juxtaglomerular complex.

Juxtaglomerular cells secrete two hormones, viz. renin and erythropoietin.

1. *Secretion and functions of renin.* Juxtaglomerular cells of the apparatus secrete renin into the blood:

- When blood pressure is decreased.
- When extracellular fluid volume (ECF) is reduced.
- When sympathetic activity is increased.

Renin is a glycoprotein. It acts on alpha$_2$-globulin called angiotensinogen of blood and converts it into angiotensin I. Angiotensin I is converted to angiotensin II by an angiotensin converting enzyme in the lungs. The overall effect of renin secretion is as follows:

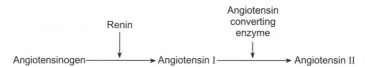

Angiotensin II has the following actions:

- It causes constriction of systemic arterioles causing elevation of blood pressure.
- It stimulates adrenal cortex to secrete aldosterone which in turn increases absorption of sodium and water by distal nephrons of kidney.
- It helps to maintain GFR and renal blood flow.

Local renin release is stimulated by decrease in the delivery of sodium chloride in the distal tubule near macula densa region. Renin is released into interstitial tissue of juxtaglomerular complex. Thus renin affects tubuloglomerular feedback and thereby plays an important role in autoregulation of GFR and renal blood flow.

2. *Secretion and function of erythropoietin.* Erythropoietin is released from kidney and its rate of synthesis depends on the level of O_2 in blood. The mechanisms of sensing O_2 deficit and production of erythropoietin appear to be located in same cells. The exact site of erythropoietin is not known but it may be a juxtaglomerular apparatus.

Erythropoietin is a glycoprotein and it stimulates the bone marrow and increases the rate of erythropoiesis.

Function of macula densa: Macula densa acts as a sensor of a tubular fluid flow and/or composition. This helps in local homeostatic response, which regulate renin secretion as well as helps in autoregulation of GFR.

Describe the afferent arteriolar vasodilation feedback mechanism for regulating GFR.

The mechanism is as follows:

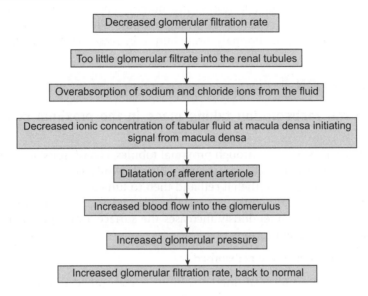

Thus, this negative feedback mechanism keeps GFR steady. It also autoregulates renal blood flow.

Describe the efferent arteriolar vasoconstrictor mechanism for regulating GFR.

The mechanism is as follows:

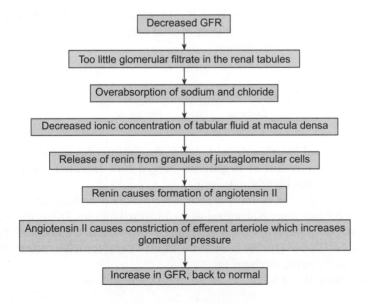

What is the effect of arterial pressure on urinary output?

There is almost no change in GFR when arterial pressure varies in the range of 75 to 160 mmHg (normal mean arterial pressure is 100 mmHg). When arterial pressure falls below 75 mmHg, it decreases urine output. A pressure of about 50 mmHg causes almost complete cessation of urinary output. When arterial pressure rises above 200 mmHg (double normal), urine output increases about sevenfold.

REABSORPTION

Describe the reabsorption taking place in the proximal convoluted tubule.

While the filtrate is passing through proximal tubules, certain substances are reabsorbed (from lumen to cell and then to blood) while certain substances are secreted (from blood to epithelial cell and then to lumen).

Proximal tubular epithelium is specially adapted for reabsorption. It has a brush border which tremendously increases the surface area. Epithelial cells are also loaded with protein carriers.

Following substances are reabsorbed:

1. *Sodium.* About 65% of filtered sodium is reabsorbed in the proximal tubules. There are two mechanisms for reabsorption.

(a) *Primary active transport or uniport mechanism.* This is the active transport of sodium through basolateral surface of epithelial cell by Na^+-K^+ pump. This causes lowering of Na^+ concentration in the epithelial cell and allows diffusion of sodium from lumen into the cell through luminal surface.

This mechanism also helps in absorption of glucose and amino acids along with sodium in Na^+-co-transport mechanisms. It also causes osmotic absorption of water.

(b) *Antiport mechanism.* This is sodium counter-transport mechanism. When sodium ion diffuses from lumen to epithelial cell, some other ion (H^+ or K^+) is transported from cell to the lumen.

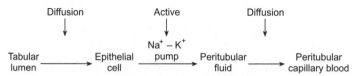

2. *Chloride and bicarbonate ions.* Active absorption of positively charged ions causes passive absorption of negatively charged ions (anions), mainly chloride and to a lesser extent bicarbonate ions.

3. *Water.* Absorption of water is secondary, mainly to sodium (osmotic absorption). About 65% of water is absorbed in the proximal tubules. This is termed obligatory water reabsorption as it cannot be changed according to the needs of the body.

4. *Glucose.* Filtered glucose is almost completely reabsorbed in proximal tubules by sodium co-transport mechanism.

5. *Phosphate.* It is actively absorbed in proximal tubules.

6. *Proteins.* Very small amount of protein is filtered, and is completely absorbed by proximal tubules by pinocytosis.

7. *Potassium.* Almost all potassium filtered is reabsorbed by proximal tubules (potassium excreted in urine comes from secretion in the distal segment of nephron).

8. *Sulphates, urates and lactates.* These are reabsorbed by active transport mechanisms.

9. *Uric acid and urea.* Uric acid is mainly reabsorbed in proximal tubules; only 10% of filtered uric acid is excreted.

Large amount of filtered load of urea is reabsorbed in proximal tubules, by passive absorption. When water is reabsorbed, there is increase in concentration of urea in the tubular fluid. This creates a high concentration gradient for urea between tubular fluid and peritubular fluid. This causes reabsorption of urea. Thus urea reabsorption depends on water and salt reabsorption. Greater is the salt and water reabsorption, greater is the gradient produced and greater is the reabsorption of urea.

Urea reabsorption also depends on the rate at which tubular fluid flows in the tubule.

Describe the reabsorption in distal tubules and collecting ducts.

Distal tubule is divided into early and late part. First half of the tubule (like thick ascending limb of loop of Henle) reabsorbs most of the ions (Na^+, K^+, Cl^-, etc.), but is virtually impermeable to water and urea. It is referred to as diluting segment as it dilutes the tubular fluid.

Second half of the distal tubules and cortical collecting ducts have similar functional characteristics. They have two distinct types of cells—principal cells and intercalated cells.

Principal cells cause reabsorption of sodium and secretion of potassium. This function depends on Na^+-K^+ pump activity in the basolateral membrane of the cell. Pump maintains intracellular sodium concentration low, which favours diffusion of sodium from lumen into the cell. Potassium enters the cell due to activity of Na^+-K^+ pump in the basolateral membrane of the cell. This increases concentration of potassium in the cell leading to diffusion of potassium down its concentration gradient from cell to lumen through luminal surface (potassium is thus secreted). The process of sodium reabsorption and potassium secretion is controlled by hormone aldosterone.

Intercalated cells contain enzyme carbonic anhydrase. This facilitates formation of carbonic acid from CO_2 and water. Carbonic acid dissociates into H^+ and ions. Hydrogen ions are secreted from cell into the tubular lumen by hydrogen-ATPase transport mechanism. For each hydrogen ion secreted into the lumen, one bicarbonate ion is reabsorbed through basolateral membrane of the cell. Hydrogen secretion which occurs by primary active transport mechanism causes secretion of hydrogen ion against a large concentration gradient (1000:1) in contrast to a small gradient (four to tenfold) for secretion of hydrogen ions by secondary active transport mechanism in proximal tubules. This greatly helps in maintenance of pH of body fluids. Intercalated cells also secrete potassium ions, mechanism of which is not yet understood.

Late distal tubules and cortical collecting ducts are impermeable to urea and their permeability to water depends on concentration of antidiuretic hormone (ADH). In the absence of ADH they are impermeable to water.

Medullary collecting ducts are permeable to urea. Urea is therefore reabsorbed which helps to raise osmolarity of medullary interstitium. Permeability of these tubules to water is controlled by hormone ADH. These ducts secrete hydrogen ions against a large concentration gradient as in case of cortical collecting ducts. This is important in regulation of pH of body fluids.

Name the substances which are reabsorbed in loop of Henle.

In the descending limb of loop of Henle, there is passive reabsorption of water (because of hypertonic interstitial fluid). It is accompanied by diffusion of sodium ions from interstitial fluid into tubular lumen.

Ascending limb of loop of Henle is impermeable to water and therefore fluid leaving ascending limb is hypotonic relative to plasma.

In thick part of ascending limb, sodium ions are actively absorbed along with chloride and K^+ ions. In thin part of ascending limb, movement of the salt is passive and it occurs passively down a concentration gradient.

Urea may be passively absorbed in the loop.

What is the glomerulotubular balance in proximal tubule?

Under normal condition, almost a constant percentage of sodium and fluid (about 65%) is reabsorbed while the filtrate is passing through proximal tubule regardless of the rate of glomerular filtration. This is called glomerulotubular balance, e.g. when GFR is 100 ml/min, tubular reabsorption is 65 ml/min. If GFR increases to 200 ml/min, tubular reabsorption also increases to 130 ml/min, thus maintaining proportional balance (65%).

What is the importance of glomerulotubular balance?

Glomerulotubular balance prevents overloading of more distal tubular segments when the GFR increases.

Glomerulotubular balance therefore acts as a second line of defence to buffer the effects of spontaneous increase in GFR on urine output.

How much is the normal rate of reabsorption in renal tubules?

Normal rate of reabsorption in peritubular capillaries is 124 ml/min. GFR, i.e. amount of filtrate entering the tubule is 125 ml/min. Volume of urine formed is therefore approximately 1 ml/min.

How much is the net reabsorptive force in peritubular capillaries?

Net reabsorptive force is calculated by deducting total force opposing reabsorption from total force favouring reabsorption.

FORCES WHICH FAVOUR REABSORPTION ARE:

- Hydrostatic pressure in renal interstitium outside the capillaries. It is 6 mmHg.
- Colloid osmotic pressure of peritubular capillary blood. It is 32 mmHg.

Thus total force favouring reabsorption is 6 + 32 = 38 mmHg.

FORCES WHICH OPPOSE REABSORPTION ARE:

- Peritubular capillary blood hydrostatic pressure. It is 13 mmHg.
- Colloid osmotic pressure (due to proteins) in renal interstitium. It is 15 mmHg.
- Total force opposing reabsorption is therefore 13 + 15 = 28 mmHg.
- Net reabsorptive force is 38 mmHg − 28 mmHg, i.e. 10 mmHg.

How much is the filtration coefficient in peritubular capillaries?

Filtration coefficient in peritubular capillaries is large due to high hydraulic conductivity and large surface area of capillaries.

As net reabsorption rate is 124 ml/min and net reabsorption pressure is 10 mmHg, filtration coefficient (K_f) is 12.4 ml/min/mmHg.

Enumerate the factors which increase reabsorption in peritubular capillaries.

The rate of reabsorption in the peritubular capillaries increases due to:

1. *Increase in colloid osmotic pressure.* Increase in colloid osmotic pressure in peritubular capillary blood is due to:
   - *Increase in plasma protein concentration of systemic blood.* This causes increase in colloid osmotic pressure in peritubular capillary blood.
   - *Increase in filtration fraction.* As filtration fraction increases, protein concentration of plasma remaining behind is increased as plasma proteins get concentrated (because of filtration of protein free plasma). Thus increasing filtration fraction causes increase in rate of reabsorption in peritubular capillaries.

2. *Reduction in peritubular capillary hydrostatic pressure.* Increase in resistance of either afferent or efferent arterioles reduces peritubular capillary hydrostatic pressure and tends to increase rate of reabsorption.

3. *Increase in peritubular capillary filtration coefficient (K_f).* K_f is a measure of capillary surface area, therefore increase in K_f increases the rate of reabsorption. But in most physiological conditions K_f remains constant.

Enumerate the factors which decrease the rate of reabsorption in peritubular capillaries.

1. *Increase in hydrostatic pressure in peritubular capillaries.* Increase in hydrostatic pressure decreases rate of reabsorption.

Increase in arterial blood pressure tends to raise peritubular capillary hydrostatic pressure. But this effect is buffered to some extent by autoregulatory mechanisms that maintain relatively constant renal blood flow as well as relatively constant hydrostatic pressure in renal vessels.

2. *Decrease in peritubular capillary K_f.* K_f is a measure of capillary surface area, therefore decrease in K_f (filtration coefficient) decreases the rate of reabsorption. But in most physiological conditions K_f remains constant.

SECRETION

Name the substances which are secreted by renal tubules.

Potassium ions are secreted in the distal tubule and collecting ducts. Potassium and hydrogen are both exchanged for sodium which is reabsorbed. Potassium secretion is modified by plasma level of aldosterone.

Hydrogen ions are secreted throughout the renal tubule but most significantly in the distal tubule.

Certain foreign substances and drugs are secreted. Para-aminohippuric acid (PAHA-foreign substance) is secreted actively by proximal tubular cells. Diodone and penicillin are also similarly secreted. Tubular secretion of foreign substances is important in clearing of the plasma of a substance in one passage through the kidney. Tubular secretion of drugs plays important role in maintaining the blood level of the drug and hence the therapeutic efficiency.

TUBULAR LOAD, TUBULAR MAXIMUM

What is tubular load?

Tubular load is the amount of substance that filters through the glomerular membrane into tubules each minute.

What is tubular maximum (T_{max}) of any substance?

For substances that are actively reabsorbed or secreted by renal tubules there is a maximum rate (limit) at which they can be transported which is referred to as 'tubular maximum' (T_{max}) for reabsorption or secretion, respectively. Limiting factor is saturation of carrier protein as tubular load increases.

T_{MAX} FOR SOME ACTIVELY REABSORBED SUBSTANCES

Substance	T_{max} value
Glucose	320 mg/min
Phosphate	0.1 mg/min
Sulphate	0.06 mg/min
Amino acids	1.5 mg/min
Plasma protein	30 mg/min

T_{MAX} FOR SOME ACTIVELY SECRETED SUBSTANCES

Substance	T_{max} value
Creatinine	16 mg/min
Para-aminohippuric acid	80 mg/min

Substances which are passively transported do not exhibit T_{max}.

What is renal threshold for a substance?

Every substance that has a transport maximum also has a specific (threshold) concentration in the plasma below which none of it appears in the urine and above which progressively larger quantities appear in urine. This concentration is

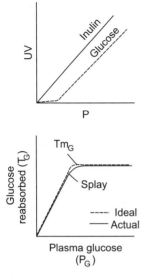

FIGURE 5.4 Relation between plasma glucose level (P_G) and amount of glucose reabsorbed (T_G) indicating splay.

called renal threshold, e.g. renal threshold for glucose is 180 mg/100 ml.

What is tubular maximum for glucose? What is splay?

Tubular maximum for glucose is 320 mg/min and is termed TmG.

Normally, measurable glucose does not appear in urine because essentially all filtered glucose is reabsorbed by proximal tubules by Na^+-co-transport mechanism. Filtered or tubular load of glucose is calculated by multiplying GFR by plasma level.

$$\text{Tubular load of glucose/min} = \text{GFR} \times \text{Plasma concentration of glucose}$$

When tubular load exceeds 320 mg/min then only ideally glucose should appear in urine, but it is observed that at tubular load of 220 mg/min (blood level of 180 mg/100 ml) glucose begins to appear in urine though T_{max} level is not yet reached. If curve of plasma glucose and glucose reabsorbed is plotted, actual curve is rounded and deviates from the ideal curve. This deviation is termed splay (Fig. 5.4). Splay occurs because all nephrons of kidneys do not have the same TmG, therefore some nephrons may excrete glucose before others have reached their T_{max}. Overall transport maximum for kidneys is reached when all nephrons have reached their maximal capacity to reabsorb glucose.

What are threshold substances? Give a few examples.

Substances which are absorbed almost totally by renal tubules till the plasma concentration is below the threshold and are excreted progressively in larger quantities in urine as plasma concentration increases above the threshold are called threshold substances, e.g. glucose, phosphate, sulphate, amino acids.

What are non-threshold substances? Give a few examples.

Substances which are excreted in urine irrespective of their concentrations in plasma are called non-threshold substances. They do not possess threshold level in plasma, e.g. urea, uric acid, sodium (in proximal tubules).

PLASMA CLEARANCE

What is plasma clearance of any substance?

Plasma clearance of any substance is the volume of plasma which contains the same amount of the substance which is excreted in urine/minute, e.g. if concentration of a substance in plasma is 0.1 g/100 ml and if 0.05 g of that substance is excreted in urine/minute, plasma clearance value is 50 ml (because 0.05 g which is the amount excreted per minute is present in 50 ml of plasma).

How is plasma clearance calculated?

Plasma clearance is calculated by the following formula:

$$\text{Plasma clearance (ml/min)} = \frac{\text{Urine flow (ml/min)} \times \text{Concentration in urine}}{\text{Concentration in plasma}}$$

What is inulin clearance used for? Why?

Inulin clearance gives the value equivalent to GFR and is therefore used for measuring GFR. Inulin is easily filtered and is neither reabsorbed nor secreted by renal tubules; therefore, its rate of filtration is equal to rate of excretion. Glomerular filtrate has virtually the same concentration of inulin as does plasma and all glomerular filtrate formed is cleared of inulin. Thus plasma clearance per minute of inulin is equal to glomerular filtration rate.

How do you measure inulin clearance?

Inulin is a soluble polysaccharide with a molecular weight of 5200 daltons. It is non-toxic and physiologically inert and therefore safe for use.

To determine glomerular filtration rate in man a large initial dose of inulin is injected intravenously. This is followed by a constant inulin infusion at a rate which compensates loss in urine. A reasonably constant plasma level is then maintained. The inulin concentration in the plasma of venous blood (P) and urinary concentration (U), and volume of urine excreted per minute (V) are determined. Inulin clearance is calculated by the formula:

$$\text{Inulin clearance} = \frac{UV}{P}$$

What is creatinine clearance?

Creatinine clearance is also used to measure GFR. Since creatinine is endogenous (present in body fluids) and its plasma concentration is steady throughout the day, it is easier to measure (no intravenous administration is required as in the case of inulin clearance test). Simply determination of plasma creatinine concentration and its amount in one minute urinary output are sufficient. In clinical practice, creatinine clearance test is therefore used for measuring GFR, though its value is sometimes lesser and sometimes greater than GFR because of reabsorption and secretion of creatinine by renal tubules, respectively.

Clearance of which substance is used to find out the plasma flow to kidneys?

Para-aminohippuric acid (PAH) clearance is a measure of plasma flow to the kidneys. After glomerular filtrate is formed, remaining PAH in the plasma is secreted into the renal tubules from the peritubular capillaries by proximal tubular epithelium. Almost all PAH that comes to the kidney is excreted (only one-tenth of the original PAH remains in the plasma by the time blood leaves the kidneys). Therefore, whatever plasma flows to the kidneys per minute is completely getting cleared of PAH, and thus PAH clearance is equivalent to plasma flow to kidney. However, as some amount of PAH still remains in the blood when it leaves the kidneys, PAH clearance is 91% and not 100%. Therefore, PAH clearance value is divided by 0.91 to get total plasma flow to the kidney.

How is the renal blood flow calculated?

Total plasma flow to the kidneys is calculated by dividing PAH clearance by 0.91. Then haematocrit is determined. If it is 45 then total blood flow is equal to:

$$\text{Plasma flow} \times \frac{100}{100} \text{ per minute}$$

Describe urea clearance test.

Two one-hourly samples of urine are collected. Blood is collected at the end of first hour, its urea content is determined. Urine samples are measured and their urea contents are determined separately. Minute output of urine is calculated.

CALCULATION OF UREA CLEARANCE

(a) *Maximum urea clearance*. If minute output of urine is 2 ml or more, the maximum urea clearance (C_m) is calculated as:

$$\text{Urea clearance} = \frac{Uu \times V}{Pu}$$

where, Uu = Urea in mg/ml of urine,
        V = Volume of urine, ml/min and
        Pu = Urea in mg/ml of plasma.

In normal adults, value of urea clearance is relatively constant. Value of 75 ml is taken as 100% efficiency of kidneys. If value decreases to 50 ml, efficiency is:

$$100 \times \frac{50}{75} = 66.6\%$$

(b) *Standard urea clearance*. If the volume of urine output is less than 2 ml/min, standard urea clearance (C_s) is calculated as:

$$\text{Urea clearance} = \frac{Uu \times \sqrt{V}}{Pu}$$

Normal C_s is 40 to 65 ml (average 54 ml). Urea clearance value varies proportionately with its filtration rate.

FORMATION OF DILUTE OR CONCENTRATED URINE

What is the counter current multiplier mechanism? What is its purpose?

Counter current multiplier mechanism is in the loop of Henle (mainly of juxtamedullary nephrons). Its purpose is to create a very high osmotic pressure (hyperosmolarity) of the medullary interstitial fluid.

Explain the counter current multiplier mechanism.

The loops of Henle of juxtamedullary nephrons dip deep into the medulla. The mechanism depends on these typical anatomical arrangements of loop of Henle. Normal osmolarity of fluid entering the loop is 300 mOsm/L.

In medullary interstitial fluid, osmolarity increases to 1200 mOsm/L (or up to 1400 mOsm/L under the effect of ADH) in pelvic tip of medulla. Three different mechanisms are responsible for this (Fig. 5.5).

(a) Active transport of sodium ions out of thick portion of ascending limb of loop of Henle. $1Na^+$, $2Cl^-$ and $1K^+$ ions are co-transported actively from tubular lumen to medullary interstitial fluid. This movement of salt is not accompanied by water reabsorption (this part of the limb is impermeable to water). So the concentration of salt in the ascending limb decreases, but its concentration in the medullary interstitial fluid rises. In renal medulla all other tubular structures (except ascending limb) are in osmotic equilibrium. The descending limb therefore acquires the increased osmolality of the surrounding fluid. The effect is multiplied as new iso-osmolar filtrate arrives at the descending limb and forces the concentrated tubular contents towards the tip of loop of Henle (hairpin band).

(b) Smaller quantities of ions are also transported from collecting ducts to medullary interstitial fluid mainly by active transport of sodium followed by electrogenic passive absorption of chloride ions.

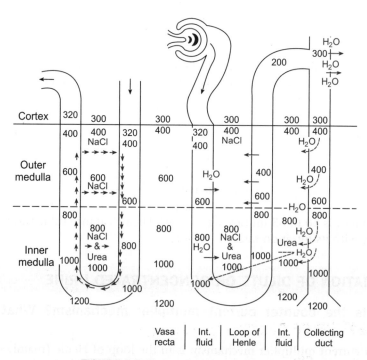

FIGURE 5.5 The counter current mechanism.

(c) When concentration of ADH is high in blood, there is further increase in osmolality of medullary interstitial fluid due to increased urea absorption by the following mechanisms:

- Increased permeability of collecting ducts to urea.
- Greatly increased permeability of collecting ducts for water. Increased water reabsorption from the collecting ducts greatly increases urea concentration inside the ducts, thereby increasing its diffusion from collecting ducts to medullary interstitial fluid.

What is counter current exchange mechanism? What is its purpose? How does it work?

Counter current exchange mechanism takes place in vasa recta. This mechanism is responsible for maintaining hyperosmolality of medullary interstitial fluid (removal of excess solute by blood is prevented).

Vasa recta are loop-shaped vessels paralleling loop of Henle. They also loop down from cortex to medulla and then back into the cortex of the kidney. The mechanism of counter current exchange works as follows:

(a) Inner medullary blood flow is very low (1 to 2% of total flow to kidney). Because flow is sluggish, removal of solutes is minimized.

(b) Vasa recta functions as counter current exchanger. In 'U'-shaped vasa recta, two arms lie in close proximity so that fluid and solutes exchange very rapidly between the two arms. Both are highly permeable to solutes. Because of rapid exchange of salts and fluid between ascending and descending arms of vasa recta, there is negligible washing out of solutes (e.g. when blood flows down in descending limb of vasa recta, sodium chloride and urea diffuse into the blood and water diffuses outward. When blood flows back in ascending limb, sodium chloride and urea diffuse back into the medullary interstitium and water diffuses into blood. Therefore, by the time blood finally leaves medulla, its osmolar concentration is only slightly greater than blood that initially enters vasa recta).

What is the effect of ADH on renal tubules?

Antidiuretic hormone increases the permeability of cortical collecting ducts, medullary collecting ducts and late distal tubules to water.

When is ADH secreted?

Antidiuretic hormone is secreted when osmolality of body fluid increases above the normal.

How is ADH secretion controlled?

Antidiuretic hormone secretion is controlled by two pathways:

1. *Osmoreceptor pathway.* There are two areas in hypothalamus, namely supraoptic nuclei and paraventricular nuclei which secrete ADH. ADH is transported

down the axons of neurons to their tips which terminate in posterior pituitary. There is another area called median preoptic nucleus along the anterolateral border of the third ventricle, AV 3V. In the vicinity of this area and supraoptic nucleus, neuronal cells are excited by minute increases in extracellular fluid osmolality and inhibited by decrease in extracellular fluid osmolality (they act as osmoreceptors). They send nerve signal to supraoptic nuclei to control ADH secretion.

2. *Cardiovascular reflexes.*
   - *Arterial baroreceptor reflex.* Fall in blood volume decreases blood pressure. This decrease in blood pressure through baroreceptor reflex causes increased secretion of ADH.
   - *Volume receptor reflex.* When there is decrease blood volume, volume receptors present in atria of heart and pulmonary artery are stimulated. Stimulation of volume receptors reflexly increases ADH secretion.

All the mechanisms described above not only cause ADH release but also stimulate the thirst centre.

What is the role of ADH in homeostasis?

Antidiuretic hormone controls and maintains osmolality and sodium concentration of the extracellular fluid. Increased sodium concentration causes increased osmolality of extracellular fluid. This excites the osmoreceptors causing release of ADH, which increases absorption of water in the renal tubules, thereby increasing the relative proportion of water in extracellular fluid and decreasing the proportion of solutes and thus bringing osmolality of extracellular fluid back to normal. Exactly reverse changes occur when there is decreased osmolality of extracellular fluid. Thus ADH controls extracellular fluid osmolality as well as sodium concentration.

How much is the concentration of urine?

Concentration of urine varies from 65 mOsm/L to 1400 mOsm/L, depending upon the concentration of ADH in blood at a given time.

What is the mechanism of formation of concentrated urine?

When there is increased osmolality of the extracellular fluid, there is excitation of osmoreceptors which causes release of ADH from posterior pituitary. This ADH increases permeability of late distal tubules, cortical and medullary collecting ducts for water causing increased conservation of water. Highest osmolality of tubular fluid or urine is equal to that of the medullary interstitial fluid. Thus concentrated urine is formed.

How and when is dilute urine formed?

When there is excess water in the body, i.e. when osmolality of extracellular fluid decreases, there is decreased ADH secretion. This makes late distal tubules, cortical and medullary collecting ducts almost impermeable to water but sodium chloride is still absorbed to a certain degree. Thus tubular fluid concentration decreases below that of plasma (it can be as low as 65 mOsm/L) and thus dilute urine is formed.

What is water diuresis?

When person drinks large quantity of water within 45 minutes, urine output increases (due to decreased ADH). This is known as water diuresis. It continues till osmolality of extracellular fluid returns back to normal.

REGULATION OF ELECTROLYTE BALANCE

How is the excretion of sodium by kidneys controlled?

Since sodium is easily filtered through glomerular membrane and is actively reabsorbed but not secreted, the amount of sodium excreted is given by:

Sodium excreted = Sodium filtered − Sodium reabsorbed.

Sodium excretion can be adjusted either by changing GFR or by changing sodium reabsorption.

1. *Control by changing GFR.* When total body sodium is decreased, it can be adjusted by changing GFR.

Increased total body sodium causes increased plasma volume and exactly opposite effects leading to increase in GFR to cause increased sodium and water loss.

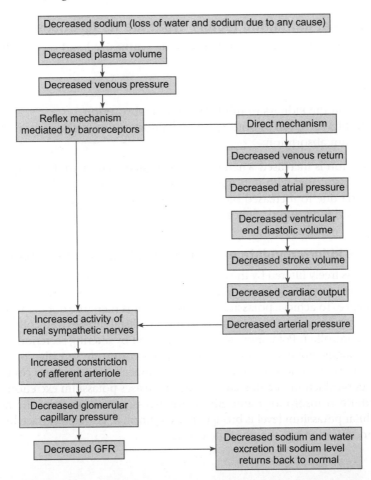

2. *Control by changing reabsorption.* Long-term regulation of sodium excretion is done by controlling sodium reabsorption. Aldosterone is the major factor determining tubular sodium reabsorption. It mainly stimulates sodium reabsorption in late distal tubules and collecting ducts. In absence of aldosterone, person excretes about 15 g of sodium, whereas excretion is almost zero when aldosterone is present in large quantities. Aldosterone secretion in turn is controlled by renin-angiotensin mechanism. Renin secreted by juxtaglomerular complex splits of angiotensin I from a large plasma protein which is then converted to angiotensin II by angiotensin converting enzyme present mostly in lungs. Renin secretion is controlled by:

(a) *Renal sympathetic nerves.* Reduction in body sodium and plasma volume lowers the blood pressure and via baroreceptors triggers increased sympathetic discharge which in turn stimulates renal sympathetic nerves leading to renin release.

(b) *Intrarenal baroreceptors.* Renin secreting cells themselves are pressure sensitive and function as intrarenal baroreceptors. They secrete more renin when low extracellular volume causes decreased renal arterial pressure.

(c) *Macula densa.* Senses the sodium chloride concentration of tubular fluid. Decreased salt concentration in tubular fluid increases renin secretion.

Thus renin-angiotensin mechanism regulates sodium balance and thereby plasma balance and hence also contributes to the control of blood pressure.

What is atrial natriuretic factor? What are its functions?

Atrial natriuretic factor is a peptide hormone synthesized and secreted by cells in the cardiac atria.

FUNCTIONS:

- Acts on the kidneys to inhibit sodium reabsorption.
- Inhibits secretion of both renin and aldosterone which results in decreased sodium absorption.

Its secretion is increased when there is increased sodium in the body. Increased sodium is associated with increased extracellular fluid volume. This causes distension of atria due to increased blood volume. Distension of atria is a stimulus for release of atrial natriuretic factor.

How does kidney regulate extracellular potassium ion concentration?

Potassium is freely filtered by the glomerular membrane. Usually, filtered potassium is reabsorbed (especially in proximal tubules) regardless of changes in body potassium balance. To achieve potassium homeostasis it is therefore not the reabsorption but the secretion of potassium mainly in the late distal tubules and collecting ducts which is controlled. Potassium secretion is altered by altering secretion of aldosterone. The aldosterone secreting cells of adrenal cortex are sensitive to potassium concentration of extracellular fluid. Increased extracellular potassium concentration stimulates production of aldosterone which increases potassium excretion (coupled with sodium reabsorption) and eliminates excess potassium from the body, and extracellular potassium level is brought back to normal. Lowered extracellular potassium concentration has the opposite effects.

How are calcium and phosphate excretions controlled by kidneys?

Calcium excretion. Calcium is filtered as well as reabsorbed by nephrons and therefore its rate of excretion can be calculated as follows:

Rate of excretion of calcium = Calcium filtered − Calcium reabsorbed.

In plasma, 50% of calcium is bound to plasma proteins and remaining 50% is ionized which therefore can be filtered by glomeruli. Normally 99% of filtered calcium is reabsorbed, only 1% is excreted. About 65% of calcium is reabsorbed in proximal tubules, 25 to 30% in the loop of Henle and about 4 to 9% in distal tubules and collecting ducts.

Excretion of calcium is adjusted to meet body's needs in the following ways:

(a) Primary controller of renal tubular calcium reabsorption is parathyroid hormone (PTH). Increased PTH levels increase reabsorption of calcium in the thick ascending limb of loop of Henle and distal tubules. This reduces calcium excretion. Reduction in PTH has the opposite effect.

(b) In the proximal tubule calcium reabsorption usually parallels sodium and water reabsorption. Therefore, when ECF volume increases (or BP rises), it leads to decreased sodium and water reabsorption as well as reduction in calcium reabsorption in proximal tubules. This increases excretion of calcium in urine.

(c) Plasma concentration of phosphate influences calcium excretion as follows: an increase in plasma phosphate stimulates secretion of PTH, which increases calcium reabsorption by renal tubules (loop of Henle and distal tubules) and decreases calcium excretion. Reduction in plasma phosphate concentration has the opposite effects.

Phosphate excretion. It is regulated as follows:

Phosphate is reabsorbed only in proximal tubules by active mechanism. This reabsorption is therefore T_{max} limited. T_{max} for phosphate is 0.1 mg per minute. When less than this amount is present in glomerular filtrate, all filtered phosphate is absorbed. When more than this amount is present in the filtrate, the excess phosphate is excreted.

Phosphate excretion is regulated by PTH as follows: PTH promotes bone reabsorption and hence pumps large amount of phosphate in ECF. PTH also decreases Tm of phosphate in renal tubules. Both these activities cause greater loss of phosphate in urine.

REGULATION OF pH OF BODY FLUIDS

Define acid and base.

Acid is a molecule or an ion that can function as a proton donor. Base is the molecule or an ion that can function as a proton acceptor.

What are strong and weak acids or bases?

Acid or base having strong tendency to dissociate into ions is called strong acid or strong base. Acid or base having weak tendency to dissociate into ions is called weak acid or weak base.

What is pH?

pH is negative log of H^+ ion concentration.

What is the normal pH of blood and of intracellular fluid?

Normal pH of arterial blood is 7.4 and that of venous blood and interstitial fluid is 7.35. pH of intracellular fluid is 7 (varies from 6 to 7.4).

Why should the pH of the body fluids be maintained?

(a) Slight changes in H^+ ion concentration causes marked alteration in the rates of chemical reactions in the cells.

(b) Acidosis depresses the neurons leading to coma, whereas alkalosis excites the neurons leading to convulsions. Alkalosis also causes tetany. Thus changes in pH can be lethal. pH of body fluids must be maintained.

Name the mechanisms which regulate pH.

The control systems in the body for regulating pH are:
- Buffer systems present in different body fluids.
- Respiratory mechanism causes changes in rate of CO_2 removal and brings H^+ ion concentration back to normal.
- Renal mechanism secreting acid or alkaline urine according to the need.

What is the importance of different control systems controlling pH of body fluids?

- Buffer system is quick to act within seconds.
- Respiratory system acts within 1 to 2 minutes to do additional acute adjustments.
- Renal system though slow (hours to days) is the most powerful of all the acid-base regulatory systems.

State the equation of Henderson–Hasselbalch.

$$pH = pK + \log \times \frac{HCO_3^-}{CO_2}$$

According to this equation, increase in HCO_3^- ion concentration causes pH to rise and increase in dissolved CO_2 causes pH to decrease.

What are the sources of hydrogen ion gain in the body?

H^+ ions are gained in the body as follows:
- Generation of hydrogen ions from CO_2.
- Production of acids during metabolism of proteins and other organic molecules.
- Gain of H^+ ions due to loss of bicarbonate ions in stool (as in diarrhoea) or in urine.

What are the ways in which H⁺ ions are lost from the body?

Loss of H^+ ions occurs due to:

- Loss of H^+ ions in vomitus when there is severe vomiting.
- Loss of H^+ ions in urine.

State the mechanism by which H⁺ ions are secreted by renal tubules.

H^+ ions are secreted by secondary active transport mechanism in proximal convoluted tubules and thick segment of ascending limb of the loop of Henle. From late distal tubule onwards, different parts of renal tubules secrete H^+ ion by primary active transport mechanism. It accounts normally for less than 5% of the total H^+ ions excreted, but it can concentrate H^+ ions to thousand-fold in contrast to four to tenfold concentration in proximal tubules (Figs 5.6a and 5.6b).

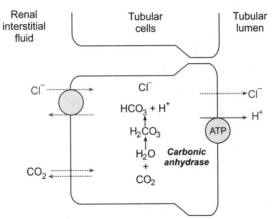

FIGURE 5.6 (a) Primary active secretion of hydrogen ions through the luminal membrane of the epithelial cells of the distal and collecting tubules.

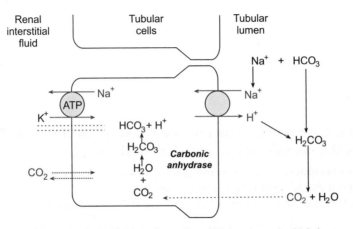

FIGURE 5.6 (b) Mechanism of secretion of H^+ ions in proximal tubules.

Describe the mechanism of secretion of H⁺ ions in proximal tubules.

H^+ ions are secreted from peritubular capillaries into the tubular lumen by secondary active transport mechanism (Na^+-H^+ counter-transport mechanism) as:

In renal tubular epithelial cell CO_2 reacts with water to form carbonic acid under the effect of carbonic anhydrase enzyme.

$$CO_2 + H_2O \rightarrow H_2CO_3 \rightarrow H^+ + HCO_3^-$$

As H_2CO_3 dissociates into H^+ and HCO_3^- ions, H^+ ion is actively secreted into the lumen (in its place Na^+ ion diffuses into the cell) and ion is reabsorbed into the peritubular capillary blood. Thus, with secretion of one H^+ ion there is reabsorption of one ion.

H^+ ions secreted in the tubular fluid react with HCO_3 (which are formed from dissociation of $NaHCO_3$ of the filtrate) forming H_2CO_3. H_2CO_3 dissociates into CO_2 and H_2O. CO_2 is absorbed in the epithelial cell where again it is reconverted into H_2CO_3 ($H^+ + HCO_3^-$).

Na^+ ions from $NaHCO_3$ of filtrate diffuse into the cell and then are actively transported into the peritubular fluid due to activity of Na^+-K^+ pump, present in basolateral membrane of the cell. This mechanism concentrates H^+ ion in tubular fluid from four to tenfold (Fig. 5.6b).

Describe the mechanism of secretion of H⁺ ions by primary active transport in distal nephron.

Primary active transport for secretion of H^+ ions occurs in late distal tubules and collecting ducts. It occurs at the luminal surface of the tubular cell, where H^+ ions are directly transported by a specific transport protein (a hydrogen transporting adenosine triphosphate-ATPase). Energy required for transport is obtained from breaking down of ATP. The mechanism is as follows (Fig. 5.6a):

- Dissolved CO_2 reacts with water inside the cell to form H_2CO_3.

    $$CO_2 + H_2O \rightarrow H_2CO_3$$

- Carbonic acid dissociates into H^+ and HCO_3^- ions.

    $$H_2CO_3 \rightarrow H + HCO_3^-$$

Intercalated cells or dark cells present in renal tubules (special type of cells present from late distal tubules onwards) are responsible for primary active transport of H^+ ions formed by dissociation of H_2CO_3. This mechanism concentrates H^+ ions up to thousandfold.

What is the factor on which the rate of secretion of H⁺ ions depends? What is the normal rate of secretion of H⁺ ions?

The rate of secretion of H^+ ions changes with changes in extracellular fluid hydrogen ion concentration and CO_2 concentration.

Normal rate of secretion of H^+ ions is about 4400 mEq/day.

What is the normal rate of filtration of HCO_3^- ions?

The normal rate of HCO_3^- ions filtered in the glomerular filtrate is 4320 mEq/day. Thus it is almost equal to the rate of H^+ ion secretion, and hence it is said that bicarbonate ions and hydrogen ions normally titrate each other in the tubules. As there is a slight excess of H^+ ions in the tubular fluid they are excreted in urine. This is essential for the excretion of non-volatile end products of metabolism.

What is the basic mechanism by which kidney corrects acidosis or alkalosis?

Kidney corrects acidosis or alkalosis by incomplete titration of H^+ ions against bicarbonate ions, leaving one of them to pass into the urine and therefore to be removed from the extracellular fluid.

Describe the renal correction of acidosis.

In acidosis, ratio of dissolved CO_2 to HCO_3^- ions in the extracellular fluid is increased. This increases the rate of hydrogen ion secretion especially in distal tubules and collecting ducts, above the rate of filtration of bicarbonate ions. As a result, excess hydrogen ions (not titrated by HCO_3^- ions) remain in the renal tubules for excretion. They combine with buffer in tubular fluid and are excreted into the urine. Each time hydrogen ion is secreted into the tubules, HCO_3^- ions formed along with it in tubular cell is reabsorbed in the extracellular fluid. Sodium ions absorbed from tubular lumen are also transported from epithelial cells to extracellular fluid.

Net effect of secretion of excess number of H^+ ions into the tubule is due to the increased rate of absorption of HCO_3^- ions into the extracellular fluid. This corrects acidosis.

How are the excess H^+ ions secreted by renal tubular cells excreted in urine?

When excess H^+ ions are secreted into the tubular lumen, pH of renal tubular fluid becomes acidic. If pH of tubular fluid reaches a critical level (pH 4.5), further hydrogen ion secretion ceases. Therefore, it is necessary to keep the tubular fluid pH above this level for continuous secretion of H^+ ions (till acidosis is corrected). This is achieved by the following mechanism:

- Phosphate buffer formed of mixture of HCO_4^- and $H_2PO_4^-$. It is a powerful buffer in the tubular fluid.
- Ammonia buffer. NH_3^+ and NH_4 form a more important buffer system. Epithelial cells of all tubules (besides those of thin segment) continuously synthesize ammonia which combines with H^+ ions in tubular fluid to form NH_4. NH_3 concentration of tubular fluid decreases causing still more ammonia to diffuse. Rate of ammonia secretion is thus controlled by amount of excess H^+ ions to be transported. 60% ammonia is synthesized by tubules from glutamine and the remaining 40% by other amino acids and amines.

- Most of the negative ions in tubular fluid are chloride ions. Only a few H^+ ions are transported in direct combination with chloride as HCl is a very strong acid and would easily lower tubular fluid pH to reach a critical value of pH 4.5 and further H^+ ion secretion will cease.

Describe the renal mechanism for correction of alkalosis.

In alkalosis, ratio of bicarbonate ions to dissolved CO_2 increases in the extracellular fluid, leading to increased bicarbonate ions filtered in the glomerular filtrate as compared to the number of H^+ ions secreted by renal tubules. No bicarbonate ion can be absorbed without first reacting with H^+ ions. Therefore, excess bicarbonate ions which are filtered pass into the urine along with sodium. Net effect is removal of excess sodium bicarbonate from extracellular fluid which corrects the pH back to normal.

What is titrable acidity?

The amount of alkali in mM/L which is required to adjust pH of a sample of urine to that of plasma (7.4) is described as a measure of titrable acidity.

What is respiratory acidosis or alkalosis?

Acidosis or alkalosis caused due to decreased or increased pulmonary ventilation (resulting into decreased and increased CO_2 loss, respectively) is called respiratory acidosis or alkalosis.

What are the causes of respiratory acidosis?

Respiratory acidosis is caused due to pathological conditions causing reduced breathing, e.g. obstruction in respiratory passage, pneumonia, etc.

What are the causes of respiratory alkalosis?

Respiratory alkalosis is caused due to increased pulmonary ventilation which rarely occurs pathologically. Physiologic type of respiratory alkalosis is produced when person ascends to high altitude.

What is metabolic acidosis or alkalosis?

Metabolic acidosis or alkalosis refers to all other abnormalities of acid-base balance, besides caused by excess or insufficient CO_2 in the body.

What are the causes of metabolic acidosis?

The causes of metabolic acidosis are:

- Failure of kidneys to excrete acids normally formed in the body.
- Formation of excess quantity of metabolic acids in the body.

- Intravenous administration of metabolic acids.
- Addition of metabolic acids by absorption from gastrointestinal tract.
- Loss of base from the body fluids.

Metabolic acidosis occurs in diabetes mellitus, uraemia and diarrhoea.

What are the causes of metabolic alkalosis?

The causes of metabolic alkalosis are:

- Administration of diuretics.
- Excessive ingestion of alkaline drugs such as sodium bicarbonate.
- Loss of chloride ions due to excessive vomiting of mainly gastric contents.
- Excessive aldosterone secretion.

RENAL FUNCTION TESTS

Enumerate the various renal function tests.

Renal function tests:

1. *Renal clearance tests.*
   - Inulin clearance test for GFR.
   - PAH clearance tests for renal plasma flow.
   - Urea clearance test.
2. *Intravenous pyelography.* Substances containing large quantities of iodine in molecules (diodrast, hippuran and iopax) are excreted into the urine, both by glomerular filtration and by active secretion. Iodine makes these compounds opaque to X-rays. Intravenous injection of one of these substances causes their excretion in urine within a few minutes. X-rays taken after 5 minutes show shadows of renal pelvis, ureters and even urinary bladder. Failure to show distinct shadows of renal pelvis within this time indicates depressed renal clearance.
3. *Radioactive clearance study.* If any of the substance, diodrast, hippuran or iopax, is prepared with radioactive iodine and its trace amount is injected intravenously, one can measure radioactivity from the renal pelvis of both the kidneys by placing appropriate radioactivity counters over the kidneys within a few minutes of intravenous injection.
4. *Blood analysis.* Measuring concentration in blood of various substances which are mainly excreted by kidneys:
   - Urea level: Normally it is about 26 mg/100 ml. It rises in renal insufficiency.
   - Creatinine level: Normal creatinine level in the blood is 1.1 mg/100 ml. It increases in renal insufficiency.
5. *Physical measurements of urine.*
   - Measurement of total volume of urine/day is important. It reduces to a great extent in acute renal failure. It increases slightly in moderate renal failure. In chronic renal failure also it is diminished.
   - Specific gravity of urine varies from 1.002 to 1.045. When a person drinks large quantities of water, specific gravity of urine shows minimal value. If a person is deprived of water for 12 hours or so, maximum concentration of the urine is obtained.

MICTURITION

What is micturition?

Micturition is the process by which urinary bladder empties when it becomes filled.

What is the function of urinary bladder?

Urinary bladder stores the urine which is transported to it from kidneys via ureters. Bladder is emptied at intervals of up to several hours.

Urine stored in the bladder remains unchanged in its chemical composition.

Describe the anatomy of urinary bladder.

Urinary bladder is formed of smooth muscle known as detrusor muscle. It mainly consists of body and neck. Neck is a funnel-shaped extension of the body that connects with urethra.

Posterior wall of the bladder shows a triangular area called trigone. At the lowermost apex of the trigone, bladder neck opens into posterior urethra; two ureters open at the uppermost angles of the trigone. Ureters enter the bladder obliquely through the detrusor. This prevents back flow of urine.

Bladder neck is 2 to 3 cm long. Muscle in this area is known as internal sphincter. Its natural tone prevents emptying of bladder until pressure in the bladder rises to a critical level. Beyond the posterior urethra, urethra passes through the urogenital diaphragm which contains a layer of muscle called external sphincter. It is formed of a voluntary (skeletal) muscle and is under voluntary control.

What are the functions of afferent nerve supply of the urinary bladder?

Afferent nerves to bladder subserve two functions:

- Indicate degree of distension of the bladder.
- Convey pain sensibility.

Describe the nerve supply of urinary bladder.

For details see Table 5.1.

What is the function of efferent nerve supply of urinary bladder?

Sympathetic efferent fibres when stimulated cause relaxation of bladder wall and constriction of internal sphincter. Parasympathetic efferent fibres when stimulated cause contraction of bladder muscle and relaxation of internal sphincter.

What is the function of efferent somatic nerve supply of the external sphincter?

Somatic efferent supply to the external sphincter muscle is responsible for voluntary control over micturition.

Table 5.1	Nerve Supply of Urinary Bladder		
	Nerve roots	**Peripheral nerves**	**Structure innervated**
1. Efferent fibres			
(a) Sympathetic	T_{11} and T_{12} L_1 and L_2	Hypogastric nerve	Detrusor muscle of the bladder and internal sphincter
(b) Parasympathetic	S_2–S_4	Nerve erigentes (pelvic nerves)	Detrusor muscle of the bladder and internal sphincter
2. Afferent fibres			
(a) Sympathetic	Dorsal roots of L_1 and L_2 and lower thoracic segments	Hypogastric nerve	Detrusor muscle
(b) Parasympathetic	Sacral roots	Pelvic nerve	Detrusor muscle
3. Somatic afferent fibres	S_2, S_3, and S_4	Pudic nerve	Urethra
4. Somatic efferent fibres	S_3 and S_4	Pudic nerve	External sphincter and distal urethra

What is the physiological capacity of urinary bladder?
Physiological capacity of urinary bladder ranges from 250 to 450 ml.

What is the anatomical capacity of urinary bladder?
Anatomical capacity of urinary bladder is 700 to 800 ml.

Describe the mechanism of filling of bladder.
The bladder is filled by urine coming from two ureters. When no urine is present in the bladder, the intravesical pressure is almost zero. When 20 to 50 ml of urine gets collected, pressure rises to 5 to 10 cm of water. Additional 200 to 300 ml of urine can be collected without much rise in pressure due to intrinsic tone of the bladder wall itself. When amount of urine collected becomes more than 300 to 400 ml, there is sudden rise in pressure.

What is micturition reflex?
When the bladder becomes full, its wall is stretched and stretch receptors in the wall are stimulated. Sensory signals are conducted to sacral segments of the cord through the pelvic nerves and then through the parasympathetic fibres in the same nerve to bladder wall to cause the contraction of detrusor muscle. Once micturition

reflex is initiated, it is self-regenerative, i.e. initial contraction of bladder wall further activates the receptors to increase sensory impulses from bladder and urethra which causes further contraction (stronger) of the detrusor muscle. This cycle repeats again and again until bladder has reached to a strong degree of contraction. After a few seconds, reflex fatigues and regenerative cycle ceases. Once a micturition reflex has occurred but not succeeded in emptying the bladder, the nervous elements of this reflex usually remain in an inhibited state for at least a few minutes to an hour before another micturition reflex occurs.

Once the micturition reflex becomes powerful enough, this causes another reflex which passes through pudendal nerves to external sphincter to cause its inhibition. If inhibition is more potent, urination will occur. If not, urination will not occur unless the bladder fills still more and micturition reflex becomes more powerful.

How is micturition controlled?

Micturition reflex is a purely spinal cord reflex but it can be inhibited or facilitated by brain, because of certain centres in the brain:

1. Strong facilitatory and inhibitory centres in the brain stem (probably in pons).
2. Several centres located in cerebral cortex that are mainly inhibitory but at times become facilitatory. These higher centres keep the micturition reflex partially inhibited all the time except when micturition is desired. Even if micturition reflex occurs, still higher centres can keep it inhibited by causing tonic contraction of external sphincter until a convenient time presents.

When convenient time presents, cortical centres facilitate sacral micturition centres to initiate micturition reflex, inhibit external urinary sphincter so that urination can occur.

What is atonic bladder? When does it occur?

Destruction of sensory nerve fibres from the bladder leads to atonic bladder. There is a lack of stretch signals from bladder preventing micturition reflex contractions. Therefore, instead of getting emptied periodically, bladder fills to its capacity and overflows. This is called overflow dribbling or incontinence. Atonic bladder occurs commonly in syphilis (tabes dorsalis). The bladder is known as tabetic bladder.

What is automatic bladder? When does it occur?

If spinal cord is damaged above the sacral segments but sacral segments are intact, it results in automatic bladder. This occurs after the person recovers from spinal shock following injury to the spinal cord.

Recovery from the spinal shock allows the sacral centres to take over the function and typical micturition reflex returns. When bladder is full, it automatically is emptied (no voluntary control).

Stimulation of skin in the genital region elicits micturition reflex.

What is uninhibited neurogenic bladder?

Frequent and relatively uncontrollable micturition occurs when there is uninhibited neurogenic bladder. This condition results due to partial damage in the spinal cord or brain stem which interrupts most of the inhibitory signals.

DIALYSIS

What is dialysis?

In certain types of acute renal failure (following poisoning, circulatory shock), dialysis is done to tide over the patient for a few weeks until the renal damage heals and kidneys resume their normal function. It is also used in patient with chronic renal failure for maintaining the health till the operation of renal transplantation is done. Lives of such patients completely depend upon dialysis.*

There are two methods of dialysis:

1. *Haemodialysis.*
2. *Peritoneal dialysis.*

---

*For details refer Vaz M, Kurpad A, Raj T, editors. *Guyton & Hall Textbook of Medical Physiology.* Elsevier: New Delhi, 2013, p. 530.

CHAPTER 6
Temperature Regulation

What is a homeothermic animal?

An animal capable of maintaining its body temperature within very narrow limits is termed homeothermic, e.g. human being.

What is the skin and core temperature?

Skin temperature is the surface temperature and it rises and falls with the temperature of the surroundings. Core temperature is the temperature of deep tissues of the body and it remains almost constant. Total heat content of the body is determined by the net difference between heat produced and heat lost. Maintaining constant body temperature implies that overall heat production must equal heat loss. Both these variations are subject to precise physiological control.

How much is normal core temperature? How is it measured?

Normal body temperature varies from 97°F to 99.5°F (36°C to 37.5°C). It is measured with the help of clinical thermometer kept either in mouth, or per rectum. Rectal temperature is 1°F greater than the oral temperature. Average oral temperature is 98°F to 98.6°F.

What are the physiological variations in the body temperature?

- Body temperature varies with exercise. During strenuous exercise, excessive heat is produced and rectal temperature can rise as high as 101°F to 104°F.
- Exposure to severe cold may reduce rectal temperature below 97°F.
- There is a characteristic circadian fluctuation in body temperature. It is lowest during sleep and highest when person is awake.
- In females, higher temperature is recorded during the last half of menstrual cycle.

Why is temperature regulation needed?

Maintaining the constant body temperature prevents biochemical reactions from fluctuating with external temperature. Large elevation in body temperature causes nerve malfunction and protein denaturation. Some people may get convulsions at body temperature of 41 °C (106 °F).

MECHANISMS OF HEAT PRODUCTION

Name the various mechanisms by which heat is produced in the body.

1. Basal rate of metabolism in all the cells of the body.
2. *Muscular activity.* Extra rate of metabolism due to muscle activity.
   - *Shivering.* Characteristic muscle response to cold is called shivering. Shivering consists of oscillating rhythmic muscle tremors occurring at a rate of 10 to 20/s. During shivering, efferent impulses to skeletal muscles are controlled by descending pathways, primarily by hypothalamus, and heat production may increase several folds within seconds to minutes. As no work is performed during shivering, all the energy liberated by muscles appears as internal heat (shivering thermogenesis).
   - *Non-shivering thermogenesis.* On chronic exposure to cold, there is an increase in metabolic rate due to increased secretion of epinephrine and to certain extent thyroid hormones. Such type of non-shivering thermogenesis is minimal in adult human beings.

MECHANISMS OF HEAT LOSS

Enumerate the mechanisms by which heat is lost.

Most of the heat is produced by deep organs (liver, brain, muscles and heart). This heat is transferred from the deep organs to the skin through blood. The surface of the body exchanges heat with the environment by:

- Radiation.
- Conduction.
- Convection.
- Evaporation of water.

Amount of heat loss is determined by two factors:

- Rapidity with which heat is conducted from the core to the skin.
- Rapidity with which heat is transferred from the skin to the surroundings.

Describe the insulator system of the body.

Skin, subcutaneous tissue and the fat of subcutaneous tissue are heat insulators for the body. Fat conducts heat only one-third as readily as other tissues. This insulation is important in maintaining core temperature even though skin temperature varies with that of the surroundings.

The skin is not a perfect insulator (if it were so, no heat would ever be lost from the core) and so the temperature of its outer surface is somewhere between that of the external environment and that of the core.

Describe the radiator system of the body.

Blood vessels penetrate fatty subcutaneous insulator tissue and are distributed profusely beneath the skin. There is a venous plexus underneath the skin which is supplied by inflow of blood from the skin capillaries. In exposed areas of the body such as hands, feet and ears, there is arteriovenous anastomosis (blood is supplied to the venous plexus directly from the small arteries). The rate of blood flow through venous plexus can be increased up to 30% of total cardiac output. When there is full vasoconstriction, rate of blood flow can be reduced to as much as 2 to 3% of cardiac output. Changing flow of blood through the skin is thus the effective mechanism of controlling heat loss. The skin is therefore an effective radiator system.

Describe the mechanism of heat loss by radiation, conduction and convection.

Radiation, conduction and convection are the mechanisms of heat loss only when the body temperature is higher than the surrounding temperature.

1. *Radiation.* Radiation is the process by which surfaces of all the objects emit heat in the form of electromagnetic waves. The rate of emission depends upon the temperature of the surface. The rate of heat loss depends upon the temperature difference between the skin surface and the environment.

2. *Conduction.* It is a gain or loss of heat due to transfer of thermal energy during collisions between adjacent molecules. Body surface loses or gains heat by conduction through direct contact with cooler or warmer objects, respectively.

3. *Convection.* It is the process by which conductive heat loss is aided by movement of air or water next to the body. Air next to the body is heated by conduction of heat from the body. This air moves away and carries away the heat and its place is taken by fresh cool air. This air when gets heated follows the same pattern. Some amount of convection is always occurring because warm air becomes lighter and therefore rises but it is greatly facilitated by external forces like wind or fan. Thus, convection aids conductive heat loss by continuously maintaining the supply of cool air.

Describe the mechanism of evaporation.

Water is evaporated from the surface of the skin and membranes of the respiratory tract. When liquid is converted to gaseous state, about 580 to 600 cal of energy is required for the transformation. When water evaporates from the skin, heat required is conducted from the surface and causes cooling of the surface. Water that evaporates by diffusion through skin (in absence of sweating) and respiratory membrane is known as insensible perspiration. It amounts to 600 ml/day. But this heat loss is not under control and therefore cannot be changed as required. Evaporation of sweat from the surface causes evaporative heat loss which is under the control of nervous system. Sweat glands are supplied by sympathetic nerves.

Stimulation of sympathetic nervous system causes sweating. Sweat is a dilute solution of sodium chloride. For cooling effect sweat must evaporate from the surface. Humidity or water vapour concentration of the air is the most important factor determining evaporation of sweat. On humid day, due to failure of evaporation, sweat simply remains on the skin. When the surrounding temperature is high, evaporation is the only means of heat loss.

What are the behavioural responses for altering heat loss by radiation and conduction?

There are three behavioural responses that alter the heat loss:

1. *Changes in surface urea*. Curling up into the bed and hunching of shoulders are the responses to cold which reduce the surface area exposed to the environment.

2. *Clothing*. Outer surface of clothes forms the true exterior of body surface. Skin loses heat directly to the air space trapped between skin and clothes. Clothes in turn pick up the heat and transfer it to the environment acting as insulators. Insulator ability of clothing depends on thickness of the trapped air layer. Clothing is also important in summer. When environment is hot, radiation and conduction acts as heat gain mechanisms. Person insulates himself against such temperature by clothing. White clothing is cooler since it reflects more radiant energy.

3. *Behavioural mechanisms*. Seeking warmer or colder surroundings is the behaviour response.

REGULATION OF BODY TEMPERATURE

Where is the temperature regulating centre?

Temperature regulating centre is present in the hypothalamus. It is also called hypothalamic thermostat.

Anterior hypothalamus and preoptic area contain large number of heat sensitive neurons and cold sensitive neurons. If preoptic area is heated, it initiates heat loss mechanisms and brings temperature back to normal. Thus, this area mainly controls heat loss mechanism.

Posterior hypothalamic area near mamillary bodies receives signals from various peripheral thermoreceptors as well as preoptic anterior hypothalamic area. Posterior hypothalamic area in turn sends signals to the periphery to provide heat producing and heat conserving mechanisms.

Temperature of 37.1 °C is called set point of the temperature control mechanism (Fig. 6.1). If temperature of the body increases beyond the set point, all mechanisms of heat loss come into play to bring body temperature back to normal. If body temperature falls below the set point, all the mechanisms of increased heat production and heat conservation are stimulated and body temperature is brought to the set point.

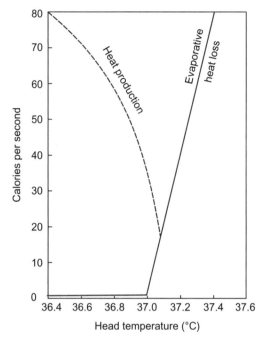

FIGURE 6.1 Effects of the hypothalamic temperature on evaporative heat loss and heat production and shivering.

Name the different thermoreceptors.

There are two groups of thermoreceptors.

1. *Peripheral thermoreceptors.* Present in skin and mucous membrane, they are either warm or cold receptors.

2. *Central thermoreceptors.* These are present in hypothalamus, spinal cord, various organs and in the great veins. Impulses from various receptors go to posterior hypothalamus at the level of mammary bodies. This area in turn sends signals to periphery for heat producing and heat conserving reactions of the body.

What are the mechanisms of heat conservation?

Mechanisms of heat conservation are the ones which decrease the heat loss from the body.

1. *Skin vasoconstriction.* It is due to stimulation of posterior hypothalamic sympathetic centres.

2. *Piloerection ('Hair standing on').* This is also due to sympathetic stimulation causing contraction of erector pili muscles attached to hair follicles of the skin. Hair become upright, thus increasing the thickness of insulated layer of air next to the skin preventing transfer of heat to the surroundings.

Enumerate the different mechanisms which bring the body temperature back to normal when body is too hot.

1. *Increased heat loss due to:*
   - Vasodilation of skin vessels.
   - Sweating.
   - Behavioural response (put on cooler clothes, switch on the fan, etc.).
2. *Decreased heat production due to:*
   - Decreased muscle tone and voluntary activity.
   - Decreased secretion of epinephrine and thyroid hormones.
   - Decreased food appetite.

Enumerate the different mechanisms which bring the body temperature back to normal when body is too cold.

1. *Decreased heat loss due to:*
   - Vasoconstriction of skin vessels.
   - Reduction of surface by curling up.
   - Behavioural responses (to put warmer clothes).
2. *Increased heat production due to:*
   - Increased muscle tone.
   - Shivering.
   - Increased secretion of epinephrine and thyroid hormones.
   - Increased food appetite.

What is the role of peripheral thermoreceptors present in the skin in temperature regulation?

Stimulation of skin receptors helps as follows:

1. Stimulation of skin receptors changes the set point of hypothalamus. Set point increases when skin temperature decreases (stimulation of cold receptors). Because set point is higher, all mechanisms for increasing body temperature set in, so that mechanisms of increased heat production and decreased heat loss are initiated in anticipation before the body temperature falls below normal.
2. Stimulation of skin receptors also causes behavioural mechanisms for control of temperature.
3. Local cord reflexes prevent excessive heat exchange. When any part of the body is kept under hot lamp, there is local vasodilatation and sweating caused through cord reflex, thus causing excessive heat loss from the local surface.

Describe the mechanism of sweat secretion.

Sweat glands have a deep subdermal coiled portion, a duct passing outward in the dermis and epidermis of the skin.

Epithelial cells lining the coiled portion secrete primary secretion. These cells are supplied by cholinergic sympathetic nerves. Stimulation of these nerves stimulates the gland to secrete primary secretion which is similar to plasma except for plasma proteins and high NaCl concentration. When this secretion passes through the duct, there is absorption of sodium and chloride. Slight stimulation of sweat glands causes this primary secretion to pass through the duct. Slowly and essentially almost all sodium and chloride is reabsorbed. This causes osmotic absorption of water which concentrates the other constituents (urea, lactic acid, potassium ions) in the sweat.

With strong sympathetic stimulation of the glands, rate of secretion is high. Primary solution quickly passes through the duct and therefore sodium and chloride ions are absorbed only slightly. Water reabsorption is greatly reduced. Other dissolved constituents are only moderately increased.

What is acclimatization of sweating mechanism?

Usually, rate of secretion of sweat is rarely more than 700 ml/hr but when person is exposed to hot weather for a few (2 to 6) weeks, rate of secretion is greatly increased (2 L/hr). This is due to direct increased capability of sweat glands themselves. Later on, there is adaptation known as acclimatization producing changes in sweat volume and composition. This is the effect of chronic exposure to hot weather. Acclimatization is due to increased secretion of aldosterone (stimulated due to slight decrease in NaCl level of body fluids because of excessive sweating before acclimatization). Aldosterone increases absorption of sodium and chloride from the duct. This reduces excretion of salt to 3 to 5 g/day as compared to 15 to 30 g/day before acclimatization.

ABNORMALITIES IN TEMPERATURE REGULATION

Describe the different abnormalities in temperature regulating mechanism.*

1. *Fever.* It is hyperthermia resulting from disturbance in temperature regulating centre, i.e. resetting of hypothalamic thermostat to level of higher temperature than the normal (37°C) as a result of bacterial infections or physical trauma.

2. *Heat stroke.* It is a grave syndrome most commonly seen in tropical countries. It also occurs as a complication of diseases causing hyperpyrexia. The symptoms are due to hyperpyrexia, salt loss and dehydration.

3. *Exposure to severe cold.*
   (a) Loss of temperature regulation at low temperature.
   (b) Frostbite.

Write a note on hypothermia.

In animals, hypothermia occurs during hibernation and the body temperature varies with that of environment over a range of 5° to 15°C.

---

*For details refer Vaz M, Kurpad A, Raj T, editors. *Guyton & Hall Textbook of Medical Physiology.* Elsevier: New Delhi, 2013, p. 861.

In man, hypothermia may be accidental or it may be used deliberately in surgery of brain and heart.

Accidental hypothermia. It may occur in healthy persons exposed to excessive cooling, e.g. immersion in cold sea water after shipwreck. The capacity of thermoregulatory mechanisms is overcome and body temperature falls. At 33°C temperature regulation fails. Death occurs at body temperature below 25°C.

Accidental hypothermia can also occur in elderly persons living in inadequately heated rooms.

Hypothermia occurs in myxoedema because the patients cannot increase their metabolic rate on exposure to cold.

Deliberately induced hypothermia. Hypothermia is deliberately induced in some patients undergoing operations on heart and brain.

Several surgical procedures of heart and brain require temporary suspension of normal circulation. This is made possible by cardiopulmonary bypass machine.

Hypothermia may cause certain harmful effects on the body such as hypocapnia and hypoxia. Impaired oxygenation of tissues may lead to metabolic acidosis. Reduction in metabolic rate reduces the activity of metabolically fuelled pumps such as sodium pump. Hence K^+ is lost and Na^+ is gained by tissues. This leads to hyperkalaemia.

In spite of all the above problems, hypothermia is used in cardiac surgery because it provides time to the surgeon for manipulating the heart without producing permanent ischaemic damage. The maximum period of circulatory arrest increases markedly at low body temperatures.

SKIN AND ITS FUNCTIONS

Describe the structure and functions of skin.

STRUCTURE OF SKIN

Skin is made up of two layers:

1. *Epidermis (outer layer).* It is made up of 5 layers:
   (a) *Stratum corneum.*
   (b) *Stratum lucidum.*
   (c) *Stratum granulosum.*
   (d) *Stratum germinativum.* New cells are constantly formed here by mitosis. Newly formed cells move continuously towards stratum corneum. From this layer some projections extent down to dermis. These projections provide anchoring and nutrition. Cells in this layer contain pigment melanin and the colour of the skin depends on amount of melanin present.
   (e) *Stratum spinosum* (prickle cell layer).
2. *Dermis (inner layer).* It is a connective tissue layer and is made up of 2 layers:
   (a) *Superficial papillary layer.*
   (b) *Deeper reticular layer.*

Hair bulbs are present in dermis; from here, hair come out which partly remains in epidermis and the rest shoots out from the skin.

Sweat glands lie in this layer and are of 2 types:

(a) Eccrine glands are simple, highly coiled tubular structures present in dermis. The rest of the duct is mostly straight and passes through superficial layer of dermis and then through epidermis, ultimately opening as a pore into the exterior. Sweat is synthesized by coiled portion. Eccrine glands are common and occur all over the body but their population is most dense over the thick skin.

(b) Apocrine glands are found in pubic region, axilla and around nipple. They are of less importance in human beings.

Sebaceous glands usually open in hair follicle except in the face where they open into the exterior directly. The secretion from these glands is rich in oily substances, which prevents evaporation of water from the skin.

FUNCTIONS OF SKIN

1. *Protective function.* Skin forms the covering of the body and protects inner organs from the following agents.

(a) *Bacteria and toxic substances.* Keratinized stratum corneum is responsible for protective functions against chemicals like acids and alkalies. Intact skin also offers resistance to many harmful agents like bacteria. If there is injury to the skin, bacteria invade from external environment.

(b) *Mechanical blow.* Skin is somewhat lose and moves over the underlying subcutaneous tissue. Therefore, mechanical impact of any blow to the skin is not transmitted to the underlying tissues.

(c) *Ultraviolet rays.* Ultraviolet rays of sun can cause damage to the skin. But melanin pigment and stratum corneum together protect from such injury. Exposure to ultraviolet rays stimulates melanin production and also increases the thickness of stratum corneum. Melanin and stratum corneum absorb light waves having wavelength of less than 360 nm. Such waves are often cancer producing.

2. *Temperature regulation.* Role of skin in temperature regulation is already explained.

3. *As a sense organ.* Skin is the largest sense organ of the body. It has many nerve endings which are specialized into receptors. Those cutaneous receptors are stimulated by touch, pain, pressure and temperature (hot and cold receptors). These sensations are conveyed to brain through afferent nerves. Thus different sensations are perceived.

4. *Storage function.* Skin can store fat and water.

5. *Synthesis of vitamin D.* Vitamin D is synthesized in skin by the action of ultraviolet rays on cholesterol.

6. *Excretory function.* Skin can excrete small quantities of waste products like urea, salts and fatty substances in its secretion.

7. *Absorption.* Skin can absorb certain soluble substances and some ointments.

8. *Secretory function.* Sweat glands secrete sweat and sebaceous glands secrete sebum. Secretion of sweat helps in temperature regulation and water balance. Sebum keeps the skin smooth and moist.

CHAPTER 7
Respiratory System

Enumerate the functions of respiratory system.

- Exchange of gases between atmosphere and blood.
- Maintenance of pH of the body fluids.
- Excretion of water vapour.
- Excretion of certain volatile substances, e.g. acetone.
- Respiratory muscles are used during laughing, singing, etc.
- Metabolic functions of lungs:
  - Formation of surfactant.
  - Protein synthesis for maintenance of structural framework.
  - Capillary endothelium has angiotensin converting enzyme (ACE) which converts angiotensin I to angiotensin II.
  - Many vasoactive substances are partially or totally inactivated, e.g. bradykinin, serotonin and some prostaglandins.
  - Secretion of immunoglobulins (IgA).

What is external respiration?

Respiration concerned with exchange of gases between environment and lungs, transfer of gases through respiratory membrane and their transport to and from the tissues is called external respiration.

What is internal respiration?

Respiration concerned with consumption of oxygen by body cells through metabolic transformation is known as internal respiration.

Describe the functional anatomy of respiratory system.

Respiratory system consists of conductive airway and lungs. Air passes through various parts of conducting airway and ultimately to alveoli of lungs as follows.

1. *Two nasal openings.* Air from atmosphere enters the nasal cavity through nasal openings. Except external nares (which are lined by skin) rest of the nasal cavity is lined by ciliated columnar epithelium with scattered goblet cells which secrete mucus. Mucous membrane of nasal cavity is continuous with that of nasal sinuses. Cilia

constantly beat outward for removal of any foreign particle outwards. Fine hair present in nasal cavity remove gross impurities in air. Nasal cavity is richly supplied by blood, therefore air entering the cavity also becomes warm (to body temperature). Thus air is warmed and purified while it passes through the nasal cavity.

2. *Pharynx.* Through posterior nasal openings air from nasal cavity enters into the pharynx. Pharynx is a common pathway for food and air. Therefore, during passage of food through it (pharyngeal phase of swallowing), laryngeal opening is closed and respiration is inhibited. Nasopharynx is lined by ciliated epithelium with scattered goblet cells. Oropharynx is lined by stratified epithelium.

3. *Larynx.* From pharynx air passes into the larynx which is commonly known as voice box. It contains vocal cords and number of cartilages. Vibration of vocal cords produces sound. Upper part of vocal cord is lined by stratified squamous epithelium. Lower part is lined by ciliated epithelium.

4. *Trachea.* From larynx air enters into the trachea which is commonly termed wind pipe. Trachea is formed of cartilaginous rings which run only half way (anteriorly), posterior parts of the rings are formed by smooth muscle. Presence of cartilaginous rings prevents total blockage of trachea. Trachea is lined by ciliated epithelium with goblet cells and deep glands.

5. *Bronchi.* Trachea divides into two bronchi, left and right, which enter the respective lung.

6. *Lungs.* Bronchus entering into the lung divides and redivides for about 20 to 23 subdivisions. Smaller division is termed bronchiole. The last portion of conducting airway is termed terminal bronchiole (so the part of the respiratory system from nose to terminal bronchiole only conducts the air and no gaseous exchange occurs through their membrane).

Terminal bronchiole onwards is the part which does the function of gaseous exchange; terminal bronchiole divides therefore in respiratory bronchioles. Each respiratory bronchiole further divides into 5 to 6 alveolar ducts. Each alveolar duct ends blindly in a dilated sac termed alveolar sac. The wall of each alveolar sac shows large number of bends which are termed alveoli (Fig. 7.1).

Epithelium of large bronchi is the same as that of trachea but in bronchioles goblet cells and deep glands are lost.

Efficiency of ciliated cells of trachea and bronchi in propelling mucus and waste products is of higher order. Cilia are not influenced by nerve impulses.

Elastic tissue. Bronchial tree is rich in elastic tissue. Most of the fibres are arranged longitudinally. Elastic membrane thus extends from trachea, bronchi and bronchioles to alveoli. It is responsible for elastic recoil of the bronchial tree during expiration.

Cartilages. In larynx cartilages support special structures necessary for attachment of vocal cords.

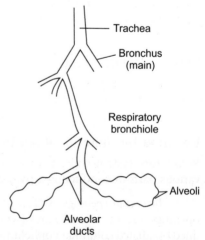

FIGURE 7.1 Diagrammatic representation of respiratory system.

Cartilaginous rings of trachea are incomplete on their posterior aspect. This allows some contraction of trachea but tracheal lumen cannot be completely obliterated easily.

Smooth muscle. Ends of cartilaginous rings of trachea are approximated by transverse smooth muscle fibres. In bronchi bands of fibres tend to become circular so that they form a sphincter in the terminal bronchiole. Muscle does not extend further.

Blood supply. Conducting airway is supplied by systemic blood, whereas respiratory part of lung (from respiratory bronchioles to alveolar sac) is supplied by deoxygenated (venous) blood coming through pulmonary arteries to lungs. Blood is oxygenated in lungs and is returned to left atrium via pulmonary veins.

Respiratory bronchiole gets systemic (through bronchial artery) as well as pulmonary blood supply.

Nerve supply. Bronchoconstrictor fibres pass through vagus nerve and bronchodilator fibres through sympathetic nerves. Afferents from lungs pass through vagi nerves.

Name the muscles of normal tidal respiration.

- Diaphragm. Major muscle responsible for 75% of tidal volume.
- External intercostal muscles (Fig. 7.2).

Name the accessory muscles of inspiration.

- Scalene.
- Sternomastoid.
- Serratus anterior and alae nasi.

Name the muscles of expiration.

- Abdominal muscles.
  - Abdominal recti muscles.
  - Transverse abdominis muscles.
  - Internal oblique muscles.
  - External oblique muscles.
- Internal intercostal muscles (Fig. 7.2).

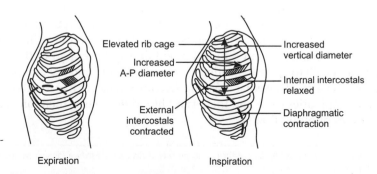

FIGURE 7.2 Expansion and contraction of the thoracic cage during inspiration and expiration.

PULMONARY CIRCULATION

Describe the pulmonary circulation.

In pulmonary circulation deoxygenated blood from right ventricle passes to lungs via pulmonary arteries. Blood is oxygenated in pulmonary capillaries which join to form pulmonary veins. Pulmonary veins carry oxygenated blood from lungs to left atrium.

Describe the characteristic features of pulmonary circulation.

CHARACTERISTIC FEATURES OF PULMONARY CIRCULATION*

1. *Compliance of pulmonary vessels.* Pulmonary arterial system is thin walled and distensible. Because of this, pulmonary arterial tree has a large compliance (distensibility per unit rise in pressure) of 7 ml per mmHg which is similar to that of entire systemic tree. This allows pulmonary arteries to accommodate about two-third of the stroke volume output of right ventricle. Pulmonary veins are as distensible as systemic veins.

2. *Pressure in pulmonary circulation.* In pulmonary artery, systemic pressure is 25 mmHg and diastolic pressure is 8 mmHg, with a pulse pressure 17 mmHg and mean pressure 15 mmHg. Pulmonary capillary pressure is 7 mmHg. The mean pressure in major pulmonary veins and left atrium is 2 mmHg in recumbent position.

3. *Blood volume of lungs.* Quantity of blood present in lungs varies from 225 to 900 ml. Failure in left side of heart causes blood to dam up in pulmonary circulation, leading to corresponding increase in pulmonary vascular pressure.

4. *Blood flow to lungs.* Blood flow to lungs is equal to cardiac output. All factors affecting cardiac output therefore control pulmonary blood flow.

5. *Effect of hypoxia.* The main function of lungs is to oxygenate blood. Blood therefore must be distributed to those segments of lungs where alveoli are best oxygenated. This occurs as follows:

When concentration of O_2 in alveoli decreases below normal, adjacent blood vessels slowly constrict within 3 to 10 minutes. This is opposite to the effect normally observed in systemic vessels which dilate in response to low O_2. This response is probably due to release of some vasoconstrictor substance from alveolar epithelial cells in response to hypoxia.

6. *Effect of hydrostatic pressure on blood flow through lungs.* In standing position, pulmonary arterial pressure in the uppermost portion of lungs is 15 mmHg less (than pulmonary arterial pressure at the level of heart), and pressure in the lowermost portion of lungs is about 8 mmHg greater (than pulmonary arterial pressure at the level of heart). This results in decreased blood flow in upper part of the lungs and greater (about 5 times) blood flow in lower part of the lungs.

Pulmonary capillaries are distended by blood pressure and are compressed by alveolar air pressure. If alveolar pressure becomes greater than capillary blood pressure, the capillaries close and there is no blood flow. Lung therefore has three different zones of blood flow.

---

*For details refer Vaz M, Kurpad A, Raj T, editors. *Guyton & Hall Textbook of Medical Physiology.* Elsevier: New Delhi, 2013, p. 336.

Zone 1. No blood flow at all during any part of cardiac cycle because local capillary pressure never rises beyond that of alveolar air pressure.

Zone 2. Intermittent flow of blood in systole of heart only as pulmonary arterial pressure rises above the alveolar air pressure only during systole.

Zone 3. Continuous blood flow because pulmonary capillary pressure remains greater than alveolar pressure during the entire cardiac cycle.

The normal lung has two zones—zone 2 and zone 3. At the apices of lungs in upright position there is flow of blood intermittently during systole (zone 2). In the lower regions of lungs there is continuous flow of blood (zone 3).

In zone 1, blood flow occurs only under abnormal conditions.

7. *Pulmonary capillary dynamics.*
   (a) Forces tending to cause movement of fluid outward from capillaries into pulmonary interstitium.
   - Capillary pressure   7 mmHg
   - Interstitial fluid colloid osmotic pressure (as pulmonary capillaries are relatively leaky to proteins)   14 mmHg
   - Negative interstitial fluid pressure   8 mmHg

   Total outward force   29 mmHg

   (b) Forces tending to cause absorption of fluid in pulmonary capillaries.

Plasma colloid osmotic pressure	28 mmHg
Total inward force	28 mmHg
Total outward force	29 mmHg
∴ Net mean filtration pressure	1 mmHg

This net pressure causes very small quantity of fluid to flow out from capillaries into pulmonary interstitium and alveoli.

Because of negative interstitial fluid pressure, if fluid enters alveoli, it is sucked into interstitium through small openings between epithelial cells of alveoli. Thus normally alveoli are kept dry except for a small quantity of fluid on their surface to keep them moist.

What is the effect of left-sided heart failure on pulmonary circulation?

When there is left-sided heart failure, blood begins to damp up in the left atrium. This causes rise of pressure in left atrium. Initial rise of pressure up to 7 mmHg has no effect on pulmonary circulation as this pressure expands pulmonary venules and capillaries. When pressure rises more than 7 to 8 mmHg in the left atrium, it causes increase in pulmonary capillary pressure leading to pulmonary oedema.

How much is the safety factor against pulmonary oedema?

Unless the pressure in pulmonary capillaries rises approximately up to colloid osmotic pressure of blood, pulmonary oedema does not develop. In normal person colloid osmotic pressure of blood is 28 mmHg. Thus, unless pulmonary capillary pressure does not rise up to 28 mmHg, pulmonary oedema does not develop. Normal pressure in pulmonary capillaries is 7 mmHg. Therefore, $28 - 7$ mmHg = 21 mmHg is the safety factor against pulmonary oedema.

State PO_2 and PCO_2 levels of pulmonary capillary blood.

$$PO_2 \quad = \quad 40 \text{ mmHg.}$$
$$PCO_2 \quad = \quad 45 \text{ mmHg.}$$

MECHANISM OF RESPIRATION

Describe the mechanism of respiration.

There are two lungs which are placed on either side of heart in the mediastinum. The entry of bronchus, blood vessels, lymph vessels, nerves, etc. occurs into the lung at the hilum of the lung which lies on medial side.

Each lung is invested by a double layer of membranes called pleura. Visceral pleura is attached to the lungs and parietal pleura is attached to the inner side of the thoracic wall. Visceral pleura is attached at the hilum, it completely invests the lung and comes back to hilum, then gets reflected to form a parietal pleura. Thus two pleural membranes actually form a closed bag surrounding each lung. The space between two pleural membranes is infinitely small and is termed intrapleural space. It is filled with a small quantity of fluid termed intrapleural fluid. Because of hydraulic pressure of this fluid, two pleural membranes are inseparable.

Lungs are attached to the body only at their hila. Rest of the surface is free to move. They are also connected to atmosphere through nose. If the thoracic cage expands the parietal pleura is taken away, the visceral pleura being inseparable also moves along with. This causes expansion of the lung leading to pressure of air in the lungs to drop below the atmospheric pressure which in turn causes atmospheric air to rush into the expanded lung—leading to inspiration.

Then after a few seconds thoracic cage reduces in size, parietal pleura and along with the visceral pleura go back to the original state, lung also becomes smaller in size. This causes pressure of air inside the lungs to increase slightly above the atmospheric pressure; therefore, air flows from lungs to atmosphere leading to expiration.

Thus alternate increase and decrease in thoracic cage dimensions causes alternate inflation and deflation of lungs leading to alternate inspiration and expiration. Increase and decrease in dimensions of thorax is caused by muscles of inspiration and expiration, respectively.

Vertical diameter of the thorax increases due to contraction and flattening of dome-shaped diaphragm lying at the boundary of thorax and abdomen. Increase in anteroposterior diameter of the thorax occurs as follows: In natural resting position the ribs slant downwards and thus allowing the sternum to fall backward towards the spinal column (so that anteroposterior diameter of the thorax is less). When the rib cage is elevated, ribs project directly forward, away from the spine increasing the anteroposterior diameter of the chest by 20%. Ribs are directly or indirectly attached to sternum; therefore lifting upward of sternum or any of the ribs causes lifting of the whole of the rib cage.

Increase in transverse diameter of the thorax occurs as follows. During expiration ribs are not only slanting downward from vertebral column but their position is like fallen bucket handle (this reduces the transverse diameter). Contraction of some inspiratory muscles raises the ribs like raising of a bucket handle. This causes increase in transverse diameter.

Describe the mechanism of tidal respiration.

MECHANISM OF TIDAL RESPIRATION

During tidal respiration, diaphragm and external intercostal muscles contract during inspiration and cause increase in all the three diameters of the thorax to a small degree. Relaxation of these muscles causes expiration and therefore tidal expiration is a passive process.

Ninety per cent of the expansion of chest is caused due to contraction of diaphragm in tidal inspiration, remaining 10% due to contraction of external intercostal muscles.

Diaphragm is a dome-shaped muscle present at the boundary of thorax and abdomen. The convexity of this dome is directed towards the thorax. Contraction of any of the fibres of diaphragm makes the dome little flatter and increases the vertical diameter of the chest. During expiration diaphragm relaxes and again becomes a dome, reducing the vertical diameter of the chest. The total excursion of diaphragm (down and up) during tidal respiration (inspiration and expiration) is about 1 cm.

External intercostal muscles are present in each intercostal space. When external intercostal muscles contract they pull the upper ribs forward in relation to lower ribs. This causes an increase in anteroposterior diameter due to lifting of rib cage upward and transverse diameter of the chest (due to raising of bucket handle like movement of the ribs). Relaxation of external intercostal muscles causes tidal expiration (Fig. 7.2).

Normal breathing is thus accomplished by active contraction of inspiratory muscles (diaphragm, external intercostal muscles which enlarge the thorax), which further lowers intrathoracic or intrapleural pressure (it is usually less than atmospheric pressure) and pulls on the lungs, enlarges alveoli, alveolar ducts and bronchioles. This expands alveolar gas and decreases its pressure below atmospheric. Air from atmosphere then flows in nose, mouth, trachea and to lungs because of pressure gradient.

During tidal expiration thoracic cavity reduces in diameter, lungs contract and reduce in their volume. This increases intra-alveolar pressure above the atmospheric and because of pressure gradient air passes from lungs to atmosphere.

Though diaphragm is a skeletal muscle, why is it not fatigued?

Diaphragm is a dome-shaped sheet of muscle separating thorax and abdomen. Contraction of only a few muscle fibres causes the dome of the diaphragm to descend. Thus, at a time only a few muscle fibres in the diaphragm contract, other fibres are resting. Therefore diaphragm does not get fatigued.

Describe the mechanism of forced respiration.

In forced respiration both inspiration and expiration are more powerful than in tidal respiration.

Forced inspiration is caused as follows:

- The diaphragm contracts more powerfully so that its total excursion during forceful inspiration and expiration can be as high as 10 cm as compared to 1 cm during tidal respiration.
- External intercostal muscles also contract more powerfully.

Accessory muscles of inspiration contract and cause the following effects.

- Sternomastoid muscles contract and lift the sternum upwards.
- Anterior serrati muscles contract and lift many of the ribs upward.
- Scaleni muscles contract and lift first two ribs.

Forced expiration is active and is caused as follows:

- Contraction of abdominal muscles causes compression of abdomen and increase in intra-abdominal pressure which pushes the diaphragm upwards, i.e. more towards the thorax thereby reducing vertical diameter of the chest.
- In addition, contraction of abdominal recti muscles pulls downwards on the lower ribs and thus causes decrease in anteroposterior diameter of the chest.
- Internal intercostal muscles are present in intercostal spaces. When they contract they pull the lower ribs downward in relation to upper ribs (the action which is exactly opposite to that of external intercostal muscles). This reduces anteroposterior as well as transverse diameter (because of action of ribs like falling of bucket handle) of the chest (Figs 7.1 and 7.2).

PULMONARY PRESSURES

INTRAPLEURAL PRESSURE

What is intrapleural pressure? How is it measured?

Pressure inside the intrapleural space is termed intrapleural pressure.

Intrapleural pressure can be recorded by inserting a needle into the intrapleural space and injecting a tiny bubble of air therein, whereupon suitable manometric recordings can be made.

Intrapleural pressure can also be measured by introducing air containing latex balloon sealed over a catheter into the lower part of oesophagus (just above the cardiac sphincter) through nostril. Other end of the catheter is connected to a pressure transducer or a recording system.

State the variation that occurs in intrapleural pressure during normal tidal respiration.

In normal tidal breathing, intrapleural pressure is always negative, i.e. below the atmospheric pressure because of continuous tendency of the lungs to collapse away from the chest wall. In normal tidal respiration, intrapleural pressure varies from -5 cm of H_2O during expiration to -7.5 cm of H_2O during inspiration.

What is the cause of negativity of intrapleural pressure?

Intrapleural pressure is negative, i.e. subatmospheric, due to two opposing forces:

- Chest wall is normally partially pulled inward (compressed) and it constantly tends to pop outward.
- Lungs have a constant tendency to collapse, i.e. recoil away from the chest wall.

Recoil tendency of the lung is due to:

- Elastic tissue in the lungs is constantly stretched and it has a tendency to recoil. One-third of recoil tendency of the lungs is due to this cause.
- Surface tension of fluid lining the alveoli tends to cause collapse of each alveolar sac. Because it occurs in all the air sacs of lungs, the net effect is to cause lungs to recoil away from the chest. Surface tension force is responsible for two-third of the total recoil tendency of the lungs.

Thus, lungs are constantly tending to move inward from their stretched position and thoracic wall is tending to move outward from its compressed position. These two opposing forces tend to cause infinitesimal enlargement of the fluid-filled intrapleural space between them. But fluid cannot expand the way air can and so even this tiny enlargement of intrapleural space drops the intrapleural pressure below atmospheric pressure. In this way elastic recoil of both lungs and the chest wall creates the subatmospheric (negative) intrapleural pressure that keeps them from moving apart more than a tiny amount.

What is surface tension? What is its effect on the lungs?

The force that tends to minimize the surface area at the interface is known as surface tension.

This is caused due to unbalanced attraction of surface molecules by the molecules below the surface. In the lungs, surface tension at the fluid-air interface of alveolus has a tendency to reduce the size of each alveolus, thus resulting in recoil tendency of the lung.

What is a surfactant? What is its action?

Surfactant is a substance which reduces the surface tension at the interface because of adsorption of surface active molecules at the interface.

Name the surfactant present in the lungs. What are its functions?

Surfactant present in the lungs is a complex mixture of several phospholipids, proteins and ions. Diapalmitoyl-phosphatidylcholine along with several other phospholipids is responsible for reducing surface tension. One portion of each phospholipid molecule is hydrophilic and dissolves in the water lining the alveoli. Lipid hydrophobic portion of the molecule is oriented toward the air. This causes spreading of surfactant molecules over the surface of fluid lining the alveoli. Apo-proteins and calcium ions are responsible for uniform and quick spreading of surfactant molecules over the surface.

Hydrophobic surface exposed to air has one-twelfth to one-half the surface tension of a pure water surface. The exact surface tension depends upon the concentration and orientation of surfactant molecules on the surface.

Normal fluid lining the alveoli has a surface tension (without surfactant) of 50 dynes/cm². Fluid lining alveoli with surfactant included has a surface tension between 5 and 30 dynes/cm².

What are the functions of surfactant?

FUNCTIONS OF SURFACTANT

1. The surface tension in a thin-walled sphere as alveolus tends to make the sphere smaller or to collapse. By reducing surface tension, surfactant reduces the tendency of alveoli to collapse.
2. Due to reduction in surface tension, the mean alveolar radius is increased (Laplace's law). This reduces the transmural pressure required for expanding the alveoli. In other words, it reduces work of breathing as alveoli are easily expanded.
3. Surfactant prevents pulmonary oedema, i.e. excess collection of fluid in alveoli and interstitial space surrounding alveoli. Surface tension is a retracting force which not only pulls alveolar wall to the centre of alveolus but also pulls fluid from capillaries which leads to pulmonary oedema. With reduction in surface tension by the surfactant, the inward force drawing fluid out of the capillaries is reduced and therefore pulmonary oedema is prevented.
4. Surfactant also causes stability of alveoli, i.e. it maintains almost uniform size of alveoli. Pulling pressure of 18 cm of H2O is reduced to 4 cm of H_2O due to surfactant.

Instability due to surface tension effect is produced as follows:

If air passages leading to alveoli are blocked and two air spaces are connected to each other, the amount of pressure generated in each is given by the following formula (Laplace's law):

$$\text{Pressure} = \frac{2 \times \text{Surface tension}}{\text{Radius}}$$

Naturally, if surface tension remains constant, smaller the radius greater will be the pressure. Between the two connected alveolar sacs if one is smaller than the other, pressure developed in the smaller will be more than that in the larger. This will cause pushing of air from smaller alveolar sac to a larger sac, resulting in smaller sac to become still smaller and larger sac to become still larger. As stated above, this will also result into air being pushed from the smaller to the larger sac. This cycle will continue till the smaller sac totally collapses leading to large distension of the other sac, thereby producing instability of alveoli (alveoli having different sizes). Effect of radius on size is as follows: smaller the alveolus greater is its tendency to collapse, whereas larger the alveolus lesser is the tendency to collapse (greater tendency to get distended).

The presence of surfactant prevents instability of alveoli in the following way.

If alveolus becomes larger in size the surfactant molecules are scattered on the larger surface (as number of molecules is limited). This causes lesser reduction in surface tension and therefore according to Laplace's law increases the tendency of alveolus to collapse by causing a rise in collapse pressure. This opposes the effect of increase in radius and prevents change in size of alveolus and alveolar sac.

If alveolus becomes smaller in size, the surfactant molecules form the thicker layer on the surface and cause greater reduction in surface tension and therefore according to Laplace's law the tendency of alveolus (or sac) to expand by causing reduction in collapse pressure. This opposes or neutralizes the effect caused by reduction in radius and helps in maintaining the size of alveolus or sac constant.

Thus, due to surfactant stability of alveoli is maintained.

What is respiratory distress syndrome?

Respiratory distress syndrome (RDS) is the condition seen in newborn babies due to inadequate formation of surfactant. In this condition, it is extremely difficult to expand the lungs. Respiratory work is greatly increased and there is inadequate exchange of gases due to alveolar instability and pulmonary oedema. This results in severe respiratory insufficiency.

What is atelectasis?

Alveolar collapse in part of the lung is known as atelectasis.

What is adult respiratory distress syndrome?

Trauma, shock and systemic infections cause abnormal surfactant function in the adults, leading to adult RDS.

What are the effects of intrapleural pressure on cardiovascular system?

When negativity of intrapleural pressure increases (during inspiration), mediastinal pressure also becomes more negative leading to expansion of thin walled structures in the thorax, especially large veins (superior and inferior vena cava), and thereby decreasing pressure in them. This causes blood to be sucked into these veins from extrathoracic regions. Thus there is increased venous return to the heart during inspiration due to suction action of respiratory pump. Descent of the diaphragm during inspiration causes a slight rise in intra-abdominal pressure, thereby further increasing the pressure gradient between abdomen and thorax. Increase in venous return to the heart during inspiration increases the cardiac output. The respiratory pump action is especially marked during muscular exercise.

During violent expiratory efforts, particularly with closed glottis (as in Valsalva manoeuvre, severe bouts of cough in old people), exactly reverse occurs. The positive intrapleural pressure which occurs in these conditions leads to marked decrease in venous return and therefore also the cardiac output. Fall in cardiac output leads to cerebral ischaemia, visual blackouts and unconsciousness.

Under what circumstances does intrapleural pressure become positive?

When expiratory muscles are working against closed glottis, intrapleural pressure can become positive (greater than the atmospheric pressure), e.g. during defaecation and coughing. It also becomes positive when there is injury to the chest causing exposure of pleural cavity to the exterior. Atmospheric air is then sucked into the cavity.

INTRA-ALVEOLAR PRESSURE

What is intra-alveolar pressure? How does it vary during normal tidal respiration?

Pressure of air inside the alveoli is called intra-alveolar pressure. When lungs expand (during inspiration), it becomes -1 cm of H_2O whereas when lungs contract (during expiration), it becomes $+1$ cm of H_2O. At the end of normal inspiration, it is zero (i.e. equal to atmospheric), at which time air is not flowing either in or out of the lungs.

When is alveolar pressure equal to atmospheric pressure?

At the end of expiration or at the end of inspiration, there is no air flow and pressure in alveoli and atmosphere is same.

TRANSPULMONARY PRESSURE

What is transpulmonary pressure?

Transpulmonary pressure is the pressure inside the lung (intra-alveolar pressure) minus the pressure just outside the lung (intrapleural pressure).

APPLIED ASPECT

What is pleural effusion?

Pleural effusion means collection of large amount of free fluid in pleural space. Common causes:

- Cardiac failure.
- Reduced plasma colloid osmotic pressure.
- Blockage of lymphatics draining from pleural cavity.
- Infection or any other cause of inflammation of pleural surfaces of pleural cavity.

What is pneumothorax?

Pressure of air in pleural cavity is known as pneumothorax. Air enters either through a rupture in lung or a hole in chest wall.

COMPLIANCE

What is compliance of the lungs? How much is it?

Compliance is change in volume of the lung per unit change in transpulmonary pressure. Normally it is 0.13 L/cm of H_2O (for lungs and thorax together). It is 0.22 L/cm of H_2O for lungs alone.

How do you measure lung compliance?

Intra-oesophageal balloon is passed in a person for recording intrapleural pressure. A person is asked to inspire in steps (taking in about 50 to 100 ml of air with each step). At the end of each step, intra-oesophageal pressure is recorded. These points are plotted on the graph of pressure against volume and inspiratory compliance curve is obtained (Fig. 7.3). Similarly, expiration is also done in steps and expiratory compliance curve is obtained.

The slope (steepness) of this pressure-volume curve denotes compliance.

$$\text{Compliance} = \frac{\Delta V}{\Delta P}$$

where, ΔV = change in volume of the lung.
ΔP = change in transpulmonary pressure.

The inspiratory and expiratory compliance curves do not coincide. This type of curve is called hysteresis curve. Difference in stretchability of lung in expiratory and inspiratory phases accounts for this type of curve. It is clear from the graph that at identical intrapleural pressure, volume of lung is less in inspiratory phase than that in expiratory phase.

The compliance measured in this way is static compliance.

Clinically, the term specific compliance is used:

$$\text{Specific compliance} = \frac{\text{Compliance}}{\text{Functional residual capacity}}$$

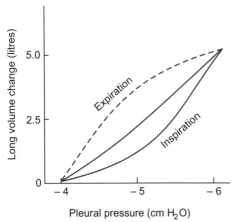

FIGURE 7.3 Compliance diagram in a normal person.

Specific compliance is therefore the compliance of the lung at relaxation volume (the point at the end of a tidal expiration) expressed per litre of functional residual capacity (FRC). For example, if static compliance is 0.2 L/cm H_2O and FRC is 2500 ml, specific compliance is 0.2/2.5, i.e. equal to 0.08 L/cm of H_2O.

Though the compliance is a measure of distensibility there is a fallacy. If in a person one lung is removed surgically, static compliance becomes half, i.e. 0.1 L/cm of H_2O though remaining lung is normal, healthy and distensible. This discrepancy becomes more important in interpreting the lung compliance of a child (lung compliance itself is less for small lungs as compared to that for large lungs, and it is less the more the lungs in the given subject are inflated). This discrepancy is removed by expressing the compliance as specific compliance as explained above. Specific compliance therefore gives a clear idea of distensibility of lungs.

How much is the compliance of the thorax?
Compliance of thorax is 0.11 L/cm of H_2O.

APPLIED ASPECT

Name the clinical conditions which reduce the compliance of the lungs.
Compliance of the lungs is reduced in lung diseases like tuberculosis, abscess, RDS (respiratory distress syndrome). These diseases result in decrease in functional lung tissue and are therefore known as restrictive lung diseases.

In which condition is compliance of the lungs increased?
Chronic obstructive lung diseases lead to increased lung compliance. This is because there is dissolution of alveolar septa which leads to increase in air space size (emphysema), but as the total surface area available for exchange of gases is reduced, it is not advantageous.

WORK OF BREATHING

How do you define work of breathing?
Energy generated by respiratory muscles to overcome the resistance in thorax and respiratory tract is known as work of breathing.

What is airway resistance?
Resistance caused by friction of gas molecules between themselves and the walls of the airways is called airway resistance.

What is tissue resistance?
Resistance offered by the tissues as they expand or contract is called tissue resistance.

Name the factors affecting airway resistance.
Airway resistance is determined by:

- *Rate of gas flow.* Greater the rate of gas flow, greater is the resistance. Resistance offered by intermediate size branch is highest because of velocity.

- *Airway diameter.* It is the most important factor. Smaller the diameter of the airway, greater is the resistance. Airway diameter increases when lungs expand (during inspiration), and it decreases when lungs contract (during expiration).
- In the body, diameter of airway is controlled by autonomic nervous system. Sympathetic system causes bronchodilation and parasympathetic system causes bronchoconstriction. Substance P, neurokinins A and B cause bronchoconstriction and may be causative agents in bronchial asthma.
- *Length of airway.* It does not show much change during respiration or in lung diseases and therefore is not an important factor.

What is the work of breathing?

Work of breathing is work done by the respiratory muscles during pulmonary ventilation. The work done by respiratory muscles is expressed as pressure multiplied by volume. During tidal expiration no work is done because relaxation of contracted respiratory muscles causes tidal expiration.

The work of inspiration is divided into three fractions (Fig. 7.4).

1. **Compliance work.** Work required to expand the lungs against the lung and chest elastic forces. As shown in Figure 7.4, it is calculated by multiplying volume of expansion times the average pressure required to cause expansion. This is equal to area of triangle represented in Figure 7.4.

$$\text{Compliance work} = \frac{\Delta P \times \Delta V}{2}$$

where ΔV is increase in volume and ΔP is the change in intrapleural pressure.

2. **Tissue resistance work.** It is the work required to overcome the viscosity of the lungs.

3. **Airway resistance work.** This is the work required to overcome the resistance to air flow through respiratory passageways.

It is clear from Figure 7.4 that during normal quiet breathing, most of the work is utilized simply to expand lungs and only small percentage of work is used to overcome tissue resistance and airway resistance.

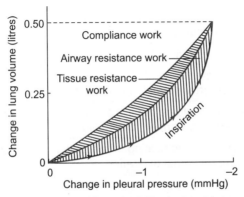

FIGURE 7.4 Graphical representation of three different types of work accomplished during inspiration.

In pulmonary diseases usually all types of work are frequently increased. Compliance work and tissue resistance work are especially increased by diseases causing fibrosis of the lungs.

Airway resistance is greatly increased in obstructive lung diseases such as bronchial asthma.

During quiet breathing no work is done during expiration. But in heavy breathing or when airway resistance and tissue resistance are high, expiratory work does occur and at times it may become more than inspiratory work.

VENTILATION

What is pulmonary ventilation?

Pulmonary ventilation is a cyclic process by which fresh air enters lungs and equal volume of air is exhaled. It is volume of air taken in or given out during normal tidal respiration.

What is the importance of recording lung volumes and capacities?

Recording of lung volumes and capacities is one of the important lung function tests (Table 7.1).

Table 7.1	Lung Volumes and Capacities (see also Fig. 7.5)	
Lung Volumes		
Name	**Definition**	**Normal Value (adult male)**
Tidal Volumes (TV)	Volume of air that is taken in or given out during normal quiet respiration	500 ml
Inspiratory Reserve Volume (IRV)	Maximum volume of air that can be taken in over and above the tidal volume	3000 ml
Expiratory Reserve Volume (ERV)	Maximum volume of air that can be expired over and above the tidal volume	1100 ml
Residual Volume (RV)	Volume of air that remains in the lungs after forceful expiration	1200 ml
Lung Capacities		
Inspiratory Capacity (IC) = TV + IRV	Maximum volume of air that can be inspired after normal tidal expiration	3500 ml
Expiratory Capacity (EC) = TV + ERV	Maximum volume of air that can be expired after normal tidal inspiration	1600 ml
Functional Residual Capacity (FRC) = RV + ERV	Volume of air remaining in the lungs after normal tidal expiration	2300 ml
Vital Capacity (VC) = IRV + TV + ERV	Maximum volume of air that can be expired after deepest possible inspiration	4600 ml

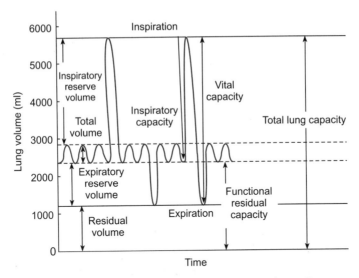

FIGURE 7.5 Spirogram: record of lung volumes and capacities.

How are volumes and capacities of the lungs recorded?

All volumes and capacities except residual volume, functional residual capacity and total lung capacity are recorded by spirometer (Fig. 7.6). Functional residual capacity is determined by nitrogen wash-out method or helium dilution method and then residual volume and total lung capacity are calculated.

Describe the recording of lung volumes and capacities by spirometry.

A spirometer (Fig. 7.6) consists of a drum inverted over a chamber of water. The drum is counterbalanced by a weight with the help of a string passing from upper part of drum over a pulley. The drum can be filled with air or O_2. It is connected outside to a mouthpiece for recording; the nose of the subject is closed by a nose-clip. Mouthpiece is put in the mouth. Thus the subject is connected to a spirometer. When a subject breathes in and out of the air chamber, the drum rises and falls. This movement is recorded on a moving sheet of paper by attaching pen to the string.

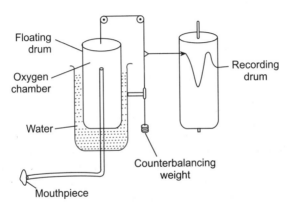

FIGURE 7.6 Spirometer.

With this simple spirometer, the recording is done for a short time because of collection of excess CO_2 in the chamber which causes suffocation. To avoid this, a soda lime tower is put in a spirometer. This tower absorbs CO_2 and therefore does not allow its excess collection in the chamber.

The spirometer records tidal volume, inspiratory reserve volume, expiratory reserve volume, inspiratory capacity, expiratory capacity and vital capacity. Recording of residual volume, functional residual capacity and total lung capacity is not possible with a spirometer.

What is the significance of residual volume or functional residual capacity?

Some amount of air is always present in the lungs because of residual volume (RV) or FRC, and therefore continuous exchange of gases is made possible and thereby concentrations of O_2 and CO_2 in blood are maintained constant.

What is the significance of vital capacity? Enumerate the factors affecting vital capacity.

Vital capacity is a very important lung function test. It is influenced by:

1. **Position in which vital capacity is recorded.** Greater reading is obtained when it is recorded in standing position as compared to when recorded in lying down position. This is because in lying down position abdominal contents push the diaphragm upwards, i.e. towards the thoracic cavity, causing lesser expansion of thorax.

2. **Sex.** In females, all volumes and capacities are 25% lesser than in males.

3. **Body build.** Vital capacity is higher in tall and thin people as compared to short and obese people.

4. **Compliance of the lung.** If by any disease, compliance of the lung is reduced, vital capacity is reduced.

Describe the methods used for measuring functional residual capacity (FRC).

Methods used for measuring FRC are:

1. *Nitrogen wash-out method.* At the end of normal expiration, the person is asked to inhale O_2 for a few minutes. During this period, expired air is collected and analysed for N_2 content and from this FRC is calculated:

$$FRC = N_2 \text{ content} \times \frac{100}{80}$$

N_2 content of air present in the lungs at the beginning of the experiment is 80%.

2. *Helium dilution method.* A spirometer of known volume is filled with a mixture of helium and air at a known concentration. If concentration of helium is C_1 and volume of spirometer is V_1.

Amount of helium in spirometer $= C_1 V_1$.

The person is connected to a spirometer at the end of normal expiration (when the volume of air present in the lungs is equal to FRC, say V_2). As the person begins to breathe from the spirometer, the gases in spirometer begin to mix with the gases in the lungs, and helium in the spirometer becomes diluted by functional residual capacity. Helium, however, does not leak out as it is a closed circuit method. After some time, degree of dilution is determined by finding out concentration of helium in spirometer. Say it is C_2.

∴ Final volume of helium is $C_2V_1 + C_2V_2$.

This final volume of helium is the same as initial volume, i.e. C_1V_1. Therefore,

$$C_1V_1 = C_2V_1 + C_2V_2$$
$$C_2V_2 = C_1V_1 - C_2V_1$$
$$\therefore C_2V_2 = V_1(C_1 - C_2)$$
$$\therefore V_2 = \frac{V_1(C_1 - C_2)}{C_1}$$
$$\therefore V_2 = V_1\left(\frac{C_1}{C_2} - \frac{C_2}{C_2}\right)$$
$$\therefore V_2 = V_1\left(\frac{C_1}{C_2} - 1\right)$$
$$\therefore V_2 = FRC = V_1\left(\frac{C_1}{C_2} - 1\right)$$

What is the maximum expiratory flow rate? What is its value? How does it change during lung diseases?

When a person takes deepest inspiration and expires with great force, the expiratory flow rate reaches the maximum, beyond which the flow rate cannot be increased with increased additional effort. During expiration when there is compression of lungs, pressure is applied to the outsides of alveoli and bronchioles. Compression of alveoli increases the expiratory flow rate but at the same time bronchioles also collapse, this reduces their diameters and increases airway resistance. When increased airway resistance totally opposes the effect of increased alveolar pressure, no further increase in expiratory flow rate can occur even if the person expires with a greater force. Thus, expiratory flow rate reaches the maximum value. The normal maximum expiratory flow rate is 400 L/min (Fig. 7.7).

In constrictive lung disease, the lung volume becomes smaller and there is reduction in total lung capacity (TLC) and residual volume (RV). Because the lung cannot expand to its normal volume, even on enlargement of lung the bronchi and bronchioles are held open partially by way of elastic pull during maximum inspiration. On expiration these partially opened bronchi and bronchioles are collapsed more easily by external pressure. This reduces maximum expiratory flow rate (Fig. 7.7).

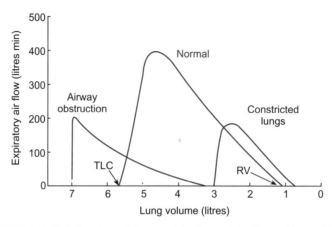

FIGURE 7.7 Expiratory flow rate in normal, in airway obstruction and in constricted lungs.

In obstructive lung diseases it is still more difficult to expire because of greater than normal tendency of bronchi and bronchioles to collapse. But during inspiration, bronchi and bronchioles get distended due to elastic pull caused by negative pleural pressure. Therefore, maximum expiratory flow rate is lesser than normal. In long standing obstructive lung diseases there is emphysema (dissolution of alveolar septa leading to larger size of alveolar sac), which causes increase in total lung capacity (TLC) and residual volume (RV). There will, however, be reduction in maximum expiratory flow rate as explained above (Fig. 7.7).

What is the forced expiratory vital capacity (FVC)? What is the forced expiratory volume (FEV)? What is their significance?

Forced expiratory vital capacity (FVC) is also termed timed vital capacity. In recording FVC, the person is first asked to take maximum inspiration and is then asked to expire in a spirometer with maximum respiratory effort as rapidly and as completely as possible. The record is obtained on a fast moving drum (Fig. 8.8). Down stroke of the record as recorded against time represents FVC.

In graphs A and B (Fig. 7.8), the total volume changes of the forced vital capacities are nearly equal. There is, however, a major difference if one calculates amount of air that comes out after first, second and third second, especially during the first second. It is therefore customary to compare the recorded forced expiratory volume during first second (FEV_1) with the normal. In a normal person, percentage of forced expiratory vital capacity (FEV_1/FVC) expired in first second is 80%. In airway obstruction it can reduce to up to 47% (Fig. 7.8).

What is respiratory minute volume (RMV)?

Volume of air that is taken in or given out per minute during normal tidal respiration is RMV.

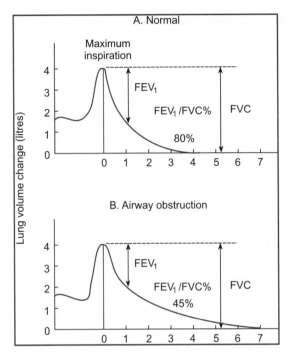

FIGURE 7.8 Recording of a forced vital capacity: (a) Normal, (b) Airway obstruction.

$$RMV = \text{Respiratory rate} \times \text{Tidal volume}$$
$$= 12 \times 500 \text{ ml}$$
$$= 6000 \text{ ml/min } (6 \text{ L/min}).$$

What is maximum ventilatory volume (MVV)?

Maximum ventilatory volume (MVV) is the maximum volume of air that can be taken in or given out per minute. It is about 120 L/min.

What is breathing reserve (BR)?

Breathing reserve is the difference between maximum ventilatory volume and respiratory minute volume.

$$BR = MVV - RMV.$$

DEAD SPACE AIR

What is dead space air?

The portion of each breath that does not take part in exchange of gases is called dead space air. It is of two types:

- Anatomical
- Physiological

What is anatomical dead space air?

Volume of air that fills the respiratory passage (from nose to terminal bronchioles) is known as anatomical dead space air. It is 150 ml in a normal adult male.

What is physiological dead space air?

Physiological dead space air is the addition of anatomical dead space air and alveolar dead space air (sometimes few alveoli are not adequately perfused with blood: V_A/Q ratio is more than normal and part of the alveolar air is not utilized for exchange of gases and forms alveolar dead space air).

In a normal person, all alveoli are supposed to be functional and therefore anatomical dead space air is equal to physiological dead space air.

How do you measure anatomical dead space air?

Anatomical dead space air is measured by single breath nitrogen wash-out test in which person is asked to inspire pure O_2 (Fig. 7.9). He expires in a nitrogen meter which continuously records nitrogen concentration in the expired air. From the graph of volume of air expired against concentration of N_2, anatomical dead space air is calculated.

In Figure 7.9, area covered by hatching (A) represents the area that has no nitrogen in it. This area is a measure of dead space air. Following formula is used for measurement.

$$V_D = \frac{\text{Area of hatching (A)}}{\text{Area of hatching (A)} + \text{Area of dots (B)}} \times V_E$$

where,

V_D = Dead space air.

V_E = Total volume of air expired.

If V_E = 500 ml, area A = 30 cm^2 and area B = 70 cm^2 then

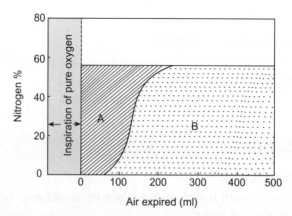

FIGURE 7.9 Continuous tracing of the change in nitrogen concentration in the expired air following a previous inspiration of pure O_2 (for calculating dead space air).

$$\text{Dead space air } (V_D) = \frac{30}{30 + 70} \times 500$$
$$= 150 \text{ ml.}$$

How do you measure physiological dead space air?

Physiological dead space air is calculated from Bohr's equation. This equation is based on the fact that inspired air contains negligible quantity of CO_2 (almost zero). Therefore, all the CO_2 in expired air is derived from functional alveoli. Equation is as follows:

Tidal volume $\times$ PCO_2 in expired air

$= (TV - X) \times$ average PCO_2 in alveolar air $+ (X \times PCO_2$ in inspired air, i.e. zero)

where, X $=$ Physiological dead space air.

ALVEOLAR VENTILATION

What is alveolar air?

Volume of air which is available for exchange of gases in alveoli per breath is called alveolar air.

$$\text{Alveolar air} = \text{Tidal volume} - \text{dead space air}$$
$$= 500 \text{ ml} - 150 \text{ ml}$$
$$= 350 \text{ ml.}$$

What is alveolar ventilation?

Rate at which alveoli get ventilated per minute is alveolar ventilation. It is 350 ml $\times$ 12 $= 4.2$ L/min.

How are alveolar air and expired air collected?

Collection of alveolar air. Alveolar air sample is collected by Haldane and Priestley's tube.
Collection of expired air. Expired air is collected in Douglas bag.

Why is composition of alveolar air different than that of atmospheric air?

Alveolar air composition is different than that of atmospheric air because:

- There is continuous exchange of gases at the respiratory membrane. This decreases O_2 concentration and increases CO_2 concentration of alveolar air.
- As air passes through respiratory passage, it gets humidified. Water vapour pressure rises to 47 mmHg. As total pressure remains the same, pressure of different gases decreases as air passes into alveoli.
- With each breath only 1/7th of the alveolar air is replaced by fresh air.

Give PO$_2$ and PCO$_2$ of alveolar air.

$$PO_2 = 104 \text{ mmHg}$$
$$PCO_2 = 40 \text{ mmHg.}$$

V$_A$/Q RATIO

What is V$_A$/Q ratio? How much is it?

V$_A$/Q ratio is the ratio of alveolar ventilation per minute to quantity of blood supplied to alveoli per minute.

$$\text{Normal ratio} = \frac{\text{Alveolar ventilation/min}}{\text{Amount of blood supplied/min}}$$

$$\frac{4 \text{ L}}{5 \text{ L}} = 0.8.$$

At this ratio (0.8), there is maximum oxygenation of blood.

What is the effect of increased V$_A$/Q ratio?

Increased V$_A$/Q ratio means rate of ventilation is more as compared to rate of blood flow. This produces alveolar dead space formation because extra air in alveoli goes waste owing to relative decrease in rate of blood flow, i.e. this air is not utilized for gaseous exchange and becomes alveolar dead space air. There will also be change in the composition of alveolar air as shown in Figure 7.8. When V$_A$/Q ratio increases to infinity, i.e. when rate of blood flow becomes zero, no exchange of gases can occur and alveolar air composition will be the same as that of humidified air composition (PO$_2$ = 149 mmHg and PCO$_2$ = almost zero). Thus increased V$_A$/Q ratio will have following effects:

- Decreased exchange of gases at respiratory membrane.
- Alveolar dead space formation.
- Change in alveolar air composition (Fig. 7.8).

What is the effect of decreased V$_A$/Q ratio?

- Decreased V$_A$/Q ratio means rate of blood flow is more as compared to rate of alveolar ventilation. The part of blood therefore will remain deoxygenated as there is not enough ventilation to provide oxygen needed to oxygenate fully the blood flowing through alveolar capillaries. The fraction or part of venous blood that does not get oxygenated while passing through pulmonary capillaries is termed shunted blood. This shunted blood plus the additional blood flowing through bronchial vessels (2% of cardiac output) forms the physiological shunt (total quantity of shunted blood per minute). When V$_A$/Q ratio becomes zero, i.e. ventilation is zero, air in alveolus comes to equilibrium with blood oxygen and carbon dioxide because these gases diffuse between blood and alveoli. As there is no ventilation, alveolar air

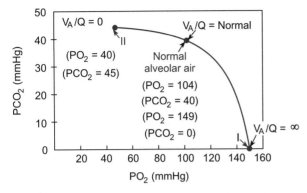

FIGURE 7.10 The normal $PO_2 - PCO_2$, V_A/Q diagram.

PO_2 and PCO_2 will be equal to those of venous blood ($PO_2 = 149$ mmHg and $PCO_2 =$ almost 0 mmHg). Exchange of gases in this situation will be zero. Thus decrease in V_A/Q ratio has following effects:

- Decreased exchange of gases at the respiratory membrane.
- Shunting of part of venous blood.
- Change in alveolar air composition (Fig. 7.10).

What are variations in V_A/Q ratio in normal lung?

In normal person in upright position, blood flow and alveolar ventilation are less in upper parts of the lungs, but blood flow is much lesser than ventilation, thus causing V_A/Q ratio to change 2.5 times more than normal value (causing moderate degree of physiologic dead space).

In lower part of the lung, there is lesser ventilation with respect to blood flow, causing the V_A/Q ratio to decrease 1.6 times the normal value and hence resulting in physiological shunt.

APPLIED ASPECT

Give examples of obstructive lung diseases.

- Emphysema.
- Bronchitis.
- Bronchial asthma.

Give examples of constrictive lung diseases.

- Asbestosis.
- Lung resection.
- Idiopathic pulmonary fibrosis.

What are the effects of chronic emphysema?*

In emphysema, which occurs on long standing obstructive lung diseases, following effects are seen:

- Increased airway resistance due to bronchiolar obstruction.
- Loss of alveolar walls causes decrease in the diffusing capacity of lung.

*For details refer Vaz M, Kurpad A, Raj T, editors. *Guyton & Hall Textbook of Medical Physiology*. Elsevier: New Delhi, 2013, p. 386.

- Abnormal V_A/Q ratio in different regions of lungs causing defective gaseous exchange.
- Pulmonary vascular resistance increases due to decrease in number of pulmonary capillaries causing pulmonary hypertension.

What are the effects of pneumonia?*

Pneumonia is an inflammatory condition of lung (pneumococci). Infection begins in alveoli and respiratory membrane becomes inflamed. Infected alveoli become progressively filled with fluid and cells. Infection spreads from one alveolus to next. There are two major pulmonary abnormalities:

- Reduction in surface area of respiratory membrane.
- Decreased V_A/Q ratio.

What are the effects of bronchial asthma?[†]

It is characterized by spastic contraction of smooth muscles in bronchioles which causes difficulty in breathing. Common cause is contractile hypersensitivity of bronchioles in response to foreign particles, substances, etc.

There is (a) localized oedema in small bronchioles and (b) spasm of bronchiolar smooth muscle. Thus airway resistance increases.

As bronchiolar diameter is reduced during expiration; there is difficulty in expiring than inspiring the air. Thus there is greatly reduced maximum expiratory flow rate and reduced timed expiratory volume. Long standing diseases result in emphysema. Chest becomes barrel shaped as FRC and residual volume are increased permanently.

DIFFUSION OF GASES

RESPIRATORY MEMBRANE

Describe the respiratory membrane.

Membranes of respiratory bronchioles, alveolar ducts and alveoli are termed collectively as respiratory membrane. The total surface area of respiratory membrane is about 70 m² in normal adult. Total quantity of blood at any given instance is 60 to 140 ml in lung capillaries. Thus small quantity of blood spreads over a large surface area allowing rapid exchange of gases.
Respiratory membrane has the following layers:

- Layer of fluid lining alveolus with monomolecular layer of surfactant.
- Alveolar epithelium.
- Alveolar basement membrane.

---

*For details refer Vaz M, Kurpad A, Raj T, editors. *Guyton & Hall Textbook of Medical Physiology*. Elsevier: New Delhi, 2013, p. 387.
[†]For details refer Vaz M, Kurpad A, Raj T, editors. *Guyton & Hall Textbook of Medical Physiology*. Elsevier: New Delhi, 2013, p. 388.

- A thin interstitial space filled with fluid between alveolar epithelium and capillary membrane.
- Capillary basement membrane (at certain places it is fused with alveolar basement membrane).
- Capillary endothelium.

Though there are many layers overall thickness of respiratory membrane is 0.6 microns.

As O_2 and CO_2 are lipid-soluble gases, they easily pass through the cell membrane. So passage of gases through respiratory membrane is equivalent to passage of gases through fluid (or water) and therefore depends upon solubility of gases in water.

The size of pulmonary capillary is about 5 microns and RBCs have to squeeze to pass through them. Red cell membrane usually touches capillary membrane, so that O_2 and CO_2 need not pass through significant amount of plasma to reach red cell. This also increases rapidity of diffusion.

FACTORS AFFECTING DIFFUSION OF GASES

Describe the factors affecting gaseous exchange at the respiratory membrane.

1. *Thickness of respiratory membrane.* Rate of diffusion is inversely proportional to the thickness of membrane. Any factor which increases thickness will therefore significantly decrease gaseous exchange, e.g.
   - *Pulmonary oedema.* Excess collection of fluid in alveoli and the surrounding interstitial fluid.
   - *Fibrosis of the lungs.* Certain lung diseases cause fibrosis of the lung at the affected site. Fibrosis increases the thickness at the site and therefore hampers exchange of gases.

2. *Surface area of respiratory membrane.* Rate of diffusion is directly proportional to the surface area, i.e. with decrease in surface area, the rate of diffusion of gases decreases, e.g.
   - Removal of one entire lung reduces surface area to half the normal.
   - Emphysema. In long standing obstructive lung diseases, lung becomes emphysematous. In obstructive lung disease, there is a greater tendency of bronchi and bronchioles to collapse. During inspiration, due to distension of lungs, bronchi and bronchioles are also distended. This causes normal quantity of air to enter into alveoli but during expiration, because bronchi and bronchioles collapse more easily than normal, greatly increased airway resistance diminishes the rate of air flow and total amount of air coming out in expiration becomes less. Thus, with each breath some amount of air is trapped in alveoli. In long standing obstructive disease, this causes dissolution of alveolar septa. Sac becomes larger and contains more amount of air but its surface area is reduced leading to emphysema.

3. *Diffusion coefficient.* The diffusion of respiratory gases is equivalent to diffusion of gases through fluid (or water) because O_2 and CO_2 (main respiratory gases) are

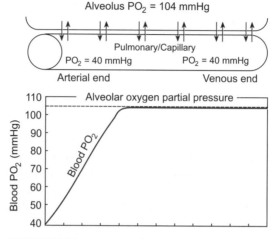

FIGURE 7.11 Uptake of O_2 by pulmonary capillary blood.

soluble in lipid and therefore can easily pass through the cell membrane. Diffusion coefficient of a gas in liquid is directly related to its solubility and inversely related to root of its molecular weight. Considering these two factors, diffusion coefficient of CO_2 through water (and therefore through fluid of respiratory membrane) is 20 times that for O_2. CO_2 therefore diffuses more easily through respiratory membrane.

4. ***Pressure gradient for gas across the respiratory membrane.*** Partial pressure of O_2 (PO_2) in alveolar air is 104 mmHg whereas that of blood is 40 mmHg. Pressure gradient therefore is 64 mmHg in the beginning, but as O_2 diffuses from alveoli to blood the PO_2 of blood goes on rising continues to increase and pressure gradient becomes lesser and lesser. When PO_2 of blood becomes the same as is equal to that in alveolar air (104 mmHg), the gradient becomes zero and no diffusion occurs. By the time blood passes one-third of distance in capillary the PO_2 of blood equals that of alveoli. This means only for one-third of blood flow in capillary there is a pressure gradient. At the beginning it is 64 mmHg as stated above and with diffusion of O_2 it becomes lesser and lesser. Average pressure gradient is therefore calculated considering the pressure gradients at various sites and the time for which particular pressure gradient was present. This time integrated average pressure gradient is 11 mmHg for O_2. PO_2 in alveoli is higher than that of blood; therefore O_2 diffuses from alveoli to blood (Fig. 7.11).

In a similar manner, time integrated pressure gradient can be calculated for CO_2 across the respiratory membrane; it is only 1 mmHg. As PCO_2 is higher in blood than in alveolar air, CO_2 diffuses from blood to alveoli.

5. ***V_A/Q ratio.*** The gaseous exchange is maximum at the normal V_A/Q ratio of 0.8, as explained earlier. Increase or decrease in ratio decreases the exchange of gases through membrane.

In which diseases diffusion of gases across the respiratory membrane would suffer?

Diseases in which respiratory membrane thickness increases (e.g. pulmonary oedema) or surface area of the membrane is reduced (e.g. emphysema).

What is venous admixture?

PO_2 in pulmonary capillary blood is 104 mmHg but PO_2 in arterial blood is about 97 mmHg. The lower systemic arterial PO_2 is due to venous admixture, i.e. mixing of venous blood with arterial blood. About 2% of blood from systemic venous blood mixes with the pulmonary capillary blood. It occurs at the respiratory bronchioles which are supplied by systemic as well as pulmonary capillaries. There is further dilution of oxygenated blood because part of the coronary venous blood flows into the chambers of the left side of the heart (through thebesian veins).

DIFFUSING CAPACITY OF LUNGS

What is the diffusing capacity of lungs for a given gas?

Amount of gas that diffuses through respiratory membrane per minute per mmHg pressure gradient is called diffusing capacity of the lungs.

How is the diffusing capacity of lungs for O_2 measured?

Diffusing capacity of carbon monoxide (CO) is measured and from that diffusing capacity of O_2 is determined by multiplying diffusing capacity of CO by 1.23 because diffusion coefficient of O_2 is 1.23 times that of CO.

Why is carbon monoxide used for determination of diffusing capacity of O_2?

For determination of diffusing capacity of any gas, pressure gradient for that gas across the respiratory membrane must be determined. This is possible when one collects alveolar air and pulmonary capillary blood and determines partial pressure of gas in both.

But it is difficult to collect pulmonary capillary blood. When CO gas is used, pulmonary blood PCO can be considered as zero because CO combines with haemoglobin very rapidly and does not allow the pressure of CO to build up in plasma. Therefore, use of CO avoids the need for collection of pulmonary capillary blood.

TRANSPORT OF GASES

TRANSPORT OF OXYGEN

Describe the transport of O_2 from atmosphere to the tissues.

O_2 is transported from lungs to tissues due to constant circulation of blood and diffusion that occurs at various sites as follows:

1. *At lungs.* The lungs are ventilated constantly and therefore new atmospheric air enters the lung. As described earlier, the alveolar air composition is different than that of atmospheric but still PO_2 is maintained because of continuous renewal. PO_2 of alveolar air is 104 mmHg and that of venous blood flowing through pulmonary capillaries is 64 mmHg; owing to this pressure gradient O_2 diffuses from alveoli into the blood.

2. *At tissues.* (a) Arterial blood which passes to tissue has PO_2 97 mmHg (because of 2% venous admixture). Tissue fluid (interstitial fluid surrounding tissue cells) has PO_2 40 mmHg. O_2 diffuses from tissue capillaries to interstitial fluid because of this pressure gradient.

(b) Intracellular PO_2 varies from 0 to 60 mmHg depending upon the rate of metabolism of the cell (i.e. rate of utilization of O_2). On an average it is 23 mmHg which is lower than that of interstitial fluid (40 mmHg). As a result of this pressure gradient, O_2 diffuses from interstitial fluid to cell.

Thus, due to constant flow of blood and diffusion occurring at different sites, O_2 from atmosphere is transported to cell.

Name the forms in which O_2 is transported in blood.

O_2 is transported through blood in two forms:

- Dissolved in plasma (3%).
- In combination with haemoglobin (97%).

What is the importance of O_2 carried in dissolved state in blood?

Though only 3% of O_2 is carried in dissolved state, it plays an important role. Partial pressure of O_2 in blood is due to dissolved O_2. PO_2 of blood determines the amount of O_2 transported by haemoglobin. At the lungs when PO_2 is high, haemoglobin gets saturated with O_2 whereas at the tissues when PO_2 of blood decreases (because of O_2 in dissolved state diffusing to tissues), haemoglobin gets desaturated providing O_2 to the tissues.

Describe the carriage of O_2 by haemoglobin.

Haemoglobin combines with O_2 reversibly, to form oxyhaemoglobin. This combination is termed oxygenation (and not oxidation). When O_2 is released from oxyhaemoglobin, it is termed reduced or deoxygenated haemoglobin.

Oxygen combines with iron ion of haemoglobin. One molecule of O_2 combines with one iron ion. Because there are four iron ions in one haemoglobin molecule (denoted as Hb4), it combines with four molecules of O_2. The reaction proceeds as:

1. $Hb_4 + O_2 \rightarrow Hb_4O_2$
2. $Hb_4O_2 + O_2 \rightarrow Hb_4O_4$
3. $Hb_4O_4 + O_2 \rightarrow Hb_4O_6$
4. $Hb_4O_6 + O_2 \rightarrow Hb_4O_8$

After each reaction, affinity of haemoglobin for O_2 increases; it is greatly increased especially after third reaction, i.e. formation of Hb_4O_6.

One gram of haemoglobin can combine with 1.34 ml of O_2 and at this stage haemoglobin is 100% saturated. If one gram of haemoglobin combines with 0.67 ml of O_2, it is said to be 50% saturated. The percentage saturation of haemoglobin is calculated as:

$$\text{Percentage saturation} = \frac{O_2 \text{ content of blood/100 ml}}{O_2 \text{ carrying capacity of blood}} \times 100$$

What is the shape of O₂ dissociation curve of haemoglobin?

Though saturation of haemoglobin with O$_2$ depends on partial pressure of O$_2$ in the surrounding fluid, relationship between PO$_2$ and haemoglobin saturation is not linear. O$_2$ dissociation curve for haemoglobin is sigmoid or 'S' shaped.

What are the advantages of sigmoid shape of O₂ dissociation curve?

O$_2$ dissociation curve has the plateau above 60 mmHg. This provides the margin of safety. PO$_2$ in the blood can vary from 60 to 300 mmHg but yet O$_2$ content of blood does not vary significantly. That means this allows great atmospheric varia- tion in PO$_2$ (60 to 300 mmHg), without affecting O$_2$ supply to the tissues.

Below 60 mmHg there is a steep portion of the curve, i.e. slight decrease in PO$_2$ will cause greater release of O$_2$ from haemoglobin (Figs 7.12 and 7.13). This allows haemoglobin to release O$_2$ readily at tissues (as PO$_2$ is low in tissues). With slight decrease in tissue PO$_2$ (due to increased O$_2$ consumption), there is greater release of O$_2$ which minimizes decrease of tissue PO$_2$ that would otherwise take place. Thus it will also regulate tissue PO$_2$ (buffering action).

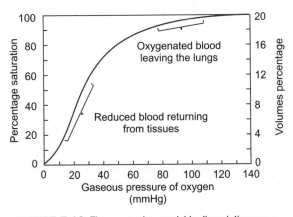

FIGURE 7.12 The oxygen-haemoglobin dissociation curve.

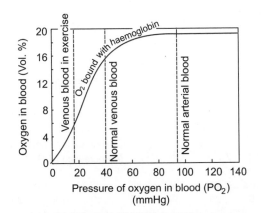

FIGURE 7.13 Effect of blood PO$_2$ on the quantity of oxygen bound to haemoglobin in each 100 ml of blood.

In summary, sigmoid shape of the curve is beneficial because:

- It allows greater uptake of O_2 at lungs despite great atmospheric variation in PO_2.
- Tissues are supplied O_2 according to their needs.
- Haemoglobin acts as a buffer and maintains tissue PO_2 at about 40 mmHg.

Why is O_2 dissociation curve sigmoid shaped?

Sigmoid shape of curve is due to:

- Presence of haemoglobin in red blood cells.
- Haemoglobin combines with four molecules of O_2. When first three molecules of O_2 combine with haemoglobin, its affinity for O_2 is greatly increased and the reaction occurs very rapidly.

What is meant by shift of O_2 dissociation curve to right? Enumerate the causes of such a shift. Is this shift advantageous?

Shifting of O_2 dissociation curve to the right means decreased affinity of haemoglobin for O_2 (Fig. 7.14).

The factors causing right shift are:

- Increased PCO_2 of blood.
- Decreased pH of blood.
- Increased temperature.
- Increased levels of 2, 3-diphosphoglycerate (2, 3-DPG).

The right shift of the curve is advantageous only to a limited extent because though at tissues, this shift would release greater O_2 from haemoglobin (at the same PO_2), at lungs it will take up less O_2 (at the same PO_2), i.e. O_2 uptake at the lungs is reduced.

What is meant by shift of O_2 dissociation curve to left? Enumerate the factors causing such a shift. Is it advantageous?

Shifting of O_2 dissociation curve to left denotes increased affinity of haemoglobin for oxygen.

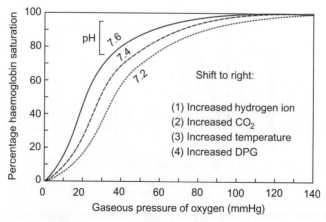

FIGURE 7.14 Shift of the oxygen-haemoglobin dissociation curve

The causes for left shift of the curve are:

- Decreased PCO_2 of blood.
- Increased pH of blood.
- Decreased temperature.
- Foetal haemoglobin.

Shift of the curve also has limited advantage because though it allows greater uptake of O_2 at lungs (at the same PO_2), it decreases release of O_2 to tissues (at the same PO_2).

What is Bohr's effect?

Shifting of O_2 dissociation curve due to changes in PCO_2 is known as Bohr's effect.

Does O_2 dissociation curve show shifting to right or left normally?

At the tissues because of increased PCO_2, O_2 dissociation curve shifts to right whereas in the lungs because of excretion of CO_2 (decreased PCO_2), O_2 dissociation curve shifts to left.

What is P_{50}? What is its significance?

Partial pressure of O_2 at which haemoglobin is 50% saturated is termed P_{50}. For a normal adult at $37°C$ body temperature and at PCO_2 of blood 40 mmHg, P_{50} value is 25 mmHg. P_{50} indicates affinity of haemoglobin for oxygen.

P_{50} value lesser than normal (Hb gets 50% saturated at lower PO_2) indicates increased affinity of haemoglobin for O_2. It is equivalent therefore to shift of O_2 dissociation curve to left.

P_{50} value higher than normal indicates that affinity of haemoglobin for oxygen is reduced (Hb gets 50% saturated at higher PO_2). It is equivalent therefore to shift of O_2 dissociation curve to right.

Foetal haemoglobin has lower P_{50} value than adult haemoglobin. Myoglobin also has lower P_{50} value than adult haemoglobin.

Presence of excess CO_2, increased acidity, increased temperature and increased levels of 2, 3-DPG causes rise in P_{50} value.

What is utilization coefficient for O_2?

Utilization coefficient for O_2 is percentage of O_2 extracted by tissues.

$$\text{Utilization coefficient} = \frac{\text{Arterial blood } O_2 \text{ content} - \text{Venous blood } O_2 \text{ content}}{\text{Arterial blood } O_2 \text{ content}} \times 100$$

$$= \frac{20 - 15}{20} \times 100$$

$$= 25\%$$

At rest, utilization coefficient of O_2 is 25%. However, it increases to 75 to 85% with exercise.

TRANSPORT OF CARBON DIOXIDE

Describe the transport of CO_2 from tissues to atmosphere.

Carbon dioxide is transported from tissues to atmosphere due to constant circulation of blood and diffusion of CO_2 that occurs at various sites as follows:

1. *In tissues.* (a) Cells constantly form CO_2 during metabolism. Intracellular PCO_2 is therefore always higher (46 mmHg) than PCO_2 of interstitial fluid surrounding the cells (45 mmHg). Due to this pressure gradient, CO_2 diffuses from cells to interstitial fluid.

(b) PCO_2 of arterial blood flowing through tissue capillaries is 40 mmHg and that of interstitial fluid is 45 mmHg; because of pressure gradient CO_2 diffuses from interstitial fluid into the blood. By the time blood reaches veins its PCO_2 raises to 45 mmHg (equal to that of interstitial fluid).

2. *At lungs.* Venous blood passing through pulmonary capillaries has PCO_2 of 45 mmHg, whereas alveolar air PCO_2 is 40 mmHg and because of pressure gradient, CO_2 diffuses from blood to alveoli. Due to constant ventilation, CO_2 from alveoli is transported to atmosphere.

State the various forms in which CO_2 is transported in blood.

Venous blood contains 52 ml and arterial blood 48 ml of CO_2 per 100 ml. Thus 4 ml of CO_2 is transported per 100 ml of blood from tissues to lungs (Fig. 7.15).

CO_2 is transported in the following three forms:

1. *Dissolved state in plasma (7%).* In venous blood with PCO_2 45 mmHg, the amount of CO_2 in dissolved state is about 2.7 ml per 100 ml. In arterial blood with PCO_2 40 mmHg, the amount of CO_2 in dissolved state is 2.4 ml per 100 ml. Thus, only 0.3 ml of CO_2 is carried per 100 ml of blood in dissolved state from tissues to lungs.

2. *In bicarbonate form (70%).* After entering the blood, CO_2 combines with water to form H_2CO_3 which dissociates into H^+ and HCO_3^- ions. This reaction occurs at a very high rate in RBCs as they contain enzyme carbonic anhydrase. H^+ ions are buffered by haemoglobin and HCO_3^- ions pass out from cell to plasma and are carried as $NaHCO_3$ (alkali reserve of blood) (Fig. 7.16).

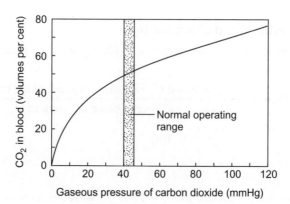

FIGURE 7.15 CO_2 dissociation curve.

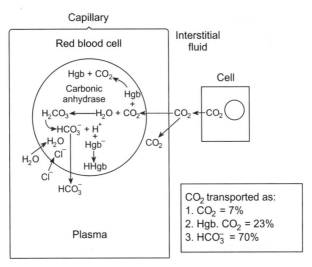

FIGURE 7.16 Transport of CO_2 in the blood.

3. *In carbamino compound form (23%).* CO_2 reacts directly with amino (NH_2) group of the proteins, haemoglobin and plasma proteins, to form carbamino compound:

$$R \bullet NH_2 + CO_2 \rightarrow R \bullet NHCOOH$$

Carbon dioxide reacting with plasma proteins is much less significant because quantity of these proteins is one-fourth that of haemoglobin. Combination of CO_2 with haemoglobin forms carbaminohaemoglobin. It is a reversible reaction that occurs with a loose bond.

Theoretically, haemoglobin and plasma protein can carry 30% of CO_2 in carbamino compound form but normally only 23% of CO_2 is carried in this form. This is because the reaction of CO_2 with amino group of proteins is much slower than the reaction of CO_2 with water in RBCs.

What is chloride shift?

At the tissues when CO_2 enters the blood, it reacts with water to form H_2CO_3 which dissociates into H^+ and HCO_3^- ions (Fig. 7.16). H^+ ions formed in the reaction are buffered by proteins (plasma proteins and haemoglobin). This leads to increased HCO_3^- inside the red cells as compared to that in the plasma. Therefore, HCO_3^- ions diffuse from RBCs to plasma. As HCO_3^- is a negatively charged ion and the red cell membrane is relatively impermeable to cations, inside of the cells becomes less negatively charged. In order to neutralize the effect, negatively charged chloride ions (Cl^-) diffuse from plasma into the red blood cells. This is called chloride shift. Reversal of this reaction occurs in blood of pulmonary capillaries.

Why are venous RBCs more fragile than arterial RBCs?

When blood passes through tissue capillaries, CO_2 enters into blood and, as described above, this causes chloride shift. According to Donnan's equilibrium this

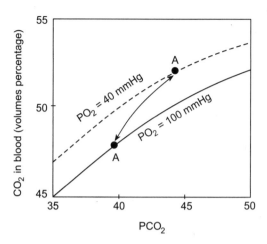

FIGURE 7.17 Haldane's effect on the transport of CO_2.

shift will continue till ratios of ions inside and outside for Cl^- and HCO_3^- become the same, i.e.

$$\frac{HCO_3^- \text{ (inside)}}{HCO_3^- \text{ (outside)}} = \frac{Cl^- \text{ (inside)}}{Cl^- \text{ (outside)}}$$

Because of chloride shift, this ratio is higher in venous blood than in arterial blood and as a result, osmotic pressure inside the RBCs becomes higher than that of plasma. This causes osmotic absorption of fluid into the RBCs. Venous RBCs contain therefore the greater quantity of fluid as compared to arterial blood RBCs. When placed in hypotonic solutions they can take lesser amount of fluid and are hence more fragile than arterial RBCs.

What is Haldane's effect? How is it beneficial?

Deoxyhaemoglobin (reduced haemoglobin) combines with more CO_2 as compared to oxyhaemoglobin. This is known as Haldane's effect (Fig. 7.17). Haldane's effect is beneficial because it almost doubles the quantity of CO_2 to be carried from the tissues to lungs and also doubles the amount of CO_2 to be excreted by lungs. Because of this effect CO_2 dissociation curve shifts to the left when blood flows in tissues and it shifts to the right when blood flows in pulmonary capillaries.

RESPIRATORY EXCHANGE RATIO

What is respiratory exchange ratio?

Ratio of carbon dioxide output to oxygen uptake is called respiratory exchange ratio (R).

$$R = \frac{\text{Rate of } CO_2 \text{ output}}{\text{Rate of } O_2 \text{ uptake}}$$

Value of 'R' can change under different metabolic conditions. When carbohydrates are exclusively used for metabolism, value of R is 1. When exclusively fats are utilised for metabolic energy, value of R is 0.7. In a person with balanced diet, with average amounts of carbohydrates, fats and proteins, the value of R is 0.825.

APPLIED ASPECT

What is carboxyhaemoglobin?

Combination of carbon monoxide gas (CO) with haemoglobin forms carboxyhaemoglobin.

Why carbon monoxide is poisonous?

Carbon monoxide gas combines with haemoglobin at the same site where O_2 combines. As haemoglobin has 250 times greater affinity for CO as compared to that for O_2, even with carbon monoxide pressure 0.4 mmHg, it competes equally with O_2 for combination with haemoglobin. Over half of haemoglobin binds with CO when its pressure is more than 0.4 mmHg. This can be lethal as it causes hypoxia.

How is CO poisoning treated?

Administration of 100% (pure) O_2 is beneficial as it increases PO_2 of alveolar air by 5 times the normal. This high PO_2 causes displacement of CO from haemoglobin far more rapidly. Secondly, it also increases the amount of O_2 carried in a dissolved state. This would maintain adequate delivery of oxygen to tissues. Addition of small quantity of CO_2 is useful because it increases the ventilation and diminishes concentration of CO in alveolar air (helps in rapid removal of CO).

What is methaemoglobin?

When iron in haemoglobin, which is in ferrous (F^{++}) state, is oxidized to ferric (Fe^{+++}) state, methaemoglobin is formed, which is incapable of carrying oxygen. It is formed in the red cells at a slow rate and is reconverted to functional haemoglobin by reducing compounds in red cells during metabolism. Many drugs (nitrites, phenacetin) can produce methaemoglobin.

REGULATION OF RESPIRATION

Describe mechanisms which control respiration.

Control or regulation of respiration involves adjustment of ventilation to match metabolic needs of the body so that arterial blood oxygen pressure (PO_2) and carbon dioxide pressure (PCO_2) are almost maintained constant whether it be during quiet breathing, sleep or muscular exercise.

There are two regulatory mechanisms:

1. *Nervous mechanism.* This mechanism regulates respiration by several groups of neurons situated bilaterally in medulla and pons. These neurons

form the respiratory centres. There are four major collections of neurons:

- Dorsal medullary group   ⎫   located in
- Ventral medullary group   ⎬   medulla
- Apneustic centre   ⎭   located in lower pons
- Pneumotaxic centre   —   located in upper pons

2. *Chemical mechanism.* It involves control of ventilation in response to changes in arterial blood PO_2, PCO_2 and H^+ ions.

NERVOUS REGULATION

What is the role of medullary centre in control of respiration?

Heart possesses the property of autorhythmicity, i.e. it generates its own rhythm. This is not the case with respiratory muscles which are skeletal and therefore require electrical stimulation via somatic nerves to initiate contraction. Respiratory muscles alternately contract and relax during inspiration and expiration, respectively. This rhythm of inspiration followed by expiration, and followed by next inspiration and expiration is generated in the medulla. The centre in the medulla is termed medullary respiratory centre. It is divided into: (i) dorsal respiratory group of neurons and (ii) ventral respiratory group of neurons (Fig. 7.18).

What are the functions of medullary respiratory centre?

1. *Dorsal respiratory group of neurons* (Fig. 7.18). Most of these neurons are located within the nucleus of tractus solitarius and some are located in adjacent reticular substance of medulla. The basic rhythm of respiration is generated by these neurons. Neurons emit repetitive bursts of inspiratory action potentials. The basic cause of this repetitive discharge is not known. From these neurons, nerve signals are transmitted to inspiratory muscles such as diaphragm and external intercostal muscles. This signal is not instantaneous but is a 'ramp' signal, i.e. it is

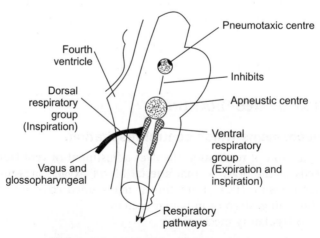

FIGURE 7.18 Organization of respiratory centres.

weak in the beginning and it steadily increases in a ramp manner for about 2 seconds. This leads to steady increase in lung volume during inspiration rather than respiratory gasps (abrupt distension). Ramp signal abruptly ceases for approximately next 3 seconds. This causes turning off of excitation of diaphragm and external intercostal muscles. These muscles therefore relax allowing elastic recoil of the chest wall and the lungs to cause expiration. After expiration again there is a ramp signal for starting another cycle. Thus cycle of inspiration/expiration, again inspiration/expiration goes on continuously to cause tidal respiration.

Ramp signal can be controlled as follows:

- Control of rate of discharge of the ramp signal—when rate of discharge increases there is active inspiration causing greater and rapid expansion of lungs.
- Control of limiting point at which ramp suddenly ceases. This controls rate of respiration. Earlier the ramp signal ceases, shorter is the duration of inspiration which also shortens duration of expiration, leading to increase in rate of respiration.

2. *Ventral respiratory group of neurons.* This group is located in nucleus ambiguus and nucleus retroambiguus. During tidal respiration neurons in the ventral group remain totally inactive. Normal quite breathing as stated above is caused by repetitive inspiratory signals from dorsal respiratory group of neurons. Ventral group of neurons play a role when there is increased pulmonary ventilation. During increased pulmonary ventilation, respiratory drive becomes greater than normal and respiratory signals spill over into ventral neurons from the dorsal respiratory area. This ventral area contributes to both inspiration and expiration and is especially important in providing powerful expiratory signals to expiratory muscles. This area operates when high levels of pulmonary ventilation are required.

What is the function of apneustic centre?

Apneustic centre is located bilaterally in lower part of pons. It sends signals to dorsal respiratory group of neurons that prevents the 'switch-off' of the inspiratory ramp signal. This leads to prolonged inspiration which is termed apneusis. It operates in association with pneumotaxic centre to control the depth of inspiration.

What is the function of pneumotaxic centre?

Pneumotaxic centres are located bilaterally in nucleus parabrachialis of the upper pons. The primary function of this centre is to control the 'switch-off' point of inspiratory ramp, thus controlling the duration of inspiration.

When pneumotaxic signal is strong, the rate of respiration increases to 30 to 40 breaths per minute, because of rapid 'switching off' of ramp signals which reduces duration of inspiration and therefore also expiration. Weak pneumotaxic signal may reduce the rate to only a few breaths per minute.

Thus, though rhythm of respiration resides in dorsal respiratory group of neurons in medulla, pneumotaxic and apneustic centres control these neurons to regulate the depth and rate of respiration.

What is the role of higher centres in respiratory control?

Normally respiration goes on absolutely unconsciously. Higher centres can cause only temporary breath holding or temporary hyperventilation.

What is Hering–Breuer reflex?

Inhibition of inspiration on inflation of lungs is called the Hering–Breuer reflex. When the lung is inflated and stretch receptors (present in the walls of bronchi, bronchioles, etc.) are stimulated, then they send impulses through vagi nerves to pontine and medullary respiratory centres to inhibit inspiration.

What is the importance of Hering–Breuer reflex?

Hering–Breuer reflex is initiated only when the tidal volume is more than 1.5 litres in human beings. In humans, therefore, it has only a protective role in preventing excessive distension of lungs (which may cause damage). It does not play any regulatory role in tidal respiration.

Other effect of Hering–Breuer reflex is to minimize the work of breathing. Ideally, regulation of respiration not only provides proper volume of alveolar ventilation but also accomplishes it with minimum expenditure of energy by muscles of respiration. Hering–Breuer reflex regulates tidal volume and respiratory rate in such a way that required level of ventilation is achieved with minimal expenditure of energy (i.e. minimal respiratory muscle work) under different conditions, e.g. exercise.

CHEMICAL REGULATION

Name the chemical factors which control respiration.

PCO_2, PO_2 and pH of blood are the chemical factors regulating the respiration (Fig. 7.19). These factors influence respiration in such a way that their own levels in the blood are maintained constant.

What are central chemoreceptors?

Central chemoreceptors are the neurons present just beneath the ventral surface of medulla. They respond to changes in H^+ ion concentration of cerebrospinal fluid and surrounding interstitial fluid.

What is the mechanism by which increase in CO_2 concentration stimulates central chemoreceptors?

Increased CO_2 concentration in blood immediately increases CO_2 concentration in CSF also, because there is no blood-CSF barrier for CO_2. In the CSF, CO_2 combines with water to form H_2CO_3 which dissociates into H^+ and HCO_3^- ions. The increase in H^+ ion concentration stimulates the neurons of chemoreceptors, leading to increase in respiratory rate and depth (about 85% of resting respiratory

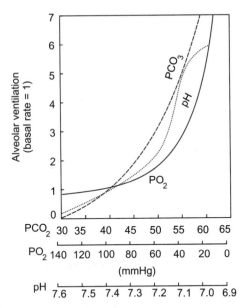

FIGURE 7.19 Effect of changing concentration of carbon dioxide, hydrogen ions and oxygen in arterial blood on alveolar ventilation when only one factor is changed and other two are maintained at normal level.

drive is due to stimulatory effect of CO_2 on the central chemoreceptors). Similar reaction also occurs in interstitial fluid of brain leading to increase in H^+ ion concentration of the fluid which in turn stimulates central chemoreceptors.

Why increased PCO_2 in CSF is more effective in stimulating central chemoreceptors than increased PCO_2 in interstitial fluid of brain?

Actual stimulus for central chemoreceptors is the increased H^+ ion concentration. In CSF, there are no buffers (proteins) to buffer H^+ ions formed from H_2CO_3. The interstitial fluid is surrounded by cells having proteins as buffers. Therefore, for the same change in CO_2 concentration, H^+ ion concentration of CSF is more than that of interstitial fluid; thus, increased PCO_2 of CSF is the more important stimulus.

Where are the peripheral chemoreceptors situated? What are the stimuli for them?

Peripheral chemoreceptors are situated in carotid and aortic bodies (Fig. 7.20). Decreased PO_2 (below 60 mmHg), increased PCO_2 (by 10 mmHg) and decreased pH (by 0.1 unit) are the stimuli for them.

Why decrease in PO_2 of blood up to 60 mmHg does not stimulate chemoreceptors?

Lack of O_2 supply is the actual stimulus for peripheral chemoreceptors. O_2 dissociation curve has a plateau between 100 mmHg and 60 mmHg, i.e. O_2

carriage to the tissues remains normal till PO_2 arterial blood falls to 60 mmHg. Secondly, peripheral chemoreceptors have rich blood supply. Therefore, unless PO_2 of arterial blood falls below 60 mmHg, chemoreceptors are not stimulated.

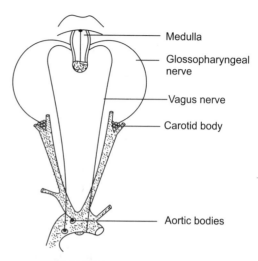

FIGURE 7.20 Carotid and aortic bodies.

What is the importance of reflex regulation of respiration caused by decreased PO_2 in blood?

Reflex regulatory mechanism initiated by decreased PO_2 is poor because it is not initiated until PO_2 drops to a low level in the blood (60 mmHg). Secondly, its effect on ventilation is neutralized by breaking effect of CO_2. But still it is important mechanism because it is the only mechanism by which decreased O_2 can stimulate ventilation and especially it is important in various respiratory diseases. It is the only respiratory drive in certain conditions.

What is the breaking effect of CO_2?

When decrease in PO_2 of arterial blood or decreased pH of arterial blood stimulates ventilation, increased ventilation causes washing out of CO_2. This leads to decrease in PCO_2 of blood and inhibits respiration through central chemoreceptors. It opposes and neutralizes the action of diminished O_2 or pH.

Why CO_2 acts as a main regulator of respiration?

CO_2 acts as a main regulator because:

1. It has a direct effect on respiratory centre (through central chemoreceptors).
2. It has no blood-brain or blood-CSF barrier, therefore, as soon as concentration of CO_2 in blood increases, almost immediately that of interstitial fluid of brain and CSF also increases. H^+ ions pass very slowly through these barriers.
3. CO_2 also has a very strong breaking effect on the action of either decreased PO_2 or pH.
4. PO_2 or pH do not have very strong breaking effect on the action of increased CO_2 on ventilation (Fig. 7.21).

How is respiration controlled by nervous and chemical mechanisms?

Respiratory centres on the basis of their PCO_2 or reflex demands or both decide how much ventilation is needed. On the basis of additional information fed to the respiratory centres from lung afferents, centres decide optimal combination of

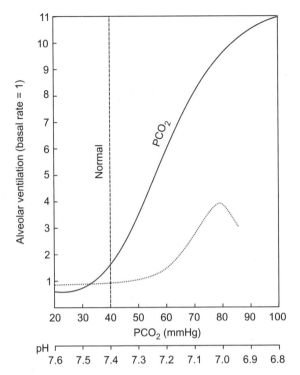

FIGURE 7.21 Effects of increased PCO_2 and decreased pH on the rate of alveolar ventilation.

rate of respiration (frequency) and tidal volume to achieve desired ventilation with minimum expenditure of energy.

If, however, thoracic or pulmonary compliance has decreased or resistance has increased, gamma loop system operates as a servo to drive main muscle fibres to develop additional tension and quickly achieve the proper ventilation.

PERIODIC BREATHING

What is Cheyne–Stokes respiration? When does it occur?

Cheyne–Stokes breathing is periodic type of breathing where there are alternate periods of respiratory activity and apnoea occurring at regular intervals. During the period of respiratory activity there is waxing and waning of tidal volume. Cheyne–Stokes respiration occurs during:

- Increased circulation time from lungs to brain as in chronic heart failure.
- Increased negative feedback gain in the respiratory centre due to brain damage.
- In infants, sometimes such type of breathing occurs during sleep. It is physiological and occurs because the centres are not yet developed.

What is Biot's breathing?

Biot's breathing is also a type of periodic breathing showing alternate periods of respiratory activity and apnoea. It differs from Cheyne–Stokes breathing in that it occurs at irregular intervals. There is no waxing and waning of tidal volume during the period of respiratory activity and it can never be physiological. It occurs due to damage to the brain.

IMPORTANT RESPIRATORY REFLEXES

What is cough reflex?

Entry of any foreign material initiates this reflex to cause removal of that material, therefore it is a protective reflex.

Bronchi and trachea are very sensitive and therefore even small amount of irritant initiates cough reflex. The larynx, carina, terminal bronchioles and alveoli are also sensitive to various chemicals.

When irritant material enters the respiratory tract, afferent signals for cough reflex pass through vagus nerve to medulla. This results in automatic sequence of events to initiate cough reflex as follows:

- First about 2.5 litres of air is rapidly inspired.
- Epiglottis closes and vocal cords are tightly shut to entrap air in the lungs.
- Abdominal muscles contract forcefully and even expiratory muscles contract forcefully.
- This causes pressure inside the lung to rise to 100 mmHg or more.
- Vocal cords and epiglottis suddenly open widely and air under high pressure in lungs explodes outward.
- Exploding air carries with it the foreign material.

What is sneeze reflex?

It is also a protective reflex and it helps to clear nasal passages.

This reflex is initiated by irritation in nasal passage. The afferent impulses pass via trigeminal (Vth cranial) nerve to the medulla. This results in same sequence of events as cough reflex but the only difference is as uvula is depressed, large amount of air passes through nose cleaning nasal passage from foreign material.

RECEPTORS IN THE AIRWAY

What is the effect of irritant receptors in airway?

Epithelium of trachea, bronchi, bronchioles, etc. are supplied with sensory nerve endings. They get stimulated by various irritants. Probably they cause bronchoconstriction in disease like bronchial asthma.

What are 'J' receptors?

'J' receptors are non-myelinated nerve fibres in alveolar walls, pulmonary capillaries, etc. These receptors get stimulated especially with pulmonary congestion, pulmonary oedema, etc. Exact functional role of 'J' receptors is not known but probably they are responsible for giving a feeling of dyspnoea to a person.

TERMS USED FOR ALTERED RESPIRATION

Term	Brief Description
Apnoea	Temporary stoppage of respiration.
Hypercapnia	Increased PCO_2 level of body fluids.
Hyperventilation	Increased rate and depth of breathing. It is defined as ventilation in excess of metabolic needs and leads to an increase in arterial O_2 tension (PO_2) and decrease in arterial CO_2 tension (PCO_2) with concomitant increase in arterial blood pH.
Hypoventilation	Decreased rate and depth of breathing. It is defined as ventilation lesser than metabolic needs and it results into decrease in arterial O_2 tension (PO_2) and increase in arterial CO_2 tension (PCO_2) with concomitant decrease in arterial blood pH.
Dyspnoea	Difficulty in breathing associated with a sense of distress. The patient is conscious of increased respiratory effort (therefore the real synonym is air hunger). Real discomfort develops when ventilation is increased four- to fivefold, this level of ventilation is called the dyspnoea point. Dyspnoea usually results when breathing reserve falls to 60%. Breathing reserve may be lowered due to decrease in MVV (maximum ventilatory volume) or rise in pulmonary minute ventilation.
Asphyxia	A condition in which hypoxia is associated with hypercapnia (increased CO_2 level).

What are the types and causes of asphyxia?

The causes of asphyxia are the same as for hypoxia (except for arterial hypoxia of high altitude as it is not associated with hypercapnia).

Asphyxia can be general or local. Local asphyxia is caused by obstruction of blood vessel or ligation of blood vessel.

General asphyxia can be acute or chronic.

Chronic asphyxia. It occurs in cor pulmonale, i.e. right ventricular failure due to lung disease.

Acute asphyxia. It occurs in strangulation, acute tracheal obstruction (due to entry of food or due to choking), paralysis of diaphragm (as in poliomyelitis). Acute asphyxia is very dangerous and if not treated death occurs within 5 minutes.

There are three stages of acute asphyxia:

Stage I. Duration of this stage is 1 minute. During this stage there is increase in rate and depth of respiration, dyspnoea. The expiratory movement is more pronounced. This stage is due to stimulation of respiratory centre on account of increased PCO_2. O_2 lack is not yet enough to stimulate ventilation.

Stage II. It lasts for 1 to 2 minutes. There is unconsciousness. Expiration becomes more pronounced. There are convulsions. All signs of central excitation such as rise in systemic blood pressure due to widespread vasoconstriction, constriction of pupils and exaggerated reflexes are seen. Vomiting and micturition may occur. This stage occurs due to excess CO_2 stimulating the centres directly and lack of O_2 stimulating the centres reflexly. Convulsions are due to excess PCO_2. This is called the stage of central excitation.

Stage III. It lasts for 2 to 3 minutes. Convulsions cease. Respiration becomes slow and finally it becomes gasping (shallow and with low frequency). There are signs of central depression such as fall in blood pressure, dilatation of pupils and abolition of reflexes. Thus it is a stage of central depression. It is due to direct effect of O_2 lack on vital centres causing their inhibition. Factors in stage II fail to excite them. The whole body lies still and finally death occurs.

HYPOXIA

What is hypoxia?

Hypoxia is inadequate oxygen supply to the tissues. It may be caused due to:

- Decreased PO_2 arterial blood.
- Decreased O_2 carrying capacity of blood.
- Decreased rate of blood flow to the tissues.

Enumerate the various types of hypoxia.

- Arterial (hypoxic).
- Hypokinetic (stagnant).
- Anaemic.
- Histotoxic.

In histotoxic, tissues are supplied with adequate oxygen but they are poisoned and, therefore, are not capable of utilizing oxygen. So histotoxic is not a true hypoxia.

What is arterial hypoxia? What are its causes?

Arterial hypoxia is the one where PO_2 of arterial blood is less than normal but O_2 carrying capacity of blood and rate of blood flow are normal.

CAUSES

1. High altitude where person is exposed to low atmospheric PO_2.
2. Breathing artificial gas mixture with low PO_2.
3. Hypoventilation due to any cause: damage to respiratory centre by drugs, paresis or paralysis of respiratory muscles as in poliomyelitis, increased airway resistance, decreased lung compliance. Hypoventilation decreases PO_2 in alveoli.
4. Diffusion limitation due to loss of surface area of respiratory membrane in various pulmonary diseases.

5. V_A/Q (ventilation-perfusion) ratio imbalance leading to physiologic shunt formation. There is low PO_2 in areas of lungs with low V_A/Q ratios. Blood from this area has less PO_2, and when it is mixed with blood from other regions in the lungs, it causes overall decrease in PO_2 of arterial blood.

6. Anatomic shunts. True venous blood enters in systemic circulation, due to abnormal connections between right and left sides of the heart caused by congenital heart disease or blood flow through atelectatic areas of lungs. Thus shunted venous blood is dumped into arterial circulation resulting in dilution of normally oxygenated blood.

What is anaemic hypoxia? What are its causes?

Anaemic hypoxia is the hypoxia resulting due to decreased O_2 carrying capacity of blood. In this, PO_2 of arterial blood and rate of flow of blood are normal.

CAUSES

1. Decreased haemoglobin content of blood, i.e. in all types of anaemia.
2. Altered haemoglobin which is not capable of carrying O_2, e.g. in CO poisoning, methaemoglobin formation.

What is stagnant hypoxia? What are its causes?

Stagnant hypoxia is due to inadequate rate of blood flow to the tissues. PO_2 of arterial blood and O_2 carrying capacity of blood are normal. It may be generalized or localized.

CAUSES

Generalized stagnant hypoxia is caused by congestive cardiac failure. Localized stagnant hypoxia is caused by abnormalities in regional vessels, such as athero-sclerosis, thrombosis or embolism.

What is histotoxic hypoxia? What is its cause?

Decreased ability of tissues themselves to utilize oxygen is called histotoxic hypoxia. It is not a true hypoxia because O_2 supply to the tissues is adequate.

It results due to metabolic poisons such as cyanide.

In which type of hypoxia, O_2 therapy would be most useful?

In arterial hypoxia, O_2 therapy is most effective.

What are the signs of hypoxia?

- Cyanosis—not a reliable sign.
- Tachycardia.
- Tachypnoea (increased rate of respiration).
- Hyperpnoea (increased depth of respiration).

Signs and symptoms of hypoxia depend on which factors?

Symptoms of hypoxia depend on the rapidity of development and severity of hypoxia.

1. *Fulminant hypoxia.* When severe hypoxia develops very fast (going at high levels above 30,000 feet in unpressurized aeroplane), it results into unconsciousness within 15 to 20 seconds due to lack of O_2 supply to the brain. Brain death may follow in 4 to 5 minutes.

2. *Acute hypoxia.* It may be produced due to exposure to low PO_2. It causes slowed reflexes, muscular incoordination, slurred speech, overconfidence and eventually unconsciousness. Death occurs in minutes to hours if compensatory mechanisms are not adequate.

3. *Chronic hypoxia.* It is due to exposure to low PO_2 (40 to 60 mmHg) for long periods. It causes severe fatigue, dyspnoea and shortness of breath. Due to lack of O_2 supply to tissues, person may be bedridden or limited to sitting and may get respiratory arrhythmias.

When, person from a sea level goes and stays at high altitude, he is exposed to low PO_2 for a long time. Various changes in body tissues occur for adjusting the body to low PO_2. This is termed acclimatization.

ACCLIMATIZATION

What is acclimatization? State the changes occurring during acclimatization.

Acclimatization refers to changes in the body tissues in response to long-term exposure to hypoxia, such as when a person living at sea level goes and stays at high altitude for a long time. With longer stay, the person gradually gets acclimatized to low PO_2.

The principal changes that occur during acclimatization are as follows:

1. *Increase in pulmonary ventilation.* Because of exposure to low PO_2, hypoxic stimulation of peripheral chemoreceptors leads to increase in ventilation, which is only 65% above normal. This is immediate compensation for the high altitude. The rise is only 65% above normal because of breaking effect of CO_2 on the action of decreased PO_2. However, when the person stays at high altitude for many days, there is a gradual increase in ventilation to an average of about five times the normal. This is because of loss of breaking effect of CO_2 due to renal correction of alkalosis, leading to decreased HCO_3^- ion concentration in CSF and brain tissue.

2. *Increase in red blood cells and haemoglobin.* Hypoxia stimulates secretion of erythropoietin by kidneys. Erythropoietin increases the rate of RBC production, thereby increasing the number of circulating RBCs. This leads to increase in haematocrit from normal value of 40% to 45% to 60% after full acclimatization. This also causes the concentration of haemoglobin to rise from normal 15 g per 100 ml to about 20 g per 100 ml. There is also increase in blood volume by 20 to 30% leading to total increase in circulating haemoglobin by 50%.

Increase in haemoglobin and blood volume starts after 2 weeks, development reaches half-way stage in a month and is fully developed only after many months.

3. *Increase in diffusing capacity of lungs.* Diffusing capacity of lungs increases due to increase in surface area of respiratory membrane. Greatly increased pulmonary capillary blood volume expands the capillaries, thereby increasing surface area. Hypoxia increases pulmonary ventilation leading to increase in lung volume which expands the surface area of alveolar membrane. Pulmonary arterial pressure is also increased, and this forces blood into greater number of alveolar capillaries than under normal conditions, especially in upper parts of lungs which are poorly perfused.

4. *Changes in cardiovascular system.* Hypoxia stimulates vasomotor centre which causes sympathetic stimulation of heart leading to increase in heart rate and force of contraction of heart. This results in about 30% increase in cardiac output as an immediate effect to compensate for hypoxia. Later on cardiac output decreases back to normal as blood haematocrit increases so that amount of O_2 supply to tissue remains about normal.

Blood pressure, however, may fall or rise or may remain normal. Vasoconstriction occurs because of stimulation of vasomotor centre due to hypoxia but is opposed by vasodilation produced by local effect of hypoxia. The resultant of these two opposing forces determines the outcome. Polycythaemia which occurs after 2 weeks of exposure to high altitude causes rise in blood pressure.

5. *Shift of O_2 dissociation curve.* Hypoxia raises the 2, 3-DPG level of blood, which in turn causes shift of O_2 dissociation curve to right and increase in P_{50} level. This may be beneficial at tissue level as shift to the right increases unloading of O_2 from haemoglobin, but it also decreases O_2 uptake at the lungs; so this effect is not of much advantage at a moderately high altitude.

There is increase in number of capillaries (increased capillary density) in the tissues as a result of hypoxia. In active tissue, chronic hypoxia stimulates angiogenesis. This effect is mainly seen in persons born and bred at high altitude.

Increased cardiac output increases the pulmonary blood flow, leading to pulmonary hypertension. In some persons it may lead to right ventricular hypertrophy.

6. *Cellular acclimatization.* In persons who are natives of high altitude of 13,000 to 17,000 feet, mitochondria and certain oxidative enzyme systems are slightly more plentiful and therefore can use oxygen more effectively than can their sea level counterparts.

MOUNTAIN SICKNESS

What is acute mountain sickness?

It is the sickness occurring in some individuals on exposure to high altitude (9000 to 10,000 feet above the sea level). There is fatigue, nausea, vomiting, loss of appetite, dyspnoea, headache, palpitation and sleep disturbances. In some cases there may be cerebral or pulmonary oedema which may be fatal.

What is chronic mountain sickness?

It is the disease occurring in long-term residents of high altitude. There is extreme polycythaemia which increases viscosity of blood and hence reducing the rate of blood flow. This causes cyanosis, fatigue and exercise intolerance. It may result in pulmonary oedema which is fatal.

HYPERBARIC OXYGEN THERAPY

What is the significance of hyperbaric O_2 therapy?

Hyperbaric oxygen has valuable therapeutic effects in several clinical conditions. Oxygen of 2 to 3 atmospheric pressure is administrated. It is believed that some oxidizing-free radicals are responsible for therapeutic benefit. It is especially useful in treating chronic wounds and ulcers. It is given in gas gangrene, leprosy, etc.

CYANOSIS

What is cyanosis? What are its causes? Describe the factors affecting degree of cyanosis.

Cyanosis is bluish discolouration of skin and mucous membrane, caused by the presence of increased amount of reduced haemoglobin in the capillaries of skin and mucous membrane. For cyanosis to occur a minimum 5 g of haemoglobin must be present in reduced form. Cyanosis is caused because red colour of oxyhaemoglobin is weak in comparison to dark blue colour of deoxygenated haemoglobin.

Clinically cyanosis may be central or peripheral. Central cyanosis occurs when central oxygenating organs (lungs) are diseased, i.e. it occurs in lung diseases which decrease oxygenation of haemoglobin. Peripheral cyanosis occurs when there is defect in O_2 transport from lungs to periphery, i.e. it occurs in circulatory failure.

FACTORS AFFECTING CYANOSIS

1. Colour of the skin. Cyanosis is more obvious in persons with fair complexion.
2. Rate of blood flow to skin and the amount of deoxyhaemoglobin present in arterial blood supplying skin.
3. Amount of O_2 removed by skin from capillary blood. Normally metabolism of skin is very low and therefore the quantity of O_2 removed (or amount of deoxyhaemoglobin formed) in skin is negligible. However, if blood flow becomes extremely sluggish, even low skin metabolism can cause cyanosis. This explains the cyanosis that occurs in very cold weather, particularly in children as they have thin skin.
4. Thickness of skin determines the intensity of colour. It is therefore more marked on lips, cheeks, earlobes, nose and fingertips.
5. Amount of haemoglobin. Cyanosis is not obvious unless 5 g of haemoglobin is in deoxygenated form in the capillaries of the skin. In a very anaemic person with low haemoglobin concentration (lower than 5 g/100 ml), cyanosis cannot occur. On the other hand, in polycythaemia there may be cyanosis because of reduced rate of blood flow due to increased viscosity. This reduces rate of blood flow in the capillaries and as a result blood stays there for a long time and haemoglobin becomes excessively reduced.

ARTIFICIAL RESPIRATION

What are the indications of artificial respiration?

The condition where heart continues beating but respiration fails, artificial respiration is indicated, e.g.

- When breathing fails due to drowning, inhalation of poisonous gases, overdose of narcotics or anaesthetics.
- Gradual paralysis of respiratory muscles as in poliomyelitis, diphtheria.

EXPOSURE TO LOW ATMOSPHERIC PRESSURE

What is decompression sickness (caisson disease, diver's paralysis or dysbarism)? What is its cause?

A diver working in deep sea for a long time when suddenly comes to sea level may develop decompression sickness.

When the diver is working in deep sea (high barometric pressure), large amount of nitrogen is dissolved in his body fluids and fats. Sudden exposure to low barometric pressure at sea level causes formation of nitrogen bubbles in body fluids and fatty tissues, leading to decompression sickness.

What are the symptoms and signs of decompression sickness?

Symptoms and signs of decompression sickness vary according to the site where the nitrogen bubbles are formed. Blood vessels in tissues at these sites are blocked due to the bubbles leading to tissue ischaemia and tissue death.

Common symptoms are pain in joints, muscles of legs and arms. When nervous system is affected, there is dizziness, paralysis, collapse and unconsciousness. Paralysis is usually temporary.

Bubble formation in lung vessels results into 'the chokes' characterized by shortness of breath and pulmonary oedema.

What is the treatment for decompression sickness?

Decompression sickness is treated by immediate recompression in a chamber and gradual decompression.

How is decompression sickness prevented?

Decompression sickness can be prevented by:

(a) Gradual ascent from sea—strictly according to standard tables.
(b) Inhalation of oxygen-helium mixture before the ascent.

EXPOSURE TO HIGH ATMOSPHERIC PRESSURE

What are the effects of high partial pressures of gases on the body?

A person is exposed to high pressures of gases when he descends beneath the sea.

The high partial pressures of gases on the body have the following effects:

1. *Nitrogen narcosis.* This is due to nitrogen dissolving in the membranes of neurons affecting electrical conductance and thereby reducing their excitability.

2. *O_2 toxicity.* At high pressures of O_2, dissolved O_2 in plasma is greatly increased, this in turn causes rise in tissue PO_2. This causes convulsions leading to coma. Convulsions are likely to be lethal to divers submerged beneath the sea. The toxicity is caused due to conversion of molecular oxygen into active oxygen (oxygen-free radicals). These radicals oxidize polyunsaturated fatty acids (essential compounds of cell membranes) and also oxidize cellular enzymes (damaging cellular metabolic systems). Nervous tissues are especially susceptible because of their high lipid content. Therefore, lethal effects are mostly related to brain dysfunction.

CARDIORESPIRATORY CHANGES DURING EXERCISE

Describe the cardiorespiratory changes during muscular exercise.

During exercise there is increase in metabolic needs of body tissues (especially muscles), and hence increased need for oxygen. Various adjustments in the body during exercise therefore aim at:

- Supplying sufficient nutrients and O_2 to the muscles and other tissues for increased metabolic needs.
- Increased excretion of CO_2 which is formed in excess.
- Prevention of increase in body temperature as large amount of heat is formed during muscular exercise.

Most of the above demands are fulfilled by changes occurring in cardiovascular and respiratory system in an integrated fashion as part of homeostatic responses.

CLASSIFICATION OF EXERCISE

Five-level classification system based on energy required by untrained men and women performing different physical activities is depicted in Table 7.2. As 5 kcal is equivalent to one litre of O_2 consumption, it is possible to present five-level classification in terms of litres of oxygen consumed per minute or METs. A MET is a multiple of resting metabolic rate. Thus one MET is equivalent to resting O_2 uptake of 250 ml per minute for an average man and 200 ml per minute for an

Table 7.2   Five-Level Classification System Based on Exercise Intensity

Level	O_2 consumption (L/min)		METs	
	Men	Women	Men	Women
1. Light	0.4 − 1.49	0.30 − 0.69	1.6 − 3.9	1.2 − 2.7
2. Moderate	1 − 1.49	0.7 − 1.09	4 − 5.9	2.8 − 4.3
3. Heavy	1.5 − 1.99	1.1 − 1.49	6 − 7.9	4.4 − 5.9
4. Very heavy	1 − 2.49	1.5 − 1.89	8.9 − 9.9	6 −7.5
5. Unduly heavy	2.5	1.9	10.0	7.6

average woman. Exercise of 2 METs requires twice the resting metabolism and twice the amount of O_2 per minute and so on.

TYPES OF EXERCISE

Exercise may be: (1) Isotonic or dynamic, (2) isometric or static.

Dynamic exercise involves isotonic muscle contractions. External work is involved in this type of exercise. It causes prompt increase in heart rate, marked increase in stroke volume and net fall in peripheral resistance. There is rise in systolic pressure and no change in diastolic pressure. Amount of heat produced is greater than in static exercise.

Static exercise involves isometric muscle contractions. There is increase in heart rate, sharp rise in both systolic and diastolic pressure and stroke volume changes relatively little. Blood flow to steadily contracting muscles is reduced as a result of compression on their blood vessels.

1. EFFECTS OF EXERCISE ON CARDIOVASCULAR SYSTEM

When cerebral cortex sends impulses to the exercising muscles at the beginning of exercise, it also causes sympathetic stimulation. Once exercise begins afferents from receptors in muscles and joints cause reflex stimulation of sympathetic system. In tournaments excitement may also cause sympathetic stimulation.

The following changes occur:

(a) *Increase in heart rate.* There is increase in heart rate during exercise—to about 180 to 185 beats per minute but only during short bursts of very vigorous exercise; it may reach 200 to 240 beats per minute.

The factors causing increase in heart rate are: (i) sympathetic stimulation as stated above—it is the most important factor, (ii) reduction in vagal tone, (iii) the circulating catecholamines (epinephrine, norepinephrine) secreted in large quantities during exercise increase heart rate and (iv) rise in body temperature stimulates the SA node directly or stimulates cardiac centres via hypothalamus.

Usually heart rate increases by 270%.

(b) *Increase in stroke volume.* There is 50% increase in stroke volume, up to 162 ml per beat.

Cardiac output is increased because of increase in stroke volume and increase in heart rate. Heart rate increase accounts by far for a greater proportion of increase in cardiac output than does the increase in stroke volume during strenuous exercise.

(c) *Cardiac output.* Cardiac output increases from normal 5 L/min to 30 L/min. As heart rate increases, diastolic period decreases and stroke volume is reduced, but reduced diastolic period is compensated by increased venous return and therefore increase in heart rate and stroke volume taken together cause spectacular increase in cardiac output.

The heart pumping effectiveness of each heart beat is 40 to 50% greater in highly trained athletes than in untrained persons because training causes hypertrophy of cardiac muscle and increases its pumping ability.

(d) *VO_2 max and its relation to cardiovascular performance.* The amount of O_2 that can be consumed by a person per minute when he/she is working maximally is called VO_2 max. During maximal exercise both heart rate and stroke volume increase to about 95% of their maximal levels, i.e. cardiac output (stroke volume × heart rate) also increases to about 90% of maximum. This is in contrast to 65% of maximum pulmonary ventilation. It means cardiovascular system is normally much more limiting on VO_2 max than in respiratory system, because oxygen utilization by the body can never be more than the rate at which cardiovascular system can transport oxygen to the tissues. Therefore, performance of a person mainly depends on cardiovascular efficiency.

(e) *Effect on blood pressure.* Because of increase in cardiac output, systolic pressure rises during exercise. Diastolic pressure mainly depends on peripheral resistance. Due to sympathetic stimulation there is vasoconstriction leading to increase in peripheral resistance. This is compensated by vasodilation that occurs due to local causes in exercising muscles. Thus, there is no change in peripheral resistance or there is a fall in peripheral resistance in strenuous exercise. The diastolic pressure therefore remains normal or falls. Pulse pressure (difference between systolic and diastolic) rises sharply. The mean pressure remains normal or falls.

(f) *Coronary circulation.* Due to indirect effect of sympathetic stimulation (increase in cardiac output) coronary blood is greatly increased during exercise. Due to relative local hypoxia there is vasodilation of coronary vessels.

(g) *Muscle blood flow (Fig. 7.22).* Exercising muscles get extra nutrients and O_2 through blood which they receive. Muscle blood flow drastically increases during exercise. It can increase to about twenty-fivefold during most strenuous exercise. During actual contractile process, blood flow decreases because contracting muscle compresses the vessels. Due to relative hypoxia local factors are released (ADP, lactic acid, etc.) and there is vasodilatation.

(h) *Blood flow to skin.* Due to increase in body temperature there is decreased sympathetic nerve discharge to skin. This causes vasodilation leading to increased heat loss.

(i) *Blood flow to GI tract and kidneys.* Due to sympathetic stimulation there is vasoconstriction, leading to decreased blood flow in kidneys and GI tract.

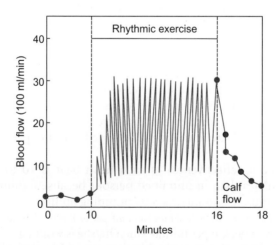

FIGURE 7.22 Effects of muscle exercise on blood flow in the calf of a leg during strong rhythmical contraction.

2. CHANGES IN RESPIRATORY SYSTEM

During heavy exercise, blood flow through lungs increases 4 to 5 times. Extra blood is accommodated in lungs by

- increasing number of open capillaries;
- distending all capillaries and increasing rate of blood flow through them; and
- increasing pulmonary arterial pressure.

First two effects are more marked.

There is twentyfold increase in O_2 consumption and CO_2 excretion during heavy exercise which produces the following effects on the system.

(a) *Increase in pulmonary ventilation.* When cortex sends excitatory impulses to exercising muscles at the beginning of exercise, through collaterals impulses are also sent to respiratory centre to cause anticipatory rise in ventilation (before starting of exercise, ventilation is increased).

When exercise actually starts the receptors from muscles and joints are stimulated, sensory impulses from them also stimulate respiratory centre to cause increased ventilation.

Thus, as stated above, the ventilation increases due to nervous factors. Usually nervous factors increase ventilation to a required level and therefore concentration of CO_2 and O_2 in the blood is maintained normal during exercise. If ventilation is not changed to desired levels, then there is change in concentration of chemical factors in blood (PO_2 and PCO_2) which through chemoreceptors make desired changes in ventilation. Thus chemical factors do the final and finer adjustment in ventilation.

(b) *Increase in diffusing capacity.* Diffusing capacity of lungs for gases increases to about 3 times during heavy exercise, e.g. diffusing capacity of respiratory membrane is normally 21 ml which can increase up to 65 ml. Increase in diffusing capacity is due to increase in surface area of respiratory membrane. With increase in ventilation, surface area on alveolar side is increased. Due to increase in blood flow, the surface area on the capillary side is increased.

(c) *Changes in V_A/Q ratio.* Gaseous exchange becomes better because of change in V_A/Q ratio to normal, especially in upper part of the lung. Normally because of decreased blood flow in this region V_A/Q ratio is higher than the normal. During exercise blood in upper part of the lungs rises and therefore V_A/Q ratio is brought to near normal. The blood normally remains in the lungs for longer time than required—blood is oxygenated completely by the time it reaches only one-third capillary distance (safety factor). Therefore, even if the rate of blood flow increases still the blood gets completely oxygenated.

(d) *Shift of O_2 dissociation curve.* Due to increase in 2, 3-DPG, O_2 dissociation curve shifts to right. This increases O_2 release from haemoglobin at the tissue level.

CHAPTER 8
Special Senses

EYE

State the functions of lacrimal secretion.

Lacrimal secretion has the following functions:

- It keeps the conjunctiva moist and clean. If any foreign body enters into the eye, there is excess lacrimal secretion which washes out the foreign body.
- Lacrimal secretion contains enzyme 'lysozyme' which kills the bacteria.

Name the different tunics (coats) of the eyeball.

There are three different tunics of the eyeball:

- Outer fibrous tunic made up of sclera and cornea.
- Middle vascular tunic made up of choroid, ciliary body and iris.
- Inner nervous tunic called retina, covers only posterior 5/6th portion of the eyeball.

What is lamina cribrosa?

A little to the medial side of the posterior pole of the eye, optic nerve enters the eyeball by piercing sclera. At this site sclera is thinned out and contains a number of perforations for passage of nerve fibres as well as blood vessels. This part of the sclera is known as lamina cribrosa. This is the weakest portion of the sclera and is the first to yield causing so-called 'cupping of the optic disc' when there is increase in intraocular pressure (IOP).

Why can cornea be successfully transplanted?

Cornea can be successfully transplanted from one person to the other because it is devoid of blood supply.

How does cornea obtain its nutrition?

Cornea obtains its nutrition mainly from aqueous humour which is the fluid present in front of the lens of the eye. Part of the O_2 supply to cornea occurs from atmosphere.

Describe the structure of ciliary body.

Ciliary body lies anterior to choroid. It is formed of three structures (Fig. 8.1):

1. *Orbicularis ciliaris.* It is a fibrous band of 4 mm breadth which completely encircles the eyeball just in front of choroid.

2. *Ciliary processes.* From orbicularis ciliaris several triangular processes project towards the interior of the eye and surround the lens. These are ciliary processes. Gap between lens capsule and ciliary processes is filled in by suspensory ligament (which suspends the lens).

3. *Ciliary muscles.* There are two types of ciliary muscle fibres:
   - *Meridional* fibres originate from sclerocorneal junction, run little backward and get inserted into the ciliary processes.
   - *Circular* fibres form circular band of muscle tissue which is called ciliary sphincter lying just in front and on the outer side of ciliary processes.

What is pupil?

Pupil is the aperture in the centre of the iris through which light passes into the eye.

What are the muscles present in the iris?

Iris contains two types of muscles:

1. *Sphincter pupillae muscle.* It forms a circular band of tissues surrounding the pupil. When it contracts, pupil constricts.

2. *Dilator pupillae muscle.* Muscle fibres run in radiating manner from periphery of iris towards the pupil and blend with fibres of sphincter pupillae muscle. When this muscle contracts, it causes dilatation of pupil.

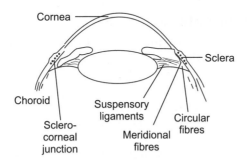

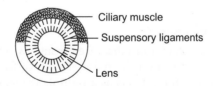

FIGURE 8.1 Ciliary body, suspensory ligaments and lens.

What is the function of the iris?

The main function of iris is to control the amount of light passing into the eye. This is done by constricting or dilating the pupil with the help of muscles. Iris cuts off the peripheral rays and avoids spherical aberration. Colour of the eyes is due to pigment cells present in the iris. Pigment cells are present in posterior epithelium and stroma of the iris. Black colour is due to pigment cells present in stroma of the iris. Sometimes stroma does not contain pigment cells, then the colour of the eyes is blue or grey because of colour of the pigment cells present in posterior epithelium as seen through unpigmented stroma.

How is the amount of light entering the eye controlled?

Amount of light entering the eye is controlled by controlling the size of the pupil. Diameter of pupil can vary from 1.5 to 8 mm. Amount of light entering the eye is proportional to the square of the diameter of the pupil. Therefore, when pupil size varies from 1.5 to 8 mm diameter, the amount of light entering the eye can vary nearly 30 times. Change in pupillary diameter is caused due to contraction of sphincter pupillae (constriction of pupil) and dilator pupillae (dilatation of pupil) muscle.

What is spherical aberration?

Parallel light rays passing through the peripheral portions of the eye lens do not exactly focus at the same point where rays passing through central portion of the lens focus. This defect is physiological and is called spherical aberration. It is minimized especially when pupil constricts because of the iris covering the peripheral portions of the lens.

What is chromatic aberration?

Refractive power of the lens of the eye is different for different colours. Therefore, the light rays of different colours get focused at different distances behind the lens. This error is also physiological and is called chromatic aberration. Light rays passing through the central portion of the lens almost pass without refraction. But rays passing through the peripheral portion of the eye lens get more and more refracted. When pupil dilates, this error increases because peripheral portions of the lens are exposed. When pupil constricts, this error is minimized as only central portion of the lens is exposed.

What is depth of focus?

Depth of focus is the maximum distance through which object can be moved but still can be clearly focused on the retina. Depth of focus is highest with smallest pupillary size because then it acts as a pinhole camera. Depth of focus decreases as size of the pupil increases.

What is diffraction of light?

Bending of the light rays as they pass over the sharp borders of the pupil is known as diffraction. It interferes with image formation when pupillary size is small. The ideal size of pupil is 2.5 mm and not 1.5 mm (smallest diameter possible) because though with 1.5 mm diameter of pupil, depth of focus is highest, diffraction of light will interfere with image.

What is cataract?

Cataract is opaque area in the lens. This is a common eye abnormality occurring in old persons. At first there is denaturation of proteins of the lens and then lens proteins are coagulated to form an opaque area. With deposition of calcium in the coagulated proteins at a later stage, there is further increase in lens's opacity. Opacity of the lens greatly hampers transmission of light and seriously affects vision.

What is the treatment of cataract?

Surgical removal of the opaque lens with replacement of another lens or glasses is the treatment of cataract.

AQUEOUS HUMOUR

What is aqueous humour? How is it formed? What is its composition?

Aqueous humour is a clear liquid which fills the anterior and posterior chambers of eye. It is formed by active transport and diffusion from capillaries in the ciliary body. It has the same composition as that of blood plasma (only protein concentration in it is much lower than that of plasma). It carries glucose, amino acids and respiratory gases. It has high content of ascorbic acid.

What are the functions of aqueous humour?

1. Supplies nutrition to lens and cornea, both of which are avascular structures.
2. Maintains intraocular pressure and therefore the shape of the eyeball.

How is aqueous humour circulated?

Aqueous humour is produced by ciliary body and enters the posterior chamber. Then through pupil it enters the anterior chamber. From here it is reabsorbed through a network of trabeculae called 'canal of Schlemm' (present at sclerocorneal junction) and goes to episcleral venous plexus and then into anterior ciliary veins. Pressure of blood in episcleral venous plexus is always lesser than the pressure of aqueous humour in the eye. This acts as a force causing continuous outflow of aqueous humour. Blinking movements of eye further increase this pressure gradient and helps the outflow of aqueous humour. There is a constant renewal of aqueous humour. Complete renewal of aqueous humour occurs once every hour.

What is intraocular pressure? How is it measured? How much is it normally?

Pressure of aqueous humour in the eye is 16 to 18 mmHg. It is called intraocular pressure and is measured with the help of an instrument known as tonometer. This pressure helps to maintain the shape of the eyeball.

What is glaucoma?

Glaucoma is the condition where there is increased intraocular pressure. It is due to obstruction of the outflow of aqueous humour. This obstruction usually occurs at 'canal of Schlemm'.

VITREOUS HUMOUR

What is vitreous humour? What is its function?

Vitreous humour is a clear gelatinous material which fills the space between lens and retina. It has high viscosity. It consists of gel like substance that contains a network of thin fibres of a highly hygroscopic protein analogous to gelatin.

The function of vitreous humour is to maintain the shape of the eyeball and to refract light.

REFRACTION

What is refractive index?

When light rays pass from one medium into the other, velocity of light changes. The substances through which light passes are known as transparent substances. The refractive index of any transparent substance is the ratio of velocity of light in air to velocity of light in the substance.

What is refraction?

Bending of light rays at an angulated interface is known as refraction. When light passes from one medium into another, if the interface between two media is plane (perpendicular to the beam of light) there is no change in the direction of light rays while passing from one medium into another (only velocity changes). But when interface between two media is angulated then light rays change their direction at the interface. Refraction depends on two factors:

- Degree of angulation of interface between two media and the beam of light rays—greater the angulation greater is the refraction.
- Difference in the refractive indices of two media—greater the difference greater is the refraction.

Enumerate the different types of lenses.

Lenses have two varieties, namely (a) spherical, and (b) cylindrical. Each one may be convex or concave. Thus there are four types of lenses:

- Convex spherical lens.
- Convex cylindrical lens.
- Concave spherical lens.
- Concave cylindrical lens.

What is the main difference between convex and concave lenses?

Convex lens converges the light whereas the concave lens diverges the light rays.

What is the difference between spherical and cylindrical lenses?

Spherical lens refracts the light in all the planes whereas the cylindrical lens refracts the light only in one plane.

What is the focal length of the lens?

In case of convex lens, parallel light rays are focused to a single point (or line in cylindrical convex lens) beyond the lens, called focal point. The distance between centre of the lens and focal point is called focal length of the lens.

How do you express the refractive power of the lens?

In case of convex spherical lens, refractive power is equal to 1 divided by focal length of the lens in metres. If focal length is 1 m, refractive power of the lens is +1 D (dioptre). If focal length is 0.5 m, refractive power will be +2 D.

In case of concave lens, light rays diverge and therefore it cannot be expressed in terms of focal distance beyond the lens. The power of concave lens is expressed by comparing it with the power of convex lens. If a concave lens diverge the same amount of light which convex lens of say +2 D is converging, the refractive power of a concave lens is said to be −2 D (i.e. it completely nullifies the effect of convex lens of +2 D).

Name the different refractive media of the eye with their refractive indices.

Light passes from air into the eye through the following refractive media:

Refractive medium		Refractive index
1. Cornea	=	1.38
2. Aqueous humour	=	1.33
3. Lens	=	1.4
4. Vitreous humour	=	1.34
5. Air	=	1

Name the different refractive surfaces of the eye and their refractive powers.

Refractive surface	Refractive power
1. Anterior surface of cornea	+48 D
2. Posterior surface of cornea	−4 D
3. Lens of the eye	+15 D

At which refractive surface in the eye maximum refraction occurs and why?

Maximum refraction occurs at the anterior surface of cornea. The reasons are:

- Anterior surface of the cornea has greater curvature.
- There is greater difference between refractive indices of air and cornea.

What is the refractive power of the lens of the eye when it is taken out? Why?

Refractive power of the lens inside the eye is +15 D and when it is taken out, its refractive power is +150 D. Lens is surrounded by two fluids inside the eye (aqueous humour in front and vitreous humour behind) and refractive indices of these two fluids do not differ much from that of the lens. But when the lens is taken out of the eye, its refractive power is much more because of the greater difference between refractive indices of the lens and the air which surrounds it.

What is reduced eye?

Reduced eye is schematic representation of the eye considering that the eye has only a single convex lens of +59 D (algebraic summation of refractive powers of different refractive surfaces of the eye) placed at a distance of 17 mm from retina.

What is nodal point? Where does it lie in normal eye?

Centre of the lens of the reduced eye is called nodal point. It lies 7.08 mm behind the cornea.

ERRORS OF REFRACTION

What is emmetropia?

Emmetropia is the condition in which with ciliary muscles completely relaxed, parallel rays coming from the distant object are focused on the retina. Normal eye is emmetropic (Fig. 8.2).

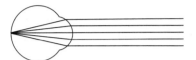

FIGURE 8.2 Emmetropia.

Name the different refractive errors of the eye.

PATHOLOGICAL ERRORS

- Myopia or near sightedness.
- Hypermetropia or far sightedness.
- Astigmatism.

PHYSIOLOGICAL ERRORS

- Spherical aberration.
- Chromatic aberration.
- Diffraction.

What is myopia or short sightedness? What are its causes?

Myopia is the refractive error of the eye in which with ciliary muscles completely relaxed, parallel rays coming from the distant object are focused in front of the retina. It is either due to too long eyeball (relative to its refractive power) or increased refractive power of the lens (Fig. 8.3).

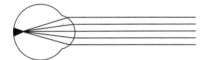

FIGURE 8.3 Myopia.

What are the far point and near point for myopic person?

With ciliary muscles completely relaxed, the parallel rays coming from the distant object are focused in front of the retina in a myopic person. There is no mechanism available in the eye to reduce the power of the lens further. Therefore, myopic person is unable to see the distant object. As the object comes nearer and nearer to the eye, a point will come at which it is focused on the retina and is seen clearly by the person. This is far point for a myopic person which is nearer to the eye as compared to in emmetropic person. When the object moves still nearer and nearer from this far point, person would contract his ciliary muscles (accommodation for near vision) till the ciliary muscles fully or maximally contract. The distance from the eye at which ciliary muscles maximally contract would be the near point. For the myopic person it is nearer to the eye as compared to in emmetropic person.

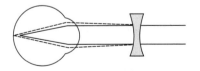

FIGURE 8.4 Correction of myopia.

How is myopia corrected?

Myopia is corrected by giving concave lens of appropriate refractive power {decided by trial and error method (Fig. 8.4)}.

What is hypermetropia or far sightedness?

Hypermetropia or far sightedness is the condition in which with ciliary muscles completely relaxed, parallel rays coming from the distant object are not refracted sufficiently by a lens system to come to a focus by the time they reach retina {i.e. parallel rays are focused behind the retina (Fig. 8.5)}.

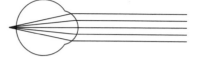

FIGURE 8.5 Hypermetropia.

What are the causes of hypermetropia?

Hypermetropia is due to too short eyeball (relative to its refractive power) or weaker lens system of the eye.

Where is the far point and near point for hypermetropic person?

Hypermetropic person cannot see the distant object clearly with ciliary muscles completely relaxed. To overcome this, his ciliary muscles slightly contract and increase the power of the lens to see the far object. Thus hypermetropic person has the same far point as emmetropic person but he uses his power of accommodation for near vision to certain extent for focusing the far objects. When the object comes nearer and nearer, there is greater and greater contraction of ciliary muscles to focus the object on the retina. A point comes at which ciliary muscles are maximally contracted. This is the near point for the hypermetropic person. It is away from the eye as compared to emmetropic person, i.e. near point recedes.

How is hypermetropia corrected?

Hypermetropia is corrected by giving convex lens of appropriate strength {decided by trial and error method (Fig. 8.6)}.

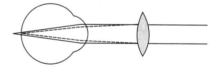

FIGURE 8.6 Correction of hypermetropia.

What is astigmatism? What is it due to?

Astigmatism is the defect in the refractive power of the lens of the eye only in one plane. It is due to oblong shape of the cornea or lens. Due to oblong shape, degree of curvature in long axis is not as great as that in short axis. Therefore, refractive power of the lens in two planes is different.

How is astigmatism corrected?

Astigmatism is corrected by giving cylindrical lens in a defective axis.

Why is cylindrical lens used for correcting astigmatism?

In astigmatic lens, the refractive error is present only in one plane of the lens and cylindrical lens refracts only in one plane. Therefore, for correction of astigmatism, cylindrical lens is given in the plane which requires correction.

How is plane of abnormal component of the astigmatic lens determined?

There is a chart having parallel black bars deviating from the centre. The person is asked to look at the chart with one eye. If there is no astigmatism, bars in all directions will be seen clearly. If there is astigmatism, bars in one plane may be out of the focus and therefore not clearly seen by the person. Same is the plane in which cylindrical lens is given for correcting astigmatism. Strength of the lens is decided by trial and error method (Fig. 8.7).

What are contact lenses? What are their advantages and disadvantages?

In recent years, either glass or plastic lenses are prepared and fitted snugly against the cornea for correcting refractive errors of eye. Such lenses are called contact lenses.

ADVANTAGES

- Lens turns with the eye and therefore gives a broader field of vision.
- Contact lens has little effect on the size of the object the person sees through the lens as compared to lens placed several centimetres away from the eye.
- The refraction from the anterior surface of cornea is totally nullified because the contact lens is snugly fitted against the anterior surface of the cornea. This is especially important in a person in whom the refractive error is caused due to abnormal shape of cornea, e.g. keratoconus—the condition in which there is bulging of the cornea.

DISADVANTAGES

Contact lens fits snugly against the cornea. Cornea being an avascular structure, a part of oxygen for it is obtained directly from the atmosphere. Due to contact lens, this supply of oxygen is affected causing damage to the cornea leading to corneal opacity at the site of damage.

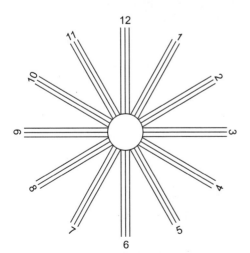

FIGURE 8.7 Chart composed of parallel black bars for determining the axis of astigmatism.

ACCOMMODATION

What is accommodation?

Ability of the eye to see near as well as far objects clearly is known as accommodation.

How is the eye accommodated for far vision?

Object can be seen clearly only when it is focused on the retina. For looking at the far object, ciliary muscles are completely relaxed, suspensory ligament is tensed, eye lens has minimum refractive power of +15 D. Therefore, parallel rays coming from the far object are focused on the retina which is placed at the focal plane of lens system of the eye.

What is the effect of contraction of ciliary muscles?

Contraction of both types of ciliary muscles causes laxation of suspensory ligament. This reduces the tension on the lens capsule and because of its elastic nature, lens assumes globular shape and its refractive power increases. With maximum contraction of ciliary muscles, the eye lens has refractive power of +29 D. With different degrees of ciliary muscles contraction, the lens power increases from +15 D to +29 D (Fig. 8.8).

How is the eye accommodated for near vision?

Light rays coming from the near object are divergent. Therefore, greater refractive power of the lens is required to focus them on the retina. This is achieved by contraction of ciliary muscles which causes laxation of suspensory ligament and makes the lens more globular. The degree of contraction of ciliary muscles depends upon the distance between the object and the eye. Lesser the distance, greater is the contraction. Thus any near object's image is focused on the retina by increasing the refractive power of the lens of the eye and the person is able to see the object clearly. Highest refractive power of the lens achieved in young person is +29 D (with maximum contraction of ciliary muscles).

How is the contraction of ciliary muscles controlled?

Ciliary muscles are supplied by parasympathetic nerves which run in third cranial or oculomotor nerve. Stimulation of these nerves causes contraction of ciliary

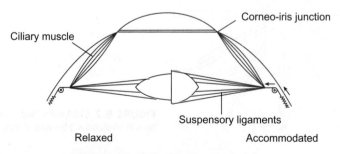

FIGURE 8.8 Mechanism of accommodation.

muscles. When the object is at a far distance, there are no parasympathetic impulses to ciliary muscles, therefore they remain in a relaxed state. But when object is brought nearer and nearer to the eye, more and more number of parasympathetic impulses impinge on ciliary muscles leading to greater and greater degree of contraction of ciliary muscles.

What is far point?

Far point is the farthest distance from the eye at which an object is seen clearly. Normally far point is supposed to be at 20 feet or 6 m distance from the eye.

What is near point?

Nearest distance from the eye at which object can be seen clearly is called near point. In a normal young person it is 25 cm (approximately 10 inches) from the eye.

What is the range of accommodation?

Distance between far point and near point is known as range of accommodation.

What is the amplitude of accommodation?

Amplitude of accommodation is the difference between the refractive powers of the lens with ciliary muscles maximally contracted (+29 D) and with ciliary muscles completely relaxed (+15 D). In normal young person amplitude of accommodation is 29 D − 15 D = 14 D.

What are the other changes occurring during accommodation for near vision in addition to increased refractive power of the lens?

In addition to increased refractive power of the lens during accommodation for near vision, there is convergence of eyes and constriction of pupil.

What is the benefit of constriction of pupil occurring during accommodation of eye for near vision?

When eye is accommodated for near vision, constriction of pupil that occurs is beneficial because it:

- Reduces spherical aberration.
- Reduces chromatic aberration.
- Increases depth of focus.
- Reduces the amount of light entering the eye.

What is presbyopia?

Presbyopia is the condition where the amplitude of accommodation is reduced. As person grows older, the lens of the eye loses its elasticity because of progressive denaturation of lens proteins. Therefore, ability of the lens to change its shape progressively decreases with age. At the age of 40 to 50 years, the amplitude of accommodation is reduced from 14 D to almost 2 D. This means that lens becomes an almost non-elastic solid mass and remains focused permanently at constant distance from the eye. It cannot be accommodated for far or near vision. It becomes almost non-accommodative.

How is presbyopia treated?

In presbyopia, person's eyes cannot be accommodated for far as well as near vision. Therefore, presbyopic person is given bifocal glasses with upper segment focused for seeing far objects and lower segment focused for seeing near objects.

During accommodation for near vision which surface of the lens becomes more globular?

During accommodation for near vision, the anterior surface of the eye lens becomes more convex. There is almost no change in the posterior surface of the lens.

VISUAL ACUITY

What is visual acuity?

Visual acuity or acuteness of vision is defined as power of the eye to resolve two stimuli separated in space. It is defined as minimum separable, i.e. minimum distance between two stimuli at which they are just resolvable (can be perceived as two separate stimuli). It is expressed as reciprocal of the angle subtended by two stimuli at the nodal point of the eye at which they are recognized as separate stimuli. In a normal person when angle subtended is '1 minute', stimuli are just resolvable (Fig. 8.9).

What is the importance of visual acuity?

Visual acuity helps us in determining outline, form or shape and other minute details of the object.

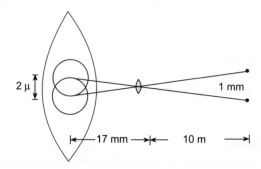

FIGURE 8.9 Maximum visual acuity for two point sources of light.

What are the factors affecting visual acuity?

- Type of stimulus.
- Illumination of the surface.
- Time exposure.
- Brightness contrast.
- Normal and abnormal errors of refraction:
  - Chromatic aberration tends to reduce visual acuity and therefore use of monochromatic light increases the visual acuity.
  - Errors of refraction such as myopia, hypermetropia and astigmatism reduce visual acuity.
- Visual acuity also depends on the site of the retina where the image is formed. Visual acuity is highest at fovea centralis where only cones are present and it tends to reduce towards the periphery of retina.

How is visual acuity tested clinically?

Visual acuity is tested clinically with the help of Snellen chart. It is tested by the ability of the subject to recognize test-letters on the chart which because of their size and distance subtend, known visual angles.

DEPTH PERCEPTION

What is monocular vision?

When only one eye is used for vision, it is called monocular vision.

What is binocular vision?

When both eyes are used for vision, it is called binocular vision.

What is depth perception?

Perceiving the distance of the object from the eye is known as depth perception.

Name mechanisms by which depth perception occurs.

Mechanisms of depth perception are:

1. *Judging the distance by sizes of retinal images.* Distance of the objects of known dimensions can be judged by sizes of retinal image. Retinal image becomes larger as the object comes nearer.

2. *Judging the distance by moving parallax.* When head is turned to one side, images of near objects move across the retina, whereas those of the far objects remain almost stationary.

3. *Stereopsis.* By using binocular vision. Images of near objects are formed on the temporal portions of the two retinae whereas images of far objects lie on nasal portions of the two retinae. This type of parallax is always there with

binocular vision which helps us to know the relative distances of the objects from the eye.

RETINA

Name the different layers of retina.

There are ten different layers of retina. From outside to inside they are as follows (Fig. 8.10):

- Pigment cell layer.
- Layer of processes of rods and cones.
- External limiting membrane.
- Outer nuclear layer of cell bodies of rods and cones.
- Outer synaptic layer—containing synapses between rods and cones and the bipolar cells.
- Inner nuclear layer—consisting mainly of bipolar cells.
- Inner synaptic layer—containing synapses between bipolar cells and ganglion cells
- Layer of ganglion cells.
- Layer of optic nerve fibres—containing axons of ganglion cells (stratum optimum).
- Internal limiting membrane.

The light has to pass through different inner layers of retina to reach the receptors (rods and cones). This definitely decreases visual acuity.

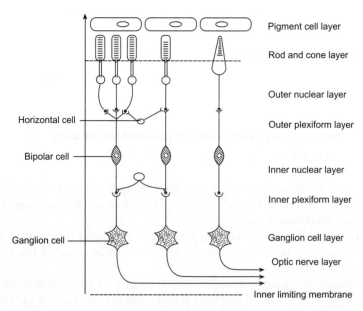

FIGURE 8.10 Layers of retina.

What are the receptors of eye?

Rods and cones are the receptors of eye.

What is the range of light to which human eye is sensitive?

Human eye is sensitive to light rays of 370 to 740 mµ (nm).

What is macula?

Macula is a small area of 1 mm^2 present in the central portion of retina. It is capable of acute and detailed vision because it contains only cones.

What is fovea or fovea centralis? Why has it the highest visual acuity?

Centre of macula (0.4 mm diameter) forms fovea centralis. Fovea is depression. Therefore this central area is depressed as compared to the surrounding area due to displacement of all outer layers of retina (nerve and vessels, ganglion cell layer, inner synaptic layer, inner nuclear layer) to one side. This allows light to pass unimpeded on the receptors (cones) which aids in acuity of visual perception.

How are the receptors rods and cones distributed over the retina?

In central portion of retina (macula) only cones are present. As one goes towards the peripheral portion, concentration of cones decreases and that of rods increases.

What is the function of cones?

Cones mainly function in bright light and are responsible for colour sensation.

What is the function of rods?

Rods mainly function in dim light and can only perceive shades of white and black.

What are the functions of pigment layer of retina?

1. Pigment layer of retina is the outermost layer. After the light passes through different layers of retina, it is absorbed by the pigment cells and reflection of light into the eye is prevented. Thus eye is converted into a dark chamber. This is essential for image formation.
2. Pigment cells also store vitamin A which is required for synthesis of photosensitive chemicals.

How does retina obtain its nutrition?

There is a central retinal artery which enters the eye along with the optic nerve. This artery supplies especially the inner layers of retina. Though retina has independent blood supply, at least outer layers of retina are partly dependent on choroid for their nutritional supply (mainly vitamin A required for formation of photosensitive chemical).

What is detachment of retina? What are its causes?

Beyond the pigment layer, different inner layers of retina form neural layers of retina. When neural layers get detached from pigment epithelium, it is called detachment of retina.

It occurs due to:

- Injury.
- Contracture of the fine collagenous fibres of vitreous humour which pull the neural retina unevenly towards the interior of the eye.

What is the treatment of retinal detachment?

Surgical replacement of retina to its normal relationship with pigment epithelium is the treatment for retinal detachment. Though retina resists degeneration because of its independent blood supply through retinal artery and diffusion of nutrients through detachment gap, it is better to operate as early as possible to obtain normal retinal function.

RECEPTORS

Describe in short the structure of rod and cone.

Basic structure of a rod or a cone is similar. Each rod or cone consists of following parts (Fig. 8.11):

- Outer segment.
- Inner segment.
- Nucleus.
- Synaptic body.

Membrane of the outer segment is thrown into large number of folds forming shelves arranged in number of discs, one on the top of the other. Photosensitive chemical is incorporated in the membrane of the disc.

Inner segment continuously synthesizes photosensitive chemical and discs which move towards the outer segment. Old discs from outer segments at their tip are destroyed by phagocytosis.

What is the photosensitive pigment (chemical) present in the rods?

Photosensitive chemical present in the rods is known as rhodopsin. It is a combination of 11-*cis* retinal (which is aldehyde of vitamin A) with a protein called scotopsin. Rhodopsin is also called visual purple.

What is the photosensitive chemical present in the cones?

Cones contain a photosensitive pigment which is formed by combination of retinal (which is absolutely same as in rhodopsin) with protein photopsin.

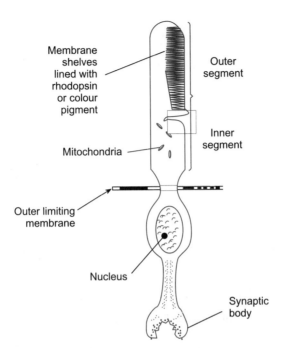

FIGURE 8.11 Functional parts of rod.

There are three different photosensitive chemicals responding to three different basic colours:

- Porphyropsin (red sensitive pigment).
- Iodopsin (green sensitive pigment).
- Cyanopsin (blue sensitive pigment).

PHOTOCHEMISTRY OF RODS

Describe rhodopsin-retinal visual cycle.

Exposure of rods to light causes retinal portion of rhodopsin to change from 11-*cis*-retinal to *all-trans*-retinal (Fig. 8.12). Reactive sites of scotopsin can no more fit into those of all transretinal and therefore it begins to split away. After forming multiple intermediate substances rhodopsin splits into all transretinal and scotopsin.

In darkness *all-trans*-retinal is converted to 11-*cis* form of retinal which automatically combines with scotopsin to form rhodopsin. *All-trans*-retinal can also be converted to *all-trans*-vitamin A, if retina is exposed to light for a long time. In darkness *all-trans*-vitamin A, is converted to 11-*cis*-vitamin A, then into 11-*cis*-retinal which combines with scotopsin to form rhodopsin.

What is night blindness or nyctalopia?

Night blindness is a disease that occurs due to vitamin A deficiency. Due to vitamin A deficiency, there is decreased amount of photosensitive chemicals in the

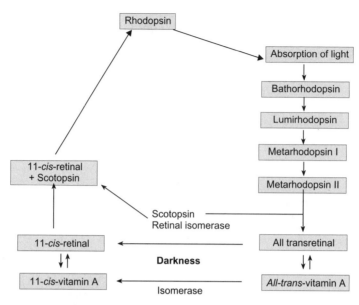

FIGURE 8.12 Rhodopsin-retinal visual cycle.

photoreceptors; bright light in day time is sufficient to stimulate them but patient has difficulty of vision in dim light (as intensity is not sufficient to stimulate receptors).

How much is the resting membrane potential of the rod or a cone?

Under-resting condition potential of a rod or a cone is –30 mV. This is because outer segment membrane is leaky to sodium under-resting condition. Inner segment constantly pumps sodium outside creating negative potential inside the receptor but sodium continuously leaks back into the receptor through membrane of outer segment, thereby neutralizing negativity on the inside of the entire cell.

How are the rods or cones excited?

When light is absorbed by the photosensitive chemicals present in outer segments of rods and cones, they get excited. Absorption of light in photosensitive chemical decreases the permeability of the membrane of outer segment for sodium. Inner segment still constantly pumps the sodium but now it does not diffuse through outer segment to the inside of the receptor. This causes greater negativity inside the receptor (hyperpolarization). Potential varies from resting -30 mv to -90 mV (with intense stimulation) (Fig. 8.13).

What are the mechanisms which cause development of receptor potential in the eye receptors?

Exact mechanism of excitation of receptors with light is not known. There are though a number of theories.

There is no direct interaction between the membrane disc containing rhodopsin and the plasma membrane of outer segment of rod which contains Na^+ channels. Some type of messenger therefore must transmit a signal from photoactivated

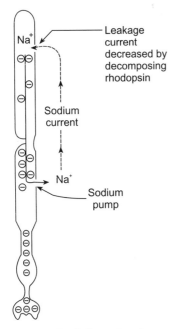

FIGURE 8.13 Generation of hyperpolarization caused by rhodopsin decomposition.

rhodopsin to the plasma membrane of outer segment causing Na^+ channels to close. c-GMP appears to be the second messenger and it regulates opening and closing of Na^+ channels. In dark there are high levels of c-GMP in the rod. c-GMP binds with protein of Na^+ channels in the rod of outer membrane to split them in open state.

In the light, photoactivated rhodopsin lowers the level of c-GMP as explained below which in turn causes closure of Na^+ channels.

- When rhodopsin absorbs a photon of light, it is converted into metarhodopsin II, which is an activated form of rhodopsin.
- Metarhodopsin II activates transducin which is a protein present in membrane of disc and plasma membrane of rod in inactive state.
- Activated transducin activates enzyme c-GMP phosphodiesterase. This enzyme degrades cyclic GMP in rod producing lowering of c-GMP level. This in turn causes closure of Na^+ channels.

Exactly similar changes occur in cones.

PHOTOCHEMISTRY OF CONES (COLOUR VISION)

Describe the mechanism of colour vision.

Cones are responsible for colour vision. There are three types of photosensitive chemicals present in three different types of cones. Spectral sensitivities of the three photosensitive chemicals are different. Each photosensitive chemical is sensitive to a small range of light wavelength and maximally sensitive to only one wavelength (colour). The cones are labelled as green, red and blue cones according to the sensitivity of their photosensitive chemicals to a particular colour (435 nm blue, 535 nm green and 575 nm red) (Fig. 8.14).

There is a trichromatic theory which explains the mechanism of colour vision. According to this theory, blue, green and red are the basic colours and different types of colour shades of spectrum can be obtained by different combinations of these basic colours. When eye is stimulated with any colour, three different types of cones are stimulated to a different extent. Ratio of stimulation of red : green : blue are responsible for recognition of a particular colour by CNS, e.g. when monochromatic orange light with wavelength 580 nm is stimulating the eye, red cones are stimulated to stimulus value of 99 (i.e. 99% of the peak stimulation at optimum wavelength), green cones are stimulated to a stimulus value of 42 and blue cones are not stimulated, i.e. their stimulus value is zero. In this case, ratio of stimulation of red : green : blue cones are 99:42:0. The nervous system interprets this set as orange colour. Likewise such multiple ratios are obtained with different wavelengths and each ratio is interpreted as a particular colour by nervous system.

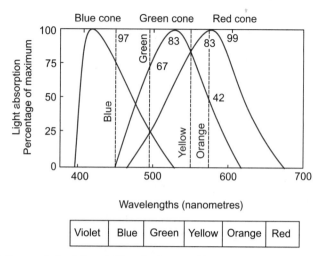

FIGURE 8.14 Degree of stimulation of different colour sensitive cones by monochromatic lights (blue, green and orange).

What is colour blindness?

Failure to differentiate some colours from the others is called colour blindness. It results due to absence of one group of colour cones. Therefore, a person may be colour blind for any one colour.

- When green cones are absent, the person is green blind. The condition is known as deuteranopia and the green colour blind person is known as deuteranope.
- When red cones are absent, the person is red blind. The condition is known as protanopia and the red colour blind person is known as protanope.

The above two defects are common and therefore if the person is red blind or green blind the condition is called red green colour blindness because protanope and deuteranope, both are unable to differentiate between red and green colours.

- When blue cones are absent, the person is blue blind. The condition is known as tritanopia. The person who is blue blind is known as tritanope. It is a very rare condition.

Why do mainly males suffer from red-green colour blindness?

Red-green colour blindness is a genetic disease. Lack of particular colour gene leads to colour blindness. Colour genes are present in X chromosome and lack of colour gene is a recessive trait. In females, there are two X chromosomes and even if colour genes are present in one of the X chromosomes, female does not suffer from colour blindness. In males, there is only one X chromosome; therefore missing of colour genes will produce colour blindness. Usually males suffer from colour blindness and it is transmitted through female.

What is colour weakness?

Sometimes person does not have colour blindness but has colour weakness for a particular colour. In this case, colour cones are not missing but they are under-represented.

There are three types of such anomalies:

- Red weakness called protanomaly.
- Green weakness called deuteranomaly.
- Blue weakness called tritanomaly.

How is colour blindness tested?

Colour blindness is tested by the following tests:

1. *Holmgren's wool test.* Wool pieces of different colours are given and the person is asked to pile pieces of the same colour in one pile. If there is no colour blindness, the person would recognize that each piece is of different colour. If he is red-green blind, he will keep yellow, green, orange, red coloured pieces in the same pile because he would recognize them as having the same colour.

2. *Ishihara chart.* This chart has a background of colour dots on which letter or number is written with different colours. The colours in the charts are arranged in such a way that only normal person can read all letters and numbers correctly. Colour blind person is either not able to read or he reads wrongly.

3. *The Edridge-Green lantern.* In this test, subject has to identify the colour of the small illuminated area, size of which can be varied. This test is done during selection of engine or lorry drivers for detecting the colour defective vision.

DARK AND LIGHT ADAPTATION

What is dark adaptation? How does it occur?

When a person remains in darkness for a long time, there is increased sensitivity of retina to light which is known as dark adaptation (Fig. 8.15).

Dark adaptation occurs due to:

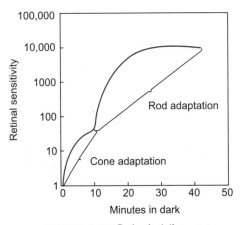

FIGURE 8.15 Dark adaptation curve.

1. *Increased sensitivity of retina to light.* Sensitivity to light is directly proportional to the antilogarithm of concentration of photosensitive chemicals in rods and cones, i.e. small change in concentration of chemicals brings about a very great change in sensitivity of retina to light. In darkness there is synthesis of photosensitive chemicals in rods and cones from retinal as well as from vitamin A. Thus concentration of photosensitive chemicals in both the receptors

increases which causes increased sensitivity of retina to light. This is the main mechanism of dark adaptation.

2. *Dilatation of pupil.* In darkness, pupil dilates and increases the amount of light entering into the eye.

3. *Neural mechanism.* It involves adaptation in the retinal neurons; the degree of adaptation is much less as compared to adaptation of photochemical system; however, this adaptation occurs in seconds, i.e. more quickly as compared to adaptation in the receptors.

How much is the time required for dark adaptation?

Moderate dark adaptation occurs in 40 minutes whereas complete dark adaptation takes about 18 hours.

What is the factor on which rate of dark adaptation depends?

Rate of dark adaptation depends on degree of previous exposure to light. If eye is exposed to light for a long time, photosensitive chemicals in the receptors not only split into retinal and opsin but vitamin A is formed from retinal. So vitamin A content of eye is high. When eye is exposed to darkness, vitamin A is first converted to retinal and then to photosensitive chemical. Interconversion of retinal to vitamin A is a slower process as compared to interconversion of retinal to photosensitive chemical. Therefore, dark adaptation takes a longer time when previous exposure of eye to light is for a long time.

What is light adaptation? How much time it takes?

When a person is exposed to light, there is decreased sensitivity of retina to light. This is called light adaptation. It occurs only in a few minutes.

Why light adaptation is quicker than dark adaptation?

Light adaptation occurs due to reduction in the concentration of photosensitive chemicals in rods and cones due to their splitting into retinal and opsin. Therefore, in light adaptation, slow reaction (interconversion between retinal and vitamin A) does not play any role and thus it occurs quickly.

What is negative after image?

When a person steadily looks at a particular scene for a long time, bright area of the scene causes light adaptation in corresponding portion of retina and dark area of the scene causes dark adaptation in corresponding retinal areas. If a person suddenly looks at a white screen, he sees the same scene but bright areas appear dark and dark areas of the scene appear bright. This is due to dark and light adaptation.

What is flicker fusion frequency?

Image of any object remains on the retina for some time so that if pictures are shown one after the other, they give an appearance of being continuous.

The critical frequency at which fusion occurs is known as flicker fusion frequency. Critical frequency is much higher in bright light as compared to in darkness.

What is the importance of light and dark adaptation?

Sensitivity of retina increases during darkness and decreases during exposure to light. Thus sensitivity of retina is automatically adjusted to changes in illumination.

What is photopic vision?

Photopic vision is the vision capable of discriminating different colours. It occurs in bright light in which cones are optimally functioning.

What is scotopic vision?

Scotopic vision is the vision capable of discriminating only between shades of black and white. It occurs in dim light in which rods are optimally functioning.

What is Purkinje shift?

In bright light, cones are optimally functioning; therefore the peak spectral sensitivity of retina is at 560 nm. In scotopic vision only rods are functional; therefore peak spectral sensitivity of retina is at 500 nm. This shift of peak spectral sensitivity when a person goes from bright to dim light is known as Purkinje shift.

NEURONAL CONNECTIONS IN RETINA

Name the neurons present in the retina and their connections.

Rods and cones are the photoreceptors. They are also modified neurons. From rods and cones the impulses pass to bipolar cells present in the inner nuclear layer and from bipolar cells the impulses pass to ganglion cells and to axons of ganglion cells from the optic nerve. In addition to bipolar and ganglion cells, there are other two types of neurons present in retina, viz. horizontal cells and amacrine cells.

What is the role played by horizontal cells?

Horizontal cells are responsible for spreading the signal horizontally (laterally on either side of stimulated area). These signals are inhibitory in nature. So, horizontal cells are responsible for lateral inhibition, i.e. zone of inhibition surrounding the excited area. This lateral inhibition is responsible for neutralizing spread of excitatory signals on either side and thus sharpening the boundary between dark and bright areas, thereby enhancing the contrast in the visual scene. This is an essential mechanism for visual accuracy in transmitting contrast borders in the visual image.

What is the role played by amacrine cells?

Amacrine cells only send transient signals when the intensity of light changes; hence, these cells probably help in detecting the rate of change of light intensity.

What are the types of bipolar cells? What are their functions?

There are two types of bipolar cells:

1. *Depolarizing bipolar cells* which are depolarized (get excited) when rods and cones are excited.
2. *Hyperpolarizing type of bipolar cells* which are hyperpolarized (inhibited) when the rods and cones are excited.

This reciprocal relationship of bipolar cells provides a second mechanism for lateral inhibition (in addition to that of horizontal cells) and helps in sharpening the contrast borders.

FUNCTIONS OF BIPOLAR CELLS

- Transmit impulses from rods and cones to the ganglion cells.
- Reciprocal relationship of two types of bipolar cells helps in enhancing the contrast in the visual scene as explained above.

What are the different types of ganglion cells?

Different types of ganglion cells are:

1. *W cells.* 40% ganglion cells are of this type. They have diameter of less than 10 nm and receive signals mainly from rods. Their main function appears to be detection of directional movement anywhere in the field of vision. They are also responsible for most of the rod vision occurring in dim light.
2. *X cells.* About 55% of ganglion cells are of this type. They have medium diameter (10 to 15 nm). They receive signals from cones and are probably responsible for colour vision.
3. *Y cells.* These are the largest cells with diameter up to 35 nm. They respond to rapid changes in the visual image. They apprise the central nervous system (CNS) almost instantaneously when an abnormal visual event occurs in the visual field but without specifying the location of the event; it gives clue to the CNS to move the eyes towards the exciting vision.

What are the responses of ganglion cells on excitation?

There is a background discharge from each ganglion cell (i.e. discharge under-resting condition). On stimulation there is increase in the rate of discharge. On inhibition there is decrease in the rate of discharge below the background level. There are different varieties of responses obtained from ganglion cells:

1. Many ganglion cells are excited by changes in the light intensity. Some of them show on-off responses and some show off-on responses.
    - *On-off response.* When light is turned on, cell is excited for a short period. Rate of discharge increases above the background level for a

short time and it comes back to normal even if the light is on. When the light is turned off, cell is inhibited for a short while and the rate of discharge decreases below the background level for a short period of time.

■ Exactly opposite is the off-on response shown by ganglion cells lying in inhibited area.

2. Many types of ganglion cells do not respond to flat areas of light but they mainly respond to contrast borders in the scene. When retina is stimulated by light in such a way that all photoreceptors are equally stimulated, contrast type of ganglion cells are not stimulated at all because of phenomenon of lateral inhibition.

3. There are a few ganglion cells which send colour information. These type of ganglion cells are stimulated by one colour and are inhibited by contrast colour, e.g. a few cells may get stimulated with green colour and inhibited by red colour and vice versa. Such type of response is also obtained because of lateral inhibition. This is the mechanism by which retina itself can differentiate the colours.

What is ERG (electroretinogram)? What is its use?

Recording of electrical activity of retina is known as electroretinogram. It is used to investigate retinal physiology and its disorders.

VISUAL PATHWAY

Describe the visual pathway.

1. Axons of the ganglion cells form the optic nerve which leaves the eye a little on the medial side of the posterior pole. At the optic chiasma all the fibres coming from nasal halves of retina cross to the opposite side and join with fibres from the opposite temporal retina to form optic tracts.

Each optic tract relays at dorsolateral geniculate nucleus. From lateral geniculate nucleus of each side, fibres run in geniculocalcarine tracts. These fibres pass by way of optic radiation to primary visual cortex present in calcarine area of the occipital lobe.

Visual pathway in short is as follows (Figs 8.16 a and b):

This pathway is called the new system of direct transmission to visual cortex. This system allows perception of all aspects of visual forms, colours and other details of conscious vision.

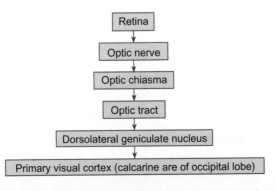

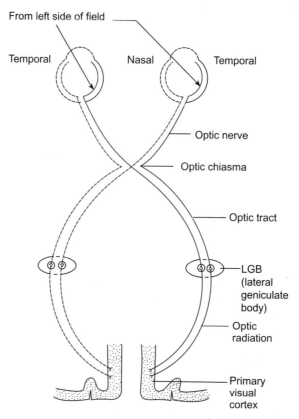

FIGURE 8.16(a) Visual pathway.

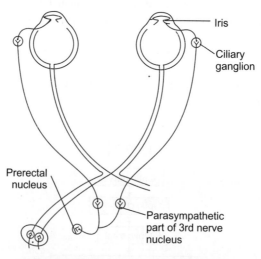

FIGURE 8.16(b) Visual pathway for light reflex.

2. Some visual fibres from optic tract go to other areas of the brain for performing different functions as follows:

- To suprachiasmatic nucleus of hypothalamus for controlling circadian rhythm which changes with day and night.
- To pretectal nucleus for activation of pupillary light reflex.
- To superior colliculus for controlling rapid directional movements of the eyes.
- To ventral lateral geniculate nucleus of thalamus to control behavioural functions.

This system which is described is the old system, which is sending impulses from receptors to midbrain and the base of the forebrain. This system does the same function as the new system in many lower animals.

How do the optic nerve fibres terminate in dorsolateral geniculate nucleus?

Optic tract which contains fibres from nasal halves of opposite retina and temporal halves of ipsilateral retina relays at dorsolateral geniculate nucleus. This nucleus has got six layers labelled as I, II, III, IV, V and VI from dorsal to ventral side. Layers II, III and V receive signals from temporal portion of ipsilateral retina whereas layers I, IV and VI receive signals from nasal halves of opposite side retina.

What are the functions of dorsolateral geniculate nucleus?

In the dorsolateral geniculate nucleus the respective retinal areas of two eyes connect with neurons that are approximately superimposed over each other in the paired layers. This helps causing comparison of images in two eyes required for depth perception, convergence and accommodation.

In the neurons of lateral geniculate body there is greater lateral inhibition caused as compared to neurons in the retina. This further enhances contrast in the visual scene. Dorsolateral geniculate nucleus relays information to the visual cortex. It acts as a 'Gate' and therefore controls the signal transmission to the cortex.

Signals from visual cortex are also transmitted to lateral geniculate nucleus through centrifugal fibres. These signals are inhibitory in nature. From dorsolateral geniculate nucleus, inhibitory signals are sent to retina to inhibit receptors. This causes filtration of retinal signals passing to the brain.

Layers I and II are called magnocellular layers because they contain large neurons. These neurons receive signals from 'Y' ganglion cells and very rapidly transmit them to the visual cortex. Layers III and IV are called parvocellular layers because they contain small sized neurons which receive signals from 'X' ganglion cells that transmit colour sensation as well as point to point spatial information.

Where is primary visual cortex located? Why is it also called striate cortex?

The primary visual cortex lies in the calcarine fissure area mostly on the medial aspect of the occipital cortex barely extending on lateral surface only at occipital pole. This is also called Brodmann cortical area 17. It shows gross striations and therefore is also called striate area.

How is the retina represented over the primary visual cortex?

Signals from macula of retina are received at the occipital pole, while signals from peripheral portions of retina terminate in concentric circles anterior to the pole and in the calcarine fissure. Upper portion of retina is represented superiorly and lower portion inferiorly. Fovea of retina has a large representation in the primary visual cortex.

How many layers does the primary visual cortex have? Where do the geniculocalcarine fibres terminate?

There are six layers in the cortex. Geniculocalcarine tract fibres terminate in layer 4 of the cortex. From layer 4, signals spread upward and downward. Signals from two eyes still remain separate.

Describe the neuronal columns of the visual cortex.

Visual cortex contains a large number of vertical columns of cells. Each column is of 30 to 50 µm diameter and represents a functional unit. Signals from dorsolateral geniculate nucleus terminate in layer 4 neurons called simple cells of the column. Then they spread outwards in layers 1, 2 and 3 and also inwards in layers 5 and 6 (formed of complex and hypercomplex cells). When signals spread into these layers, signals from two eyes do not remain separate. Separation is lost because of the lateral spread of the visual signals. Corresponding points of the two retinae fit with each other and there is fusion of images. This information is responsible for mechanism of stereopsis.

What is the function of primary visual cortex?

Visual cortex is only concerned with the contrasts in the visual scene rather than the flat areas. The degree of stimulation is proportional to the gradient of contrast. It also detects the orientation of contrast borders. This allows one to detect sizes and shapes of various objects in the visual scene.

Colour is also detected by colour contrast. Initial details of colour contrast are detected by simple cells whereas more complex colour contrasts are detected by complex and hypercomplex cells.

Where are secondary or association areas of visual cortex located? What is their function?

Association visual areas lie anterior, superior and inferior to primary visual cortex, i.e. surrounding the visual cortex from all the sides. This is called Brodmann's area 18. Located anterior to areas 17 and 18 is another association visual area, known as Brodmann's area 19.

Association areas receive signals mainly from primary visual cortex and are responsible for detection of more complex visual patterns.

What is the effect of removal of primary visual cortex?

Removal of primary visual cortex in human beings causes loss of conscious vision.

What is the effect of stimulation of primary and association visual cortex?

Stimulation of areas 17, 18 or 19 causes a person to have optic auras, i.e. he sees flashes of light, colours or simple forms such as lines, triangles.

What is the effect of destruction of areas 18 and 19?

Widespread destruction of areas 18 and 19 decreases person's ability to interpret the shapes and sizes of the different objects. If the destruction is in dominant hemisphere, it leads to 'word blindness', i.e. person can read but cannot interpret the meaning of the words.

FIELD OF VISION

What is field of vision? How is it plotted?

The field of vision is the area seen by an eye at a given instance. The area of nasal side is nasal field of vision, on lateral side is temporal field of vision, on upper side is superior field of vision and on the lower side is inferior field of vision.

Temporal field of vision represents nasal part of retina and vice versa, whereas superior field of vision represents inferior part of retina and vice versa. Field of vision is plotted on the charts with the help of perimeter (Fig. 8.17).

What is blind spot?

At the entry of optic nerve into the eye, receptors are absent and therefore this spot is blind. In the field of vision this spot lies 15° lateral to the centre because optic

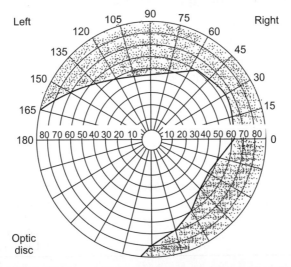

FIGURE 8.17 Perimetry chart showing the field of vision of the left eye.

nerves enter the eye through an area lying a little medial to the posterior pole. This blind spot can be determined in a person with perimetry.

What are scotomata? When do they occur?

In addition to blind spot stated above, blind spots occurring in other areas of retina are termed scotomata. They are seen in allergic reactions, tobacco poisoning, lead poisoning, etc.

What is retinitis pigmentosa?

It is the condition where retina degenerates and melanin gets deposited in degenerated retinal areas, leading to blindness detected by perimetry.

What is the use of perimetry?

Perimetry is the process by which field of vision of both eyes are plotted with the help of perimeter. It is useful in diagnosing condition like retinitis pigmentosa and scotoma. It is also useful in determining the site of lesion in the visual pathway by observing the pattern of blindness in the visual fields.

Describe the effects of lesions at different sites in the optic pathway on the field of vision.

Temporal field of vision represents nasal half of retina and vice versa because of optical system forming inverted image of the object on the retina. Superior field of vision represents inferior half of retina and vice versa.

Plotting of field of vision is useful in diagnosing site of lesion in the visual pathway from patterns of blindness in field of vision (Table 8.1).

Table 8.1	Effects of Lesions at Different Sites on the Field of Vision	
Site of lesion	**Effect on field of vision**	**Common causes**
Central portion of optic nerve on one side	Unilateral central scotoma (loss of vision in the centre of the field of vision)	• Retrobulbar neuritis leading to demyelination of optic nerve • Local disease of retina in the neighbourhood of macula mostly due to vascular disease
Central portion of optic nerve on both sides	Bilateral central scotoma	• Alcohol toxicity • Tobacco poisoning • Deficiency of vitamin B_{12} • Lesion in visual cortex

Table 8.1	Effects of Lesions at Different Sites on the Field of Vision—cont'd	
Site of lesion	**Effect on field of vision**	**Common causes**
Peripheral constriction	Concentric constriction of visual fields	• Optic atrophy • Long-standing papilloedema • Bilateral lesion of visual cortex • Retinitis pigmentosa
Damage of optic nerve	Total blindness in the corresponding eye; at first peripheral field of vision becomes blind, then the central field is affected	• Optic nerve atrophy (increased intracranial pressure)
Optic chiasma • Uncrossed fibres on one side damaged	Blindness in the nasal field of vision on the same side	• Aneurysmal dilatation of internal carotid artery Atherosclerotic internal carotid artery
• Damage to uncrossed fibres on both the sides	Blindness in nasal field of vision in both the eyes, called binasal hemianopia	• Bilateral lesions confined to uncrossed optic fibres • Open angle glaucoma
• Damage to crossed fibres (inferior half)	Blindness in both superior temporal field, called superior quadrantic bitemporal hemianopia; it gradually extends and involves whole of the temporal field	• Pituitary tumour • Traumatic or inflammatory lesions of optic chiasma
• Damage to crossed fibres (superior half)	Blindness in inferior temporal field of vision called inferior quadrantic bitemporal hemianopia	• Dilated third ventricle • Pituitary stalk tumour • Traumatic or inflammatory • Lesions of optic chiasma
Optic tract	Blindness in the temporal field of one side and nasal field of the opposite side, called homonymous hemianopia, e.g. in right optic tract lesion, left fields of vision of both eyes are blind	
Geniculocalcarine tract	Homonymous hemianopia	
Visual cortex	Homonymous hemianopia	

Loss of vision in one-half of visual field is known as hemianopia. When similar halves of both the fields are blind, it is called homonymous hemianopia. When dissimilar halves of fields of vision are blind, it is called heteronymous hemianopia. It is of two types: bitemporal (both temporal fields are blind) and binasal (both nasal fields are blind).

Any other blind spot than the normal blind spot is known as scotoma. If scotoma is in the periphery it does not affect the vision much but central scotoma (in macular region) definitely affects the vision.

When there is homonymous hemianopia, to judge whether lesion is in the optic tract or higher up, there are two tests:

- Light reflex—Fibres for light reflex leave optic tract and go to pretectal nucleus (PTN). If optic tract is damaged before these fibres leave to PTN, light reflex will be absent (when light is shown to blinded half of retina, no response is obtained). If the lesion is higher up, light reflex is present.
- Central or macular vision is spared in one sided visual cortical lesion because macula of each eye is represented bilaterally.

MUSCLES OF EYE AND EYE MOVEMENTS

What is strabismus or squint?

Lack of fusion of eyes in one or more coordinates is called strabismus or squint. These may be horizontal, vertical or torsional.

Name the extrinsic muscles of the eye.

There are three pairs of extrinsic muscles of the eye:

- Medial and lateral recti.
- Superior and inferior recti.
- Superior and inferior oblique.

What is the nerve supply of eye muscles?

Three sets of eye muscles are reciprocally innervated. Superior oblique is supplied by trochlear or IVth cranial, lateral rectus is supplied by abducent or VIth cranial nerve. Rest of the eye muscles are supplied by oculomotor or third cranial nerve. Nuclei of IIIrd, IVth and VIth cranial nerves are connected to each other through medial longitudinal fasciculus.

Describe the actions of various extrinsic muscles of the eye.

- Medial rectus: moves the eye medially (adduction).
- Lateral rectus: moves the eye laterally (abduction).
- Superior rectus: causes elevation (upward movement), adduction and intorsion (medial rotation) of the eye.
- Inferior rectus: causes depression (downward movement), adduction and extorsion (lateral rotation) of the eye.

- Superior oblique: causes depression, abduction and intorsion of eye.
- Inferior oblique: causes elevation, abduction and extorsion of the eye.

Describe the control of eye muscles.

Eye muscles are controlled by occipital visual areas through occipito-pectoral and occipito-collicular tracts going to pretectal and superior collicular areas of brain stem. Frontal cortex also controls the movements through frontotectal tracts passing from frontal cortex to pretectal nucleus. From pretectal and superior collicular areas signals go to nuclei of IIIrd, IVth and VIth cranial nerves. Signals are also transmitted to these nuclei from vestibular nuclei through medial longitudinal fasciculus.

Describe the fixation movements of eyes.

Fixation movements of the eyes are the ones by which eyes fix on the discrete portion in the visual field. It consists of two mechanisms:

1. Voluntary fixation mechanism by which person moves his eyes voluntarily to find object upon which he wishes to fix his vision. It is controlled by bilateral premotor cortical regions of the frontal lobes.
2. Involuntary fixation mechanism by which eyes are fixed on the object (image of the object is not allowed to leave fovea). It is controlled by area 19 of the occipital cortex.

What are the saccadic movements of the eyes?

Fixation of eyes on continuously moving visual scene is called saccadic movement, e.g. they occur when visual scene is constantly moving. When a person sitting in a moving train is looking out of the window, the movements of the eyes are called opticokinetic movements. In this, as the visual scene is moving, eyes keep on jumping from one point of fixation to other (2 to 3 jumps/sec). These jumps are called saccades. Similar type of saccadic movements takes place while reading.

What is the pursuit movement of eyes?

Movement of the eyes that occurs when they are fixed on moving object is called pursuit movement of the eyes, e.g. movement of eyes when they are fixed on a ball moving up and down. This type of movement occurs due to highly developed cortical mechanism.

What are the conjugate movements of eyes? How are they controlled?

Moving both the eyes simultaneously in one direction is called the conjugate movement. It is mainly controlled by superior colliculi.

Describe the autonomic nerve supply to the eye.

Eye is supplied by parasympathetic and sympathetic nerves. Parasympathetic preganglionic fibres arise from Edinger–Westphal nucleus (visceral nucleus of the third cranial nerve) and pass through the third cranial nerve to ciliary ganglion which lies behind the eye. Here the fibres synapse and postganglionic fibres pass through ciliary nerves into the eyeball. These nerves supply ciliary muscles and sphincter pupillae muscle of iris.

Sympathetic nerves to the eye originate in intermediolateral horn of first thoracic segment of the spinal cord. Preganglionic fibres arising from here relay at superior cervical ganglion and postganglionic sympathetic fibres from the ganglion spread along the carotid artery and its successive small branches. They enter the eye along with its arterial supply. These sympathetic fibres supply dilator pupillae muscle and many extraocular structures.

What is miosis?

Constriction of pupil is known as miosis. Stimulation of parasympathetic nerves to eye causes miosis.

What is mydriasis?

Dilatation of pupil is known as mydriasis. It occurs on sympathetic nerve stimulation.

PUPILLARY REFLEXES

What is pupillary light reflex?

When light is shown into the eye, pupil constricts. This is known as pupillary light reflex.

What is direct and indirect (consensual) light reflex?

When light is shown into the eye there is constriction of pupil. This is called direct light reflex. When light is shown in one eye, pupil on the other side constricts. This is known as indirect or consensual light reflex, occurring due to crossing over of nerve fibres in the visual pathway mainly at optic chiasma.

Describe the pathway of light reflex.

Pathway of light reflex is as follows:

Receptors (of retina) → optic nerve → optic chiasma → optic tract → pretectal nucleus → Edinger–Westphal nucleus → oculomotor nerve (parasympathetic fibres) → ciliary ganglion → short ciliary nerves → sphincter pupillae muscle causing constriction of pupil.

What is the function of light reflex?

Function of light reflex is to help the eye adapt rapidly to changing light condition.

Describe the pathway for accommodation reflex.

Pathway for accommodation reflex is as follows:

Receptors (of retina) → optic nerve → optic chiasma → optic tract → lateral geniculate body → visual cortex → frontal eye field (area 8) → internal capsule to opposite side Edinger–Westphal nucleus → oculomotor nerve → ciliary ganglion → ciliary nerves → ciliary muscles and sphincter pupillae muscle.

How is accommodation regulated?

Accommodation of lens is regulated by a negative feedback mechanism that automatically adjusts the focal power of the lens for highest degree of visual acuity. Different types of clues help to change the strength of the lens in the proper direction as follows:

- Chromatic aberration—Red light is focused posterior to blue. Depending on which of the two colours is better focused, lens is made stronger or weaker.
- During accommodation for near vision, there is convergence of eyes. Convergence mechanism causes simultaneous signals to increase the power of the lens of the eye.
- Fovea lies a little posterior than rest of the retina. So depending on clarity of focus in the depth of the fovea or that at the edge of the fovea, the clue to change the power of the lens is obtained.
- Degree of accommodation of lens oscillates slightly all the time. If visual image becomes clearer when strength of the lens increases, the lens strength will change in the same direction and vice versa.

What is Argyll Robertson pupil?

Pupil that fails to respond to light but does respond to accommodation and also is very small is called Argyll Robertson pupil. It is the diagnostic sign of central nervous system syphilis.

HORNER'S SYNDROME

What is Horner's syndrome?

When the sympathetic nerves to the eye are interrupted and interruption occurs at cervical sympathetic chain, it results into Horner's syndrome. This syndrome is characterized by the following:

- Pupil on that side remains persistently constricted (smaller in size).
- Superior eyelid droops on the corresponding side (partial ptosis).
- Blood vessels on the corresponding side of face and head become persistently dilated.
- Sweating cannot occur on the affected side of face and head.

HEARING

INTRODUCTION

What is the sound frequency range to which human ear is sensitive?

Human ear is sensitive to sound frequencies between 20 and 20,000 cycles/second.

Name the different parts of the ear.

Ear is divided into 3 parts:

1. External ear—pinna and external auditory meatus.
2. Middle ear.
3. Inner ear.

STRUCTURE AND FUNCTIONS OF EXTERNAL (OUTER) AND MIDDLE EAR

What is the function of pinna of the ear?

Pinna collects and reflects the sound waves into the external auditory canal. Pinna is more important in lower animals in whom it is movable.

What is the function of external auditory meatus or canal?

External auditory meatus conducts the sound waves to the tympanic membrane which shuts the external auditory canal medially.

What are the advantages of tortuosity of external auditory canal?

- Mechanical injury to the tympanic membrane is prevented.
- Helps in maintaining favourable temperature and humidity for normal functioning of tympanic membrane.

What is the shape of tympanic membrane?

Tympanic membrane shuts the external auditory canal medially. It is cone shaped with concavity directed towards the external auditory canal. Point of maximum convexity is called umbo.

Describe the walls of middle ear.

Middle ear is an air-filled cavity. Its lateral wall is formed of tympanic membrane. Its posterior wall communicates with air cavities in the mastoid process. Anterior wall contains two canals; upper one lodges the tensor tympani muscle and lower one lodges the Eustachian tube. Medial wall contains two windows. Oval window above in which footplate (faceplate) of stapes is put and round window below which is closed by a thin membrane.

What is the function of Eustachian tube?

Eustachian tube opens in middle ear by one end and its other end opens in the pharynx. Air can therefore pass through this tube. It does the function of equalization of pressure on two sides of the tympanic membrane.

What does middle ear contain?

Middle ear contains three small ossicles (malleus, incus and stapes) and two muscles (tensor tympani and stapedius).

Describe the arrangement of middle ear ossicles.

Ossicles in the middle ear are attached to each other by ligaments and form a chain. Handle of the malleus is attached to the umbo (convexity of tympanic membrane at its centre). At the other end of malleus, incus is attached and at the opposite end of incus, stem of stapes is attached. The faceplate of stapes lies in the oval window to which it is attached loosely by annular ligament.

What is the function of tensor tympani muscle?

Tensor tympani muscle constantly pulls the handle of malleus inwards and thus keeps the tympanic membrane tensed. Due to this, vibrations on any portion of the tympanic membrane are transmitted to the malleus.

What are the functions of middle ear?

1. Transmission of sound from external ear to inner ear through ossicular chain. When tympanic membrane vibrates with sound, ossicular system also vibrates and conducts the vibrations to fluid filled inner ear. While doing it, middle ear does the function of impedance matching.
2. Attenuation of sound by attenuation reflex. When ear is stimulated with a loud sound, it is attenuated, thus preventing damage which might be caused to inner ear because of loud sound.

What is impedance matching? How is it done?

Impedance is any obstacle in the pathway of sound and is expressed as amount of sound energy lost when sound passes in a medium. Impedance in a medium depends on acoustic resistance of the medium, which in turn depends on density and elasticity of the medium. When the sound is passing from one medium to the other of same acoustic resistance, sound wave will pass easily from one medium into the other. But if acoustic resistances of two media widely differ (i.e. their impedances do not match), most of the sound waves will be reflected back from the interface between two media. In the ear, sound is to be conducted from air-filled middle ear into the fluid-filled inner ear. Acoustic resistance of fluid is much more than that of air. Therefore, greater pressure is required to produce vibrations in fluid of inner ear. Unless fluid of inner ear vibrates, receptors are not stimulated and also the sound is not heard.

Pressure of sound wave is increased at the junction between middle and inner ear, i.e. oval window, by two mechanisms. Thus there are two mechanisms by which impedance matching is obtained.

(a) Surface area of tympanic membrane (55 mm^2) is 17 times larger than that of faceplate of stapes (3.2 mm^2). Therefore, though the same force is applied by the sound wave force per unit area, the pressure is increased by 17 times at the faceplate of stapes.

(b) Ossicles in chain act as lever system. This lever does not increase the amplitude of movement but increases pressure at faceplate of stapes by 1.3 times (compared to that at tympanic membrane).

Total increase in pressure at faceplate of stapes is equal to 17 × 1.3, i.e. 22 times. This increase is sufficient to overcome the impedance (inertia) of fluid and therefore it creates vibrations in the fluid of inner ear. Impedance matching is 50 to 75% for sound frequencies between 300 to 3000 cycles/sec.

What is attenuation reflex?

When very loud sound is transmitted through ossicular system to CNS, reflex is initiated with a latent period of 40 to 80 ms. This reflex causes contraction of tensor tympani muscle and the stapedius muscle. Contraction of tensor tympani muscle pulls the malleus inwards whereas contraction of stapedius muscle pulls stapes outward. These two opposing forces make the ossicular system very rigid and therefore it fails to vibrate with the sound wave. Thus sound is not allowed to enter inner ear (it is attenuated) or its intensity is reduced by 30 to 40 decibels.

What are the advantages of attenuation reflex?

1. Attenuation reflex occurs when loud sound enters the ear. It reduces its intensity (loud voice is converted to whisper). Thus it protects cochlea (inner ear) from damaging vibrations caused by excessively loud sound.
2. It attenuates and masks all the low frequency environmental sounds and allows the person to concentrate on the sounds above 1000 cycles/second, where most of the pertinent information in voice communication is transmitted.
3. When a person is talking loudly, it decreases person's hearing sensitivity to his own speech.

But because attenuation reflex has a latent period of 40 to 80 ms, sudden loud sound is likely to cause damage to the cochlea.

STRUCTURE AND FUNCTIONS OF INNER EAR (COCHLEA)

What is a resonant frequency of any vibrating system?

Any vibrating system that has inertia and an elastic component has a natural frequency at which it vibrates most easily. This frequency is called resonant frequency. Resonant frequency of ossicular system is 700 to 1400 cycles/sec.

What are the ways in which sound waves are transmitted to cochlea or inner ear?

1. Cochlea is embedded in bony cavity in the temporal bone and hence vibrations of the entire skull can cause fluid vibrations in cochlea. Therefore, tuning fork or electronic vibrator placed on the bony prominences of the skull, especially the mastoid process make the person to hear the sound. Energy available in air is not sufficient to cause hearing through bone.
2. Normally the sound waves are transmitted from tympanic membrane through ossicular system to oval window and then to the fluid of cochlea (air condition).

What is cochlea? Describe the structure.

Cochlea is a coiled bony tube, like shell of a snail, lying in the cavity of petrous part of the temporal bone. There is a central bony pillar called modiolus which has internal auditory canal containing auditory nerve. Bony canal of cochlea winds round the modiolus for two and a half turns tapering from base to the apex. A bony ledge osseous spiral lamina projects into the bony canal of cochlea. It winds round the modiolus like the thread of a screw. From the tip of osseous spiral lamina, basilar membrane arises which extends to the wall of cochlea. Another thin membrane called vestibular (Reissner's) membrane arises from upper surface of modiolus and extends up to the wall of cochlea. These two membranes divide cochlear bony canal into three tubes: (i) scala vestibule, above the vestibular membrane, (ii) scala media, between vestibular and basilar membrane, (iii) scala tympani, below the basilar membrane. Scala media is blind at both the ends. Scala vestibuli and scala tympani are connected at the apex through helicotrema. At the base, scala vestibuli opens at oval window where footplate of stapes lies. Scala tympani opens at round window at the base of the cochlea. Round window is covered by a thin membrane. Scala media is filled with endolymph composition of which is like intracellular fluid, and on the basilar membrane it contains organ of Corti which is the receptor organ. Scala vestibuli and tympani are filled with perilymph, composition of which is like extracellular fluid (Fig. 8.18).

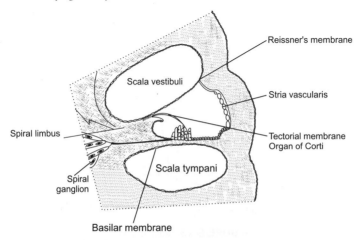

FIGURE 8.18 A section through one of the turns of cochlea.

Describe in short the structure of organ of Corti.

The main features of organ of Corti are the inner and outer rods of Corti forming a single row. These are based on the basilar membrane. Their upper ends converge and join forming part of lamina reticularis (Fig. 8.19).

Receptor cells in the organ of Corti are inner and outer cells. Their bases lie on the basilar membrane and their upper ends are embedded in lamina reticularis.

Inner hair cells form a single row on the inner side of inner rod of Corti. Outer hair cells form 3 to 4 rows on the outer side of outer rod of Corti. Hair coming out from upper end is covered by tectorial membrane. These cells are supplied by network of cochlear nerve endings. They lead to spiral ganglion present in modiolus.

Describe the basilar membrane.

Basilar membrane is a fibrous plate containing about 20,000 to 30,000 basilar fibres. Each fibre projects from the tip of osseous spiral lamina to the wall of the cochlea. These fibres are stiff, elastic and hair-like and are not fixed at their distal ends. Distal ends are embedded in the loose basilar membrane. These fibres vibrate like reeds of harmonica. The length of basilar fibres increases progressively from base to apex of cochlea (from 0.04 to 0.5 mm). Thus there is twelvefold increase in length. Diameter of the fibres decreases from base to the apex of cochlea. Therefore, there are stiff short fibres at the base which can vibrate with high frequency and thin long fibres at the tip which vibrate with low frequency.

Describe the transmission of sound wave in the cochlea.

Sound wave enters the cochlea at oval window. Each sound wave causes inward and outward movement of stapes. When stapes move inwards because of the movement of fluid, basilar fibres bulge towards the round window. This initiates a wave in the basilar membrane which travels from base to apex. Each wave is weak in the beginning. It becomes stronger and stronger as it passes from base to apex and ultimately becomes the strongest when it reaches the portion of the

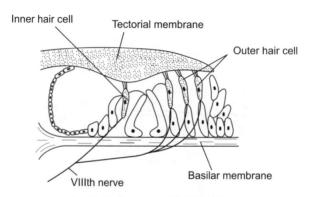

FIGURE 8.19 Organ of Corti.

basilar membrane with same resonant frequency (as that of stimulating sound wave). Basilar membrane vibrates at this site with a great ease so that the energy in the wave is dissipated and wave fails to travel further. Thus high frequency sound wave travels only short distance along the basilar membrane. Medium frequency travels about halfway whereas low frequency sound wave travels the entire distance along the membrane (Fig. 8.20).

Initially, wave travels faster and progressively it becomes slower. Therefore, high frequency sounds (at the base of basilar membrane) get spread out and therefore get easily discriminated from one another.

Inward and outward movement of stapes (one sound wave) actually causes development of four waves as follows:

- When stapes moves inwards.
- When stapes moves back to original position.
- When stapes moves outwards.
- When stapes comes back to original position.

Extent of movement of basilar membrane during one complete vibratory cycle (due to 4 waves as described above) is called the amplitude pattern of vibration of basilar membrane for a particular sound frequency. Basilar membrane vibrates up and down with each sound wave (Fig. 8.21a).

How is sound frequency analysis done?

Sound frequency is determined by place principle. Low frequencies of sound cause maximal activation of basilar membrane near the apex of cochlea. Sounds of high frequency activate the basilar membrane near the base of the cochlea and

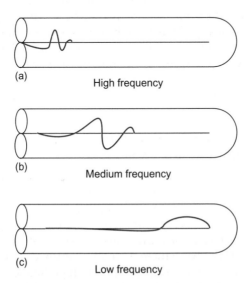

(a) High frequency

(b) Medium frequency

(c) Low frequency

FIGURE 8.20 Travelling waves along the basilar membrane for (a) high, (b) medium and (c) low frequency sound.

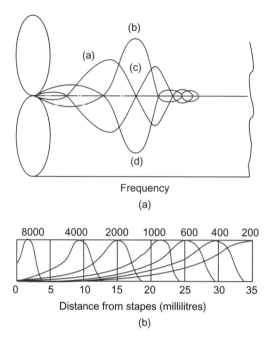

Frequency

(a)

Distance from stapes (millilitres)

(b)

FIGURE 8.21 (a) Amplitude pattern of vibration of basilar membrane for a medium frequency sound. (b) Amplitude pattern of sounds of different frequencies.

intermediate frequencies activate the membrane at intermediate distances (Fig. 8.21b). So, different portions of basilar membrane are activated by different frequencies of sound. There is also a spatial organization of nerve fibres in the auditory pathway all the way from basilar membrane to the auditory cortex. With each sound frequency, therefore, specific neurons are activated. This is the major method by which nervous system detects the frequencies of sound (by determining the portion of basilar membrane which is most stimulated). This is called the place theory. For very low frequencies of sound, there is synchronization between frequency of sound and rate of discharge through cochlear nerve. Low sound frequencies between 20 and 200 cycles/second are detected by this way.

Why basilar fibres near base vibrate at high frequency and those near the apex vibrate at low frequency?

Basilar fibres near the base are short and stiff whereas those at apex are thin and long. Therefore, basilar fibres near base vibrate with high frequency and those at apex vibrate with low frequency. In addition, the fibres are differentially loaded. The sound wave enters the cochlea through oval window at the base. Therefore, movement of activated basilar membrane also moves fluid between it and the oval window. For fibre near the base, there is small quantity of fluid to move between it and the oval window, so that it can vibrate with high frequency. Fibre at the apex has a large quantity of fluid to be moved between it and the oval window. Therefore, fibres at the apex vibrate with low frequency.

Name the potentials recorded from the ear at rest.

Under-resting condition (when ear is not stimulated with sound), two different potentials are recorded as follows:

1. Endocochlear potential. Electrical potential of $+80$ mV exists between endolymph of scala media and perilymph of scala vestibuli and tympani. This is called endocochlear or endolymphatic potential. It is due to some metabolic activity of stria vascularis (highly vascular structure present on the outer wall of scala media).
2. Resting potential of the hair cells. Each cell has a negative resting membrane potential. Therefore, intracellular fluid is at a potential of -70 mV with respect to perilymph. At the upper end of hair cell the potential difference between intracellular fluid and endolymph is therefore 150 mV (70 + 80). This high potential makes the cell very sensitive. Slightest movement of hair stimulates the cell.

How are hair cells excited?

When basilar membrane vibrates up and down with the sound wave, rods of Corti and lamina reticularis also vibrate up and down alongwith it. This causes sheering of hair of hair cells back and forth against the tectorial membrane. This excites the hair cells.

Name the potentials which are recorded from ear on stimulation.

When ear is stimulated with sound, two types of potentials are recorded:

- Cochlear microphonic potential.
- Action potential in the auditory nerve.

Describe the cochlear microphonic potential.

Cochlear microphonic potentials are produced by transformation of mechanical energy into electrical energy in much the same manner as pressure on a quartz crystal induces piezoelectric potential. These are produced at the upper ends of inner hair cells at the level of lamina reticularis, and are recorded by placing one electrode in scala media and one electrode in scala tympani. By recording cochlear microphonic potentials, it is found that basal turns of cochlea respond to all frequencies of sound stimuli. Only low frequencies cause a microphonic response from apical turn. Potentials recorded have the same form and polarity as that of the sound wave which is stimulating the ear. Increase in current flow associated with the cochlear microphonic stimulates terminal non-medulated auditory nerve endings. The excitatory phase of cochlear microphonic (i.e. increasing negativity in scala media) is associated with a current flow outwards across the membrane of the nerve fibres (Fig. 8.22).

State the properties of cochlear microphonic potential.

When cochlear microphonic potentials were first recorded, they were mistaken for action potential because they were first recorded from auditory nerve. But later on,

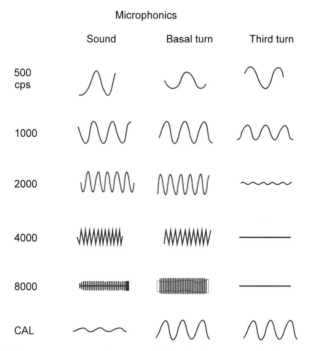

FIGURE 8.22 Relation between intensity of sound (left column) and microphonic responses recorded from basal turn (middle column) and the third turn (right column) of cochlea.

it was found that they differ in many properties from action potentials. They have the following properties:

- Resistant to ischaemia or anaesthesia.
- Do not show any latency or refractory period.
- Similar in wave form and polarity to the sound wave stimulating the ear.

Describe the action potentials in auditory nerve.

As anywhere else, action potentials in auditory nerve fibre show refractory period, obey all or none law. At threshold intensity, the nerve endings respond to only a narrow range of frequencies. As intensities are increased the nerve endings respond to an increasingly wide range of sound frequencies. The refractory period of auditory nerve fibre is 1 ms. Therefore, maximum rate of discharge through fibre can be only 1000 impulses/second. At a very low frequency (20 to 200 cycles/sec), there is synchronization between sound frequency and the rate of discharge.

How is the intensity of the sound perceived?

Intensity of the sound is perceived in three different ways:

1. As sound becomes louder, amplitude of vibration of basilar membrane increases. This increases the rate of discharge through auditory nerve fibres.

2. As amplitude of vibration increases, it causes more and more hair cells on the fringes of the resonating portion of the basilar membrane to become stimulated. This increases the number of hair cells stimulated and in turn more number of auditory nerve fibres is stimulated.
3. Certain hair cells (outer hair cells) are not stimulated unless the sound is very loud. Stimulation of these cells therefore apprises nervous system that sound is very loud.

Why is it possible for us to discriminate over a very large range of intensity?

For hearing sensation, interpreted intensity changes with the cube root of actual intensity. Intensity scale is thus greatly compressed by the perception mechanisms. This allows the person to discriminate over an extremely wide range of intensity.

What is the unit for intensity of the sound?

Sound intensity is expressed as a logarithm of actual intensity. The unit used is known as bel (tenfold increase in intensity is 1 bel because log of 10 is 1). One-tenth of a bel is a decibel which is the unit commonly used because decibel is the smallest difference in sound audible to the ears.

AUDITORY PATHWAY

Describe the auditory pathway.

Nerve fibres supplying hair cells of organ of Corti go to the spiral ganglion present in modiolus. Axons of spiral ganglion pass to ventral and dorsal cochlear nuclei located in upper part of medulla. All the fibres synapse here. Then second order neurons mainly pass to opposite side to superior olivary nucleus by crossing through trapezoid body. A few fibres go to ipsilateral superior olivary nucleus. From superior olivary nucleus, fibres pass through lateral lemniscus to inferior colliculus. Some fibres synapse in nucleus of lateral lemniscus. Some fibres of one side cross to the other side forming commissure of Probst. Many fibres bypass this nucleus and go to inferior colliculus where almost all of them synapse. Some fibres pass from inferior colliculus of one side to the other forming inferior collicular commissure.

From inferior colliculus, fibres pass to medial geniculate body where all the fibres synapse and from medial geniculate body fibres pass through auditory radiation to the auditory cortex located in superior temporal gyrus (Fig. 8.23).

What are the peculiarities of auditory pathway?

1. Impulses from each ear are transmitted to both the sides of the brain with slight preponderance to contralateral side. This is because of crossing over of fibres at three places:
   - Trapezoid body.
   - Commissure of Probst.
   - Inferior collicular commissure.

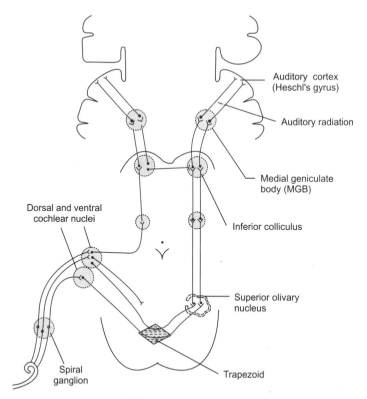

Auditory cortex
(Heschl's gyrus)

Auditory radiation

Medial geniculate
body (MGB)

Inferior colliculus

Superior olivary
nucleus

Trapezoid

Dorsal and ventral
cochlear nuclei

Spiral
ganglion

FIGURE 8.23 Auditory pathway.

2. Collateral tracts from auditory pathway also pass to reticular activating system.
3. Collaterals from auditory pathway also pass to vermis of cerebellum, which is activated instantaneously in the event of a sudden noise.
4. There is a spatial orientation in the pathway from basilar membrane, all the way to the cerebral cortex.
5. Some tracts going to cortex are more direct as a few fibres do not synapse at superior olivary nucleus, nucleus of lateral lemniscus or inferior colliculus. These fibres have only four neurons in their pathway instead of six. This means that some information is relayed earlier to cortex than the other though the impulses originate in the ear at the same time.
6. For low frequencies of sound, rate of discharge through auditory nerve fibres synchronizes with the sound frequency.
7. Auditory nerve fibres have background discharge, i.e. low rate of impulse discharge even in the absence of sound. Because of this, positive (increase in rate of discharge above the background when basilar membrane moves upwards) information as well as negative information (decrease in rate of discharge below the background) can be relayed to the CNS.

What are the various areas of auditory cortex?

Auditory cortex mainly lies in the supratemporal plane of the superior temporal gyrus but also extends over the lateral border of the temporal lobe, over much of the insular cortex and to lateral most portion of the parietal operculum.

There are two separate areas:

1. Primary auditory cortex which is directly excited by signals from medial geniculate body (areas 41, 42).
2. Secondary auditory cortex or auditory association areas which are excited by signals from primary auditory cortex and thalamic association areas (area 22).

What is the function of auditory cortex?

Auditory cortex does the following functions:

- Perception of sound frequency, i.e. discrimination of different pitches of sound.
- Judging the intensity of the sound.
- Analysis of different properties of sound.

What is the effect of removal of primary auditory cortex in human beings?

Total destruction of primary auditory cortices greatly reduce one's ability of hearing whereas removal of primary auditory cortex only on one side has little effect on hearing because there are many cross-connections.

What is the effect of lesions of auditory association areas?

Removal or lesion only of auditory association areas (but not of primary auditory cortex) decreases person's ability to discriminate different tones and to interpret simple patterns of sounds. Person can hear the sound but is unable to interpret the meaning.

What is Wernicke's area? What is the effect of lesion in this area?

Wernicke's area is a confluence of different sensory interpretative areas (somatic, visual auditory, etc). It lies in posterior part of the superior temporal gyrus. It is highly developed in dominant hemisphere. When there is damage to this area, it is difficult for the person to interpret the meanings of the words he hears though he is even able to repeat them perfectly.

DEAFNESS

What is deafness? What are the different types of deafness?

Inability to hear is called deafness. Deafness is of two types:

1. Conduction deafness which is due to impairment in transmission of sound into the cochlea.
2. Nerve deafness which is due to impairment of cochlea or auditory nerve. When either cochlea or nerve is completely destroyed, the person is permanently deaf.

Name the tests used for differentiating between nerve deafness and conduction deafness.

There are three tests to differentiate between nerve and conduction deafness:

- Rinne's test.
- Weber's test.
- Audiometry.

Enumerate the causes of conduction deafness.

- Foreign body or wax in the external ear.
- Otitis media which damages the tympanic membrane and/or ossicles.
- Pathological fixation of stapes to oval window (osteosclerosis).

Enumerate the causes of nerve deafness.

- Degenerative.
- Hereditary.
- Toxic due to quinine, measles, etc.
- Acoustic trauma.
- Meningitis.
- Acoustic neuroma.

Describe Rinne's test.

Rinne's test is done to compare air conduction and bone conduction of sound. Normally air conduction is better (remains audible for a longer time) than bone conduction. In conduction deafness, air-conducted sounds are less well perceived than the bone-conducted sounds. This is the basis of Rinne's test.

In the Rinne's test, base of the vibrating tuning fork of 256 cycles per second is first placed on the mastoid process. When person stops hearing the sound, it is placed in front of the ear. Normal person hears the sound when the fork is held in front of the ear because air conduction is better than bone conduction. This is called Rinne's negative test.

In person having conduction deafness, bone conduction is greater (remains audible for a longer period of time), i.e. the Rinne's test is positive.

In person having nerve deafness both air-conducted and bone-conducted sounds are less perceived.

Describe Weber's test.

In Weber's test, vibrating tuning fork of 256 cycles/second is placed on the vertex in the midline. Normally sound is heard equally in both the ears. In unilateral conduction deafness the sound is better heard in the "affected" ear because there is no masking of air-conducted sounds in the affected ear (because of conduction deafness). If there is nerve deafness on one side, sound is heard louder on normal side.

What is audiometry? What is its use?

Audiometry is a test conducted in a soundproof room. One ear is tested at a time. Audiometer used is an electronic oscillator to which earphone is connected. Oscillator is capable of emitting pure tones of different frequencies. The audiometer is so calibrated that zero intensity is the threshold intensity for all different frequencies. Intensity (loudness) at each frequency can be increased or decreased from the zero level.

In conduction deafness, audiogram is normal when tested through bone conduction device, but when tested through air conduction device, hearing losses will be obtained especially for low frequencies of sound.

In nerve deafness there will be hearing losses when tested by both air and bone conduction. Hearing losses are mostly for sounds of high frequencies. Thus audiometry is used for determining hearing disabilities (Fig. 8.24).

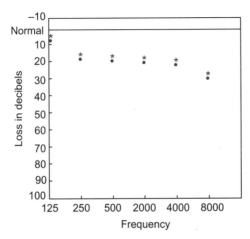

FIGURE 8.24 Audiogram of old-age type of nerve deafness.

TASTE

What is the importance of taste sensation?

Taste allows the person to separate undesirable or even lethal food from nutritious food. Taste thus determines the quality of food the person takes. Usually food is selected according to needs of the body, e.g. adrenalectomized animals automatically select water with high concentration of sodium chloride in preference to pure water.

What are the receptor organs for taste? Where are they situated?

Receptor organs for taste are the taste buds which contain hair cells known as taste cells. Taste buds are mainly situated over the surface of the tongue in tongue papillae. Additional taste buds are located on the palate, tonsillar pillars and epiglottis and even on the proximal oesophagus.

Describe the location of taste buds over the tongue.

There are three different types of tongue papillae, each containing variable number of taste buds:

1. *Circumvallate papillae* arranged in the form of a 'V' on the surface of posterior part of tongue.
2. *Fungiform papillae* present over the anterior surface of the tongue.
3. *Filiform papillae* located in the folds along the lateral surface of the tongue.

Name the different primary taste sensations.

Different primary taste sensations are sour, salty, sweet, bitter and umami.

What is taste blindness?

Many people are taste blind to certain substances, especially the thiourea compounds—commonly phenylthiocarbamide. About 15 to 30% of people exhibit taste blindness for this substance.

What is the function of saliva in tasting the food?

Taste is a chemical sense. A substance can be tasted only when it is in dissolved state. Saliva acts as a solvent for the taste substances.

Which primary taste has lowest threshold? What is the significance?

Bitter taste has the lowest threshold. Bitter taste when occurs in high intensity causes person to reject food. This has an important protective function. Many toxins found in poisonous plants are alkaloids which are bitter.

Which are the receptor cells present in taste buds?

Each taste bud contains about 7 to 10 taste cells. Each taste cell is

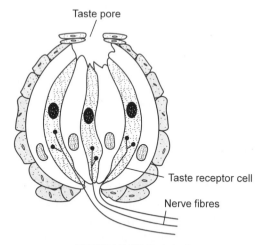

Taste pore

Taste receptor cell

Nerve fibres

FIGURE 8.25 Taste bud.

spindle shaped and provided with fine hair like projections which project on the surface of the tongue. Taste cells are modified epithelial cells and are constantly being replaced by new cells (Fig. 8.25).

What is the mechanism of stimulation of a taste cell?

Single taste bud responds to two or more primary taste stimuli. Application of taste substance to the hair of taste cell stimulates it and receptor potential is developed. Taste chemical binds with the protein receptor molecules that are present in membrane of the hair. This opens the ion channels allowing entry of sodium ions to cause depolarization of cell. Taste substance is gradually washed away by saliva and thus taste stimulus is removed.

Receptor potential generated in the taste cell initiates action potential in the nerve fibres supplying the taste cell.

Describe the pathway for taste sensation.

From anterior two-third of the tongue, taste sensation is carried through chorda tympani branch of facial (seventh cranial) nerve to tractus solitarius in the brain stem. From posterior region of the tongue the taste sensation is carried by glossopharyngeal (ninth cranial) nerve to tractus solitarius at a lower level. From base of the tongue and other parts in the pharyngeal region, taste sensations are carried by vagus (tenth cranial) nerve to tractus solitarius. From tractus solitarius, fibres pass to ventral posteromedial nucleus of thalamus located slightly medial to facial regions of dorsal column.

From thalamus, impulses pass to lower tip of postcentral gyrus in the parietal cortex adjacent to opercular insular area and in Sylvian fissure. This lies lateral and ventral to somatic sensory area for tongue (Fig. 8.26).

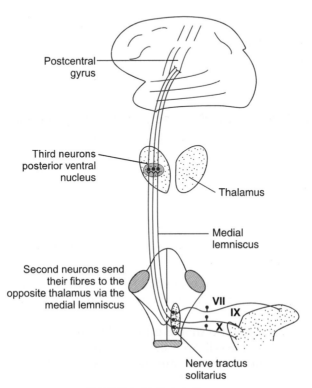

FIGURE 8.26 Taste pathway.

SMELL

What is the significance of smell sensation?
Smell sensation along with the taste allows us to separate undesirable food from nutritious food.

What is anosmia?
Loss of sense of smell is known as anosmia.

What is hyposmia?
Hyposmia is diminished olfactory sensitivity.

What is dysosmia?
Dysosmia is distorted sense of smell.

What is hyperosmia?
Hyperosmia is increased sense of smell.

What are the receptors for smell sensation? Where are they situated?
Receptors for smell sensation are olfactory cells. They lie in olfactory epithelium present in small area of 2.4 cm^2 at the roof of the each nostril. Mucosal end of olfactory cell (dendrite) forms a knob called olfactory vesicle which contains tuft of cilia. These olfactory cilia project to the surface of epithelium (Fig. 8.27).

How does odourous material reach olfactory epithelium?
Olfactory epithelium lies high up in the nose, therefore odourous material reaches it either by diffusion or by development of eddy currents.

Eddy currents constitute the most effective factor in stimulation of olfactory endings and a deep inspiration is the most effective means by which such currents are set up.

What should be the properties of odourous substance to have stronger odour?
1. Olfactory epithelium is lined by fluid secreted by Bowman's glands. Therefore, odourous material should be water soluble and should get dissolved in surface water.
2. Odourous material also should get dissolved in lipid of olfactory hair before it stimulates the cell. So it should be lipid soluble.
3. Odourous material must emit odourous particles, so it should be volatile.

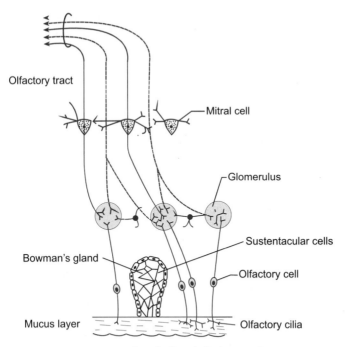

FIGURE 8.27 Organization of olfactory membrane.

What are the different primary smell sensations?

Physiologists have tried to classify primary smell sensations but they have not been totally successful in doing it. So far the following primary smell sensations are known:

- Camphoraceous
- Musky
- Floral
- Pepperminty
- Ethereal
- Pungent
- Putrid

Describe the mechanism of stimulation of olfactory cells.

Olfactory cell cilia have large number of protein molecules protruding all the way through their membrane. These proteins are odorant binding proteins. There are two theories explaining the excitation of olfactory cells:

1. Odorant material binds with odorant binding protein to open sodium channels. Sodium ions diffuse into the cell causing development of receptor potential.

2. Binding of odorant material to odorant binding protein activates adenyl cyclase at its inner end. This catalyzes formation of cyclic AMP which acts on other membrane proteins to cause opening of sodium channels. Through

these channels sodium ions diffuse into the cell producing receptor potential. This receptor potential generates action potential in the axons of olfactory cells (which are themselves neurons). Membrane potential of unstimulated olfactory cell is -55 mV generating continuous action potentials at a low rate. On stimulation, it becomes as low as -30 mV or even less. This increases the number of action potentials in the axons.

Do olfactory receptors adapt rapidly?

Yes. Olfactory cells adapt up to 50% in one second after stimulation and thereafter they adapt slowly. There is a psychological adaptation to strong odour to a far greater degree than receptor adaptation. Most of the adaptation occurs in CNS and there is extinction of sensation of smell within a minute or so.

What is electro-olfactogram?

When an odourous substance gets absorbed on to the olfactory mucosa, electrical changes are set up. Monophasic negative potential is recorded which lasts for 4 to 6 seconds. This recorded response is known as electro-olfactogram.

Describe the pathway of smell sensation.

Axons of bipolar cells present in olfactory epithelium form about 20 strands of olfactory nerves. These nerves enter the skull through perforations of cribriform plate. They enter olfactory bulb which lies just above the cribriform plate.

The axons terminate in multiple globular structures of olfactory bulb called glomeruli. Each glomerulus contains dendrites of 25 large mitral cells and about 60 smaller tufted cells (cell bodies lie above the glomeruli). These cells send their axons through olfactory tract into CNS.

Olfactory tract divides into two pathways—one goes to medial olfactory area and another to the lateral olfactory area. Medial olfactory area (very old olfactory area) consists of group of nuclei located in midbasal portions of brain, anterior and superior to hypothalamus. They in turn, send impulses to hypothalamus and other portions of brain's limbic system (Fig. 8.28). It is responsible for more primitive responses to olfaction such as licking the lips, salivation and other feeding responses caused by smell of food.

Lateral olfactory area (old olfactory area) consists mainly of prepyriform, pyriform cortex and cortical portion of amygdaloid nuclei. From these areas, signals pass to almost all portions of limbic system especially hippocampus which is important in learning process—learning of likes and dislikes of certain foods depending upon previous experiences about the food. This lateral olfactory area sends signals to older type of cortex (paleocortex) present in anteromedial portion of the temporal lobe. This is the only area of the cortex where signals pass directly to cortex without passing through the thalamus. In addition there is a newer olfactory pathway.

The newer olfactory pathway passes through thalamus (dorsomedial thalamic nucleus) to lateroposterior quadrant of orbitofrontal cortex. This system is responsible for conscious perception of olfaction.

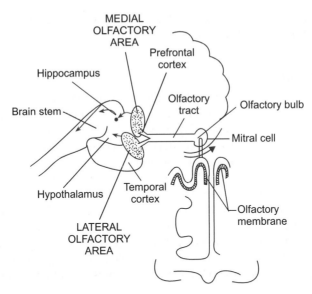

FIGURE 8.28 Neural connections of olfactory system.

EQUILIBRIUM

STRUCTURE AND FUNCTIONS OF VESTIBULAR APPARATUS

Name the different parts of vestibular apparatus.

Vestibular apparatus consists of three bony semicircular canals (in which membranous semicircular canals lie) and vestibule which contains utricle and saccule (membranous parts inside the vestibule).

What are the sense organs present in vestibular apparatus?

Sense organ present in each semicircular canal is called crista. Sense organ present in utricle and saccule is known as macula.

What are the stimuli for sense organs in vestibular apparatus?

Gravitational pull and rotational movements are stimuli for vestibular apparatus.

What is the function of maculae of utricle and saccule?

Maculae of utricle and saccule are responsible for maintenance of equilibrium under static condition. They also help in detecting linear acceleration.

What is the function of crista of semicircular canal?

Semicircular canals are stimulated due to angular acceleration. Therefore, they are stimulated during rotational movements. They play important role in maintaining posture under dynamic condition. They predict ahead of time that the person might fall off balance and do the adjustments to prevent the fall. Thus semicircular canals have predictive function.

Describe macula.

Sense organ of utricle and the saccule is called macula. Macula consists of hair cells covered by otolith membrane, a gelatinous material containing calcium carbonate crystals (called otoliths or statoconia) embedded in it. Each macula contains thousands of hair cells. Cilia (called stereocilia) from hair cell project into the gelatinous layer. The longest cilium, known as kinocilium, is located to one side of the cell and the stereocilia become progressively shorter towards the other side of the cell. When stereocilia move towards the direction of kinocilium, the cell gets depolarized and when it moves in opposite direction, the cell is inhibited. Thus kinocilium gives directional sensitivity to the hair cell. In each macula, hair cells are oriented in different directions, therefore different groups of cells are stimulated by bending of head in different directions. Thus pattern of excitation changes with each position of head. This pattern of excitation apprises brain of the head's position.

What are the functions of macula?

1. As described above, the pattern of excitation of macular cells apprises CNS of the position of head with respect to gravity. In turn reticular, vestibular and cerebellar motor systems excite the appropriate muscles to maintain proper equilibrium. Thus macula helps in maintaining static equilibrium.
2. Macula also helps in detecting linear acceleration. It does not detect the linear speed. It is not stimulated if the person is running at a constant speed but it is stimulated when the speed increases or decreases. Thus only rate of change of linear speed (i.e. linear acceleration) is detected by macula.

Describe the positions of semicircular canals.

On each side in the vestibular apparatus (in petrous portion of temporal bone) there are three bony semicircular canals. They are known as anterior, posterior and horizontal semicircular canals. They are arranged at right angles to each other. When head is bent forward approximately 30°, the horizontal semicircular canals on two sides are located approximately horizontal to the surface of the earth. The anterior canals are located in vertical plane that projects forward and 45° outward and the posterior canals are located also in vertical plane that projects backward and 45° outward. Thus anterior canal of each side is in plane parallel to that of the posterior canal of the opposite side, whereas horizontal canals of both sides are in the same plane (Fig. 8.29).

Describe the sense organ present in semicircular canals.

Each bony semicircular canal has a membranous semicircular canal which has an enlargement at one of its end, called ampulla. This ampulla contains a small crest, *crista ampullaris*. On top of *crista ampullaris*, there is a dome-shaped gelatinous mass called cupula. There are hair cells located on the crest. They project their cilia into the cupula. Each hair cell also has the longest cilium, kinocilium, directed towards the same side of cupula as the others. Therefore, bending of cupula in that

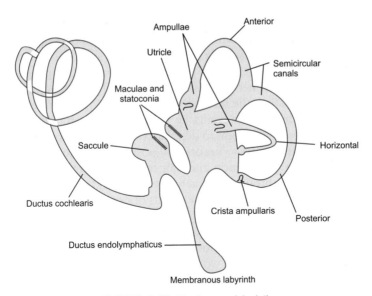

FIGURE 8.29 Membranous labyrinth.

direction causes stimulation of the hair cells whereas bending in the opposite direction causes inhibition of the hair cells. The hair cells are supplied by fibres of vestibular nerve (Fig. 8.30).

How is the sense organ in semicircular canals stimulated?

The hair cells of the horizontal canals are oriented with the kinocilium located closest to the utricle. Head movements that bend stereocilia towards the utricle cause the hair cells to depolarize, while movements that bend the stereocilia away from the utricle cause hyperpolarization. When head begins to rotate (say towards the left), the fluid within the semicircular canals lags behind the head movement (because of inertia) and pushes the cupula in the left horizontal canal towards the utricle (i.e. cupula moves towards the right) causing hair cells to depolarize. At the same time the hair cells within the right horizontal canal are pushed away from the utricle and

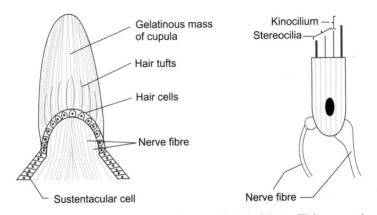

FIGURE 8.30 The hair cell of the membranous labyrinth of the equilibrium apparatus.

hyperpolarize. This information is sent to the CNS. After 15 to 20 seconds of continuous movement at a constant velocity, the velocity of fluid catches up to that of the head and cupula returns to its resting position. This causes stereocilia to return to their upright position and hair cells to return to their resting membrane potential and the rate of discharge through the nerve fibres comes back to the background level.

When head stops rotating, the fluid continues to move (in the direction of rotation) causing exactly the opposite events, i.e. hair cells in the left horizontal canal to hyperpolarize and those in the right to depolarize. After a few seconds, endolymph stops moving and cupula comes to the original position. Then the stereocilia of hair cells return to their upright position and hair cells return to their resting position and the rate of discharge through their nerve fibres return to the background level.

Thus, the semicircular canals transmit signals of one polarity when head begins to rotate and signals of opposite polarity when head stops rotating. Thus semicircular canals signal changes in motion (angular acceleration) and are insensitive to movements at a constant angular velocity.

Vertical semicircular canals also work in pairs. When anterior canal of one side is stimulated, the posterior vertical canal of the other side is inhibited. In the vertical canal, the kinocilium of the cell is located on the side of the hair cells away from the utricle.

Because each pair of the three semicircular canals is oriented in a different plane, movement of head in any direction causes a unique pattern of activity to be generated by semicircular canals. This information is used by CNS to interpret the change in speed and direction of head movement and to make appropriate adjustments in posture and eye position.

What is the function of semicircular canals?

Semicircular canals are stimulated only when the speed of rotation changes. Therefore, they detect angular acceleration and not the speed of rotation. They can predict ahead of time that person might fall off balance. Appropriate corrections are made to prevent fall, e.g. when person is running fast and suddenly wants to turn to right he might fall off balance. Maculae cannot detect off-balance until it actually occurs. Here when person wants to turn to right while running as he turns his head to right, semicircular canals would be stimulated and they predict ahead of time that person might fall on right side. Appropriate adjustments are done to prevent fall. Thus, semicircular canals have a predictive function in maintenance of equilibrium.

VESTIBULAR PATHWAY

Describe the vestibular pathway.

Fibres supplying hair cells of maculae and crista ampullaris form vestibular nerve. Most of the vestibular nerve fibres end in vestibular nuclei present at the junction between pons and medulla. Some fibres of vestibular nerve pass without synapsing at vestibular nuclei to reticular nuclei of brain stem and fastigial nuclei, uvula, flocculonodular lobes of cerebellum. Fibres ending in vestibular nuclei are relayed to:

- Same areas of cerebellum as described above as well as to cortex of cerebellum.
- Into vestibulospinal tracts.

- Into medial longitudinal fasciculus.
- Other areas of brain stem—particularly reticular nuclei.

Primary pathway for reflexes of equilibrium begins in vestibular nerve, passes to vestibular nuclei and cerebellum which are connected to and fro. From these areas, signals are sent to reticular nuclei of the brain stem and then through reticulospinal tract and vestibulospinal tract to spinal cord to control interplay between facilitation and inhibition of antigravity muscles, thus controlling the equilibrium.

Flocculonodular lobes of cerebellum mostly get information from semicircular canals and have predictive functions as that of semicircular canals. Impulses from maculae mostly go to uvula of cerebellum which plays a role in the maintenance of static equilibrium.

Signals transmitted through medial longitudinal fasciculus cause corrective movements of the eyes when head rotates. Signals from vestibular nuclei also pass to cerebral cortex, to primary equilibrium centre present deep in sylvian fissure in parietal lobe. These signals apprise the psyche of the equilibrium status of the body.

Vestibular nuclei on either side are divided into four groups as follows:

Superior and *medial* vestibular nuclei receive signals mainly from semicircular canals and in turn send signals to medial longitudinal fasciculus (for causing corrective movements of eyes) and medial vestibulospinal tract to cause appropriate movements of neck and head.

Lateral vestibular nuclei receive signals mainly from utricle and saccule and in turn send signals to spinal cord through lateral vestibulospinal tract to control body movements.

Inferior vestibular nuclei receive signals from semicircular canals and utricle and in turn send signals to cerebellum and reticular formation of brain stem.

NYSTAGMUS

What is nystagmus? What are the types?

Characteristic jerky movements of eyes which occur when they are fixed successively at different fields is called nystagmus. It occurs either when visual scene is moving (opticokinetic nystagmus) and person is stationary or when person is rotating but the visual scene is stationary (vestibular nystagmus). At both these times nystagmus is occurring physiologically. If nystagmus occurs in a person where neither visual scene nor person is rotating, it is called pathological nystagmus.

VESTIBULAR FUNCTION TESTS

Name the tests used for detecting integrity of vestibular apparatus.

- Bárány's test.
- Caloric stimulation of semicircular canals by instilling either hot or cold water in the ear.
- Balancing test. Individual is asked to stand perfectly erect with eyes closed.

CHAPTER 9
Endocrinology

Why are endocrine glands called ductless glands?

Endocrine glands are called ductless glands because they do not possess ducts. They pour their secretion directly into the blood stream.

Enumerate the functions of endocrine glands.

Endocrine glands secrete hormones which regulate metabolic functions of the cells but they do not initiate cellular reactions.

Hormones regulate biochemical reactions. They stimulate or inhibit the rate and magnitude of biochemical reactions by controlling enzymes. Thus they regulate energy producing process and also circulating levels of nutrients or energy yielding substances like glucose and fatty acids.

Hormones regulate different bodily processes as growth, maturation, differentiation, regeneration, reproduction and behaviour. Thus, main function of endocrine glands is to maintain homeostasis in internal environment.

Name the various hormone secreting tissues.

Hormone secreting tissues are as follows:

1. Principal endocrine glands:
   - Pituitary gland (hypophysis).
   - Hypothalamus.
   - Thyroid gland.
   - Adrenal gland.
   - Parathyroid gland.
   - Gonads—testes or ovaries.
   - Islet of pancreas.
2. Other organs with endocrine function are:
   - Heart—secretes atrial natriuretic factor.
   - Kidneys—secrete 1,25-dihydroxycholecalciferol.
   - Liver—secretes 25-hydroxycholecalciferol and somatomedin.
   - Pineal gland—secretes melatonin.
   - Skin—secretes calciferol (vitamin D).
   - Gastrointestinal tract—secretes hormones acting locally, e.g. gastrin, secretin, vasoactive intestinal peptide.

Describe the nervous control of endocrine glands.

Nervous system controls the secretion of endocrine glands through hypothalamus. Hypothalamus controls secretory activity of anterior pituitary gland by secreting various hypothalamic releasing hormones which pass to anterior pituitary gland through hypothalamo-hypophysial portal system. Posterior lobe of pituitary and hypothalamus are connected by hypothalamo-hypophysial nervous tract.

1. *Hypothalamo-hypophysial portal system.* Median eminence of hypothalamus is located beneath the inferior portion of the third ventricle. This is the centre for different releasing hormones of hypothalamus. Median eminence has a poorly developed blood-brain barrier. Small blood vessels penetrate into the substance of the median eminence and then return to the surface and coalesce to form hypothalamo-hypophysial portal vessels. They run downward along the pituitary stalk and supply blood to anterior pituitary sinuses. Special neurons in the median eminence secrete the hypothalamic releasing and inhibitory hormones or factors which pass to anterior pituitary gland through these portal vessels and control secretion of anterior pituitary hormones.

Releasing hormones are produced for all the hormones of anterior pituitary, except prolactin. For prolactin an inhibitory factor is produced which inhibits prolactin secretion.

2. *Hypothalamo-hypophysial nervous tract.* This tract joins hypothalamus with posterior pituitary gland. Hormones of posterior pituitary are actually synthesized in the hypothalamus (supraoptic and paraventricular nuclei) from where the neural tracts originate. Neural tract then passes hypothalamus through hypophysial (pituitary) stalk to posterior pituitary. Endings of nerves contain many secretory granules which enter the adjacent capillaries by exocytosis.

Hypothalamus receives neuronal connections from many regions of central nervous system. This is the way by which the nervous system can affect the endocrine secretions of anterior and posterior pituitary glands. Anterior pituitary gland in turn affects the secretion of most of the other endocrine glands.

HORMONES

What is a hormone?

Hormone is a chemical messenger secreted by endocrine glands. It is secreted directly into the blood and is transported to specific target tissue where it elicits physiological and biochemical responses, but some hormones act locally.

What is the difference between a hormone and a vitamin?

Hormones do not have any nutritive role as vitamins have in responsive tissues. They are also not incorporated as a structural moiety into another molecule.

What is target tissue?

Some hormones affect only specific tissues. These tissues are called target tissues because only these tissues possess specific receptors which can bind with the hormones for initiation of their action.

What are local hormones?

The hormones which have specific local effects are called local hormones, e.g. secretin, cholecystokinin.

What are general hormones?

The hormones which affect almost all the tissues of the body are called general hormones, e.g. thyroid hormone, growth hormone.

What are hormones chemically?

There are three major classes of hormones:

- *Steroids.* Adrenal cortical hormones, male and female sex hormones.
- *Proteins or polypeptides.* Hypothalamic hormones, posterior pituitary hormones, parathyroid hormone, calcitonin, insulin, etc.
- *Amino acid derivatives.* Thyroid hormones, adrenal medullary hormones.

Name the physical characteristics of hormones.

Physical characteristics of hormones are:

1. Concentration of the hormones in the plasma is low because of low rate of their secretion from the endocrine glands.
2. Latent period (time interval between administration of hormone and initiation of its effect) for the action of hormone is usually long. It may be as long as seconds, minutes, hours or even days.
3. Hormones are circulated in plasma by binding with protein. Protein binding of hormones has the following effects:
   - Excretion of circulating hormones in urine is prevented.
   - Slows rate of degradation by the liver, thus providing circulating reserve of hormones.
4. Only small amount of hormone is in unbound form which passes through capillaries to produce its effect.
5. Target tissue has got the receptors for hormones. The specificity of hormone depends on formation of a strong covalent bond with hormone receptor.
   Hormone receptors can be present on the surface of cell membrane, cell cytoplasm, cell nucleus, etc.
6. Most of the hormones are metabolized quickly after secretion especially the peptide hormones.
7. Interaction of hormones with their target cells is followed by intracellular degradation.
8. Only small portion of circulating hormone is degraded by target tissue. The hormones are degraded mainly in liver and kidney by enzymatic

mechanisms. Very small fraction (less than 1%) of hormone is excreted in urine or faeces without degradation.

9. Chemically hormones are steroids, proteins and polypeptides or amino acid derivatives.

Name the mechanisms of hormonal action.*

Mechanisms of hormonal action are as follows:

- Change in membrane permeability.
- Activation of intracellular enzyme when hormone combines with membrane receptor.
- Activation of genes by binding of hormone with intracellular receptors.

Describe the mechanisms of control of hormone synthesis and release.

Rate of secretion of hormone is controlled by one of the following mechanisms.

1. *Negative feedback mechanism.* It is the main mechanism controlling hormone level. Usually there is a tendency of endocrine gland to over secrete its hormone. This results into increased effect of hormone on target tissue (increase in the function of target tissue). Some factors of the function feedback to endocrine gland causing a negative effect on hormone secretion from it.

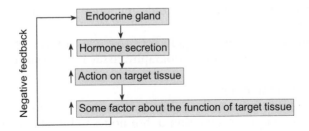

Hormones such as thyroxine and cortisol are controlled by hypothalamus and pituitary glands. Hypothalamus secretes releasing hormone which acts on pituitary to cause release of tropic hormone. Tropic hormone in turn acts on target endocrine gland to cause release of its hormone. In a long loop negative feedback, rise of circulating hormone (or some factor due to its action) inhibits hypothalamus pituitary system. There is a negative feedback for release of releasing hormone from hypothalamus. This in turn reduces release of tropic hormone from anterior pituitary which results in inhibition of release of hormone from the target endocrine gland.

In a short loop negative feedback rise in tropic hormone from anterior pituitary inhibits release of releasing hormone from hypothalamus.

2. *Positive feedback mechanism.* Secretion of some hormones is controlled by positive feedback mechanism, e.g. release of oxytocin at the time of delivery of a baby.

*For details refer Vaz M, Kurpad A, Raj T, editors. *Guyton & Hall Textbook of Medical Physiology.* Elsevier: New Delhi, 2013, p. 542.

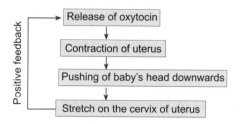

3. *Direct control.* In a few instances, hormone secretion is regulated by blood concentration of a substance which is controlled by the hormone, e.g.
   ▪ Secretion of insulin from pancreas is promoted by rise in blood glucose level and vice versa.
   ▪ Secretion of parathyroid hormone is controlled by blood levels of calcium.

What is metabolic clearance rate of hormone?

The rate of removal of hormone from the blood is called metabolic clearance rate of hormone.

What are the methods used for hormonal assays?

1. *Biological assays.* These are not very sensitive. However, with developments in separation techniques such as solvent extraction, chromatography and molecular sieving, biological assays of steroids, peptides and catecholamines have become very sensitive.
2. *Chemical assay.* This is highly sensitive, e.g. fluorescence method for catecholamines, gas-liquid chromatography, assay of thyroid hormones using radioactive isotope[131]I.
3. *Immunochemical assay.*
   (a) Radioimmunoassay is a highly sensitive technique for measuring physiological concentration of hormones in blood and body fluids.
   (b) In place of antibody, specific carrier globulin of plasma which is a natural binding agent for some specific hormone is used, e.g. plasma-binding globulin for plasma cortisol assay. The assay is then carried out in the same way as the radioimmunoassay procedure.
4. Enzyme-linked immunosorbent assay (ELISA).*

Describe the procedure of radioimmunoassay.*

1. Antibody for hormone to be measured is prepared in a lower animal.
2. Then following mixture is prepared:
   ▪ Small quantity of fluid in which hormone level is to be determined (unknown).
   ▪ Small quantity of antibody.

---

*For details refer Vaz M, Kurpad A, Raj T, editors. *Guyton & Hall Textbook of Medical Physiology.* Elsevier: New Delhi, 2013, p. 548.

- Appropriate quantity of purified standard hormone tagged with a radioactive isotope.

Antibody should be too little to bind completely with both radioactively tagged hormone and hormone present in fluid to be assayed. Therefore, natural hormone and tagged hormone compete for binding sites on the antibody. Quantity of natural and tagged hormones that binds is proportional to its concentration.

3. After binding has reached equilibrium, antibody-hormone complex is separated. Then the quantity of radioactive hormone bound is measured by radioactive counting technique.
4. To make assay quantitative, the above procedure is performed for standard solutions of untagged hormone at several different concentrations. Then comparing radioactive counts and standard concentrations of hormone, a standard curve is obtained. Radioactive counts obtained for unknown (fluid in which level of natural hormone is to be determined) are compared by using this standard curve and concentration of the hormone in the fluid is measured.

ANTERIOR PITUITARY GLAND

Enumerate the cells present in anterior pituitary gland and hormones secreted by them

Cells present in anterior pituitary gland	Hormones secreted
Somatotropes (30 to 40%)	Growth hormones (GH)—somatotropic hormone (SH), somatotropin
Corticotropes (20%)	Adrenocorticotropic hormone (ACTH)
Thyrotropes (3 to 5%)	Thyroid stimulating hormone (TSH) or thyrotropin
Gonadotropes (3 to 5%)	Luteinizing hormone (LH), Follicular stimulating hormone (FSH)
Lactotropes (3 to 5%)	Prolactin

Name the releasing and inhibitory hormones (factors) secreted by hypothalamus.

Hypothalamus (median eminence) secretes the following factors:

1. *Thyroid stimulating hormone releasing factor (TRH)*. Causing release of TSH from pituitary.
2. *Corticotropin releasing hormone (CRH)*. Causing release of ACTH.
3. *Growth hormone releasing hormone (GHRH)*. Causing release of growth hormone and also growth hormone inhibitory hormone (GHIH) which is the same as hormone somatostatin and it inhibits release of growth hormone.

4. *Gonadotropin releasing hormone (GnRH)*. Causing release of FSH and LH.
5. *Prolactin inhibitory factor (PIF)*. Causing inhibition of prolactin secretion.

GROWTH HORMONE

Describe the synthesis and chemistry of growth hormone.

Growth hormone is synthesized by acidophils of anterior pituitary. It is a single un-branched polypeptide containing 191 amino acids. It is highly species specific. Growth hormone shows large diurnal fluctuations. A regular nocturnal peak level occurs 1 to 2 hours after the onset of deep sleep. The plasma GH concentration in the growing child is not significantly higher than that in the adult whose growth is ceased.

What is the general effect of the growth hormone?

Growth hormone causes the growth of almost all the tissues of the body that are capable of growing. It promotes mitosis in the cells, thus increasing their number. It also increases the size of each cell.

What is the effect of growth hormone on protein metabolism?

Growth hormone has got anabolic effect, i.e. it stimulates protein synthesis. The effect is predominantly seen in skeletal and cardiac muscles. Growth hormone promotes protein synthesis and deposition by the following series of effects:

- Enhances the transport of amino acids through the cell membrane and increases the amount of amino acids in the cells.
- Increases RNA translation.
- Also stimulates transcription of DNA in the nucleus leading to increased formation of RNA.

Growth hormone decreases the breaking down of cell protein by making fatty acids available for energy purpose. It reduces circulating levels of amino acids and urea leading to positive nitrogen balance.

What is the effect of GH on fat metabolism?

Growth hormone has catabolic effect on adipose tissue. It stimulates mobilization of fatty acids from adipose tissue leading to decreased triglyceride content of adipose tissue and increased fatty acid levels in blood.

In all the tissues of the body, GH promotes conversion of fatty acid to acetyl CoA with subsequent utilization for energy. GH increases hepatic oxidation of fatty acids to ketone bodies, acetoacetic acid and beta-hydroxybutyrate. Thus GH has got ketogenic effect. It causes release of ketone bodies (acetoacetic acid, acetone, beta-hydroxybutyrate) from liver into the blood.

What is the effect of GH on carbohydrate metabolism?

GH is a diabetogenic hormone. It causes hyperglycaemia.

ACTIONS OF GH

1. Reduces utilization of glucose by the cells. This is mainly because GH favours utilization of fatty acids. Utilization of fatty acids produces larger quantity of acetyl CoA which causes feedback effects to block glycolytic breakdown of glucose by inhibiting pyruvate kinase enzyme.
2. Enhances glycogen deposition in the cell. Glucose that enters the cell is polymerized to glycogen and is deposited because of decreased glucose utilization.
3. Increases blood glucose level due to decreased utilization by the cells. Therefore, pituitary diabetes results which is insulin resistant.
4. GH increases basal plasma levels of insulin—increased glucose concentration caused by GH stimulates beta cells of islet of Langerhans to release insulin. GH also has a direct stimulatory effect on beta cells. Secretion and overstimulation of beta cells results into literally 'burning out' of these cells.
5. Inhibits glucose transport in adipose tissue (required for triglyceride synthesis) because of anti-insulin effect. Thus, GH antagonizes insulin-stimulated lipogenesis.

Describe the effects of growth hormone in bone and cartilage growth.

Effects of growth hormone on bones and cartilages are mediated by a family of polypeptides called 'somatomedins' which are synthesized in liver. Growth hormone stimulates liver cells to synthesize many types of somatomedins, four of which have been isolated. Of these somatomedin 'C' is important. GH is weakly attached to the plasma proteins in the blood. Therefore, it is released into the tissues rapidly (with a half-time of 20 min) but somatomedin strongly binds with a carrier protein in blood and slowly enters the tissues with a half time of 20 hours. This is important because it prolongs growth promoting effects. Through somatomedin, GH has the following effects:

1. Increased deposition of proteins by chondrocytes and osteogenic cells. There is also increased rate of reproduction of these cells. It also converts chondrocytes into osteogenic cells.
2. Long bones grow in length at epiphyseal cartilage. This growth causes deposition of new cartilage which is converted into new bone thus elongating the shaft and pushing the epiphyseal cartilages apart. At the same time epiphyseal cartilage is progressively used up. So by adolescence no additional epiphyseal cartilage remains to provide further growth. At the same time bony fusion occurs between shaft and each end of epiphysis, so that no further growth in length is possible. Thus at this stage, GH has no further ability to lengthen the bones.
3. Thickness of the bone increases. Osteoblasts in the bone periosteum and medullary cavities deposit new bone on the surface of older bone. Simultaneously, osteoclasts in the bone remove old bone. When the rate of bone deposition is greater than that of resorption, thickness of the bone increases.

Growth hormone strongly stimulates the osteoblasts. Therefore, bone can continue to enlarge throughout life under the effect of GH.

How is the growth hormone secretion regulated?

The normal concentration of growth hormone in plasma is 1.5 to 3 ng/ml in adults and about 6 ng/ml in children and adolescents. Rate of growth hormone secretion changes with the state of person's nutrition or stress, e.g. starvation, hypoglycaemia, low fatty acids level, exercise excitement, trauma. GH level increases during first 2 hours of sleep. Under acute conditions hypoglycaemia is the most potent stimulator for growth hormone secretion.

Under chronic conditions, growth hormone secretion is correlated more with the degree of cellular protein depletion than with glucose insufficiency. Decreased cellular protein stimulates growth hormone. The factors discussed above control growth hormone secretion through hormones of hypothalamus. Hypothalamus secretes two factors, viz. growth hormone releasing hormone (GHRH) and growth hormone inhibitory hormone (GHIH) or somatostatin. GHRH is released by ventromedial nucleus in response to hypoglycaemia and GHIH is released by nearby area. These are carried by hypothalamo-hypophysial portal system to hypophysis (anterior pituitary) to cause the respective effects.

STIMULATION OF GH SECRETION

Hypothalamic signals depicting emotions, stress and trauma can affect hypothalamic control of growth hormone. Catecholamines, dopamine and serotonin released by different neuronal systems in hypothalamus also increase the rate of growth hormone secretion through release of GHRH.

INHIBITION OF GROWTH HORMONE SECRETION

- Somatostatin inhibits the synthesis and release of GH. Growth hormone can inhibit its own secretion via a short feedback loop mechanism that operates between anterior lobe of pituitary and median eminence of hypothalamus, causing release of somatostatin which inhibits synthesis and release of GH.
- Glucocorticoids can also decrease GH secretion.

APPLIED

Describe the various disorders associated with increased secretion of growth hormone.*

Disorders of increased GH secretion:

1. Gigantism. Oversecretion of GH before adolescence results into gigantism. All the body tissues grow rapidly including bones. There is excessive increase in length of long bones. So the person becomes a giant. He may grow to a height of 8 to 9 feet and face the problem of hyperglycaemia. Both hyperglycaemia and growth hormone stimulate beta cells of islets of Langerhans to become overactive. Later they degenerate. Usually, gigantism results due to tumour of the acidophilic cells of pituitary gland.

---

*For details refer Vaz M, Kurpad A, Raj T, editors. *Guyton & Hall Textbook of Medical Physiology.* Elsevier: New Delhi, 2013, p. 556.

2. *Acromegaly.* This results due to excessive growth hormone secretion in adulthood, i.e. after adolescence (after epiphysis of long bones have fused with the shafts). Because of this, the person cannot grow taller but bones continue to grow in thickness.

Enlargement is especially marked in the membranous bones (cranium, nose, bosses on forehead, supraorbital ridge, lower jaw, portions of vertebrae) as their growth does not cease at adolescence. Therefore, in a person with acromegaly lower jaw protrudes forward, forehead slants forward and because of excessive development of supraorbital bridges, nose is large. Change in vertebrae causes kyphosis. Many soft tissue organs (tongue, liver, kidneys) also get greatly enlarged.

Describe the disorders associated with decreased secretion of growth hormone.

1. *Dwarfism.* This results due to decreased secretion of growth hormone during childhood (before adolescence). There is a stunted physical growth but features of the body develop in appropriate proportions. In some dwarfs, amount of growth hormone secreted is normal but there is hereditary inability to synthesize somatomedin C in response to growth hormone. The mental growth of a pituitary dwarf is normal.

2. *Panhypopituitarism.* This is due to decreased secretion of all the hormones of anterior pituitary. If it develops during childhood, then such dwarfs never pass through puberty and never secrete sufficient quantity of gonadotropic hormones to develop adult sexual functions. In one-third of the dwarfs there is deficiency of growth hormone alone. Such individuals do mature sexually and occasionally reproduce.

3. *Thrombosis of pituitary blood vessels.* Effects of panhypopituitarism in adults are:
   - Hypothyroidism.
   - Depressed function of glucocorticoids.
   - Suppressed secretion of gonadotropic hormones to such an extent that sexual functions are lost. The person is therefore lethargic (thyroid hormone lack), gains weight, with loss of sexual functions.

Treatment. Dwarfs having pure growth hormone deficiency can be completely cured by giving human growth hormone.

Panhypopituitarism in adults is treated by administration of adrenocortical and thyroid hormones.

POSTERIOR PITUITARY GLAND

Name the hormones released by posterior pituitary. Where are they synthesized?

Hormones of posterior pituitary are *antidiuretic hormone (ADH)* and *oxytocin.* ADH is secreted by cells of supraoptic nuclei of hypothalamus called magnocellular neurosecretory neurons. This hormone passes through hypothalamo-hypophysial nervous tract to the posterior pituitary gland and is stored there. Oxytocin is synthesized in cells of paraventricular nuclei of hypothalamus (magnocellular) and through hypothalamo-hypophysial nervous tract passes to posterior pituitary. It is stored in posterior pituitary gland.

What are ADH and oxytocin chemically?

Both are polypeptides containing nine amino acids.

Describe the role of ADH.

Antidiuretic hormone increases the permeability of late distal tubules and collecting ducts of kidneys to water. This increases water reabsorption by kidneys, leads to decreased urine formation, increased extracellular fluid volume. If ADH is not there, late distal tubules and ducts remain totally impermeable to water and kidneys excrete large volume of urine. Thus ADH controls water excretion by kidneys and helps in maintaining osmolality of body fluids.

At high concentration ADH causes constriction of arterioles thereby increasing the blood pressure. That is why it has been given another name, vasopressin.

What is the mechanism of action of ADH?

The exact mechanism by which ADH changes the permeability of late distal tubules and collecting ducts of kidneys to water is not known. Probably ADH causes special structural changes in the apical membranes of the tubular epithelial cells. This provides temporarily many new pores in the membrane for absorption of water.

How is ADH secretion controlled?

Antidiuretic hormone secretion is mainly controlled by osmolality of body fluids. Osmoreceptors are located in the hypothalamus. Increase in plasma osmolality by 1 to 2% stimulates osmoreceptor neurons in supraoptic and paraventricular nuclei. They send signals to posterior pituitary to release greater amount of ADH in circulating blood. This in turn increases water absorption from kidneys and bring osmal concentration of plasma back to normal. Conversely decreased osmolality of plasma causes complete cessation of impulses and therefore of release of ADH. This results in decreased water absorption, increased water loss and then osmal concentration of plasma is brought back to normal. The solutes to which cells are impermeable are usually more effective in increasing osmotic pressure and more effective in causing ADH release. When extracellular fluid becomes more concentrated (increased osmolality) water is absorbed by osmosis from the osmoreceptor cells, size of the cells become smaller and they initiate appropriate signals to posterior pituitary gland to release ADH. Dilution of extracellular fluid has the opposite effect.

In addition there are certain non-osmotic stimuli for ADH release, e.g. decreased effective circulating blood volume (10 to 50% decrease) causes release of ADH. Thus it participates in the maintenance of blood pressure. Decreased blood volume decreases the stretch on volume receptors located in left atrium, vena cava, aortic arch, etc. and cause increase in ADH secretion.

Certain drugs (barbiturates, acetylcholine, chlorpropamide, angiotensin II are the other non-osmotic stimuli for ADH release. Conversely increased arterial pressure secondary of increased ECF (extracellular fluid) volume inhibits ADH release.

What is diabetes incipidus?

Diabetes incipidus is a disease caused by decrease or lack of ADH. It is characterized by increased formation of urine of low specific gravity.

What are the effects of oxytocin?

1. *On gravid uterus.* Oxytocin powerfully stimulates the gravid uterus especially towards the end of gestation. The sensitivity of the myometrium to exogenous oxytocin increases as pregnancy advances. Therefore, it is believed that oxytocin plays a role in labour and is shown to be effective therapeutic agent in induction of labour.

During labour, there is a positive feedback cycle which increases the level of oxytocin as follows:

- Stretch on the cervix of uterus causes nervous signals to the brain to cause release of oxytocin.
- Released oxytocin causes strong contraction of uterus which pushes the baby downward. This causes baby's head to move down and stretch the cervix of uterus.
- Stretch on the cervix of uterus further enhances the release of oxytocin.

2. *Effect on lactating mammary glands.* Oxytocin causes contraction of myoepithelial cells of lactating mammary glands. This causes milk to be expressed from the alveoli into the ducts so that baby can obtain it by suckling.

Mechanism. Suckling stimuli from the nipple of the breast cause signals to travel along the sensory nerves to the brain to supraoptic and paraventricular areas of hypothalamus and cause release of oxytocin. Oxytocin released passes through blood to mammary glands where it causes contraction of myoepithelial cells that lie outside the alveoli. Thus within a minute after the beginning of suckling, milk begins to flow. This mechanism is called milk let-down or milk ejection.

Name the different stimuli for release of oxytocin.

- Stimulation of tactile receptors in the areolar region of the female breast during suckling.
- Genital tract stimulation during coitus and parturition.
- Stretch on cervix at the time of labour.

Name the factors inhibiting release of oxytocin.

- Emotional stress and psychic factor as fright can inhibit milk let-down.
- Ethanol inhibits endogenous oxytocin release.
- Enkephalins also inhibit oxytocin release.

THYROID GLAND

Name the hormones secreted by thyroid gland.

- Tri-iodothyronine (T_3).
- Tetra-iodothyronine (T_4) or thyroxine.
- Calcitonin.

Describe the structure of thyroid gland.

Thyroid gland consists of about 3 million of follicles (acini). Each follicle or acinus is lined by epithelial cells and is filled with colloid. Colloid is mainly made up of a glycoprotein termed thyroglobulin. Thyroglobulin contains 10% carbohydrate. It is synthesized by epithelial cells and is secreted into colloid by exocytosis of granules. T_3, T_4 hormones are formed by iodination and condensation of tyrosine molecules bound in peptide linkage in thyroglobulin molecule. T_3, T_4 hormones remain bound to thyroglobulin until their secretion.

Between basement membrane of follicle and living follicular epithelial cells, there are special cells called parafollicular or 'C' cells. They secrete hormone calcitonin.

Which mineral is required for synthesis of thyroid hormones? How much is its requirement?

Iodine is required for synthesis of thyroid hormones. It is ingested in the form of iodides. The requirement of iodine is 1 mg/week. Iodide is added to the table salt to prevent iodine deficiency.

What is the fate of dietary iodide?

Most of the iodides absorbed from gastrointestinal tract are rapidly excreted through kidneys but one-fifth is selectively removed from circulation by cells of thyroid gland. The basal membrane of thyroid gland cell has a specific ability to pump iodide actively into the interior of the cell. This is called iodide pump. Due to this, iodide can be concentrated in the thyroid gland as much as about 30 times its concentration in the blood.

Describe the synthesis of thyroid hormones T_3 and T_4.

Endoplasmic reticulum and Golgi apparatus secrete a large glycoprotein, known as thyroglobulin, into the follicles. Each thyroglobulin molecule contains about 70 molecules of amino acid tyrosine. From tyrosine, thyroid hormones are formed within the molecule of thyroglobulin and are also stored there. Formation of thyroid hormones occurs as follows:

1. *Oxidation of iodide ion.* Iodide is oxidized to iodine by enzyme peroxidase and its accompanying hydrogen peroxide. Peroxidase is located at the apical membrane of cell. At this site, iodide gets oxidated to iodine and then through membrane it passes into the stored colloid. Binding of iodine with thyroglobulin is known as organification.
2. *Iodination of tyrosine.* Oxidized iodine binds with amino acid tyrosine rapidly due to enzyme iodinase. Tyrosine is first iodized to monoiodotyrosine and then to diiodotyrosine. Then one molecule of monoiodotyrosine couples with one molecule of diiodotyrosine to form triiodothyronine (T_3). Two molecules of diiodothyronine couple to form tetraiodothyronine (T_4 or thyroxine).
3. *Storage of hormone.* After formation, T_3 and T_4 are stored in the thyroglobulin molecule. Each thyroglobulin molecule stores 1 to 3 molecules of T_4 and one molecule of T_3 per ten molecules of T_4. Stored hormones can supply normal body requirement for 2 to 3 months.

How are thyroid hormones released into the blood?

Thyroid hormones are cleared from thyroglobulin and released into the blood as follows:

- Apical surface of follicular cells ingests small part of colloid by pinocytosis forming pinocytic vesicle.
- Lysosomes fuse with the pinocytic vesicle and converts it into digestive vesicles.
- Proteinases of lysosomes digest the thyroglobulin molecule to release T_3 and T_4.
- T_3 and T_4 are released into the blood of surrounding capillaries through base of cells.
- Monoiodo and diiodotyrosines are also cleared from thyroglobulin but they are not released into the blood. Their iodine is separated by enzyme deiodinase. Iodine recycles to form additional thyroid hormones.

What is the rate of secretion of T_3 and T_4?

Over 93% of the hormone released from thyroid gland is T4 and less than 7% of hormone released is T_3. But in the target tissue T_4 is converted to T_3 which is the hormone finally delivered to the tissues. About 35 µg of T_3 is delivered to the tissues per day.

How are the thyroid hormones transported in blood?

T4 and T3 combine with plasma proteins on entering the blood as follows:
- About 80% of hormone with thyroxine-binding globulin (TBG).
- About 10 to 20% of hormone with thyroxine-binding prealbumin (TBPA).
- Remaining hormone with albumin.

Affinity of TBG for T_4 is six times than that for T_3, therefore blood level of T_4 is much greater than that of T_3.

How are T_3 and T_4 released into the tissues?

Because of high affinity of binding protein (especially for T_4), hormones are slowly released into the tissues. Half of T_4 in the blood is released into the tissues approximately every 6 days while half of T_3 is released on each day.

What is the duration of action of T_3 and T_4?

After injecting T_4, there is a latent period of 2 to 3 days before action of hormone on metabolic rate can be seen. After this latent period, activity begins and reaches its peak in 10 to 12 days and then it decreases with half-life of 15 days. Activity thus persists for $1^{1}/_{2}$ to 2 months.

T_3 has a latent period of only 6 to 12 hours with peak activity within 2 to 3 days. Latency is due to slow release of hormones from their binding with proteins.

ACTIONS OF THYROID HORMONES

Explain the effect of thyroid hormones on transcription of genes.

Most of the T_4 is converted to T_3 before acting on genes. There are receptors for thyroid hormones on DNA strands or in close proximity to them.

About 90% of the hormone that binds with receptors is T_3 and remaining is T_4. After thyroid hormones bind with DNA receptors, there is activation and initiation of transcription process resulting in a large number of messenger RNA molecules within a few minutes. This causes process of RNA translation on the cytoplasmic ribosomes within a few hours. A large number of new proteins are formed, most of them are enzymes.

What is the effect of thyroid hormone on metabolic activity?

1. T_3 and T_4 increase the metabolic activities of almost all the cells of different tissues in the body to increase BMR (basal metabolic rate) to as much as 60 to 100% above normal. This results into:
   - Increased utilization of food.
   - Increased rate of protein synthesis simultaneously with increased rate of protein catabolism.
   - Increased growth rate in young person.
   - Excitation of mental processes.
   - Increased activity of almost all the endocrine glands.
2. T_3, T_4 also increase the number and activity of mitochondria in the cells of the body. These increase the rate of ATP synthesis. Extremely high concentration of thyroid hormone causes uncoupling of the oxidative phosphorylation process. As a result, a large amount of heat is produced but little ATP.
3. Due to thyroxine, the enzyme Na^+-K^+ ATPase increases causing increased Na-K pump activity. This process utilizes energy. Therefore, amount of heat produced is increased. It is suggested that this is one of the mechanisms responsible for increase in BMR caused by thyroid hormones.

What is the effect of thyroid hormone on growth?

Thyroid hormone causes skeletal growth in children. Bones also mature rapidly and epiphyses close at an early age. Thyroid hormones also promote growth and development of brain during foetal life and for first few years after birth.

What is the effect of thyroid hormone on carbohydrate metabolism?

Overall increase in enzymes caused by thyroid hormone leads to the following effects on carbohydrate metabolism:

- Increased rate of absorption of glucose from gastrointestinal tract.
- Rapid uptake of glucose by the cells.
- Enhanced glycolysis.
- Enhanced gluconeogenesis.
- Increased insulin secretion and its effects on carbohydrate metabolism.

What is the effect of thyroid hormones on fat metabolism?

1. Cause mobilization of fat from adipose tissue.
2. Increase level of fatty acids in the blood and also enhance oxidation of free fatty acids by the cells.

3. Decrease the quantity of cholesterol, phospholipids and triglyceride in plasma. Plasma cholesterol lowering effect is due to its excess excretion in bile.

What is the effect of thyroid hormones on vitamin metabolism?

Thyroid hormones increase the quantity of enzymes. Vitamins are the essential parts of some of the enzymes and coenzymes. Therefore, thyroid hormone causes increased need for vitamins leading to relative vitamin deficiency.

What is the effect of thyroid hormones on BMR?

Increase BMR in almost all the cells of the body.

What is the effect of thyroid hormones on body weight?

Greatly increased thyroid hormones cause reduction in body weight (but this effect may not occur because the thyroid hormones increase the appetite).

What is the effect of thyroid hormones on protein metabolism?

In moderate concentration thyroid hormones have anabolic effect causing increase in RNA and protein synthesis. In high concentration of hormones there is catabolic effect on proteins leading to negative nitrogen balance.

What is the effect of thyroid hormones on cardiovascular system?

Thyroid hormones have the following effects on cardiovascular system:

1. *Vasodilatation and increased blood flow to tissues.* Thyroid hormones cause rapid utilization of oxygen and also formation of increased quantities of metabolic end products because of increased BMR. Both these effects cause vasodilatation and increase in blood flow in most of the tissues. Rate of blood flow to the skin increases because of increased need for heat elimination.

2. *Cardiac output.* As a result of increased blood flow to the tissues, cardiac output increases up to 60% above normal.

3. *Heart rate.* Thyroid hormones increase the excitability of the heart thereby causing increase in the heart rate. Increased heart rate is an important physical sign, which is used by clinicians in assessing the function of thyroid gland.

4. *Strength of heart beat.* Moderate increase in thyroid hormones increases the strength of contraction of the heart due to increased enzymatic activity. Marked increase in thyroid hormones because of excessive protein catabolism causes decrease in heart muscle strength. In thyrotoxic patients this may lead to myocardial failure due to increased cardiac load imposed by increased output (patient may die of cardiac decompensation).

5. *Blood volume.* Due to vasodilatation, there is increased volume of blood in circulation.

6. *Arterial pressure.* Due to increased strength of heart beat and increased stroke volume there is increase in systolic pressure whereas due to peripheral

vasodilatation there is decreased diastolic pressure. This results into increased pulse pressure, but the mean arterial pressure usually remains unchanged.

What is the effect of thyroid hormones on respiration?

There is increase in rate and depth of respiration. This results due to increased utilization of O_2 and increased formation of CO_2 by tissues due to increased BMR under the effect of thyroid hormones.

What is the effect of thyroid hormones on GI tract?

- Increased appetite and therefore increased food intake.
- Increased rate of secretion of digestive juices.
- Increased motility of the GI tract. This often causes diarrhoea.

What is the effect of thyroid hormones on central nervous system?

- Rapid cerebration.
- In hyperthyroidism, there is extreme nervousness, psychoneurotic tendencies, anxiety, complexes, worries, etc.
- Irritability of autonomic nervous system causes severe sweating, gastrointestinal tract hypermotility and vasomotor instability.

What is the effect of thyroid hormones on muscles?

1. Slight increase in thyroid hormones makes the muscles react with vigour but excessive quantity of thyroid hormones weakens the muscles because of increased protein catabolism.
2. Lack of thyroid hormones causes sluggishness in muscles. In hyperthyroidism there are tremors of muscles occurring very rapidly at a rate of 10 to 15 times per second because of increased reactivity of neuronal synapses in the areas of spinal cord that control muscle tone. Tremors can be observed easily by placing a sheet of paper on the extended fingers and noting the vibration of the paper.

What is the effect of thyroid hormones on sleep?

There is a feeling of constant tiredness in hyperthyroid subject due to its exhausting effects on muscles and CNS. But it is difficult for a person to get the sleep because of excitable effects on synapses of CNS.

Describe the effect of thyroid hormones on other endocrine glands.

Increased thyroid hormone not only increases the rate of secretion of almost all the other endocrine glands, but it also increases the need of the tissues for the hormones.

Describe the effects of thyroid hormones on sexual functions.

In males, lack of thyroid hormones causes complete loss of libido and excess of hormones causes impotence.

In females, lack of thyroid hormones have varying effects:

- Menorrhagia and polymenorrhagia.
- In some women lack of thyroid hormones causes irregular periods or even amenorrhoea.
- In hyperthyroid women, there is oligomenorrhoea (reduced bleeding). Therefore, action of thyroid hormones on the gonads cannot be pinpointed to a specific function. The effects of hormones on gonads are due to direct metabolic effects on the gonads as well as effects operating through anterior pituitary.

REGULATION OF THYROID HORMONES

Describe the effects of thyroid stimulating hormone (TSH) on thyroid gland.

1. Increased proteolysis of thyroglobulin with resultant release of thyroid hormones into the blood.
2. Increased activity of iodide pump, increasing rate of trapping of iodide in the glandular cells.
3. Increased iodination of tyrosine and increased coupling leading to increased synthesis of thyroid hormones.
4. Increased size and secretory activity of the thyroid cells.
5. Increase in number of thyroid cells. Change from cuboidal to columnar cells and infolding of epithelium into the follicles.

What is the mechanism of action of TSH?

1. TSH binds with the specific receptors on the basal membrane surface of thyroid cells.
2. This activates adenylcyclase enzyme in the membrane which in turn increases formation of cyclic AMP in the cell.
3. Cyclic AMP acts as a second messenger and activates protein kinase which causes multiple phosphorylations in the cell. This in turn causes immediate increase in secretion of thyroid hormones and prolonged growth of glandular tissue.

How is TSH secretion regulated?

Hypothalamic hormone, thyrotropin releasing hormone (TRH), which is secreted by nerve endings of median eminence of hypothalamus passes through hypothalamo-hypophysial portal blood to anterior pituitary.

Thyrotropin releasing hormone is a tripeptide amide. It binds with receptors present on membrane of cells of anterior pituitary. This activates phospholipase second messenger system to produce large amounts of phospholipase C, followed by many other second messenger products (calcium, diacyl glycerol) which lead to TSH release.

Exposure of animal to severe cold is the most important stimulus for TRH and therefore TSH release. Various emotional reactions also affect TRH and TSH release. Effects are mediated through hypothalamus.

How is thyroid hormone secretion regulated?

There is a negative feedback mechanism which regulates thyroid hormone level in body fluids.

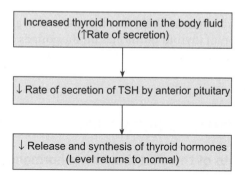

Probably feedback effect is due to reduction in number of TRH receptors on the cells that secrete TSH. Therefore, stimulating effect of TRH is greatly reduced.

There is also slowly acting feedback effect of increased thyroxine level on hypothalamus. This effect is partly caused by changes in body heat and its effect on body temperature controlling centres or hypothalamus which in turn controls pituitary gland.

THYROID FUNCTION TESTS

Describe the tests for assessment of thyroid function.

1. Determination of basal metabolic rate. In hyperthyroidism, it is increased from +30% to +60% and in hypothyroidism it ranges from −30% to −50%.
2. Measurement of concentration of free T_4 and T_3 in the plasma using radio-immunoassay procedures.
3. Measurement of concentration of TSH in plasma by radioimmuno assay. In hyperthyroidism TSH concentration is greatly reduced due to suppression of its secretion by high T_3, T_4 plasma levels. In hypothyroidism, TSH level is high and greatly increases after giving TRH.
4. Concentration of TSAb (thyroid antibodies) is measured by radioimmuno-assay. Usually, it is high in thyrotoxicosis. TSAb are immunoglobulins present in plasma that bind with the same receptors as those for TSH. They induce continuous activation of cyclic AMP with resultant development of hyperthyroidism. They have prolonged (12 hours) stimulatory effect on thyroid gland, as compared to one hour effect caused by TSH. Thus in such person antibodies are developed against the thyroid tissue and hyperthyroidism that develops in an autoimmune disease.
5. Estimation of protein bound iodine (PBI).
6. Thyroid biopsy.
7. Measurement of thyroidal radioiodine accumulation.
8. Tests that assess turnover and release of thyroidal iodine.

APPLIED

Enumerate the different diseases of thyroid gland.

1. *Hyperthyroidism.* Increased secretion of thyroid hormones.
   - Toxic goitre or thyrotoxicosis or Graves's disease.
   - Thyroid adenoma causing hyperthyroidism.
2. *Hypothyroidism.* Decreased levels of thyroid hormones. It is of the following types:
   - Endemic colloid goitre.
   - Idiopathic non-toxic colloid goitre.
   - Cretinism—Extreme hypothyroidism in foetal life, infancy and childhood.
   - Myxoedema—Extreme hypothyroidism after puberty (in adults).

What are the causes of hyperthyroidism?

1. Graves' disease is due mostly to development of thyroid-stimulating antibodies (TSAb) in the blood. It is an autoimmune disease, as patient develops antibodies against its own thyroid tissue. TSAb has the same effects on thyroid gland as those of TSH.
2. Localized adenoma or tumour of the thyroid tissue causes large amount of thyroid hormone secretion. There is no evidence of autoimmune disease.

What are the symptoms and signs of hyperthyroidism?

- Intolerence to heat.
- Increased sweating.
- Mild or extreme weight loss.
- Diarrhoea.
- Muscular weakness.
- Nervousness.
- Extreme fatigue.
- Inability to sleep.
- Tremors of the hands.
- Increased BMR.
- Soft, moist and flushed skin.
- Increased heart rate and systolic blood pressure.
- Eye signs—exophthalmos; retraction of upper eyelid due to infiltration of fat in levator palpebral muscle.

What is exophthalmos? What is it due to?

Exophthalmos is protrusion of eyeballs. It is seen in only some hyperthyroid people. Sometimes protrusion becomes severe and stretches the optic nerve enough to damage vision. But damage to the eye more commonly occurs because the person is not able to close his eyes completely leading to epithelial surfaces of eyes to become dry and irritated. They get infected and corneal ulcers result.

Exophthalmos is due to oedematous swelling of retrobulbar tissues and degenerative changes in the extraocular muscles. Probably, it is also an autoimmune disease. In most of the patients antibodies that react with eye muscles are found in blood. Concentration of these antibodies is highest in people having very high concentrations of thyroid-stimulating antibodies.

Exophthalmos is ameliorated with treatment of hyperthyroidism.

Name the various antithyroid drugs.

Drugs which suppress thyroid secretion are called antithyroid drugs. They are:

1. *Thiocyanate ions.* These ions cause competitive inhibition of iodide transport through cell membrane and thus inhibit iodide trapping mechanism.
2. *Propylthiouracil.* This blocks the peroxidase enzyme required for iodination of tyrosine and also blocks coupling of two iodinated tyrosines to form T_3 or T_4.
3. *Iodides.* When iodides are present in blood in high concentration they cause the following effects only for a few weeks:
   - Decreased rate of iodide trapping.
   - Decreased rate of iodination of tyrosine.
   - Endocytosis of colloid by thyroid cells is diminished. This decreases the release of thyroid hormones into the blood.
   - Size of thyroid gland decreases because of decrease in all the phases of thyroid activity. Its blood supply also decreases. Because of these effects, iodides are administered to patient 2 to 3 weeks prior to surgical removal of thyroid gland.

What are the characteristic features of hypothyroidism?

Characteristics of hypothyroidism:

1. Fatigue and extreme somnolence with sleeping up to 14 to 16 hours.
2. Muscular sluggishness.
3. Depressed growth of hair, scaliness of skin, development of frog-like husky voice.
4. Myxoedema. There is bagginess under the eyes and swelling of face. It is probably due to greatly increased quantities of proteins mixed with hyaluronic acid and chondroitin sulphate which form excessive quantity of tissue gel in interstitial spaces and increase in total quantity of interstitial fluid. Because of gel, excess fluid is immobile and therefore oedema is of non-pitting type.
5. Development of arteriosclerosis, due to increased blood cholesterol level. Arteriosclerosis results into peripheral vascular diseases.

What is cretinism? What are its features?

Cretinism is the condition caused by extreme hypothyroidism during foetal life, infancy and childhood.

A newborn baby has normal appearance but later on the characteristic features are seen. They are:

- Delayed milestones.
- Stunted skeletal growth with short club-like fingers, deformed bones and teeth.

- Rough, thick, dry and wrinkled skin with scanty hairs.
- Idiotic look with thick parted lips, large protruding tongue, broad nose with depressed bridge.
- Abdomen is pot-bellied and umbilicus is protruding.
- Growth of sex organs, sex glands retarded.
- Mental growth is retarded.
- Appetite is reduced because of low BMR.
- There is low blood sugar, high cholesterol and low blood iodine levels.
- Child is susceptible to cold.

Unless the child is treated within few weeks of birth, there is permanent mental retardation. Physical growth returns to normal by treating the cretin at any time.

ADRENAL CORTEX AND MEDULLA

Name the different parts of adrenal gland and the hormones secreted by them.

There are two adrenal glands lying at the superior poles of the kidneys. Central 20% portion of the gland is adrenal medulla. It is related functionally to sympathetic nervous system. Peripheral portion of the gland is called adrenal cortex. Adrenal medulla secretes two hormones, viz. epinephrine (adrenaline) and norepinephrine (noradrenaline).

Adrenal cortex secretes three types of hormones—glucocorticoids, mineralocorticoids and androgens. Adrenal cortex shows three layers (Fig. 9.1).

- Zona glomerulosa—the outermost layer which secretes mineralocorticoids (mainly aldosterone).
- Zona fasciculata—middle layer which secretes glucocorticoids (mainly cortisol) and adrenal androgens.
- Zona reticularis—deepest layer which secretes glucocorticoids and adrenal androgens.

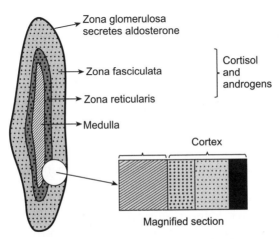

FIGURE 9.1 Different zones of adrenal cortex.

ADRENAL MEDULLARY HORMONES

Name the hormones secreted by adrenal medulla.

Adrenal medulla contains two types of chromaffin cells. One type of cells secrete norepinephrine (noradrenaline) and other type of cells secrete epinephrine (adrenaline). These hormones are stored in the form of chromaffin granules. In human, 80% of chromaffin granules contain epinephrine and 20% of granules contain norepinephrine. These two hormones are dihydroxylated phenolic amines or catecholamines.

Describe the synthesis of catecholamines.

1. L-tyrosine is hydroxylated to L-dopa (i.e. 3,4-dihydroxyphenylalanine).
2. Dopa is converted in the cytosol to dopamine by decarboxylase.
3. Dopamine enters into the chromaffin granules where it is converted to L-norepinephrine by dopamine beta-hydroxylase present exclusively in granules.
4. In 20% of cell, norepinephrine is the end product. In 80% of chromaffin cells norepinephrine diffuses back to the cytoplasm and is N-methylated by phenylalanine-N-methyltransferase to form L-epinephrine.

How is secretion of adrenal medullary hormones controlled?

1. Adrenal medulla is innervated by preganglionic sympathetic nerves emerging mainly from lower thoracic segments of ipsilateral intermediolateral grey column of the spinal cord. Therefore, the main physiological stimulus for release of hormones is acetylcholine from preganglionic sympathetic nerve endings innervating the chromaffin cells. Acetylcholine depolarizes the chromaffin cells. This results into calcium influx and release of catecholamines into the blood by exocytosis.
2. Gland is also activated in response to stress called the fight-or-flight reaction. Fear, anxiety, pain, trauma, haemorrhage, fluid loss, asphyxia, hypoxia, severe hypoglycaemia, hypotension—all these factors stimulate sympathetic nervous system and also adrenal medulla to release catecholamines. During hypoglycaemia adrenal medulla is stimulated independently. Also anger, state of anxiety stimulate the gland independently.

How are catecholamines inactivated?

Half-life of plasma catecholamines is very short (10 to 15 s). Therefore, their biologic effects are rapidly terminated. Catecholamines are metabolized by both enzymatic and non-enzymatic pathway.

1. Sympathetic nerve endings rapidly take up catecholamines from circulation which are inactivated by non-enzymatic or enzymatic (mono-amine oxidase (MAO) way).
2. Circulating catecholamines are mainly taken up by liver and kidneys. MAO is present in liver, kidneys, stomach and intestine. It catalyzes oxidative deamination of catecholamines and form 3-methoxy-4-hydroxy-mandelic acid (vanillylmandelic acid-VMA). About 2 to 3% catecholamines are excreted directly in urine.

Name the various adrenergic receptors.

There are two types of adrenergic receptors:

1. *Alpha.* Alpha receptors are activated by both epinephrine and norepinephrine and are mostly associated with excitatory functions of the body.
2. *Beta.* Beta adrenergic receptors respond to mainly epinephrine and are associated mainly with inhibitory functions.

Describe the physiological effects of catecholamines through alpha and beta receptors.

Effects of catecholamines are the same as those of sympathetic stimulation except that effects are of longer duration and produced on the tissues which are not innervated by sympathetic nerves.

EFFECTS OF CATECHOLAMINES THROUGH ALPHA RECEPTORS

Effector Organ	Response
• Dilater pupillae muscle of eyes	• Contraction (mydriasis)
• Blood vessels	• Constriction of arterioles and veins
• Intestine	• Decreased motility
• Sphincters	• Contraction
• Trigone and sphincter of urinary bladder	• Contraction
• Piloerector muscles of skin	• Piloerection
• Uterus	• Contraction
• Liver	• Glycogenolysis
• Pancreatic islets	• Inhibition of insulin release

EFFECTS OF CATECHOLAMINES THROUGH BETA RECEPTORS

Effector Organ	Response
• Ciliary muscle of eyes	• Relaxation (accommodation for far vision)
• Sinoatrial node of heart	• Increased heart rate
• Atrioventricular node	• Increase in conduction velocity
• Atria of heart	• Increase in contractility
• Ventricles of heart	• Increase in contractility
• Blood vessels	• Dilatation (mainly present in skeletal muscle)
• Bronchial muscle	• Relaxation (bronchodilation)
• Stomach	• Decrease in motility
• Intestine	• Decrease in motility
• Detrusor muscle of bladder	• Relaxation
• Uterus	• Relaxation
• Muscle	• Glycogenolysis
• Pancreatic islets	• Stimulation of insulin secretion

Describe the effects of catecholamines on carbohydrate metabolism.

Metabolic effects of catecholamines are mainly through epinephrine. Norepinephrine has little effect (except its action on pancreatic islets to inhibit insulin secretion as stated above).

Actions are as follows:

1. *Effect on liver.*
   (a) Glycogenolysis in liver—Epinephrine increases glycogenolysis in liver via Ca^{++} activated glycogen phosphorylase and inhibition of glycogen synthetase. This causes increase in blood glucose level.
   (b) Epinephrine also increases glucose production from lactate, amino acids and glycerol which are gluconeogenic substances.
2. *Effect on muscles.* Epinephrine stimulates glycogenolysis in muscles by beta adrenergic receptor mechanism involving stimulation of adenyl cyclase and cyclic AMP induced stimulation of glycogen phosphorylase.

Describe the effects of epinephrine on fat metabolism.

Epinephrine stimulates lipolysis by activating triglyceride lipase via beta adrenergic receptors. Also mobilizes free fatty acids stored in adipose tissue supplying substrate for ketogenesis in liver. Acetoacetate and beta hydroxybutyrate formed are transported from liver to peripheral tissues and are utilized for energy purpose. Especially cardiac muscle uses fatty acids and acetoacetate in preference to glucose for energy purpose. Resting skeletal muscle also uses fatty acids.

What is the difference in the action of epinephrine and norepinephrine?

Epinephrine, because of its greater effect in stimulating beta receptors has a greater effect on cardiac stimulation. It causes weaker constriction of blood vessels compared to strong vasoconstriction caused by norepinephrine. Therefore, in cases of shock, norepinephrine is given to increase the blood pressure. Epinephrine has 5 to 10 times greater metabolic effects as compared to metabolic effects of norepinephrine. Epinephrine also increases the metabolic rate of the body as much as 100% above normal.

APPLIED

What are the effects of hyposecretion and hypersecretion of adrenal medullary hormones?

Hyposecretion of catecholamines, as it occurs in tuberculosis or malignant destruction of adrenal glands or following adrenalectomy, produces no symptoms or any clinical features.

There is a dual mechanism of sympathetic stimulation: (i) Stimulation of the sympathetic nerves supplying different tissues, (ii) stimulation of adrenal medulla to increase circulating catecholamines. This dual mechanism provides a safety factor; if one mechanism is missing the other mechanism substitutes.

Hypersecretion of catecholamines occurs in chromaffin cells tumour called phaeochromocytoma. In this condition, there is a sustained paroxysmal hypertension associated with headache, sweating, palpitations, chest pain, anxiety, pallor of the skin due to vasoconstriction, blurred vision.

If epinephrine is secreted primarily heart rate is increased, and if norepinephrine is secreted predominantly pulse rate decreases (reflex effect of hypertension). Urinary excretion of catecholamines and VMA is increased. Treatment is surgical removal of the tumour.

ADRENOCORTICAL HORMONES

What are adrenocortical hormones chemically?

Chemically adrenocortical hormones are steroids.

Describe the synthesis of adrenocortical hormones.

Steps in synthesis of adrenocortical hormones are:

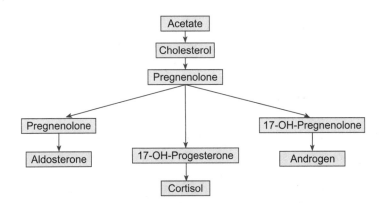

Name the different mineralocorticoids.

- Aldosterone—Very potent; accounts for 90% of mineralocorticoid activity.
- Deoxycorticosterone—One-fifth as potent as aldosterone. It is secreted in small quantities.
- Cortisol—Very slight mineralocorticoid activity, but is secreted in large amounts.
- Cortisone (synthetic)—Slight mineralocorticoid activity.

Name the different glucocorticoids.

- Cortisol—Very potent glucocorticoid and is responsible for 95% of the glucocorticoid activity.
- Corticosterone—Less potent and is responsible for 4% of glucocorticoid activity.
- Cortisone (synthetic)—As potent as cortisol.
- Prednisone (synthetic)—Four times as potent as cortisol.
- Methylprednisolone (synthetic)—Five times as potent as cortisol.
- Dexamethasone (synthetic)—Thirty times as potent as cortisol.

How are adrenal cortical hormones transported in blood?

Cortisol combines with a globulin called cortisol-binding globulin or transcortin and to a lesser extent with albumin in the plasma. Ninety-four per cent cortisol is in the bound form and remaining is free.

Only 50% of aldosterone is in the bound form and 50% is free. These hormones are transported throughout the extracellular fluid and become fixed to the target tissue within an hour or two.

What is the fate of adrenal cortical hormones?

Adrenal steroids are degraded mainly in liver and are conjugated to form glucuronides and sulphates. Twenty five per cent are excreted in bile and faeces and remaining 75% in urine.

Give the rate of secretion and concentration of aldosterone and cortisol.

Rate of secretion of aldosterone is 150 to 250 mg/day and its blood concentration is 6 nanogram/decilitre (100 ml) of blood.

Rate of secretion of cortisol is 15 to 20 mg/day and its concentration in blood is 12 microgram/decilitre of blood.

MINERALOCORTICOIDS

Describe the functions of mineralocorticoids (aldosterone).

Mineralocorticoids are essential to life. Without them, death would result due to decreased extracellular fluid and blood volume, diminished cardiac output and shock.

Ninety per cent of mineralocorticoid activity is due to aldosterone. Deoxycorticosterone has the same effect with a potency of 1/50th to that of aldosterone. Corticosterone has some mineralocorticoid effect but is less potent.

FUNCTIONS OF ALDOSTERONE

1. *Effect on renal tubules.* Aldosterone causes increased absorption of sodium with simultaneous excretion of potassium by renal tubular epithelial cells. This effect is seen in late distal tubules and collecting ducts. Thus aldosterone increases total quantity of sodium in the extracellular fluid by decreasing rate of sodium excretion in urine.

2. *Effect on extracellular fluid volume.* Absorption of sodium from renal tubules causes simultaneous osmotic absorption of water. This increases the extracellular fluid volume. Thus sodium is retained without much change in its concentration.

3. *Effect on muscles.* Excessive loss of potassium from extracellular fluid into urine under the effect of aldosterone causes hypokalaemia, i.e. decreased potassium concentration in blood (1 to 2 mEq/L). This causes severe muscular weakness due to decreased excitability of nerves and muscles.

4. *Effect on heart.* Deficiency of aldosterone causes hyperkalaemia (increased concentration of potassium ions in blood). This causes serious cardiac toxicity. There is weakness of heart contraction, arrhythmia. Even death may result due to cardiac cause.

5. *Effect on pH of blood.* Though aldosterone mainly causes secretion of potassium in exchange for sodium absorption, to a lesser extent it also causes tubular secretion of hydrogen ions. This causes decrease in H^+ ion concentration of extracellular fluid, leading to mild degree of alkalosis.

6. *Effect on sweat glands and salivary glands.* Both these glands form primary secretion which contains large amount of sodium chloride. This sodium chloride is absorbed as the secretion passes through the ducts. Aldosterone greatly increases the absorption of sodium and chloride from the ducts and in turn potassium and bicarbonate ions are excreted. Thus sodium chloride loss in these secretion (sweat and saliva) becomes less.

Aldosterone also increases absorption of sodium by the intestines (colon).

What is the mechanism of action of aldosterone?

1. Aldosterone because of its lipid solubility easily passes through the cell membranes into the interior of tubular epithelial cells.
2. Aldosterone combines with specific cytoplasmic receptor protein.
3. Aldosterone receptor complex diffuses into the nucleus and induces specific portions of DNA to form a type or types of messenger RNA.
4. Messenger RNA diffuses into the cytoplasm and stimulates protein formation in ribosomes. These proteins are enzyme proteins, receptor proteins and membrane transport proteins required for transport of sodium, potassium and hydrogen through the cell membrane (e.g. Na^+-K^+ ATPase required for Na^+-K^+ pump).

Thus aldosterone does not have immediate effect. Approximately 30 minutes are required before new RNA appears in the cell and 45 minutes before the rate of sodium transport begins to increase.

What is aldosterone escape?

Increased aldosterone secretion causes increased amount of extracellular fluid (as a result of increased sodium and water absorption by renal tubules). This leads to increase in blood pressure. Increased arterial blood pressure causes increased water and salt excretion by kidneys (pressure diuresis). Thus after 10 to 15% increase in extracellular fluid volume, secondary increase in water and salt excretion by kidneys returns renal output of salt and water to normal despite of excess aldosterone. This is called aldosterone escape.

REGULATION

How is aldosterone secretion regulated?

There are four factors regulating the secretion of aldosterone:

- Potassium ion concentration of extracellular fluid is the most potent factor in regulating aldosterone secretion. Slight increase in potassium concentration causes several fold increase in aldosterone secretion.

- Renin-angiotensin system is also a very potent mechanism. Decreased blood flow to the kidney activates renin-angiotensin system to increase aldosterone secretion several fold.
- Sodium ion concentration in extracellular fluid. Decrease in sodium ion concentration in ECF stimulates aldosterone secretion and vice versa. This regulates sodium ion concentration in ECF. But effect on aldosterone is minor.
- Adrenocorticotropic hormone (ACTH) effect on aldosterone secretion is usually minor. But total absence of ACTH can significantly reduce aldosterone secretion.

GLUCOCORTICOIDS

What is the effect of glucocorticoids on carbohydrate metabolism?

Glucocorticoids (mainly cortisol) have following effects on carbohydrate metabolism:

1. *Gluconeogenesis.* Glucocorticoids stimulate gluconeogenesis, i.e. formation of glucose from non-carbohydrate substances. This is due to the following reasons:
   - All the enzymes required for conversion of amino acids to glucose in liver cells are increased due to cortisol. Cortisol activates DNA transcription in liver cells with formation of messenger RNA leading to synthesis of protein enzymes for gluconeogenesis.
   - Cortisol mobilizes amino acids from extrahepatic tissues (mainly muscle) thereby increasing amino acids levels in plasma. Thus more amino acids are made available for liver cells for formation of glucose.

Increased glucose synthesis in liver increases glycogen storage by liver cells.

2. **Utilization of glucose by the cells.** Cortisol decreases the rate of utilization of glucose by all the cells of the body. This effect is due to depressed oxidation of NADH (nicotinamide adenine dinucleotide) by cortisol. NADH must be oxidized for rapid glycolysis. Thus glucose utilization by cells is diminished.

3. *Blood glucose level.* Cortisol causes increased gluconeogenesis and decreased utilization of glucose by the body cells as described above. Both these effects cause increase in blood glucose concentration. Occasionally it is great enough to cause adrenal diabetes.

What is the effect of glucocorticoids on protein metabolism?

Glucocorticoids cause decreased protein synthesis, increased catabolism of proteins in all the body cells except the liver cells. This effect of cortisol is due to decreased transport of amino acids and depression of formation of RNA in the extrahepatic tissues (especially muscle and lymphoid tissue). Great excess of cortisol decreases immunity functions of lymphoid tissue.

Cortisol increases the transport of amino acids into the liver cells and also enhances enzymes required for protein synthesis. Thus cortisol mobilizes amino acids from the extrahepatic tissue, increases blood level of amino acids and increases transport of amino acids into the liver cells. Due to this, there is increased utilization of amino acids by liver cells, e.g. increased deamination, increased protein synthesis, increased formation of plasma protein and increased conversion of amino acids to glucose.

What is the effect of glucocorticoids on fat metabolism?

Glucocorticoids promote the mobilization of fatty acids from the adipose tissues. This causes increase in free fatty acids level in blood. Glucocorticoid also increases the utilization of fatty acids for energy (effect is secondary because of reduced availability of glucose for metabolism under the effect of glucocorticoids). Increased mobilization of fatty acids from adipose tissue is due to the following mechanism.

Alpha glycerophosphate is derived from glucose and glucocorticoid decreases the transport of glucose into the fat cells. Alpha glycerophosphate is required for deposition and maintenance of triglycerides in fat cells. Therefore, its absence or decrease causes release of fatty acids.

Increased utilization of fatty acids for energy purpose causes increased formation of ketone bodies and ketosis. Thus glucocorticoids have ketogenic effect. This effect occurs only if insulin is deficient.

Glucocorticoids cause development of a peculiar type of obesity. There is excess deposition of fat in chest and head regions of the body giving rise to rounded face known as 'moon face'. This obesity is due to excess stimulation of food intake. Therefore, fat is generated at a greater rate than the rate of its mobilization and oxidation.

Describe the anti-inflammatory effects of cortisol.

When tissues are damaged by trauma or infection, they become inflamed, i.e. there is increased blood flow, leakage of large quantities of plasma out of capillaries (non-pitting oedema), infiltration of leucocytes and healing by fibrosis. Cortisol has anti-inflammatory effects. It blocks early stages of inflammation and causes rapid resolution of the inflammation if it has already begun. These effects occur due to following mechanisms:

1. Stabilizes lysosomal membranes and thus prevents rupture of lysosomes and reduces the release of proteolytic enzymes from damaged tissue.
2. Decreases capillary permeability preventing loss of plasma into the tissues. This is secondary to decreased release of proteolytic enzymes.
3. Decreases migration of WBCs into inflamed area and phagocytosis of the damaged cells. This is also due to decreased release of lysosomal enzymes and other substances from damaged cells.
4. Suppresses immune system, decreasing lymphocyte reproduction markedly (especially T lymphocytes). Both T cells and antibodies are decreased which would have promoted inflammatory process.
5. Reduces release of interleukin-1 from WBCs which principally excites hypothalamic temperature control system to cause fever. Thus cortisol lowers the fever.
6. Even after inflammation is established, cortisol causes its resolution. As stated above, most of the factors promoting inflammation are blocked, the

rate of healing is enhanced. This is due to increased mobilization of amino acids for repair and increased amount of fatty acids and glucose for cellular energy. Such anti-inflammatory effect of cortisol is useful in combating certain diseases like rheumatic fever, rheumatoid arthritis and acute glomerular nephritis.

How do glucocorticoids help during stress?

Glucocorticoids help in various types of stress such as trauma, infections, intense heat or cold and surgical operations. Variety of such non-specific stimuli causes greater release of cortisol.

Cortisol causes rapid mobilization of amino acids and fats from stores and makes them available for energy. It also causes synthesis of compounds (especially glucose). Newly available amino acids are used by damaged tissues to form new proteins, intracellular substances, like purines, pyrimidines and creatine phosphate necessary for cell-life and reproduction.

What is the effect of cortisol on allergy?

Basic allergic reaction between antigen and antibody is not affected by cortisol but it blocks inflammatory response to allergic reactions. Inflammatory response is responsible for serious and lethal effects of allergic reaction. So administration of cortisol is lifesaving in cases of anaphylaxis.

What is the effect of cortisol on blood cells and immunity?

Cortisol decreases eosinophils and lymphocytes in the blood. Giving large doses of cortisol causes significant atrophy of all the lymphoid tissues, decreasing output of T cells and antibodies. Level of immunity for all foreign invaders is decreased. This can lead to fulminating infections and death from diseases which would not be lethal. But this ability of cortisol is useful in preventing immunologic rejection of transplanted tissues. Cortisol increases production of RBCs.

REGULATION

How is cortisol secretion regulated?

Secretion of cortisol is entirely controlled by adrenocorticotropic hormone (ACTH) secreted by anterior pituitary (Fig. 9:2). ACTH also enhances the production of adrenal androgens. It activates adenylcyclase enzyme in the adrenocortical cell membrane which induces formation of cyclic AMP. Cyclic AMP in turn activates intracellular enzymes that cause formation of adrenocortical hormones. ACTH converts cholesterol to pregnenolone.

Secretion of ACTH in turn is controlled by corticotropin releasing factor (CRF) from hypothalamus. CRF is secreted by neurons in the paraventricular nuclei of hypothalamus. It passes through hypothalamo-hypophysial portal system to anterior pituitary to stimulate secretion of ACTH. Without CRF, rate of secretion of ACTH by anterior pituitary is very small.

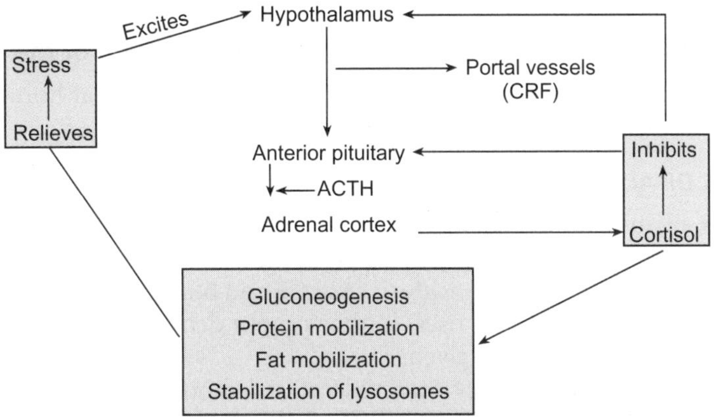

FIGURE 9.2 Regulation of glucocorticoid secretion.

Paraventricular nuclei of hypothalamus receive many connections from limbic system and lower brain stem.

Cortisol has direct negative feedback effects on both—on hypothalamus to decrease formation of CRF and on anterior pituitary to decrease formation of ACTH. This feedback regulates plasma level of cortisol. Physical or mental stress increases ACTH secretion. Physical stress stimulates perifornical area of hypothalamus and then the impulses to paraventricular nuclei and to median eminence where CRF is secreted in portal system. This CRF causes ACTH release to cause increased glucocorticoids secretion within minutes.

Mental stress is due to increased activity of limbic system (amygdala and hippocampus) and transmission of signal to posterior medial hypothalamus to cause ACTH secretion.

OTHER HORMONES

What is melanocyte stimulating hormone? How is it secreted? What is its action?

ACTH formation from anterior pituitary initially causes formation of 'preprohormone' which is a large protein molecule which contains ACTH, MSH, beta-lipotropin and beta-endorphin. Under normal condition only ACTH is secreted and others are not secreted in enough quantities to have any effect on the body. But when ACTH is secreted in large quantities, MSH is secreted. It causes melanocytes present in dermis and epidermis of skin to form black pigment melanin which is dispersed in the cells of epidermis causing intense darkening of the skin.

What are the functions of androgens secreted by adrenal cortex?

Most important adrenal androgen is dehydroepiandrosterone. Progesterone and oestrogen are also secreted in minute quantities. Adrenal androgens may be partly responsible for development of male sex organs in childhood. In females, pubic and axillary hair growth occurs due to adrenal androgens. Some adrenal androgens are converted to testosterone in the extra adrenal tissue, accounting for androgenic activity.

APPLIED

What is Addison's disease? What are the main features of the disease?

Addison's disease is due to decreased secretion of adrenocortical hormones. Frequently the cause is atrophy of adrenal cortex.

FEATURES OF ADDISON'S DISEASE

1. Lack of mineralocorticoids causes excessive loss of sodium chloride and water in urine leading to decreased volume of extracellular fluid and blood, hyperkalaemia and mild acidosis. As ECF and blood volume decrease, RBC concentration markedly rises, cardiac output decreases and patient dies of shock if no treatment is given.
2. Glucocorticoid deficiency causes decreased mobilization of fats, proteins and failure to maintain normal blood glucose between meals (because of decreased gluconeogenesis). Thus there is sluggishness of energy mobilization when cortisol is not available. Muscles become very weak. Person is highly susceptible to stress.
3. Depressed cortisol secretion causes increased rate of ACTH secretion by usual negative feedback. There is simultaneous increase in MSH secretion. This causes pigmentation of the skin. Person, if not treated, dies within a few weeks. Treatment is to give small quantities of mineralocorticoids and glucocorticoids.

What is Addisonian crisis?

In Addison's disease, concentration of glucocorticoids does not increase in stress like trauma, disease and surgery. Lack of glucocorticoids at such times leads to severe debility which is called Addisonian crisis.

What is Cushing's syndrome?

Hypersecretion of cortisol causes Cushing's syndrome. There is mobilization of fat from lower part of the body and deposition in thoracic and upper abdominal region giving rise to so-called 'buffalo hump' and 'moon face'. There is hypertension due to increased mineralocorticoid activity.

Increased glucocorticoids secretion causes increased blood glucose level causing constant stimulation of islets of Langerhans of pancreas. Occasionally these islets burn out because of overstimulation leading to pancreatic diabetes mellitus.

Protein catabolic effects on extrahepatic tissues cause severe muscular weakness, suppressed immune system, osteoporosis (lack of protein deposition in bones) and weakness of bones.

Cushing's syndrome can be treated by removing the adrenal tumour or bilateral partial adrenalectomy, followed by therapy of adrenocorticoids if deficiency results.

What is primary aldosteronism?

Small tumour of zona glomerulosa cells leading to excess aldosterone secretion causes primary aldosteronism. It leads to muscular paralysis due to hypokalaemia, increased sodium concentration of ECF, increased EC fluid and blood volume. Treatment is surgical removal of the tumour.

What is adrenogenital syndrome?

When adrenocortical tumour secretes excessive quantities of androgens, they cause intense masculinizing effects on the body. In females there is change in voice, growth of beard, baldness, masculine distribution of hair, growth of clitoris, deposition of proteins in skin and muscles to give typical masculine appearance.

In males, tumour in prepubertal life causes all the above effects with rapid development of male sex organs and male sexual desires. In the adult male such a tumour is obscured by normal virilizing characteristics of testosterone which makes the diagnosis difficult.

PANCREAS

Name the hormones of pancreas.

Hormones of pancreas are insulin and glucagon. They are secreted by beta and alpha cells of islets of Langerhans respectively. Delta cells of islets of Langerhans secrete 10% of total somatostatin (Fig. 9.3).

INSULIN

What is insulin chemically?

Insulin is a protein consisting of two amino acid chains connected to each other by disulphide linkage. If the two chains are split apart, functional activity of insulin is lost.

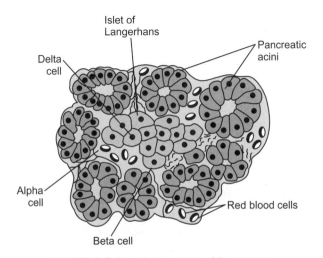

FIGURE 9.3 Physiologic anatomy of the pancreas.

Describe synthesis of insulin.

Beta cells of islets of Langerhans synthesize insulin by usual protein synthetic machinery. First insulin preprohormone is formed with molecular weight 11,500. It is cleaved to form proinsulin with molecular weight 9,000. This is further cleaved in Golgi apparatus to form insulin before formation of secretory granules.

How is insulin circulated in blood?

Insulin is circulated in blood in unbound form with plasma half-life of 6 minutes and is cleared from circulation within 10 to 15 minutes.

How is insulin degraded?

Except for the insulin that combines with receptors in the target cells, remainder is mainly degraded by enzyme insulinase in the liver and to a lesser extent in the kidneys.

Describe the mechanism by which insulin affects the target cells.

Membrane of target cells contains insulin receptors. This insulin receptor is a protein formed of four subunits held together by disulphide linkage. Two alpha subunits lie entirely outside the membrane and two beta subunits penetrate through the membrane with the ends protruding into the cell cytoplasm. Insulin binds with alpha subunits due to which beta subunits become autophosphorylated. They become activated protein kinase which in turn causes phosphorylation of multiple other cytosol enzymes and have the following effects:

- Membrane becomes highly permeable to glucose which is immediately phosphorylated.
- Membrane also becomes more permeable for many amino acids, potassium, magnesium and phosphate ions.
- Slower effects occurring in the next 10 to 15 minutes cause activation of more intracellular enzymes.
- Still much slower effects continue for hours or for several days. They change the rate of translation of messenger RNAs in ribosomes to form new proteins.
- As a still slower effect, rate of transcription of DNA in the cell nucleus changes causing remoulding of the enzymatic machinery to achieve required metabolic effects.

ACTIONS OF INSULIN

Describe the effects of insulin on carbohydrate metabolism.

1. *Effects on skeletal muscles.* During exercise, permeability of muscle membrane to glucose increases even in the absence of insulin. Under-resting state muscle membrane takes in glucose only during a few hours after meals. This is due to increased amount of insulin secreted after meals. Insulin increases permeability

of muscle membrane for glucose. It has a direct effect on the muscle cell membrane to transport glucose. It can increase rate of transport by ten- to twentyfold.

In between meals, amount of insulin secreted is not sufficient to promote the entry of glucose into the muscle. Glucose that is taken is mostly converted to glycogen in the muscle.

2. *Effects on liver.* Insulin increases the amount of glycogen in the liver as follows:
   - Insulin inhibits liver phosphorylase enzyme which causes splitting of liver glycogen to glucose.
   - By increasing activity of enzyme glucokinase, insulin increases the uptake of glucose by liver cells. Glucokinase enzyme causes initial phosphorylation of glucose. After its entry phosphorylated glucose cannot diffuse back.
   - Insulin enhances the activity of enzymes promoting glycogen synthesis, e.g. phosphofructokinase, glycogen synthetase. Between meals when blood glucose level drops and insulin secretion decreases all the above effects are reversed. Synthesis of glycogen and uptake of glucose by liver cells almost stops. Lack of insulin (alongwith increase in glucagon) activates phosphorylase enzyme causing splitting of glycogen to glucose phosphate. Glucose phosphatase also becomes activated and splits phosphate radical from glucose. Thus free glucose diffuses back into the blood.
   - Other effects. When the quantity of glucose entering the liver cells is more than can be stored in the form of glycogen, insulin promotes conversion of all excess glucose into fatty acids. Insulin also inhibits gluconeogenesis by decreasing activity of liver enzymes required for gluconeogenesis.

3. Insulin increases glucose uptake by most of the cells (except brain cells, which are permeable to glucose).

What is the effect of insulin on fat metabolism?

Insulin leads to fat storage in adipose tissue due to several reasons:

1. Insulin increases transport of glucose through liver cells and synthesis of glycogen from glucose. But when glycogen concentration increases from 5 to 6%, glycogenesis is inhibited and then additional glucose entering is converted to fat in liver cells.

First glucose is split to pyruvate (in glycolytic pathway) and pyruvate is converted to acetyl CoA which is a substrate for fatty acid synthesis.

2. Increased citrate and isocitrate formed by citric acid cycle (when excess glucose is being used for energy) activate acetyl CoA carboxylase to form malonyl CoA which is the first stage of fatty acid synthesis.
3. Fatty acid synthesized in liver cells are used by them for triglyceride synthesis. Triglyceride is the usual form of fat storage. Triglycerides formed in liver cells are released to the blood.
4. Insulin activates lipoprotein lipase in the capillary wall of adipose tissue which splits triglyceride into fatty acids. They are absorbed by fat cells and converted to triglycerides (glycerol is obtained from glucose in adipose tissue and glucose transport through adipose tissue cell membrane is increased by the action of insulin).

5. Insulin inhibits action of hormone-sensitive lipase which causes hydrolysis of fat in fat cells. Thus formation and release of fatty acids into the circulating blood is inhibited.

Describe the effects of insulin on protein metabolism.

Insulin causes storage of proteins in the cells as follows:

1. Increases the transport of many amino acids into the cells (especially amino acids valine, leucine, isoleucine, tyrosine and phenylalanine).
2. Increases the translation of messenger RNA on the ribosomes forming new proteins. In the absence of insulin, ribosomes stop working.
3. Over a longer period, insulin also increases the rate of transcription of selected DNA genetic sequences in cell nuclei. This results into formation of increased quantities of RNA causing still more protein synthesis mainly enzymes for storage of fats, proteins and carbohydrates.
4. Insulin inhibits catabolism of proteins and decreases rate of amino acid release from the cells.
5. In liver, insulin decreases rate of gluconeogenesis and thus conserves amino acids for protein synthesis.

Thus insulin promotes protein synthesis and inhibits its degradation. Because of this action, insulin is essential for growth. The growth hormone and insulin function synergistically to promote growth.

REGULATION

How is insulin secretion controlled?

Insulin secretion is mainly controlled by level of blood glucose. Acute elevation of glucose causes increase in concentration to about tenfold within 3 to 5 min due to release of preformed insulin in the blood. But this level of insulin returns to normal in another 5 to 10 minutes.

After 15 minutes, insulin secretion rises second time and remains high for 2 to 3 hours. The rise of level is greater than the initial phase. This increase in insulin is due to additional release of preformed insulin and activation of the enzyme system which synthesizes and releases new insulin from the cells. There is feedback relationship between blood glucose concentration and the rate of insulin secretion. When concentration of blood glucose rises above 100 mg/100 ml of blood, rate of insulin secretion rises rapidly to a high level. This in turn reduces blood glucose concentration to fasting level. Reduction in blood glucose causes rapid turning off of insulin secretion.

The other factors stimulating insulin secretion are:

- Amino acids. Increase of amino acids in blood (especially arginine and lysine) causes stimulation of insulin secretion. But as compared to glucose, they cause only slight rise on insulin secretion. Secreted insulin promotes transport of amino acids into the cells and also formation of cell proteins.
- Gastrointestinal hormones like gastrin, secretin, cholecystokinin and gastric inhibitory polypeptide (most potent) cause moderate increase in insulin secretion. These GI tract hormones are released after meals so they cause anticipatory rise of insulin before actual absorption of glucose and amino acids.

- Other hormones like growth hormone, cortisol, glucagon and to a lesser extent progesterone and oestrogen also stimulate insulin secretion. Prolonged secretion of any of these hormones can cause burning out of islets of Langerhans thereby causing diabetes mellitus.
- Under some conditions stimulation of sympathetic or parasympathetic nerves to pancreas increase insulin secretion.

What is the importance of blood glucose regulation?

Glucose is the only nutrient which is used by certain tissues like brain, retina, germinal epithelium, etc. It is important therefore to maintain blood glucose level to provide nutrition to the tissues.

Most of the glucose formed by gluconeogenesis in interdigestive period is used for metabolism of brain. It is important therefore that pancreas does not secrete insulin during this period because the supply of glucose will go to peripheral tissues leaving brain without a nutritive source.

Name the other hormones affecting blood glucose level.

Hormones (other than insulin) affecting blood glucose level are:

- Growth hormone
- Cortisol (glucocorticoid)
- Epinephrine
- Glucagon

All these increase the blood glucose level.

APPLIED

What is glycosuria?

Presence of glucose in urine is known as glycosuria.

What is renal glycosuria?

Presence of glucose in urine due to lowering of renal threshold is known as renal glycosuria. Normally renal threshold for glucose is 180 mg/100 ml of blood.

If blood sugar is below this level, glycosuria does not occur. But in case of renal glycosuria, renal threshold is less than normal and therefore even at blood concentration below 180 mg/l00 ml, glycosuria occurs.

What is diabetes mellitus?

Diabetes mellitus is a disease which results from diminished secretion of insulin.
There are two general types of diabetes mellitus:

- Type I diabetes or insulin dependent diabetes caused due to lack of insulin secretion.
- Type II diabetes or non-insulin dependent diabetes caused due to decreased sensitivity of target tissues to action of insulin (tissues become insulin resistant).

What are the probable causes of diabetes mellitus?

Probable causes of diabetes mellitus are:

1. *Heredity.* It usually plays a major role. It increases susceptibility of beta cells to viruses or it favours development of autoimmune antibodies against beta cells leading to their dysfunction.

2. *Obesity.* In obesity, beta cells of islets of Langerhans become less responsive to stimulation by increased glucose. Obesity also reduces the number of insulin receptors in the target cells.

Enumerate the various signs and symptoms of diabetes mellitus and their physiological basis.

1. *Increase in blood glucose concentration.* This is due to decreased utilization of glucose by the cells. Blood glucose may vary from 300 to 1200 mg/100 ml.

2. *Arteriosclerosis.* Increased mobilization of fats from fat storage areas causes abnormal fat metabolism and deposition of cholesterol in arterial walls.

3. *Depletion of proteins in the tissues.*

4. *Loss of glucose in urine.* When the level of glucose in blood rises above the critical level (i.e. 180 mg/100 ml which is a renal threshold) excess glucose spills in urine. Glucose present in urine also retains water along with it, i.e. there is osmotic diuresis (increased urinary output).

5. *Dehydration of tissue cells.* In untreated diabetes mellitus, high glucose concentration increases osmotic pressure of extracellular fluid and osmotic transfer of water from cells to the extracellular fluid leading to dehydration of cells. In addition to it, osmotic diuresis causes increased loss of water from the body thereby reducing extracellular fluid volume which also causes compensatory dehydration of cells. Both these effects contribute to circulatory shock.

6. *Lack of insulin causes use of fat instead of carbohydrate.* Because of this, fat is utilized for energy purpose. This increases the levels of keto acids (beta-hydroxybu-tyric acid and acetoacetic acid) in the body fluids from 1 mEq/L to 10 mEq/L (ketosis). This extra acid leads to acidosis which causes rapid and deep breathing called Kussmaul breathing. It is characterized by washing out of CO_2 and marked decrease in bicarbonate content of body fluids. In untreated diabetes, acidic coma and death may result.

7. *Polyuria.* Excessive urine formation due to osmotic diuresis as stated above.

8. *Polyphagia.* Excessive eating due to failure to use glucose.

9. *Polydipsia.* Excessive drinking of water due to cellular dehydration.

10. *Loss of weight.*

11. *Asthenia.* Lack of energy. It is mainly due to loss of body proteins.

What are the investigations done to diagnose diabetes mellitus?

1. *Urine examination.* Presence of glucose indicates diabetes because in a normal person glucose is not excreted. Amount of glucose excreted depends on severity of the disease.

2. *Fasting blood glucose level.* Fasting blood glucose level (in the early morning) is normally between 80 and 90 mg/100 ml and 110 mg/100 ml is

considered the upper limit of normal. Fasting blood sugar above this level indicates diabetes mellitus, adrenal diabetes or pituitary diabetes.

3. *Glucose tolerance test.* For this test one ensures that there is normal intake of carbohydrate (100 g/day), eight days prior to the test. In the early morning, fasting blood and urine samples are collected. Then person is given glucose (1 g/kg body weight), and every half an hour blood and urine samples are collected for $2\frac{1}{2}$ to 3 hours. In a normal person, fasting blood glucose is about 100 mg/100 ml. After glucose intake it reaches the peak after one hour or so; it rises up to 140 mg/100 ml. Then it returns to fasting level within 2 to $2\frac{1}{2}$ hours. Urine does not show the presence of glucose.

In diabetes mellitus, glucose tolerance curve is abnormal. Fasting glucose level is high, peak is high and blood sugar does not return to fasting level for a long time (4 to 6 hours). This slow fall of glucose level indicates failure to control due to lack of insulin secretion following sugar ingestion. This test is called oral glucose tolerance test. Rarely, intravenous glucose tolerance test is done.

4. *Acetone in urine.* Keto acids in blood increase which are excreted in urine because of greater utilization of fat for energy. So in urine, acetone may be present. Acetone is also excreted by lungs as it is volatile and sometimes diabetes is diagnosed by smelling acetone on the breath of a patient.

How is diabetes mellitus treated?

Type I diabetes is treated by giving enough insulin. Insulin is available in different forms. Regular insulin has duration of action of 3 to 8 hours.

Other forms of insulin (precipitated with zinc or with various protein derivatives) are absorbed slowly from the site of injection and therefore have duration of action of 10 to 48 hours. Usually patient is given a single dose of long acting insulin with additional doses of regular insulin if required, when blood glucose tends to rise, e.g. at meal time. In the past, insulin derived from animal pancreas was used. Recently human insulin is also available.

Type II diabetes is treated by dietetic restrictions and exercise so as to reduce weight and to reverse insulin resistance.

GLUCAGON

What is glucagon chemically? From where is it secreted?

Glucagon is a large polypeptide secreted by alpha cells of islets of Langerhans.

ACTIONS OF GLUCAGON

Describe the effects of glucagon.

Glucagon increases the blood glucose level by the following mechanisms:

1. *Increased glycogenolysis.* Glucagon causes breakdown of liver glycogen (glycogenolysis) in the following way:

Glucagon activates adenylcyclase enzyme in hepatic cell membrane which causes formation of cyclic AMP. Cyclic AMP activates the 'protein kinase regulator protein' which activates protein kinase. Protein kinase activates phosphorylase 'b' kinase which converts phosphorylase 'b' to phosphorylase 'a'.

Phosphorylase 'a' promotes degradation of glycogen into glucose phosphate. This is dephosphorylated and glucose is formed.

2. *Increased gluconeogenesis.* After the glycogen in the liver is exhausted glucagon increases the rate of gluconeogenesis. It activates multiple enzymes in gluconeogenesis especially the enzyme system converting pyruvate to phospho-pyruvate (rate limiting step in gluconeogenesis). It also increases the entry of amino acids from blood to liver cells and make them available for gluconeo-genesis.

3. *Increased fatty acids.* Glucagon activates adipose lipase making increased quantity of fatty acids available for energy. It also inhibits synthesis of triglyc-erides in liver so that the removal of fatty acid by liver (from the blood) is reduced.

In very large concentration, glucagon enhances the strength of the heart, bile secretion and inhibits gastric secretion.

REGULATION

How is glucagon secretion regulated?

Glucagon secretion is regulated as follows:

1. *Blood glucose level.* It is the most important controller. Decrease in blood glucose level increases the glucagon secretion and vice versa. This is one of the important mechanisms correcting hypoglycaemia.

2. *Amino acids.* Increased amino acids level (after protein meal) stimulates the glucagon secretion.

3. *Muscular exercise.* Muscular exercise increases glucagon secretion. The mechanism is not yet understood but increased amino acid level or nervous stimulation of islets of Langerhans may be playing a role.

SOMATOSTATIN

What is somatostatin? What are its effects?

Somatostatin is the hormone secreted by delta cells of islets of Langerhans. It is a polypeptide containing 14 amino acids. After ingestion of food, somatostatin se-cretion is increased because increased blood glucose, amino acids, fatty acids and GI tract hormones stimulate the secretion.

Somatostatin has following effects:

- Acts on the islets of Langerhans and inhibits secretion of insulin and glucagon.
- Decreases the motility of stomach, duodenum and gall bladder.
- Decreases secretion and absorption in the GI tract.

PARATHYROID

CALCIUM AND PHOSPHATE METABOLISM

Describe the intestinal absorption of calcium and phosphate.

Calcium is poorly absorbed from the intestine because of formation of insoluble salts with many compounds and also because it is a bivalent cation (bivalent cations are poorly absorbed).

Phosphate on the other hand is absorbed easily except when calcium is present in the diet to form insoluble calcium phosphate.

How are calcium and phosphate excreted?

Nine-tenth of calcium is excreted in faeces and only one-tenth is excreted in urine. Except the phosphate in combination with calcium (which is excreted in faeces) almost all the dietary phosphate is absorbed into the blood and later on is excreted in urine. Phosphate is a threshold substance, therefore when its concentration in the plasma is below the critical value (1 mmol/L), no phosphate at all is lost in urine, but above this critical concentration, rate of phosphate loss is directly proportional to the additional increase.

What is the role of vitamin D in calcium and phosphate absorption?

Vitamin D is first converted to its active form. The most important of sterols is vitamin D (cholecalciferol). It is mostly formed in the skin from 7-dehydrocholesterol by ultraviolet rays of the sun. This is converted to active compound (1,25-dihydroxy-cholecalciferol) as follows:

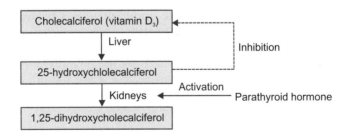

This 1,25-dihydroxycholecalciferol acts as a hormone and increases the absorption of calcium from intestine by increasing the quantity of calcium-binding protein in the intestinal epithelial cells. This protein remains in the cells for several weeks and therefore has prolonged effect on calcium absorption. It also increases calcium stimulated ATPase in the brush border of intestinal epithelial cell and formation of alkaline phosphatase in these cells. These two effects also promote calcium absorption in yet unknown way.

Vitamin D also increases absorption of phosphate but it is much less important because usually phosphate is absorbed relatively easily. Effect on phosphate absorption is probably secondary from its action on calcium absorption (calcium acts as a transport mediator for phosphate).

What are the various forms in which calcium is present in plasma? State the concentration of calcium in plasma.

The average concentration of calcium in plasma is 9.4 mg/100 ml, normally varying between 9 and 10 mg/100 ml. This is equivalent to 2.4 mmol/L or 5 mEq/L. It is regulated within very narrow limits.

Calcium is present in plasma in three different forms:

- About 40% calcium is bound to plasma protein (mainly albumin). Calcium-protein complex is a non-diffusible form as the complex cannot pass through the capillary membrane.
- Ten per cent of calcium (0.2 mmol/L) is diffusible and is combined with citrate, phosphate, etc. in plasma and interstitial fluid.
- Fifty per cent of calcium in the plasma is both diffusible and ionized. This ionic calcium does most of the functions of calcium in the body.

What are the various forms of inorganic phosphate in plasma? State the concentration.

Inorganic phosphate in the plasma is in two forms:

$$HPO_4^- \text{ and } H_2PO_4^-$$

$$\text{Concentration of } HPO_4^- = 1.05 \text{ mmol/L}$$

$$\text{Concentration of } H_2PO_4^- = 0.26 \text{ mmol/L}$$

When pH of the blood becomes more acidic, there is a relative increase in quantity of $H_2PO_4^-$ and decrease in that of HPO_4^- whereas alkaline pH has opposite effects. Thus the average total quantity of phosphate is expressed in terms of phosphorus in mg (as it is difficult to measure the quantity of phosphates in the blood chemically). Average phosphorus level is 4 mg/100 ml and varies between 3 to 4 mg/100 ml in adults and 4 to 5 mg/100 ml in children. Change in phosphate level does not cause any immediate effect on the body.

COMPOSITION AND FORMATION OF BONE

Name the various substances which form the bone.

Bone is composed of:

1. *Organic matrix.* It contains 90% to 95% collagen fibres. Remainder is a homogenous medium called ground substance. Collagen fibres extend along the lines of tensional force. They give tensile strength to the bone. Ground substance consists of extracellular fluid with proteoglycans, chondroitin sulphate and hyaluronic acid.

2. *Bone salts.* Crystalline salts are deposited in the bone matrix, principally of calcium and phosphate. Major salt is hydroxyapatite $Ca_{10}(PO_4)_6(OH)_2$; others are magnesium, sodium, potassium. Carbonate ions are also present in bone salt.

Collagen fibres give tensile strength and calcium salts give compressional strength to the bone similar to that of concrete.

What is the ratio of calcium to phosphorus in bone?

Ratio of calcium to phosphorus in bone is 1.7:1.

Describe the mechanism of bone calcification.

Osteoblasts first form collagen molecules called collagen monomers and the ground substance (mainly proteoglycans). Then collagen monomers polymerize to collagen fibres forming cartilage like osteoid tissue. Some osteoblasts become entrapped in osteoid tissue and these are called osteocytes.

Within a few days calcium salts begin to precipitate on the surfaces of collagen fibres. At first, minute nidi are formed at intervals along collagen fibres which rapidly multiply and grow in weeks to form the final product, namely hydroxy-apatite (initial calcium salts are not hydroxyapatite but amorphous salts). Osteoid tissue probably secretes a substance which neutralizes the inhibitor that normally prevents hydroxy-apatite crystallization. Due to this, normal affinity of collagen fibres for calcium salts causes their precipitation in osteoid tissue.

What is exchangeable calcium?

About 1% of the total calcium in the body consists of labile bone, i.e. calcium pool is readily exchangeable because of its physiochemical equilibrium with extracellular fluid. Calcium is in the form of calcium phosphate salts and it provides immediate reserve for sudden change in blood calcium preventing excessive rise or fall of levels of calcium in extracellular fluid. In addition to bone, small portion of exchangeable calcium is present in all the tissues; especially cells of liver and GI tract are highly permeable.

What is non-exchangeable calcium?

About 99% of total calcium consists of stable or mature bone. This is not readily exchangeable and therefore is not available for rapid mobilization.

Describe the process of deposition and absorption of bone.

Bone is continually being deposited by osteoblasts and is continually being absorbed by osteoclasts.

Osteoclasts are large phagocytic cells which are multinucleated. They are derived from monocytes or monocyte-like cells formed in the bone marrow. Osteoclasts are normally active on less than 1% of bone surfaces. Bone absorption occurs immediately adjacent to the osteoclasts. Osteoclasts send projections like villi which secrete proteolytic enzymes released from lysosomes of osteoclasts and several acids (citric acid, lactic acid, etc.) released from mitochondria of osteoclasts. The enzymes digest and dissolve organic matrix of the bone and acids cause dissolution of bone salts.

Normally except in growing bones, the rate of bone deposition and absorption are equal, therefore total mass of bone remains normal. Osteoclasts exist in small but concentrated masses. They usually eat away the bone within 3 weeks forming a small tunnel (1 mm diameter) of several millimetres in length. Then osteoclasts disappear and the tunnel is invaded by osteoblasts to continue bone deposition for several months. Bone is laid down in concentric circles known as lamellae on the inner surfaces until the tunnel is filled. New bone formation stops when it begins to encroach on blood vessels supplying the area. Blood vessels are present in haversian canals, therefore are the ones which remain of the original cavity. New area deposited in this way is called osteon.

What is the physiological significance of continuous remodelling of bone?

Continuous remodelling of bone has some physiological functions:

1. Bone adjusts its strength in proportion to degree of bone stress.
2. Even shape of bone can be rearranged for proper support of mechanical forces in accordance with the stress.
3. Old bone becomes relatively weak and brittle. The development of new bone matrix maintains the toughness of bone.

Bone is deposited in proportion to the compressional load that the bone must carry, e.g. bones of athletes become considerably heavier than non-athletes. Continuous physical stress stimulates calcification and osteoblastic deposition of bone and it also determines the shape of the bone. Fracture of bone activates all periosteal and intraosseous osteoblasts involved in break. New osteoblasts are immediately formed causing large bulge of osteoid tissue to be developed where new bone matrix is formed and bone salts get deposited (callus).

How is the rate of bone deposition indicated?

Increased level of alkaline phosphatase in blood indicates high rate of bone deposition because osteoblasts secrete large quantities of alkaline phosphatase and some of it is released into the blood.

PARATHYROID HORMONE

What is parathyroid hormone chemically?

Parathyroid hormone secreted by the parathyroid glands (four small glands located behind the thyroid gland) is a polypeptide containing 84 amino acids. It is first secreted as a larger molecule containing 110 amino acids as preprohormone. Preprohormone is cleaved to form prohormone which is packaged in secretory granules.

ACTIONS

What is the effect of parathyroid hormone on concentrations of calcium and phosphate in extracellular fluid?

Parathyroid hormone (PTH) increases the concentration of calcium in ECF due to increased absorption of calcium from the bones and reduced excretion through the kidneys.

Parathyroid hormone causes decrease in phosphate concentration of ECF because of excessive phosphate excretion through the kidneys (enough to over-ride increased phosphate absorption from bone).

Explain the effect of parathyroid hormone on the bones.

Parathyroid hormone causes increased absorption of calcium and phosphate from bones. This is done in two phases, rapid and slow.

1. *Rapid phase.* Osteocytes are osteoblasts buried in bone matrix. Long filmy processes extend from osteocyte to osteocyte throughout the bone structure. These processes also connect with the surfaces of osteocytes and osteoblasts. This extensive system is called osteocytic membrane system. It provides a membrane that separates bone from ECF. This membrane pumps calcium ions from bone fluid into ECF till calcium ion concentration falls to one-third of that of ECF. When this osteocytic pump is activated and calcium ion concentration of bone fluid falls, calcium phosphate salts are absorbed from the bone. This effect is known as osteolysis and it occurs without absorption of bone matrix. Inactivation of osteocytic pump has reverse effects. Parathyroid hormone activates osteocytic calcium pump.

2. *Slow phase.* Slow calcium release occurs because of long-term effect of PTH on bone. Parathyroid hormone produces this effect by increasing osteoclastic system in two ways:

- It causes immediate activation of osteoclasts which are already formed.
- It stimulates formation of new osteoclasts.

Thus long term effect causes increased osteoclastic resorption of bone.

Explain the action of parathyroid hormone on kidneys.

Parathyroid hormone has the following effects on kidneys:

1. Promotes active reabsorption of calcium in distal portion of nephrons, i.e. ascending limbs of loop of Henle, distal tubules, collecting ducts (and not in proximal tubules).
2. Inhibits phosphate reabsorption in the proximal tubules, i.e. lowers the renal threshold for HPO_4^- and decreases T_{max} for phosphate causing increased excretion of phosphate in urine.
3. Also increases urinary excretion of Na^+, K^+, HCO_3^-. It decreases urinary excretion of $NH4^+$ and H^+ ions.

Explain the effect of parathyroid hormone on the intestine.

Parathyroid hormone greatly enhances both calcium and phosphate absorption from the intestine by increasing 1,25-dihydroxycholecalciferol (from vitamin D).

What is the mechanism of action of parathyroid hormone?

Most of the actions of parathyroid hormone are mediated through cyclic AMP because PTH increases cyclic AMP concentration in the osteoclasts, renal cortex and other target cells.

REGULATION

How is parathyroid hormone secretion regulated?

Parathyroid hormone secretion is regulated by concentration of calcium in the blood. Increase in calcium concentration inhibits the secretion whereas decrease in concentration stimulates the secretion.

VITAMIN D

What is the action of vitamin D on bone formation, on intestine and on kidneys?

The principal active product of vitamin D is 1,25-dihydroxycholecalciferol (calcitriol).

1. *Effect on bones.* Calcitrol with PTH increases the mobilization of calcium and phosphate from the bone. Paradoxically by raising serum calcium and HPO_4^-, it also causes bone deposition. Calcitriol activates calcium-binding protein in the bone. The antirachitic action of calcitriol is due to its indirect effect, i.e. stimulation of intestinal calcium absorption (though the direct effect is bone resorption). Thus calcitriol acts synergistically with PTH to cause bone dissolution.

2. *Effect on intestine.* Calcitriol increases absorption of calcium by intestine by the induction of calcium-binding protein. It also causes increase in phosphate absorption by intestine.

3. *Effect on renal tissue.* Calcitriol promotes calcium reabsorption in distal tubules of the kidneys. It promotes phosphate reabsorption but in pharmacologic doses it does have phosphaturic (increased phosphate excretion) effect.

CALCITONIN

What is calcitonin? What is its effect on serum calcium level?

Calcitonin is a large polypeptide (32 amino acids) synthesized by parafollicular cells present between the thyroid follicles. It decreases serum calcium level (effect opposite to PTH).

Describe the mechanism by which calcitonin reduces blood calcium level.

Calcitonin decreases the absorptive activity of osteoclasts. It also inhibits osteo-lytic effect, thus shifting the balance in favour of bone deposition. This effect is significant in young animals because of rapid interchange of absorbed and depos-ited calcium.

Long term effect of calcitonin is to reduce formation of new osteoclasts. Since osteoclasts resorption of bones leads to secondary osteoblastic activity, decrease in number of osteoclasts as the influence of calcitonin also reduces osteoblastic ac-tivity. This means that over a long period calcitonin decreases both osteoclastic and osteoblastic activities. Therefore, effect on blood calcium concentration is transient. Calcitonin thus has very weak effect on plasma concentration of cal-cium in human adults.

What is the effect of changes of serum calcium level on calcitonin secretion?

Increase in serum calcium level stimulates secretion of calcitonin which provides sec-ond feedback mechanism for regulating serum calcium concentration which works exactly opposite to that of PTH. But it is different from PTH feedback in two ways:

- Operates very rapidly reaching peak within less than hour in contrast to 3 to 4 hours required for peak activity of PTH.
- Mainly acts as a short-term regulator.

CONTROL OF CALCIUM ION CONCENTRATION

Name the different mechanisms which control calcium ion concentration.

Mechanisms controlling calcium absorption are:

1. *Buffer function of bone.* Certain amorphous calcium salts (exchangeable calcium) are loosely bound and are in reversible equilibrium with the calcium and phosphate ions of ECF. Total quantity available for exchange is 5 to 10 g (1% of total calcium). Increased concentration of these salts in ECF causes immediate deposition of them in bone and vice versa. This provides buffer system to main-tain calcium and phosphate levels of ECF.

2. *Action of PTH.*
3. *Action of calcitonin.*

TETANY

What is tetany? When does it occur?

When extracellular fluid calcium concentration decreases, nervous system becomes highly excitable and peripheral nerve fibres begin to discharge spontaneously causing passage of impulses to skeletal muscle and elicit tetanic contractions of the muscles. This condition is known as tetany. Tetany occurs when plasma calcium level falls to approximately 6 mg/100 ml and it is lethal when the level falls to 4 mg/100 ml.

What are the other effects of hypocalcaemia?
1. Marked dilatation of heart.
2. Changes in cellular enzyme activity.
3. Increased cell membrane permeability in other cells in addition to nerve cells.
4. Impaired blood clotting.

What is carpopedal spasm in tetany?
In tetany, the peculiar position of the hand which develops is called carpopedal spasm. The elbow and the wrist are flexed; fingers are flexed at metacarpophalangeal joints but extended at interphalangeal joints. Thumb is in the palm and fingertips are drawn together. This is also called Trousseau's sign.

What are the other signs of tetany?
1. Laryngeal stridulus. Spasm of the glottis with inspiratory stridor.
2. Chvostek's sign. Tapping the facial nerve near the styloid process precipitates to cause facial spasm.
3. General convulsions in children.

What are the causes of hypocalcaemia and tetany?
Tetany is produced by hypocalcaemia occurring due to:

1. *Alkalosis.* It is due to different causes such as increased breathing, profuse vomiting, etc. Alkalosis disturbs the ionic balance and decreases amount of ionic calcium without much affecting the total calcium.
2. *Rickets.* Due to vitamin D deficiency calcium absorption is lowered.
3. *Renal failure.* Reabsorption of calcium in renal tubules is decreased.
4. *Hypoparathyroidism.* Decreased secretion of parathyroid hormone.
5. *Impaired absorption of calcium from the intestine.*

HYPERCALCAEMIA

What is hypercalcaemia? What are its effects?
Increased level of calcium in body fluids is called hypercalcaemia. Effects appear when blood level rises above 12 mg/100 ml.

EFFECTS OF HYPERCALCAEMIA
1. Nervous system is depressed.
2. Reflex activities of CNS become sluggish.

3. There is decreased 'QT' interval in ECG.
4. Constipation and loss of appetite due to decreased motility of intestine.
5. When calcium level rises above 17 mg/l00 ml, calcium phosphate is likely to precipitate throughout the body such as in alveoli of lungs, renal tubules, thyroid gland, acid producing stomach mucosa, walls of arteries.

HYPO- AND HYPERPARATHYROIDISM

What is hypoparathyroidism?

Insufficient secretion of PTH causes hypoparathyroidism.

What are the effects of hypoparathyroidism? How is it treated?

EFFECTS OF HYPOPARATHYROIDISM

1. Decreased osteocytic reabsorption of exchangeable calcium.
2. Osteoclasts become almost totally inactive.
3. Level of calcium in body fluid decreases because of decreased calcium reabsorption from the bones. Bones usually remain strong because calcium and phosphate are not absorbed from them.

For treating hypoparathyroidism, PTH is rarely used because it is expensive and its effect lasts only for a few hours. In most of the patients it is treated with high dose of vitamin D and calcium.

What is hyperparathyroidism? What are its effects?

Increased secretion of parathyroid hormone causes hyperparathyroidism. It is due to tumour in one of the parathyroid glands. Effects of hyperparathyroidism are:

1. There is increased osteoclastic activity. In the bones, this in turn increases the osteoblastic activity but is not sufficient to make up for increased bone resorption. This leads to extensive decalcification of bones leading to bone fracture.
2. There is increased level of alkaline phosphatase due to secondarily increased osteoblastic activity. This is the important diagnostic test in hyperparathyroidism.
3. There is increased blood calcium level up to 12 to 15 mg/100 ml or sometimes even higher. When calcium level of blood is above 17 mg/100 ml, it causes metastatic deposition of calcium in various tissues. When calcium level is high, phosphate concentration of blood also becomes high because of inability of kidneys to excrete excess phosphate absorbed from the bone.
4. Elevated blood calcium level tends to precipitate crystals of calcium phosphate or calcium oxalate in kidneys leading to formation of renal stones.

RICKETS

What is rickets?

Rickets is a disease occurring in children as a result of calcium and phosphate deficiency. It results due to lack of vitamin D. Ordinarily in rickets plasma concentration of calcium is slightly depressed but that of phosphate is greatly depressed.

What are the effects of rickets?

During prolonged rickets, there is compensatory increase in PTH secretion, causing increased osteoclastic activity and absorption of bone. Bone becomes weaker progressively and marked physical stress increases osteoblastic activity leading to formation of new osteoid tissue which does not become calcified because of lack of calcium. Thus uncalcified weak osteoid tissue gradually takes the place of bone.

In early stages of rickets, tetany is not produced because excess secretion of PTH maintains calcium level. But in later stages, when bone calcium is reduced then blood calcium concentration may fall below 7 mg/100 ml and tetany may result.

Treatment is to supply vitamin D and adequate calcium and phosphate.

What is renal rickets?

Osteomalacia or rickets caused due to prolonged kidney damage is called 'renal rickets'. It is mainly caused because damaged kidney fails to form 1,25-dihydroxycholecalciferol (active form of vitamin D).

OSTEOMALACIA

What is osteomalacia?

Osteomalacia is adult rickets produced due to dietary deficiency of vitamin D and calcium.

OSTEOPOROSIS

What is osteoporosis?

Osteoporosis is a disease seen in old age. It is different from osteomalacia or rickets because it results due to diminished organic bone matrix rather than abnormal bone calcification. Diseases causing increased protein catabolism or deficiency of protein metabolism cause osteoporosis.

CHAPTER 10
Reproduction

MALE REPRODUCTIVE SYSTEM

MALE SEX ORGANS

Describe the anatomy of male sex organs.

Testes are normally situated in the scrotum, where they are maintained at 2°C lower temperature than the normal body temperature. Each testis is surrounded by a fibrous connective tissue called tunica albuginea which in turn is surrounded by a serous membrane called tunica vaginalis. By puberty the testes have developed sufficiently to perform the function (between 12 and 14 years).

Testis, an ovoid gland, consists of about 900 coiled tubules known as seminiferous tubules; each is about 1 m in length. Basic tubular components are the germinal cells and the non-germinal (Sertoli) cells. Sperms are formed in these tubules and then empty into epididymis which is also a coiled tube of about 6 m in length. Epididymis leads into vas deferens which enlarges into ampulla of vas deferens immediately before the vas enters the body of the prostate gland. Seminal vesicle, one located on each side of the prostate gland empties into the prostatic end of ampulla and contents from both ampulla and seminal vesicles pass into an ejaculatory duct leading through the body of the prostate gland to empty into an internal urethra. Prostatic ducts from the prostate gland in turn empty into the ejaculatory duct. Finally urethra is a final connecting link from testis to the exterior. Urethra is supplied with mucus secreted by large number of minute urethral glands located along its entire extent and from bulbourethral glands (Cowper's glands) located near the region of urethra.

SPERMATOGENESIS

What is spermatogenesis?

The process of formation of sperms is known as spermatogenesis.

Describe the process of spermatogenesis.

Germinal epithelial cells of the seminiferous tubules are known as spermatogonia. They are located in two or three layers along the border of the tubular epithelium. They form the sperms through different stages (Fig. 10.1).

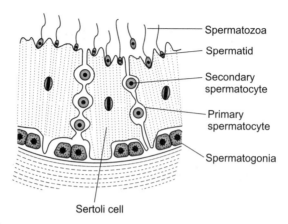

FIGURE 10.1 Cross section of a seminiferous tubule.

STAGES OF SPERMATOGENESIS

1. Primordial spermatogonia located immediately adjacent to the basement membrane of the germinal epithelium are called type A spermatogonia. They divide four times to form slightly different cells called type B spermatogonia, and migrate centrally. Sertoli cells extend through the entire thickness of germinal epithelium from basement membrane to the lumen. They form a barrier to passage of spermatogonia as they are tightly adherent to each other. Yet the spermatogonia penetrate this barrier and become totally enveloped within infolding cytoplasmic processes of Sertoli cells.

This close relationship between spermatogonia and Sertoli cells continues throughout the entire remainder development of spermatogonia.

2. Spermatogonia which cross the Sertoli cell barrier and come into the lumen enlarge to form primary spermatocytes within a period of 24 days. Primary spermatocytes are diploid cells (as DNA of chromosome is replicated).

3. Primary spermatocyte divides to form two secondary spermatocytes. This division is called meiotic division. In this process, each of 46 chromosomes becomes two chromatids that remain bound together at the centromere, the two chromatids having duplicate genes of that chromosome. When primary spermatocyte divides into secondary spermatocyte, each pair of chromosomes separates out so that each secondary spermatocyte contains 23 chromosomes (each chromosome containing two chromatids). This is first meiotic division.

4. Within 2 to 3 days, secondary spermatocyte divides to form 4 spermatids from each secondary spermatocyte. In this division, two chromatids of each of 23 chromosome split apart forming two sets of 23 chromosomes. During division one set passes into one daughter spermatid and another set into another daughter spermatid.

Thus due to two meiotic divisions, each spermatid that is finally formed has only 23 chromosomes having only half the genes of original spermatogonium (i.e. spermatids are haploid cells). Thus eventual spermatozoon that fertilizes ovum provides half of the genetic material to fertilized ovum, other half is provided by the ovum.

5. Within a few weeks, matured spermatozoa are formed from spermatids via metamorphosis. This process called spermiogenesis is characterized by absence of

cell division. Spermatids only mature and are physically reshaped by enveloping Sertoli cells to form spermatozoa (sperms). There are following changes during spermiogenesis:

- Loss of some cytoplasm.
- Reorganization of chromatin material to form a compact head.
- Collecting the remaining cytoplasm and cell membranes at one end of the cell to form a tail.

All the stages of final conversion occur in spermatocytes and spermatids which are actually embedded in the Sertoli cells.

The Sertoli cells control the spermatogenesis process. The entire period of spermatogenesis from germinal cell to sperm takes about 74 days and each spermatogonial cell gives rise to 64 sperm cells.

Enumerate the functions of the Sertoli cells during spermatogenesis.

1. Provide the mechanical support for maturing gametes.
2. Have high glycogen content and hence supply energy during spermatogenesis.

Describe the pair of sex chromosomes present in spermatogonium. How does it divide during the process of spermatogenesis?

In each spermatogonium, one of the 23 pair carries the genetic information that determines the sex of the eventual offspring. This pair is composed of 'X' chromosome or female chromosome and 'Y' chromosome or male chromosome. During meiotic division when chromosomes divide among the secondary spermatocytes, half the sperms contain male chromosome and become male sperms and the remaining half become female sperms containing 'X' chromosome. The sex of offspring is determined by the type of sperm which fertilizes the ovum.

Describe the structure of the sperm.

Spermatids first formed have the usual characteristics of epithelioid cells. Soon, each spermatid elongates into a spermatozoon having head and tail (Fig. 10.2). The head is composed of condensed nucleus within very thin cytoplasmic cell membrane layers around it. On the outside portion of two-third of head there is a thick cap called acrosome formed mainly from Golgi apparatus containing a number of enzymes (hyaluronidase, proteolytic enzymes) which play role in allowing sperm to fertilize the ovum.

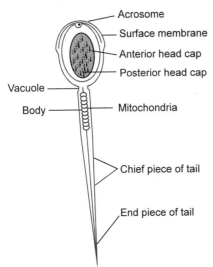

FIGURE 10.2 Structure of the human sperm.

Tail of the sperm is called the flagellum. It has three components:

- Axoneme—Central skeleton constructed of 11 microtubules. This structure is similar to that of cilia.
- Cell membrane covering axoneme.
- Collection of mitochondria surrounding the axoneme in the proximal portion of the tail.

To and fro movement of tail provides motility for the sperm. It results due to rhythmic longitudinal sliding motion between anterior and posterior tubules that make up axoneme. Energy is supplied by ATP synthesized by mitochondria. Normal sperm moves in a straight line at a velocity of 1 to 4 mm/min.

Describe the hormonal regulation of spermatogenesis.

1. Testosterone. It is secreted by interstitial cells of Leydig of testis. It is essential for growth and division of germinal cells in forming sperm.
2. Luteinizing hormone (LH). It stimulates cells of Leydig to secrete testosterone.
3. Follicle stimulating hormone (FSH). It stimulates cells of Sertoli helping in conversion of spermatids to sperms.
4. Oestrogen. Formed from testosterone by the Sertoli cells (when stimulated by FSH) and is essential for spermatogenesis.
5. Growth hormone and most of the other hormones are necessary for controlling background metabolic functions of testis. Growth hormone promotes early division of spermatogonia. In its absence the spermatogenesis is severely deficient.

If spermatogenesis proceeds rapidly, cells of Sertoli release hormone inhibin (glycoprotein) which has a strong effect on inhibiting the secretion of FSH and also a slight effect on hypothalamus to inhibit secretion of GnRH.

What is maturation of the sperm? Where does it occur?

Sperms require several days to pass through epididymis. In the early portion of epididymis, sperms are completely non-motile and cannot fertilize the ovum. Within 18 to 24 hours after the entry into epididymis, they develop the motility, even though several inhibitory proteins in the epididymal fluid still prevent actual motility until after the ejaculation. The sperms also become capable of fertilizing the ovum. This process is called maturation. Sertoli cells and the epithelium of the epididymis secrete special nutrient fluid, enzymes, which are essential for sperm maturation.

How are the sperms stored?

About 120 million sperms are formed each day. A small quantity of them is stored in the epididymis but most of them are stored in vas deferens and ampulla of vas deferens. They can remain stored maintaining their fertility for about a month.

Enumerate the factors affecting motility of sperms.

Motile and fertile sperms show flagellated movement through fluid media at a rate of 1 to 4 mm/min and they tend to travel in a straight line.

The factors affecting motility are:

- Activity is greatly enhanced in neutral and alkaline medium, but is greatly depressed in even mildly acidic medium. Strong acids cause rapid death of sperms.
- Activity of sperms increases with increasing temperature but the life span of the sperms is shortened.
- Life of sperms in female genital tract is only 1 to 2 days.

SEMINAL VESICLES AND PROSTATE

Enumerate the functions of seminal vesicles.

1. Secrete a mucoid material containing fructose and other nutrients which supply nutrition for ejaculated sperms until one of them fertilizes the ovum.
2. Secrete prostaglandins which aid fertilization by making cervical mucus more receptive to sperm and by causing reverse peristaltic contractions in uterus and fallopian tubes to move the sperms towards the ovaries.
3. Secretion of seminal vesicles also adds greatly to bulk of the ejaculated semen.

What are the functions of prostate gland?

Prostate gland secretes thin milky alkaline fluid. This fluid adds to the bulk of semen during emission due to contraction of prostatic capsule.

Alkaline characteristics of fluid help in keeping the sperm motile for successful fertilization. It also helps in neutralizing acidic fluid present in vas deferens and vagina.

SEMEN

What is the composition of semen?

Semen consists of fluid and sperms ejaculated from vas deferens (10%), fluid from seminal vesicle (60%) and fluid from prostate gland (30%). In addition, small amount of mucus is present which is secreted by bulbourethral glands. pH of semen is 7.5; appearance is milky (due to addition of prostatic fluid) and consistency is mucoid. Clotting enzyme present in prostatic fluid causes fibrinogen from seminal vesicle fluid to form weak coagulum which holds semen in deeper regions of vagina for 15 to 30 minutes (after this it is lysed by fibrinolysin formed from prostatic profibrinolysin). In ejaculated semen maximum life span of sperm is 24 to 48 hours at body temperature. When spermatozoa are first expelled in semen they are not active and are not able to fertilize the ovum because they are still held in check by multiple inhibitory factors secreted by genital duct epithelia. When they come in contact with female genital tract they are activated.

What is the normal sperm count?

Normal sperm count is about 120 millions/ml of semen. In addition to number of sperms, sperm morphology and motility is also important for fertility.

CAPACITATION

What is the capacitation of spermatozoa?

Multiple changes taking place to activate spermatozoa (sperms), when they enter female genital tract, are collectively known as capacitation of the spermatozoa. It takes 1 to 10 hours for changes to occur; these are:

1. There is washing away of different inhibitory factors suppressing sperm activity by uterine and fallopian tube fluids.
2. Sperms swim away from cholesterol vesicles covering sperm acrosome. They pass upward into uterine fluid. Because of loss of cholesterol membrane of the head becomes weaker and release of enzymes from it becomes easy.
3. Membrane of the sperm also becomes more permeable to calcium ions. Entry of calcium makes the sperm active. Powerful activity of flagellum gives it powerful whiplash motion. Entry of calcium also allows release of enzymes from acrosome as sperm penetrates the granulosa cell mass surrounding the ovum and also when it penetrates zona pellucida of the ovum itself.

FERTILIZATION OF OVUM

Explain the function of enzymes present in the acrosomes of the sperm.

Acrosomes of the sperms contain large quantities of hyaluronidase and proteolytic enzymes. Hyaluronidase depolymerizes the hyaluronic acid polymers in the intercellular cement that holds granulosa cells together. Proteolytic enzymes digest structural elements of the tissues. Thus acrosome enzymes help in causing penetration of sperm through granulosa and zona pellucida of ovum to cause fertilization. On reaching zona pellucida the anterior membrane of the sperm binds with a receptor protein in zona pellucida. Entire anterior membrane of acrosome dissolves releasing acrosomal enzymes which open penetrating pathway for passage of sperm head through zona pellucida. Within 30 min the membrane of head of the sperm and oocyte fuse. Sperm's genetic material enters the oocyte to cause fertilization.

Why does only one sperm enter the oocyte?

First of all only a few sperms get as far as zona pellucida. Within a few minutes after the first sperm penetrates zona pellucida, calcium ions diffuse into the oocyte membrane and multiple cortical granules are released from oocyte into perivitelline space. Substances present in the granules permeate all portions of zona pellucida, preventing the binding of additional sperms and sperms that have already bound to fall off. After the oocyte membrane fuses with the sperm, there is electrical depolarization which also helps in preventing entry of subsequent sperm.

EFFECT OF TEMPERATURE ON SPERMATOGENESIS

What is the effect of temperature on spermatogenesis?

Increasing the temperature of testes can prevent spermatogenesis by causing degeneration of most cells of seminiferous tubules. Dangling scrotum maintains temperature of testes 2°C below the normal body temperature.

What is cryptorchidism?

Failure of testes to descend from abdomen into the scrotum is known as cryptorchidism. Testes are derived from the genital ridges in abdomen and during late stages of gestation they descend through the inguinal canal into the scrotum. If testes remain in abdominal cavity for a long-time, tubular epithelium degenerate and testes become totally non-functional. Cryptorchidism is due to abnormally formed testes and lack of testosterone secretion from them in most of the cases.

HORMONES OF TESTIS

Which cells secrete testosterone?

Testosterone is secreted by interstitial cells of Leydig of testes. In normal man about 4 to 9 mg of testosterone is secreted daily.

What are the other hormones secreted by testis?

In addition to testosterone, testis also secretes androstenedione which is a precursor of blood oestrogen in man. Dihydrotestosterone is also synthesized in testis probably by action of 5-alpha reductase from Sertoli cells on testosterone secreted by Leydig cells. Only 20% conversion occurs in testes. Remaining conversion of testosterone into dihydrotestosterone occurs in the peripheral tissues. Dihydrotestosterone has more than twice the biologic activity of testosterone.

Androgens (testosterone and dihydrotestosterone) are synthesized from cholesterol or directly from acetyl-CoA in both testes and adrenal cortex.

How is testosterone carried in blood?

Most of the testosterone is bound loosely with plasma albumin and more tightly with a beta globulin called gonadal steroid-binding globulin. At the target tissues it is converted to dihydrotestosterone. Some actions of testosterone are dependent on this conversion.

How is testosterone degraded and excreted?

Testosterone that does not become fixed to the tissues is rapidly converted into androsterone and dihydroepiandrosterone in liver and is immediately conjugated as glucuronides and sulphates. They are excreted through gut (in the bile) or in urine.

Describe the functions of testosterone.

During foetal life testes are stimulated to secrete testosterone in moderate amount by chorionic gonadotropin from placenta, even after ten or more weeks after birth. Thereafter no testosterone is secreted during childhood until up to the age of 10 to 13 years. After this the testosterone secretion increases rapidly and lasts throughout the life. Beyond the age of 50 it starts decreasing and reduces to 20 to 50% of peak at the age of 80.

FUNCTIONS OF TESTOSTERONE

1. In foetal life testosterone is responsible for development of penis, scrotum, prostate gland, epididymis, vas deferens and seminal vesicles. It also suppresses formation of female genital organs. It also stimulates descent of the testes.

2. At puberty, it has following functions:
   - Causes growth of penis, seminal vesicles, scrotum and prostate gland.
   - *Distribution of body hair.* It causes growth of hair over the pubis, upward along the linea alba to the umbilicus or above, on face, chest and less often on the back. So on most of the portions it causes proliferation of hair (except on the top of head—testosterone decreases growth of hair on the top of head and is one of the factors causing baldness).
   - *Effect on larynx.* It causes hypertrophy of laryngeal mucosa and enlargement of the larynx. This results into cracking of voice but it gradually changes into typical adult masculine voice (probably it is due to protein anabolic effect).
   - *Effect on skin.* It increases the thickness of the skin. It also increases the secretion by sebaceous glands. Excess secretion of sebaceous glands on face causes development of acne.
   - *Effect on musculature.* Because of increased protein synthesis, muscles are developed causing increase in muscle mass.
   - *Effect on bones.* It causes bones to increase in thickness and also increases deposition of calcium salts. It increases the quantity of bone matrix due to protein anabolic effect.

     Testosterone has a specific effect on pelvis. It narrows the pelvic outlet, lengthens it making the pelvis funnel shaped. It also greatly increases the strength of the entire pelvis for load bearing.

     However, testosterone causes the epiphyses of long bones to unite with the shafts at an early age in life. Therefore, in spite of rapidity of growth, uniting of epiphyses prevents the person from growing as tall as he would have grown if testosterone had not been secreted at all.
   - *Effect on BMR.* It increases BMR during adolescence by 5 to 10%. Increased BMR is the indirect effect of increased protein anabolism causing increased quantity of enzymes.
   - *Effect on RBCs.* It causes increase in RBC count partly due to increased metabolic rate and partly due to direct effect of testosterone in red cell formation.
   - *Water and electrolytes.* It causes minor increase in salt and water retention by kidneys.

In adults, testosterone stimulates spermatogenesis and also stimulates prostatic secretion.

What is the mechanism of action of testosterone?

Testosterone increases rate of protein formation in the target cells. After entering the target cell, testosterone is converted to dihydrotestosterone which binds with cytoplasmic receptor protein. Hormone protein complex migrates to the nucleus and binds with nuclear protein, where it induces DNA-RNA transcription process. Within 30 minutes RNA concentration begins to increase. There is progressive increase in cellular protein. After several days, quantity of DNA is also increased.

Some target tissues do not possess the enzyme that converts testosterone to dihydrotestosterone. In such tissues testosterone has a direct effect usually with half the potency, e.g. in the male foetus for development of epididymis, vas deferens and seminal vesicles and in adults effect on skeletal muscles, larynx.

How is testosterone secretion controlled?

The cells of arcuate nuclei of hypothalamus secrete gonadotropin releasing hormone (10 amino acids peptide). Endings of these neurons terminate in median eminence of hypothalamus. From here gonadotropin-releasing hormone passes through hypothalamo-hypophysial portal system to anterior pituitary where it stimulates secretion of luteinizing hormone (LH) and follicular stimulating hormone (FSH). Gonadotropin-releasing hormone (GnRH) is secreted intermittently a few minutes at a time once every 1 to 3 hours. GnRH mainly controls LH secretion. LH and FSH are glycoproteins. Both these hormones affect target cells by activating cyclic AMP second messenger system, which in turn activates specific enzyme system in respective target cells.

Luteinizing hormone stimulates interstitial cells of Leydig in testes to secrete testosterone which has a reciprocal effect on pituitary to inhibit LH secretion in two ways:

(a) Greater part of inhibition of LH secretion results from direct effect of testosterone on decreasing GnRH secretion (negative feedback effect).
(b) Testosterone also has a weak negative feedback effect on anterior pituitary to inhibit secretion of LH.

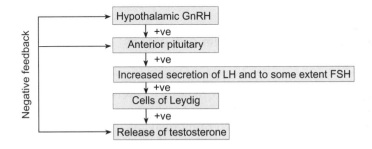

There is also a negative feedback control of seminiferous tubule activity (rate of spermatogenesis) through hormone inhibin on release of FSH and to a certain extent on release of GnRH.

What is the role of human chorionic gonadotropin (HCG)?

Human chorionic gonadotropin is secreted by placenta and has almost the same role as LH. It stimulates the secretion of testosterone by cells of Leydig.

PUBERTY AND MALE CLIMACTERIC

What is puberty? Describe how is onset of puberty regulated?

Gonads of both the sexes are quiescent until they are activated by gonadotropins from pituitary for causing final maturation of the reproductive system. This period of final maturation is known as adolescence or puberty. But puberty actually is a period when endocrine and gametogenic functions of gonads have first developed to the point where reproduction is possible. The age at the time of puberty is variable (9 to 14 years in males). At puberty there is also increase in secretion of adrenal androgens.

Control of onset of puberty. During childhood hypothalamus does not secrete significant quantities of GnRH (probably because slightest secretion of sex steroid hormones exerts strong inhibitory effect on hypothalamus). At puberty because of release of GnRH from hypothalamus there is secretion of gonadotropins from pituitary glands and this process lasts remainder of life. These gonadotropins act on testes to cause secretion of testosterone as well as spermatogenesis. Testosterone causes growth of external genitalia and accessory sex organs. The effects of testosterone are described earlier in detail.

What is male climacteric?

Decrease in male sexual function in old age is termed male climacteric. It is associated with symptoms of hot flushes, suffocation and psychic disorders. It is related to decrease in testosterone secretion.

FEMALE REPRODUCTIVE SYSTEM

FEMALE SEX ORGANS

Describe the anatomy of female sex organs.

Principal organs of female reproductive tract are ovaries, fallopian tubes, uterus and vagina.

During foetal life the outer surface of ovary is covered by a germinal epithelium (derived directly from epithelium of germinal ridges).

During development of foetus, primordial ova differentiate from germinal epithelium and migrate into the substance of ovarian cortex. Each ovum collects around it a layer of granulosa cells.

Ovum surrounded by single layer of granulosa cells is known as primordial follicle. At 30th week of gestation there are about 6 million ova, most of them degenerate and at birth only one million are present in two ovaries and only 300,000 to 400,000 of ova are present at puberty. During reproductive life, at each month a single ovum develops. This ovum is expelled into the abdominal cavity and enters through the fallopian tube in the uterus. During reproductive life (13 to 46 years) about 400 follicles develop enough to expel ova (once each month). The remainder degenerate. At the end of reproductive capability (menopause), a few primordial follicles remain in the ovaries and these also degenerate soon thereafter.

Uterus is hollow, thick walled and muscular, situated between urinary bladder and rectum. Into its upper part, fallopian tubes (one on each side) open. Below, it continues into vagina. A little below the uterine midpoint there is a slight constriction corresponding to narrowing of cavity at internal os. The part above is called the body of the uterus and part below is the cervix. Part of the body above the entry of fallopian tubes is called fundus. Cervix is 2.5 cm in length and it bulges into the anterior vaginal wall. Circular external os connects the cavity of the cervix to vagina. Uterine wall has external serosal (perimetrium), middle muscular (myometrium) and inner mucosal (endometrial) layers. Endometrium is divided into 2 layers:

- *Stratum basalis.* Functions as regenerative layer. Blood supply is through basal arteries (straight arteries).
- *Stratum functionalis.* Superficial layer which is shed during menstruation. Blood supply of this layer is through spiral (coiled) arteries.

Vagina is a fibromuscular tube lined by stratified epithelium. It opens to the exterior as vaginal orifice lying posteroanterior to the urethral orifice.

Female external genital organs include mons pubis, labia majora and minora, clitoris, vestibule, vestibular bulb and the greater vestibular glands. The term vulva includes all these parts.

HORMONES

Enumerate the hormones of female hormonal system.

- Gonadotropin releasing hormone (GnRH) or luteinizing hormone releasing hormone (LHRH) from hypothalamus.
- Follicular stimulating hormone (FSH) from anterior pituitary.
- Luteinizing hormone (LH) from anterior pituitary.
- Oestrogen from ovaries.
- Progesterone from ovaries.

These hormones are secreted at different rates during different parts of female monthly sexual cycle.

MENSTRUAL CYCLE

What is monthly ovarian cycle?

In the female, normal reproductive years are characterized by monthly rhythmic changes in the rates of secretion of the female hormones and corresponding changes in the ovaries. This rhythmic pattern is called ovarian cycle. The duration of cycle varies from 20 to 45 days. But on an average, duration of cycle is 28 days. During each cycle, a single mature ovum is released from ovary.

What is endometrial cycle?

Along with the rhythmic changes that occur in ovaries, rhythmic changes also occur in endometrium of the uterus each month. These rhythmic changes constitute endometrial cycle. Its duration is the same as that of the ovarian cycle (28 days). The rhythmic changes occurring every month in ovaries and sexual organ together constitute the female sexual cycle (or menstrual cycle).

What is menarche?

Menarche refers to the onset of menstruation which normally occurs between the ages of 12 and 14 years. Prior to menarche, minimal amounts of oestrogen are produced (by peripheral conversion of androgens).

Describe the ovarian cycle.

The ovarian cycle has following three phases:

- Preovulatory phase.
- Ovulation.
- Postovulatory phase (luteal phase).

Ovarian changes occurring during the sexual cycle completely depend on the go-nadotropic hormones, FSH and LH secreted by anterior pituitary gland (Fig. 10.3). Both FSH and LH stimulate ovarian target cells by combining with highly specific FSH and LH receptors present in their membranes. FSH and LH activate cyclic adenosine monophosphate cAMP second messenger system in the cell cytoplasm. However, some effects of the hormones cannot be attributed entirely to cAMP system.

1. *Preovulatory phase.* This phase generally lasts for 8 to 9 days but may vary from 10 to 25 days. During this phase, there is a growth of the primordial follicle of the ovary. At first, there is moderate enlargement of the ovum itself and then there is growth of additional layers of granulosa cells after which follicle is called primary follicle. Primary follicle begins as an oocyte (ovum) surrounded by a single layer of granulosa cells. Growth is accelerated in 6 to 12 such follicles each month but full maturation of only one follicle occurs.

Growth of the follicles occurs due to secretion of FSH and LH from anterior pituitary. In the beginning, mainly FSH secretion increases which causes proliferation of granulosa cells of the follicle. In addition to granulosa cells, many spindle-shaped cells develop from ovarian interstitium collected outside

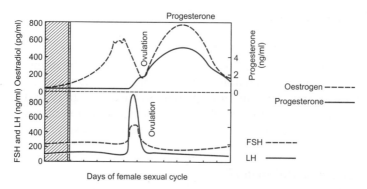

FIGURE 10.3 Plasma concentration of gonadotropins and ovarian hormones during normal female sexual cycle.

the granulosa cells. These cells are called theca cells which lie in two sublayers: (a) theca interna and (b) theca externa. Theca cells are separated from granulosa cells by basal lamina called lamina propria.

After early proliferation, granulosa cells secrete a follicular fluid. This causes cavity to be formed in the granulosa, which is called antrum. Once it is formed, granulosa and theca cells proliferate even more rapidly. Up to this stage, follicular growth is mainly stimulated by FSH alone.

Accelerated growth of antral follicle leads to much larger follicles called vesicular or Graafian follicles to develop. Growth is accelerated due to:

- Oestrogen secreted by granulosa cells into the antral fluid. The oestrogen causes granulosa cells to form increasing number of FSH receptors leading to a positive feedback effect because it makes granulosa cells more sensitive to FSH.
- FSH and oestrogen also promote LH receptors on the original granulosa cells. LH starts acting on the follicles.
- Increasing oestrogen and LH (from pituitary) act together to cause proliferation of theca cells as well as increase of the secretion from theca cells. Increase in their secretion causes further growth.

After a week one of the follicles begins to outgrow all others which begin to involute (atresia). The single outgrowing follicle reaches a size of 1 to 1.5 cm at the end of the preovulatory phase.

During preovulatory phase, dominant gonadotropic hormone is FSH and the dominant steroid is oestrogen.

2. *Ovulation.* Just prior to ovulation, the primary oocyte present in the growing follicle completes first meiotic division and forms secondary oocyte with a haploid nucleus and the first polar body. Release of this secondary oocyte from the follicle into the abdominal cavity is called ovulation which usually occurs 14 days after the onset of menstruation (in a normal 28-day cycle).

Shortly before ovulation, outer wall of the follicle swells and protrudes forming a stigma which protrudes like a nipple. Within half an hour, fluid begins to ooze from stigma. About two minutes later, the stigma ruptures widely allowing expulsion of viscous fluid along with ovum surrounded by several granulosa cells (corona radiata). For final follicular growth and ovulation, hormone LH is essential. FSH and LH synergistically cause rapid swelling of follicle several days before ovulation. LH converts granulosa and theca cells to more progesterone secreting cells and less oestrogen secreting cells. Therefore, before ovulation, secretion of oestrogen begins to fall and progesterone begins to be secreted. Two days prior to ovulation secretion of LH increases six to tenfold (LH surge). FSH secretion also increases two to threefold. Both these cause the following changes:

- Theca externa cells begin to release proteolytic enzymes from lysosomes. They cause dissolution of capsular wall and its weakening results in further swelling of the entire follicle and degeneration of stigma.
- There is rapid growth of new blood vessels into the follicle wall and prostaglandins are secreted in the follicular tissue. Both these cause diffusion of plasma into the follicular fluid and further swelling of the follicle. Simultaneous degeneration of stigma causes follicle to rupture with discharge of the ovum.

3. *Postovulatory phase.* After the expulsion of ovum, granulosa cells of the follicle rapidly change to lutein cells. They enlarge in diameter and become filled with lipid inclusions which give them a yellowish appearance. This process is called luteinization and the total mass of cells is called corpus luteum. Lutein cells form large amounts of progesterone and also oestrogen to a lesser extent. Seven days after ovulation, corpus luteum grows to about 1.5 cm in diameter. If there is no fertilization, it begins to involute and approximately 12 days after ovulation, it is converted to corpus albicans which is replaced by connective tissue during next few weeks. LH is responsible for luteinization of theca cells. Progesterone secreted by these cells has a strong negative feedback effect on the anterior pituitary gland to decrease secretion of both LH and FSH. Lutein cells also secrete hormone inhibin which inhibits secretion of especially FSH. LH and FSH blood levels begin to fall to low concentration. This makes corpus luteum to degenerate completely (on 12th day after ovulation). Therefore, on 26th day of the normal female sexual cycle, levels of oestrogen, progesterone and inhibin fall. This removes feedback inhibition of the anterior pituitary. FSH and within a few days LH secretion begins to initiate new ovarian cycle.

Describe the endometrial cycle.

Associated with cyclic changes in production of oestrogen and progesterone (during ovarian cycle) by the ovaries is an endometrial cycle which operates through the following stages:

- Proliferative phase (preovulatory or oestrogen phase).
- Secretory phase (secretory or postovulatory or progestational phase).
- Menstrual phase.

1. *Proliferative phase.* At the beginning of each monthly cycle most of endometrium is desquamated by the process of menstruation. After menstruation, only thin layer of endometrium remains at the base of original endometrium. During proliferative phase, oestrogens are secreted in large quantities in the preovulatory phase from ovaries.

Following changes takes place in the endometrium:

- Oestrogens stimulate mitosis of stratum basalis which causes regeneration of stratum functionalis. The endometrial surface is re-epithelialised within 4 to 7 days after menstruation. Until ovulation the thickness of endometrium is greatly increased (up to 3 to 4 mm thickness). Endometrial glands in cervical region secrete thin mucus in large volume. This mucus lines the cervical canal which helps to guide the sperm in the proper direction into the uterus.
- Oestrogens stimulate angiogenesis in stratum functionalis. The blood vessels become the spiral arteries that perfuse stratum functionalis.
- Oestrogens also cause growth of the endometrial glands. The glands contain glycogen but they are non-secretory. This phase lasts for about 14 days.

2. *Secretory phase.* During later half of the cycle, both progesterone and oestrogen are secreted in large quantities by corpus luteum. Oestrogen causes slight additional cellular proliferation whereas progesterone causes the following changes:

- Progesterone promotes differentiation of the endometrium causing elongation and coiling of mucous glands. These glands become secretory and secrete thick viscous fluid containing glycogen.

- The blood supply of endometrium further increases as progesterone promotes spiraling of blood vessels.

At the end of secretory phase, the thickness of endometrium increases to 5 to 6 mm. Thus the endometrium with large amounts of nutrients provides appropriate condition for implantation of ovum.

3. *Menstruation*. If fertilization does not occur, two days before the monthly cycle, levels of ovarian hormones—oestrogens and progesterone, decrease sharply and menstruation follows: The various changes are as follows: Twenty-four hours preceding the onset of menstruation, spiral arteries leading to mucosal layer become vasospastic probably by release of vasoconstrictive substances (prostaglandins). Vasospasm and loss of hormonal stimulation cause beginning of necrosis in the endometrium. Necrotic walls of the spiral arteries rupture resulting in haemorrhages. Haemorrhagic areas grow over a period of 24 to 36 hours. Necrotic outer layer of endometrium gradually separates from uterus at the site of haemorrhage. The mass of desquamated tissue and blood in the uterine cavity and prostaglandins initiate contractions of uterus. These contractions expel the uterine contents. This phase lasts for 4 to 5 days during which approximately 40 ml of blood and 35 ml of serous fluid is lost. Menstrual fluid is normally non-clotting because a fibrinolysin is released along with the necrotic endometrial material. If excessive bleeding occurs, fibrinolysin is not sufficient to prevent clotting. Presence of blood clots therefore indicates excessive bleeding and is a clinical evidence of uterine pathology.

Describe the regulation of the female monthly rhythm.

Basic rhythmic mechanism that causes cyclic variations is as follows:

Hypothalamus secretes gonadotropin releasing hormone (GnRH) and luteinizing hormone releasing hormone (LHRH). GnRH is released from arcuate nuclei and preoptic area of hypothalamus. This in turn stimulates secretion of LH and FSH from anterior pituitary. Oestrogen and progesterone levels when increase cause feedback inhibition on secretion of LH and FSH from anterior pituitary and also GnRH secretion from hypothalamus. Hormone inhibin secreted by corpus luteum inhibits secretion of FSH and to a lesser extent secretion of LH also.

Two days before menstruation, corpus luteum involutes and this results into decreased secretion of oestrogens, progesterone and inhibin. This stimulates secretion of FSH from anterior pituitary, also LH secretion a little later and to a lesser extent. These hormones cause growth of the follicle and release of greater and greater quantities of oestrogens from it. Oestrogen level reaches at peak on 13th day or so. For reasons not completely understood, anterior pituitary secretes greatly increased amounts of LH 1 to 2 days prior to ovulation (LH surge). This is probably due to positive feedback effect of rising oestrogen level on the gonadotropins especially LH. Due to LH, there is luteinization of granulosa cells which start secreting small quantity of progesterone which also possibly increase LH secretion from anterior pituitary. Without preovulatory LH surge, no ovulation can occur.

After ovulation, corpus luteum begins to secrete increasing quantities of progesterone, oestrogen and inhibin. These three hormones combined together, have negative feedback on anterior pituitary gland to suppress both secretion of FSH and LH. Their levels are decreased to a low value, 3 to 4 days prior to

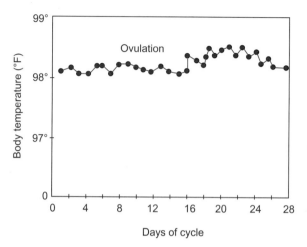

FIGURE 10.4 Body temperature recorded during menstrual cycle.

menstruation. This causes involution of corpus luteum and lowering of levels of oestrogens, progesterone and inhibin which cause shedding of endometrium (menstruation) (Fig. 10.3).

Secretion of progesterone during later half of cycle raises the body temperature by about 0.5°F, the temperature rise coming abruptly at the time of ovulation (Fig. 10.4).

What are unovulatory cycles?

The female sexual cycles during which ovulation does not occur are called unovulatory cycles. If LH surge occurring prior to ovulation is not of sufficient magnitude, ovulation does not occur. First few cycles after puberty may be unovulatory.

What are the changes that occur at puberty in females?

As in the cases of males, in females also because of release of GnRH from hypothalamus at puberty, pituitary gonadotropins are secreted. These gonadotropins in turn stimulate ovary to secrete oestrogen and progesterone.

The following changes occur at puberty:

1. *Thelarche.* It is the development of breast and is the first event.
2. *Pubarche.* It is the development of axillary and pubic hair and it follows thelarche.
3. *Menarche.* It is the first menstrual period and it follows pubarche. The initial periods are usually unovulatory. Regular ovulation appears about a year later.

The age at the time of puberty in females is 8 to 13 years.

In addition to above changes at puberty, there is development of typical female distribution of hair (over pubis and in axilla). There is also a sudden spurt of somatic growth for a short time. There is fat deposition leading to feminine shape. Pelvic girdle becomes roomy and bigger than pectoral. Thus there is development of sex and accessary sex organs and secondary sexual characteristics (for detail, see effects of oestrogen).

What is menopause?

The period during which the female sexual cycles cease and the female sex hormones diminish rapidly to almost none at all is termed menopause. It occurs between 40 and 50 years.

Which is the fertile period of female sexual cycle?

Ovum remains viable and is capable of being fertilized for a period of 24 hours after it has been expelled from the ovary. The sperms can remain fertile in the female reproductive tract for 72 hours. So, one day prior to ovulation to one day after the ovulation is the fertile period.

What is the rhythm method of contraception?

Avoiding intercourse near the time of ovulation is used as a method of contraception. The difficulty with this method is the impossibility of predicting exact time of ovulation. The interval from ovulation to the next succeeding onset of menstruation is 13 to 15 days. So, one can calculate ovulation time according to the duration of the cycle. Avoidance of intercourse for four days prior to the calculated day of ovulation and three days afterwards prevents the conception.

Describe the role of hormones in suppression of fertility.

Administration of either oestrogen or progesterone in appropriate quantity during first half of monthly female cycle can prevent preovulatory LH surge and thus also prevents ovulation (as LH surge is essential for ovulation). Pills containing combination of synthetic oestrogen and synthetic progesterone are available. The medication is usually begun in the early stages of monthly cycle and continued beyond the time that ovulation normally would have occurred. Then the medication is stopped allowing menstruation to occur and a new cycle to begin. This method of suppression of fertility is almost 100% successful.

OVARIAN HORMONES

Name the ovarian hormones.

- Oestrogen.
- Progestins (most important progesterone).

Name the important oestrogens and progestins.

There are three main oestrogens:

- Beta oestradiol.
- Oestrone.
- Oestriol.

Important progestin is progesterone. Small amount of other progestin, 17-alpha hydroxyprogesterone is also present.

Describe the synthesis of oestrogen and progesterone.

Oestrogen and progesterone are synthesized from cholesterol derived from blood and to slight extent from acetyl CoA. During synthesis, progesterone and male sex hormone testosterone are synthesized first and during follicular phase of ovarian cycle, all testosterone and much of progesterone is converted to oestrogen by the granulosa cells. During luteal phase, larger amount of progesterone is formed and secreted.

How are oestrogen and progesterone transported in blood?

Oestrogen and progesterone are transported in the blood, bound mainly with plasma albumin, specific oestrogen-binding and progesterone-binding globulins.

What is the fate of oestrogen?

Large quantities of both oestradiol and oestrone are hydroxylated (in liver) to form oestriol and then are conjugated with glucuronic acid and sulphates in liver. About one-fifth of the conjugated products are excreted in bile and remaining are excreted in urine.

What is the fate of progesterone?

Progesterone is degraded to other steroids within a few minutes after secretion. Degradation mainly occurs in liver. Major important end product of degradation is pregnanediol.

Describe the actions of oestrogen.

1. *Effect on uterus and external sex organs.* During childhood only small quantity of oestrogens are secreted but at puberty under the effect of gonadotropic hormones of anterior pituitary secretion of oestrogens increases up to twentyfold. At the same time sex organs start developing to that of adulthood. Oestrogens have protein anabolic effects. They therefore cause growth of fallopian tubes, uterus, vagina and external genitalia, all of which increase in size. Uterus increases two to threefolds. There is increase in amount of contractile proteins in myometrium and increase in spontaneous muscular contractions. Oestrogens also sensitize myometrium to the action of oxytocin which promotes uterine contractility.

Oestrogens stimulate regeneration of stratum functionalis of endometrium during proliferative phase of endometrial cycle. They cause marked proliferation of endometrial stroma and endometrial glands. The water content of and blood flow to the endometrium are increased markedly. Spiral arteries of stratum functionalis are sensitive to oestrogens and they grow very rapidly under their influence. Oestrogens have similar effects on the mucosal lining of fallopian tubes to those on uterine endometrium. There is proliferation of glandular tissue and increase in number of ciliated epithelial cells. Activity of cilia also increases which helps to propel the ovum towards the uterus.

Under the effect of oestrogens, cervix of the uterus secretes thin watery mucus in large amount which is used as an index of endogenous oestrogen secretion.

Oestrogens change the vaginal epithelium from a cuboidal type to a stratified type which is more resistant to trauma and infection. External genitalia enlarge under the effect of oestrogens with deposition of fat in the mons pubis and labia majora. There is also an enlargement of labia minora.

2. *Effect on the breast*. Oestrogens cause:

- Development of stromal tissue of the breast.
- Growth of an extensive duct system.
- Deposition of fat in the breast.

The lobules and alveoli of breast develop mainly due to the action of progesterone and prolactin. Oestrogens act synergistically with progesterone in stimulating growth of these structures.

3. *Effect on skeleton*. Oestrogens like androgens cause an increase in osteoblastic activity, which results in a growth spurt at puberty.

Oestrogens hasten bone maturation and promote the closure of epiphysial plates in the long bones more effectively than does testosterone. Therefore, female skeleton is usually shorter than the male skeleton. Oestrogens are responsible for oval and roundish shape of the female pelvic inlet. To a lesser degree than testosterone, oestrogens also promote deposition of bone matrix by causing Ca^{++} and HPO_4 retention.

4. *Effect on protein deposition*. Oestrogens cause increase in protein content of the body and a slightly positive nitrogen balance due to their effects on sexual organs, bones and other tissues. But the effect of testosterone is much more general and many times powerful.

5. *Effect on metabolism and fat deposition*. Oestrogens produce slight increase in metabolic rate; less as compared to testosterone. They cause increased deposition of subcutaneous fat thereby decreasing overall specific gravity of the body. The deposition of fat in breasts, buttocks and thighs gives rise to the characteristic feminine figure.

6. *Effect on hair distribution*. There is development of hair in the pubic region and in axillae after puberty but androgens from adrenal glands are mainly responsible for these changes.

7. *Effect on the skin*. Oestrogens cause skin to develop a soft texture and to become more vascular.

8. *Effect on electrolyte balance*. Oestrogens cause retention of sodium and water by the kidney tubules. But this effect is usually slight and is rarely of significance except in pregnancy.

9. *Intracellular effects*. Oestrogen causes protein anabolic effect but only on a few specific target organs (uterus, breasts, skeleton) whereas testosterone causes more generalized effect. Circulating oestrogens enter the target cells and combine with receptor protein molecules in the cytoplasm. This combination interacts with specific portions of DNA to initiate the process of transcription. Therefore, within minutes, production of RNA begins (over many hours DNA also may be produced, resulting into division of the cell). RNA diffuses into the cytoplasm and causes increased protein formation, thereby altering the cellular function.

Describe the actions of progesterone.

1. *Effect on uterus*.
   - *Effect on endometrium*. Progesterone stimulates secretory changes in the uterine endometrium. Endometrial glands become elongated and coiled

and secrete a glycogen rich fluid. Thus endometrium is prepared for the implantation of ovum.

- *Effect on myometrium.* Progesterone decreases the frequency and amplitude of myometrial contractions.
- *Effect on cervix.* Under the effect of progesterone, mucus secreted by cervical glands is reduced in volume and becomes thick and viscid. Consistency of cervical mucus provides presumptive evidence that ovulation and luteinization have occurred.
- *Effect on fallopian tubes.* Progesterone promotes secretory changes in the mucosal lining of fallopian tubes. These secretions provide nutrition to fertilized ovum as it passes through the fallopian tube.

2. ***Effect on the breast.*** Progesterone causes development of lobules and alveoli of the breast. Alveolar cells proliferate and become enlarged, thus causing breasts to swell. The alveoli do not secrete milk unless prolactin from anterior pituitary acts on them.

3. ***Effect on electrolyte balance.*** In large quantities progesterone enhances sodium chloride and water absorption from the distal tubules of the kidneys. There is competition between progesterone and aldosterone for receptor sites in the epithelial cells of renal tubules. Blockage of receptor sites for aldosterone by progesterone results into diminished action of the aldosterone. This results into net loss of sodium and water from the body.

PREGNANCY

How does fertilization of ovum occur?

After ejaculation, a few sperms are transported through uterus to the ampulla in the ovarian ends of fallopian tubes within 5 to 10 minutes, aided by contraction of uterus and fallopian tubes stimulated by prostaglandins in the seminal fluid and oxytocin released during female orgasm. Fertilization of ovum usually takes place soon after the ovum enters the ampulla. The fertilized ovum is transported to uterine cavity within 3 to 4 days.

How does fertilized ovum get implanted in the uterus?

While the fertilized ovum is transported through the fallopian tube, several stages of division do occur and the ovum is called blastocyst. Blastocyst with about 100 cells enters the uterine cavity, remains there for 2 to 4 days and then gets implanted. Implantation results from the action of trophoblast cells that develop over the surface of the blastocyst. These cells secrete proteolytic enzymes that digest and liquefy the cells of the endometrium. The fluid and nutrients released are transferred to trophoblast cells for their further growth. Thus blastocyst gets implanted.

How is the placenta developed?

Trophoblastic cords from blastocyst are attached to the endometrium of the uterus. Blood vessels grow into these cords from the vascular system of embryo and blood begins to flow on 16th day of fertilization. Simultaneously, blood sinuses from mother develop around the trophoblastic cords. Trophoblastic cells are arranged in two layers:

- Inner cytotrophoblast.
- Outer syncytiotrophoblast.

Trophoblast cells send more and more projections which become placental villi into which foetal capillaries grow. Thus villi carrying foetal blood get surrounded by maternal sinuses. Under the effect of progesterone secreted by corpus luteum, uterine endometrium is transformed into decidua which is a maternal portion of the placenta. Foetal blood flows through the umbilical arteries to capillaries of villi and then it comes back to foetus through umbilical vein. Mother's blood flows from the uterine arteries into large maternal sinuses surrounding villi and returns into uterine veins of the mother. Total surface area of villi is a few square metres. Within 21 days after fertilization, placenta is fully functional.

Enumerate the hormones secreted by placenta and their physiologic role.

1. *Human chorionic gonadotropin (HCG).* It is a glycoprotein with molecular weight of 39,000. It is secreted by syncytiotrophoblast soon after fertilization. Its peak is reached within 60 to 90 days. It is detectable in maternal blood 8 to 9 days after conception. Its detection in urine forms the basis for immunologic pregnancy test. Level of HCG in maternal blood is also the index of functional status of trophoblast. Biologic actions of HCG are almost same as those of LH.

FUNCTIONS

- Maintains the corpus luteum until placenta becomes autonomous in terms of hormone synthesis (about 6 to 7 weeks after conception).
- Converts corpus luteum of menstruation to corpus luteum of pregnancy thereby extending its life span.
- Stimulates corpus luteum to secrete 17-alpha hydroxyprogesterones.
- Stimulates foetal testes to secrete testosterone prior to foetal pituitary LH secretion.
- Serves as a tropic hormone for foetal adrenal cortex.

2. *Progesterone.* It is mainly synthesized by maternal cholesterol. Eighty five per cent of the progesterone formed is secreted into maternal compartment. Its level steadily rises through the gestation and reaches a maximal plateau at 36 to 40 weeks. Progesterone circulates to foetal adrenal cortex where it is converted to aldosterone and cortisol. Beyond 10 weeks, foetal adrenal cortex no longer depends on placental progesterone for synthesis of its hormone.

FUNCTIONS

- Decreases uterine motility by causing hyperpolarization of uterine myometrium.
- Converts endometrium to decidua.

- Synergistic action of progesterone with oestrogen prepares the breast for lactation.
- Contributes to growth and development of foetus by acting as a precursor for foetal corticoid secretion.
- Promotes renal excretion of sodium. This antagonizes the effect of increased aldosterone level found in pregnancy.

3. *Oestrogens.* Oestrogens are synthesized by placental trophoblasts. Oestriol (major hormone) concentration rises steadily throughout the gestation, reaching a maximal plateau at 36 to 40 weeks (similar to progesterone). Plasma oestriol concentration reflects functional status of the foetoplacental unit. Falling levels indicate impending foetal death.

FUNCTIONS

- Causes growth and development of the maternal reproductive organs. Uterus increases in size and weight, lengthens from 7 to 30 cm.
- Stimulates hepatic synthesis of thyroxine-binding globulin and steroid hormone-binding globulin, angiotensinogen as well as renal renin secretion.
- Stimulates development of ductal system in the mammary gland.
- Just before term, ratio of oestrogens to progesterone increases and the uterus is dominated by oestrogens.

4. *Relaxin.* It is secreted by corpus luteum and placenta. It causes relaxation of pelvic ligaments and ligaments of symphysis pubis.

5. *Human chorionic somatomammotropin.* It is a protein that begins to be secreted from about fifth week of intrauterine life and increases progressively throughout the remainder of the pregnancy. It has weak actions similar to those of growth hormone.

Describe the functions of placenta.

1. Endocrine functions of placenta are as described above.

2. Diffusion of food stuffs from mother's blood to foetal blood—Glucose passes by facilitated diffusion. Fatty acids diffuse slowly because of their lipid solubility. Amino acids, calcium, inorganic phosphates are actively absorbed by the placental membrane. K^+, Na^+, Cl^- ions also diffuse.

3. Diffusion of excretory products from the foetus into the mother's blood especially urea, creatinine, uric acid, etc.

4. Diffusion of oxygen—Mean PO_2 in the mother's blood in maternal sinuses is about 50 mmHg and that in foetal blood to be oxygenated is 30 mmHg. Because of pressure gradient, O_2 diffuses from the mother's blood to foetal blood. Foetal haemoglobin has higher affinity for O_2 than adult haemoglobin. Haemoglobin concentration is also more in the foetus (about 50% greater than that of mother). Foetal blood coming to placenta carries large quantities of CO_2 which is released into maternal blood. pH of foetal blood becomes alkaline, PCO_2 of foetal blood decreases to that below the maternal blood. So O_2 dissociation curve of foetal haemoglobin shifts to left and that of maternal blood shifts to the right. All these factors help the foetus to receive sufficient O_2.

5. Diffusion of CO_2—PCO_2 of foetal blood is 2 to 3 mmHg higher than that of maternal blood (as CO_2 is formed continuously in the foetus and only means by which it is excreted is through placenta). This causes CO_2 diffusion from the foetal blood to maternal blood.

Describe the maternal changes occurring during pregnancy.

Average duration of pregnancy is 40 weeks or 280 days. The following maternal changes occur during pregnancy:

1. *Maintenance of corpus luteum.* After implantation of fertilized ovum, chorionic gonadotropin secretion commences. This helps to maintain corpus luteum (known as corpus luteum of pregnancy) which continues to secrete oestrogen and progesterone. As a result, ovulation and menstruation are prevented.

2. *Changes in uterus.* There is enlargement of uterus. Its weight increases from 50 g to 1000 g at full term. Enlargement is mainly due to hypertrophy of pre-existing muscle but to some extent there is hyperplasia, i.e. formation of new fibres. Muscle fibre increases 2 to 7 times in diameter and about 7 to 11 times in length. There is also increase in amount of connective tissue and elastic tissue of uterus. For first two to three months hypertrophy is due to action of oestrogen but in later months it is due to pressure exerted by growing products of conception. Uterine wall becomes thicker in early months but later on it becomes thinner (5 mm) and therefore foetus can be easily palpated.

3. *Changes in blood.* There is increase in blood volume by 30% due to increase in plasma volume as well as in erythrocytes. But there is greater increase in plasma volume (haemodilution) which leads to physiological anaemia of pregnancy. As it is due to disproportionate changes in plasma volume and cell volume, it is not real anaemia, and red cells are normochromic and normocytic.

Increase in plasma volume is because of increased water absorption and salt absorption by kidneys (due to oestrogen and aldosterone). Red cells increase due to increased erythropoiesis. The bone marrow becomes hyperplastic.

Plasma iron levels fall because there is a great demand for iron during pregnancy. Diet must therefore contain extra iron.

Plasma fibrinogen level rises and as a result ESR increases during pregnancy. Plasma albumin level falls but alpha and beta globulin levels rise. There is decrease in total plasma proteins level.

Increase in total blood volume meets demands of the enlarged uterus and its vastly increased blood supply, increased blood supply to skin (for elimination of extra heat), increased blood flow to kidneys (for elimination of additional waste products from foetus).

4. *Changes in heart.* There is change in position of heart due to enlarging uterus pressing upwards on the diaphragm. Cardiac output increases because of increase in stroke volume and increase in heart rate.

5. *Changes in circulation.* Systolic and diastolic pressure decreases. Femoral venous pressure is raised due to pressure by enlarged uterus on pelvic veins.

Blood flow to uterus is considerably increased.

6. *Changes in respiration.* Due to growing uterus, diaphragm is pushed upwards which tends to reduce vital capacity but it is compensated by increase in width of the chest. There is increase in tidal volume and pulmonary ventilation

due to increase in sensitivity of respiratory centre to CO_2 (probably due to increase in progesterone level).

Oxygen consumption is increased to satisfy needs of foetus, increased demands from uterus, increased cardiac and respiratory work. Increased demands from placenta and breast tissue are also responsible for increasing oxygen consumption.

7. *Changes in alimentary tract.* Stomach motility and acid level decrease. Frequently there is nausea and vomiting in the morning in the first two or three months, the cause of which is not known.

8. *Changes in kidneys.* There is increase in renal blood flow and GFR. Increase in GFR increases tubular load of solutes which may cause glycosuria.

9. *Effects on endocrine glands.*
   - *Placenta.* Placenta secretes hormones already described.
   - *Thyroid.* There is slight enlargement of thyroid gland with hyperplasia. There is increased secretion of thyroxine but because of simultaneous increase in thyroxine-binding protein there are no symptoms of hyperthyroidism.
   - *Adrenal cortex.* There is enlargement of the gland especially zona glomerulosa. This causes increase in secretion of cortisol. As plasma cortisol is bound with transcortin which also increases during pregnancy, there are no symptoms of hypercorticism.

10. *Changes in nervous system.* Craving for unusual articles of diet and alterations in mood are very common effects. In a few, psychosis may develop. The cause of these mental changes is not known.

11. *Changes in skin.* Increased secretion of ACTH or melanophore stimulating hormone causes pigmentation of nipple and areola of breast. Linea alba also becomes pigmented.

12. *Metabolic changes.*
   - *Gain in weight.* There is average increase in weight by 12 kg during 40 weeks period, as follows:
   - Increase in maternal stores — 3 kg
   - Increase in tissue fluid — 1 kg
   - Increase in blood volume — 1 kg
   - Increase in size of uterus and breast — 2 kg
   - Foetus, placenta and amniotic fluid — 5 kg
   - If diet is inadequate there is decreased weight gain.
   - *Water metabolism.* There is increase in sodium and water retention due to steroid hormones. Total water increases by about 3.5 litres (increase in blood volume + increase in tissue fluid + amniotic fluid).
   - *Protein metabolism.* When diet is balanced and adequate there is nitrogen retention with positive nitrogen balance.
   - *Carbohydrate metabolism.* There is tendency of glycosuria as stated above. There is lowering of renal threshold for glucose.
   - *Fat metabolism.* There is increase in blood levels of cholesterol, phospholipids and neutral fat. There is increase in adipose tissue fat which provides a large store of energy for use in later stages of pregnancy and during lactation.
   - *Mineral metabolism.* Calcium content of foetus at term is 25 gram. Iron content is 375 mg.

What is the normal quantity of amniotic fluid?

Volume of amniotic fluid varies from 0.5 to 1.0 litre. Water of amniotic fluid is completely replaced every 3 hours and electrolytes every 15 hours.

What is toxaemia of pregnancy?

If there is rapid rise in arterial pressure associated with large amount of protein in urine during later few months of pregnancy, the condition is known as toxaemia of pregnancy or pre-eclampsia.

PARTURITION

What is parturition? How is it caused?

Process by which baby is born is known as parturition. It is caused by hormonal and mechanical factors.

Hormonal factors increase contractility of uterus.

- Oestrogens increase the degree of contraction, whereas progesterone inhibits the uterine contractility. From 7th month of pregnancy, oestrogen secretion continues to increase while progesterone secretion remains normal. Therefore, ratio of oestrogen to progesterone rises.
- Oxytocin increases contractility of uterus. Rate of oxytocin secretion considerably increases at the time of labour. Effect of stretching of uterine cervix occurs during labour and can cause neurogenic reflex which causes greater secretion of oxytocin from posterior pituitary.
- Foetal hormones (oxytocin and cortisol) also increase contractility of uterus.

Mechanical factors also increase contractility of uterus, e.g. stretch of uterine musculature, stretch and irritation of cervix.

Labour is initiated due to stretching of cervix by foetal head which in turn causes reflex contraction of the body of the uterus. Cervical stretching also causes release of oxytocin from posterior pituitary in greater and greater amounts (due to positive feedback effect).

LACTATION

Describe the effects of hormones on the mammary glands during pregnancy.

During pregnancy various hormones which are secreted prepare the mammary glands for doing the function of lactation as follows:

1. *Development of ductal system.* Large quantities of oestrogens are secreted by the placenta. They act on the breast tissue and cause ductal system of the breast to grow and branch. Stroma of the breast also increases in quantity and large amounts of fats are laid down in the stroma.

Growth of ductal system is also caused by the action of other hormones especially growth hormone, prolactin, adrenal glucocorticoids and insulin.

2. *Development of lobule.* Progesterone acting synergistically with oestrogens and other hormones causes the growth of lobules, budding of alveoli and development of secretory characteristics in the cells of alveoli.

Thus oestrogens and progesterone cause the physical development of the breasts during pregnancy but they inhibit the actual secretion of milk.

How is lactation initiated?

Oestrogens and progesterone actually inhibit the secretion of milk. The hormone prolactin promotes milk secretion. This hormone is secreted by mother's pituitary gland from 5th week of pregnancy. Its level steadily increases so that at the end of pregnancy the level of prolactin is very high. Human chorionic somatomammotropin also has a mild lactogenic effect. But because of high levels of oestrogens and progesterone secretion of milk is suppressed almost throughout the pregnancy. In the last few weeks of pregnancy, only small quantity of fluid called colostrum is secreted. Immediately after the birth of the baby, there is sudden decrease of progesterone and oestrogens secretion which allows lactogenic effect of prolactin and within next 1 to 7 days breasts begin to secrete milk. Secretion of adequate amounts of growth hormone, cortisol and parathyroid hormone is also necessary to provide amino acids, fatty acids, glucose and calcium required for milk formation.

Prolactin secretion is controlled by hypothalamus through two factors:

- Prolactin inhibitory hormone (PIH) which is the dominant hormone under normal conditions.
- Prolactin releasing factor (PRF) which intermittently increases prolactin secretion (under special condition when baby suckles).

Why are ovarian cycles suppressed during lactation?

Prolactin secretion inhibits release of gonadotropin-releasing hormone from the hypothalamus which in turn inhibits pituitary gonadotropin secretion. This results into suppression of ovarian cycle and ovulation during lactation.

How is the milk ejected?

Ejection or let-down of milk occurs due to secretion of hormone oxytocin. When baby suckles, sensory impulses from the nipple are transmitted through somatic nerves to hypothalamus which cause secretion of oxytocin and prolactin. Oxytocin is carried to the breasts via blood. Oxytocin causes myoepithelial cells surrounding the alveoli to contract. This causes milk expression from alveoli into the ducts at a pressure of 10 to 20 mmHg. Suckling of one breast causes milk flow in breasts of both the sides.

CIRCULATORY CHANGES AT BIRTH

Describe the circulatory adjustments at birth.

In foetus because the lungs are non-functional, foetal heart pumps the blood to placenta in large quantities. Blood returns through umbilical veins from placenta to ductus venosus (by passing the liver). Blood collected in right atrium from inferior vena cava passes to left atrium through foramen ovale. Thus oxygenated blood from placenta enters the left atrium and is pumped by left ventricle to head and forelimbs. Blood coming to the right atrium through superior vena cava passes to the right ventricle. From here it is pumped into the pulmonary artery. Through ductus arteriosus the blood passes from pulmonary artery to descending aorta and through two umbilical arteries to placenta (where it is oxygenated).

At birth various changes that occur are:

- There is loss of blood flow to placenta. This doubles the systemic vascular resistance. Thereby increasing aortic pressure and pressure inside the left atrium and ventricle.
- The pulmonary vascular resistance greatly decreases due to expansion of lungs. This reduces pulmonary arterial pressure, pressure in right atrium as well as in right ventricle.
- Low right atrial and high left atrial pressure causes closure of foramen ovale.
- Ductus arteriosus also closes due to increased aortic pressure and decreased pulmonary arterial pressure. Blood begins to flow backward from aorta into pulmonary artery (opposite is the flow during foetal life). After a few minutes muscular wall of ductus constricts and within 1 to 8 days the constriction is sufficient to stop the blood flow (functional closure).
- Closure of ductus venosus.

CONTRACEPTION

What is contraception? What are the methods of contraception?

Preventing conception (pregnancy) is termed contraception. There are various methods of contraception. They are classified as:

1. Temporary methods
2. Permanent methods

1. TEMPORARY METHODS

(a) **Barrier methods**
  (i) Mechanical barriers
    - *Condom:* It is non-porous latex covering placed over the penis during intercourse to prevent entry of sperms in female genital tract.
    - *Diaphragm:* It is dome-shaped structure made up of rubber which fits over the cervix of the uterus. It prevents entry of sperms into the cervix and uterus.
    - *Chemicals:* Creams, jelly, foam, tablets or sponge are placed in vagina of a female.

(b) **Natural contraception**
  (i) *Safe period (rhythm method):* Avoiding intercourse near the time of ovulation is used as a method of contraction. The difficulty with this method is the impossibility of predicting exact time of ovulation. The interval from ovulation of the next succeeding onset of menstruation is 13 to 15 days. So, one can calculate ovulation time according to

the duration of the cycle. Avoidance of intercourse for 4 days prior to the calculated day of ovulation and 3 days afterwards prevents the conception.

(ii) *Coitus interruptus:* Withdrawal of penis shortly before ejaculation.

(iii) *Complete abstinence* from intercourse.

(c) **Intrauterine devices**—These prevent implantation of zygote in uterine mucosa by altering endometrial function. They are copper T 200; multiload Cu-250, Lippe's loop, vaginal ring.

(d) **Hormonal mechanism (pills)**

(i) *Combined pills:* These are oral contraceptive pills containing large amount of progesterone and small amount of oestrogen. Pill is taken at bed time for 21 days starting from 5th day of menstrual cycle and then stopped allowing menstruation. Pills inhibits release of LH surge and therefore prevent ovulation. This method is 100% successful for contraception.

(ii) *Sequential pills:* For first 15 days of cycle large doses of oestrogen followed by combination of oestrogen and progesterone for a week are given. This also prevents ovulation.

(iii) *Postcoital pills:* Pills are given after coitus but before 72 h. These are called morning after pills. They are prepared by hormonal combinations. They prevent implantation of fertilized ovum in uterine wall.

(iv) *Slow releasing subcutaneous implants:* Six capsules containing progesterone are implanted subcutaneously. Hormone is released slowly and is effective for 3 to 5 years. Release of hormone inhibits ovulation.

(e) **Postconception**

(i) *Endometrial aspiration:* It is done by introducing a small plastic catheter into the uterus through cervix. Aspiration of lining of uterus is done by suction. Method is safe and does not require anaesthesia. It is done also before the pregnancy is established.

(ii) Medical termination of pregnancy by using following methods:
- Dilatation and curettage (D and C).
- Vacuum aspiration.
- Introducing intrauterine hypertonic saline solution (20% saline or 40% urea) or prostaglandin (D4F2).
- Pitocin drip with 5% glucose.

2. PERMANENT METHODS

(a) Vasectomy in male.

(b) Tubectomy in females.

CHAPTER 11

Nerve and Muscle

INTRODUCTION AND CLASSIFICATION

How much is the resting membrane potential of the nerve fibre?

Resting membrane potential of the nerve fibre is –90 mV.

Give the classification of nerve fibres.

Nerve fibres are classified in various ways:

1. STRUCTURALLY

- Medullated or myelinated fibres.
- Non-medullated or unmyelinated fibres.

2. DEPENDING ON THEIR ORIGIN

- Cranial fibres, originating from brain.
- Spinal fibres, originating from spinal cord.

3. FUNCTIONALLY

- Afferent fibres, carrying impulses towards the brain.
- Efferent fibres, carrying impulses away from the brain.

4. DEPENDING ON THE NEUROTRANSMITTER THEY SECRETE AT THEIR ENDINGS

- Cholinergic fibres secreting acetylcholine.
- Adrenergic fibres secreting adrenaline.
- Dopaminergic fibres secreting dopamine.

5. GENERAL CLASSIFICATION

The general classification is based on the diameter of the fibres. There are three major types, viz. A, B and C. A and B groups of fibres are myelinated and C group fibres are unmyelinated.

The diameters and velocities of conduction of different types of fibres are given in Table 11.1.

The majority of sensory fibres belong to type C. Though the rate of conduction is low, because of smaller diameters, a large number of type C fibres are

	Diameter (in micron)	Velocity of conduction (m/sec)
Table 11.1	**Diameters and Velocities of Conduction of Different Types of Fibres (Erlanger–Gasser Classification)**	
Type		
• A alpha	12–20	70–120
A beta	6–12	30–70
A gamma	3–6	15–30
A delta	2–5	12–30
• B type	1–2	3–10
• C type	0.3–1.5	0.5–2

accommodated in a small space, thus making it possible for spinal cord to have a small size.

6. SENSORY CLASSIFICATION

Physiologists have classified sensory nerve fibres into following four groups:

(a) *Group I*. These fibres are further classified into Ia and Ib. They correspond to group A alpha of general classification.

Group Ia fibres are 17 micron in diameter. They are annulospiral endings of muscle spindle receptors present in skeletal muscles.

Group Ib fibres are 16 micron in diameter. They supply Golgi tendon organ receptors present in tendons of skeletal muscles.

(b) *Group II*. These fibres are about 8 micron in diameter and correspond to A beta and gamma type of fibres, examples:

    i. Flower spray or secondary endings supplying muscle spindle receptors.
    ii. Hair receptors present in skin.
    iii. Receptors carrying vibration sense.
    iv. Some discrete touch receptors of skin.

(c) *Group III*. These fibres are about 3 micron in diameter and correspond to A delta type of fibres. Some fibres carrying pain, pressure and temperature sensations from skin are of this variety.

(d) *Group IV*. These fibres are less than 2 micron in diameter and belong to C group fibres. These fibres carry touch, pain, temperature, crude touch, itch, etc. from the skin.

STIMULUS

What is stimulus?

Stimulus is defined as any change in the external environment that elicits response from the excitable tissue.

What are the different types of stimuli?

- Thermal
- Mechanical
- Chemical
- Electrical

Which type of stimulus is used in the experimental study? Why?

Usually electrical stimulus is used in different experimental studies because:

- It can be easily quantified, i.e. strength and duration of stimulus can be controlled.
- It causes least damage to the tissues.
- Phenomena of excitation and impulse propagation are themselves electrical in nature.

Which is the type of current used for stimulating the excitable tissue? Why?

Faradic current is used for the purpose of stimulation because it is short lived and hence causes little damage to the tissue. Galvanic current on the other hand is a continuous current which causes damage to the tissue.

INITIATION OF ACTION POTENTIAL

What is action potential?

On application of threshold stimulus abrupt change that occurs in membrane potential of the excitable tissue for 1 ms is termed action potential. Action potential gets self-propagated along the axon.

Name the phases of action potential.

- Depolarization
- Repolarization

How does nerve fibre get depolarized?

Under-resting condition nerve fibre has got resting membrane potential of -90 mV. This is called polarized state. At the site of threshold stimulus the membrane permeability for sodium increases. Sodium ions diffuse from extracellular fluid into the fibre. This increases the voltage at the site. Change in voltage to threshold level initiates positive feedback cycle for opening of more and more number of voltage-gated sodium channels (Fig. 11.1), due to which permeability of membrane for sodium increases to 5000 times as compared to that at resting level. This allows entry of more positive charges into the fibre (in the form of sodium ions) than the number leaving the fibre (in the form of potassium ions).

Diffusion of large number of sodium ions to the interior of the fibre causes development of positivity inside the fibre (reversal potential) and negativity outside the fibre. This is known as depolarization. At this time, potential at the site rises abruptly from −90 mV to +45 mV for a short period of time (Fig. 11.5).

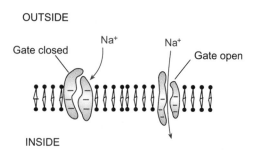

FIGURE 11.1 Na^+ channel.

What is repolarization? How does repolarization occur?

After depolarization, returning of membrane potential of the fibre back to the resting level is known as repolarization. When fibre is depolarized its potential rises from −90 mV to +35 mV. At the same time, sodium channels are closed and potassium channels (Fig. 11.2) open up. So now nerve membrane is more permeable to potassium ions. More number of potassium ions dif-

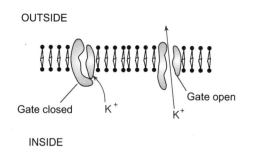

FIGURE 11.2 K^+ channel.

fuses from interior of the fibre to exterior than the number of sodium ions diffusing in. This brings the potential of the fibre back to resting level rapidly (Fig. 11.5).

PROPAGATION OF ACTION POTENTIAL

How is action potential propagated?

PROPAGATION OF ACTION POTENTIAL IN UNMYELINATED NERVE FIBRE

Once generated, action potential does not itself travel along the membrane. Rather each action potential triggers (by creating a local circuit of current) a new action potential at the adjacent areas of the membrane. Local current flow is great enough to depolarize adjacent areas and new action potential occurs here. This new action potential in turn produces local current of its own that depolarizes the regions adjacent to it, producing action potential at the next site. This is the way in which depolarization is propagated. Depolarization remains at any site for the same length of time. Therefore, portion which depolarizes first also repolarizes first. Thus the repolarization is also propagated following the depolarization (Figs 11.3a and b).

PROPAGATION IN MYELINATED NERVE FIBRE

Myelin sheath acts as an insulator and does not allow the current flow. Therefore, local circuit of current flow only occurs from one node of Ranvier to the adjacent node, i.e. the impulse jumps from one node of Ranvier to the next. This is known as saltatory conduction (Fig. 11.3c).

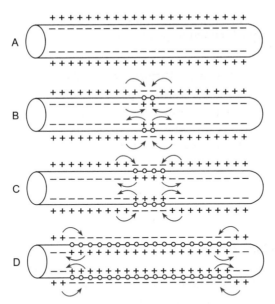

FIGURE 11.3 (a) Propagation of action potential (depolarization) in both directions along conductive fibre.

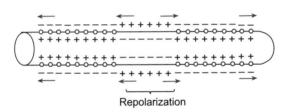

Repolarization

FIGURE 11.3 (b) Propagation of repolarization in both directions along a conductive fibre.

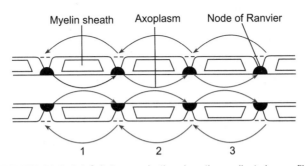

FIGURE 11.3 (c) Saltatory conduction along the myelinated nerve fibre.

What are the advantages of saltatory conduction?

1. Occurs at a faster rate as impulse jumps from one node to the next node of Ranvier.
2. Requires lesser energy. Ions diffuse only at nodes of Ranvier. Therefore, changes in ionic concentration with single impulse are very low. A number

of impulses can pass before recharging is required (recharging is done by Na^+-K^+ pump which requires energy).

What is orthodromic and antidromic conduction?

When any axon is stimulated at its centre by a threshold stimulus, action potential is initiated at that site and it travels in either direction by local circuit of current flow, i.e. two impulses travelling in opposite directions are set up. In living animal impulses normally pass in one direction, i.e. from synaptic junction or receptors along axons to their terminations. Such a conduction is termed orthodromic conduction.

Conduction in opposite direction is termed antidromic conduction. Since synapses permit conduction in one direction only, antidromic impulses which are set up fail to pass the first synapse they encounter, i.e. they die out at this point.

What is recharging? How is it done?

After the passage of impulses along the nerve fibre, bringing the ionic concentration of the fibre back to normal is called the recharging process.

With every impulse, there is diffusion of Na^+ ions inside and diffusion of K^+ ions outside the fibre. After a few impulses, concentrations of these ions inside and outside change to a sufficient degree to initiate Na^+-K^+ pump activity. Recharging is done by activation of Na^+-K^+ pump.

RECORDING OF ACTION POTENTIAL

Describe the instrument used for recording action potential.

Action potential takes place in less than one millisecond (in large myelinated nerve fibre), and hence recording meter should be capable of responding extremely rapidly, i.e. instrument must be inertia less. For practical purposes, the only available instrument for recording action potential is *cathode ray oscilloscope* (CRO). Its moving part is a stream of electrons which possess practically no mass and therefore cathode ray oscilloscope is almost an inertia less instrument (Fig. 11.4).

How is action potential recorded monophasically?

Monophasic recording of action potential is done in two ways:

1. *One electrode inside and other electrode outside surface.* We can record action potential on stimulation by placing one microelectrode inside the fibre and the other electrode on the outside surface and connecting these electrodes to cathode ray oscilloscope.

Record obtained shows spike potential, negative after potential and positive after potential (Fig. 11.5).

- *Spike potential.* It is the record showing rapid change in membrane potential from −90 mV to + 35 mV (depolarization) and rapid returning of potential to −70 mV (rapid repolarization). Spike potential is over 0.4 ms in myelinated nerve fibre. Potential change from −90 mV to +35 mV occurs due to greater permeability of membrane for Na^+ ions and entry of

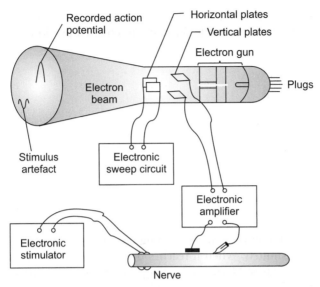

FIGURE 11.4 Cathode ray oscilloscope (CRO).

Na$^+$ ions into the fibre. Rapid repolarization from +35 mV to −70 mV is due to increased permeability of membrane for K$^+$ ions (Na$^+$ channels are closed and K$^+$ channels open at the end of depolarization) and diffusion of K$^+$ ions from inside to outside the nerve fibre.

■ *Negative after potential.* It is the slow phase of repolarization from −70 mV to −90 mV (RMP). This is due to slower diffusion of K$^+$ ions to the exterior because of decreased K$^+$ gradient across the membrane. K$^+$ ions diffusing out during rapid phase of repolarization are collected on the outside surface of membrane, and gradient of K$^+$ ions across the membrane is thus reduced.

■ *Positive after potential.* After negative after potential is reached to RMP, the record shows that potential becomes more negative from RMP (−90 mV) for some milliseconds. This is hyperpolarization. It is due to non-closing of K$^+$ channels even after complete repolarization which allows diffusion of K$^+$ ions from inside to outside of the fibre.

2. **Both the recording electrodes on outside surface of the nerve fibre.** It is recorded by placing one electrode on the crushed end of nerve and the other placed on the intact part of the nerve fibre. The crushed portion of the fibre is permanently negatively charged outside. Therefore, under the resting state current flow (upstroke) is recorded when the electrodes are connected to cathode ray oscilloscope.

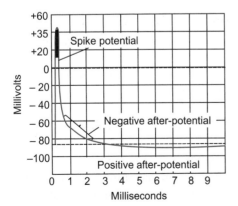

FIGURE 11.5 Action potential showing spike potential followed by a negative and a positive after potential.

This is called the *current of injury.* Current of injury is recorded. Electrode A placed on intact portion, electrode B placed on crushed portion.

(a)

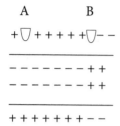

On stimulation of the fibre with stimulating electrodes beyond A, the impulse is generated and transmitted. When it reaches the membrane under electrode A, the membrane gets depolarized (negatively charged on the outside surface). At the time there is no current flow between the electrodes and the record will come to baseline:

When the impulse passes away from electrode A and membrane gets repolarized, again the current of injury will be received.

(b)

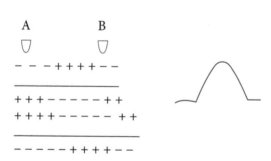

How is biphasic record of action potential obtained?

Before the introduction of intracellular electrodes it was possible to record biphasic action potential as follows:

Two recording electrodes are placed on the outside surface of the nerve fibre and they are connected to a cathode ray oscilloscope (Fig. 11.6).

What is compound action potential? How is it recorded?

It is the monophasic recording of action potential from the nerve trunk which contains many fibres. The fibres in the nerve may vary in diameter.

When the nerve is removed, it is placed in a trough and immersed in paraffin oil. Stimulating electrodes are placed at one end of the nerve and the recording electrodes at several centimetres away from the stimulating electrodes. One electrode is placed on intact nerve trunk and the other on the crushed nerve trunk.

The nerve is then stimulated with a sufficient strength of stimulus so that many nerve fibres in the nerve are stimulated simultaneously (Fig. 11.7).

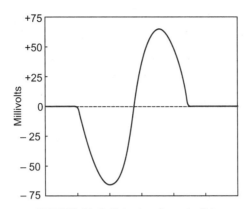

FIGURE 11.6 Biphasic action potential.

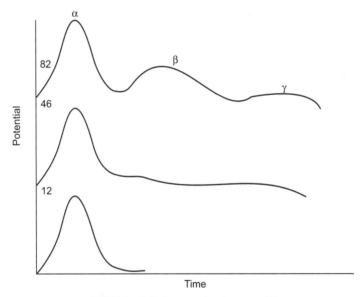

FIGURE 11.7 Compound action potential.

PROPERTIES OF NERVE FIBRE

Name the properties of the nerve fibre.

- Excitability.
- Conductivity.
- Accommodation.
- Action potential in nerve fibre obeys all or none law.
- Absolute and relative refractory period.

What is absolute and relative refractory period?

Short period following action potential during which nerve fibre has completely lost its excitability is called the absolute refractory period.

Short period following absolute refractory period is called the relative refractory period. During which excitability of the nerve fibre is less than normal.

Why nerve fibre cannot be stimulated during absolute refractory period?

During action potential, the sodium channels in the membrane of the nerve open due to opening of their activation gates. Within fraction of a millisecond, channels are closed by closure of inactivation gates of the sodium channels. These gates do not open unless potential comes back to resting level, i.e. sodium channels remain closed due to closure of inactive gates. Therefore, the fibre is not stimulated during this phase.

Why is excitability of the nerve reduced in relative refractory period?

In relative refractory phase the nerve fibre is in hyperpolarized state and therefore, the excitability is reduced.

Name the factors affecting excitability of the nerve fibre.

FACTORS INCREASING EXCITABILITY OF THE NERVE FIBRE:

- Increased potassium ion concentration in extracellular fluid.
- Reduced Ca^{++} ion concentration in extracellular fluid.

FACTORS REDUCING THE EXCITABILITY OF THE NERVE FIBRE:

- High extracellular fluid Ca^{++} ion concentration.
- Low extracellular fluid potassium ion concentration.
- Local anaesthetics like procaine, tetracaine.

What is rheobase?

The least strength of current (when allowed to pass through the excitable tissue for infinite length of time) which excites the excitable tissue is called a rheobase.

What is chronaxie?

Minimum time required to stimulate the excitable tissue when strength of the current used is double the rheobase is called chronaxie (Fig. 11.8).

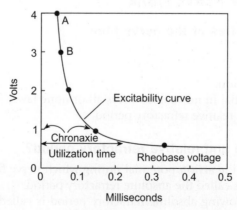

FIGURE 11.8 Excitability curve of a large myelinated nerve fibre.

What is the significance of finding out chronaxie?

Chronaxie is a measure of excitability of the tissue. More excitable the tissue lesser is the chronaxie.

Which is the most excitable tissue in the body?

Large myelinated nerve fibre is the most excitable tissue in the body.

DEGENERATION OF NERVE

What is Wallerian degeneration?

After the nerve is sectioned the nerve degenerates. The various functional and morphological changes that occur in the part of the nerve distal to the injury are called Wallerian degeneration. Though nerve continues to conduct impulses for three days (after third day ability to conduct impulses is deteriorated and after fifth day nerve fails to conduct any impulse), morphological changes start appearing in about 24 hours. Various changes are as follows:

- Axis cylinder along the whole length breaks into short lengths.
- Myelin sheath breaks and begins to bead into oily droplets.
- Macrophages from endoneurium invade the degenerating myelin sheath and axis cylinder.
- Macrophages phagocytoze the debris formed by remnants of myelin sheath and axis cylinder. They also secrete certain enzymes which aid in the destruction of myelin sheath. Thus only empty endoneural tubes remain.
- Degenerating fibre can be stained with Marchi's stain. It appears black after staining (between 8 and 21 days after injury).
- While degenerative changes are taking place, the cells of sheath of Schwann divide mitotically and form the cords of cells lying within the endoneural tube. This process is completed within three months. At the distal cut end these growing Schwann cells differentiate into thin elongated cells which grow in all directions from cut distal stump at a rate of 1 mm/day.

What is the effect of sectioning of nerve in the part of the nerve proximal to the site of injury?

The changes taking place in the part of the nerve proximal to the site of injury are termed retrograde degeneration. Changes occurring are the same as Wallerian degeneration but they occur for a variable distance from the site of injury. They may occur up to the first node of Ranvier.

What is the effect of sectioning of the nerve on nerve cell bodies?

Within 48 hours after the section of the nerve, Nissl's granules of the nerve cells begin to disintegrate into a fine dust (known as chromatolysis) because protein synthesis processes are mobilized to help the neuron to survive.

The Golgi apparatus fragments, the cell swells and becomes rounded. Neurofibrils disappear. Nucleus is displaced to the margin of the cell and may be extruded completely, in which case cell atrophies and dies. In cases of severe injury death of cells usually results. If cell does not die, repair process begins within 20 days of injury. Nissl's granules and Golgi apparatus gradually reappear. Cell regains its usual size and nucleus returns to the central position. Cell repair may occur even if the axon does not regenerate.

Describe the process of regeneration in the nerve.

If neurilemma is absent no regeneration is possible. Nerve fibres of CNS therefore once degenerated never regenerate as these nerves have no neurilemma.

If the neuron survives the nerve fibre regenerates as follows:

Central axon (proximal cut end) elongates and gives out fibrils up to 100 in number in all directions from the cut end. These fibrils are looking for the peripheral endoneural tubes for entry. During this, fibril must reach the correct address, i.e. it must enter in its own endoneural tube. The regenerating fibrils are guided by strands of Schwann cells from the distal cut end for entering into their own endoneural tube. Neurotropic factor of chemical nature is also involved in giving proper direction to the growing fibrils. Varying number of developing fibrils (0 to 25) enter into the single endoneural tube. Eventually all those fibres degenerate except one which has reached its correct address. This fibre then grows and enlarges.

Daily rate of growth of fibre is low in junctional area (0.25 mm) but once it enters the endoneural tube, it becomes higher (3 to 4 mm). Within about 15 days, medullary sheath starts developing. The Schwann cells filling the endoneural tube form the medullary sheath around the successful fibre. Completion of medullary sheath formation takes one year. But regenerated fibres attain diameters of about 80% of original diameters. This is anatomical regeneration. Functional (physiological) recovery takes longer time, because sometimes fibres do not enter the appropriate tubes, and thus there are faulty connections. This results into functional complications, requiring retraining (rehabilitation) and therefore functional recovery is delayed.

What is neuroma?

If during the regeneration of the nerve fibrils, sprouting from proximal cut end, not find their way or if the gap is too large, the fibrils turn round in search of endoneural tubes in a whorl-like mass known as neuroma. Neuroma may be quite painful.

What is phantom limb?

When the limb is amputated, neuroma developed at the site which gives the unpleasant sensation of phantom limb, i.e. excitation at the site of amputation causes the patient to feel that lost limb is still present.

REACTION OF DEGENERATION

What is reaction of degeneration?

Reaction of degeneration is the altered response of the neuromuscular apparatus to electric stimulation obtained when the nerve supplying the muscle is cut.

What is an electrotonus?

When constant current is passed through the nerve it alters the properties of the nerve in respect to excitability, conductivity and electrical state. These changes are referred to as electrotonus.

What is anelectrotonus and catelectrotonus?

When the constant current is passed through the nerve, there is decreased excitability and conductivity of the nerve at anode which is known as anelectrotonus and increased excitability and conductivity at cathode which is known as catelectrotonus.

Anelectrotonic and catelectrotonic effects spread along the nerve on either side of the electrode. The changes are exactly reversed on stoppage of current which is called resolution of anelectrotonus and catelectrotonus.

MUSCLE

INTRODUCTION

What is muscle?

Muscle is a contractile tissue with a chemically stored energy which can be transformed into mechanical energy.

Name the different types of muscles.

There are three types of muscles in the body:

- Skeletal or striated or voluntary muscle.
- Cardiac muscle.
- Smooth muscle.

Approximately 40% of the body is composed of skeletal muscle and 10% is cardiac and smooth muscle.

Which is the most excitable muscle?

Skeletal muscle is the most excitable muscle amongst the three types as its chronaxie is lowest.

STRUCTURE OF SKELETAL MUSCLE

What is a sarcomere?

Sarcomere is the fundamental contractile unit of the muscle fibre.

Name contractile proteins present in the skeletal muscles.

Actin and myosin are the contractile proteins present in the skeletal muscles.

Explain isotropic and anisotropic in connection with I and A bands?

A band is located in the middle of each sarcomere and it is made up of myosin. It is anisotropic to polarized light. I band is made up of actin and is isotropic to polarized light.

Enumerate the different muscle proteins.

Different muscle proteins in the thin filaments are:

- Actin
- Tropomyosin
- Troponin
- Alpha actinin

Different muscle proteins in thick filaments are:

- Myosin
- C-protein

Describe the structure of muscle fibre and sarcomere.

Muscle fibre is long, slender and cylindrical, its average length is 3 cm (1 to 4 cm), and the diameter varies from 10 to 100 microns.

The muscle fibre is enclosed by a cell membrane called plasma membrane (sarcolemma). Cytoplasm present inside the fibre, called sarcoplasm, contains various organelles such as nuclei, myofibrils, Golgi apparatus, mitochondria, sarcoplasmic reticulum, ribosomes, etc. There are multiple nuclei lying just beneath sarcolemma.

The muscle fibre contains a large number of myofibrils formed of muscle filaments or myofilaments.

Myofilaments are of two types—myosin filaments and actin filaments. Myosin filaments are thick, about 1,500 in number. Actin filaments are thin, around 3000 in number. These filaments lie side by side. They partially interdigitate forming alternate dark and light bands. The light band contains only actin filaments and is termed 'I' band, because it is isotropic to polarized light. The dark band contains myosin filaments as well as ends of actin filaments overlapping the myosin filament. This band is termed 'A' band because it is anisotropic to polarized light. There are small projections from the sides of myosin filament which are called cross bridges. They protrude from the surfaces of myosin filaments along the entire extent of filament except in the centre.

At regular intervals, Z discs or Z membranes composed of filamentous proteins divide the entire muscle into sarcomeres as they pass across the muscle fibre. The portion of myofibril (or whole muscle) which lies between two successive Z membranes is termed sarcomere. In a sarcomere, actin filaments are attached to Z membranes and they overlap the myosin filaments present in the centre of the sarcomere. When the length of sarcomere is two microns, actin filaments completely cover the myosin filaments and begin to overlap each other (Fig. 11.9).

Describe the structure of actin and myosin filaments.

1. *Actin filament.* Actin filament is formed of three types of proteins—actin, troponin and tropomyosins.

Actin. Actin filament is made up of double helix of 300 to 400 actin molecules. Actin molecule (F-actin) is a polymer of small globular proteins called G-actin, having a molecular weight of 42,000. There are about 13 G-actin molecules in each revolution of each strand of helix. Attached to each G-actin molecule is one ADP molecule. ADPs are active sites of actin filament with which cross bridges of myosin filament interact to cause muscle contraction.

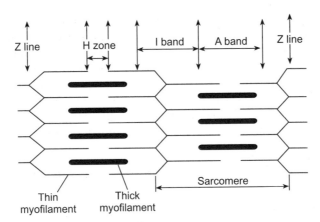

FIGURE 11.9 Structure of sarcomere.

Actin filament is 1 μm long. The bases of actin filaments are inserted strongly into the Z discs, while the other ends protrude in both the directions into the adjacent sarcomeres to lie in space between myosin molecules.

Troponin. Attached to one end of tropomyosin molecule, there is complex of three loosely bound protein subunits, called troponins I, T, C:

Troponin I—attached to F-actin.

Troponin T—attached to tropomyosin.

Troponin C—having strong affinity for calcium ions.

Tropomyosin. There are about 40 to 60 molecules of tropomyosin (molecular weight 70,000) situated along the strands of double helix of actin filament. Tropomyosin is also present in the form of double helix. It is spirally wrapped around the F-actin helix and is loosely connected to the F strand. In the resting state tropomyosin molecules physically cover the active sites of actin filament so that no interaction can occur between them and heads of myosin filaments.

2. *Myosin filament.* Myosin filament is formed by 200 myosin molecules. Each myosin molecule (molecular weight 480,000) is composed of six polypeptide chains, two heavy and four light chains.

The two heavy chains (molecular weight of each 200,000) wrap around each other to form a double helix. One end of each of these chains is folded into a globular protein mass, called myosin head. Thus there are two myosin heads at one end of double helix myosin molecule.

The four light chains each having a molecular weight of 20,000 are parts of myosin heads—two light chains for each head. These are supposed to control function of head during muscle contraction.

Myosin molecule has tail and body formed of double helix of heavy chain. A part of helix portion of each molecule extends to the sides along with heads, providing an arm that extends the heads outward from the body. The protruding arms and heads, together are called cross bridges. Each cross bridge is believed to be flexible at two points, called hinges—one where arm leaves body of the myosin filament, and the other where the two heads are attached to the arm. The hinged arms allow the heads either to be extended outward from the body of myosin filament or to be brought close to the myosin body. Hinged heads participate in the process of contraction.

For forming myosin filament, half of myosin molecules are oriented in one direction and the remaining half in the opposite direction. Because of this the central portion of the filament does not possess cross bridges as it is only composed of tails of myosin molecules. From the central part myosin filament (which is devoid of cross bridges) hinged arms extend towards both ends of myosin filament away from the centre. Myosin filament itself is twisted so that each successive set of cross bridges is axially displaced from previous set by 120°. Thus cross bridges extend in all directions around the filament. Myosin head functions as ATPase enzyme.

What is the role of regulatory proteins in the skeletal muscle contraction?

Troponin and tropomyosin are called regulatory proteins because they regulate actin-myosin interactions.

Under-resting state, calcium concentration of sarcoplasm is low and troponin-C is not bound with calcium ion. Troponin-tropomyosin complex physically covers active sites of actin filaments. This prevents interaction between heads of myosin and active sites of actin.

On excitation calcium ion concentration of sarcoplasm rises above the resting level which causes troponin-C to react with calcium. This reaction causes conformational change in tropomyosin molecule and it moves deeper into the groove between two actin strands. This uncovers the active sites of the actin filament allowing heads of myosin to combine with them to initiate muscle contraction.

What are cross bridges?

Cross bridges are the portions of the myosin molecules that extend from the surface of the thick filaments towards the thin filaments. They are force generating sites in the muscle cells.

What is sarcoplasmic triad?

Sarcoplasmic (endoplasmic) reticulum is formed of longitudinal tubules lying parallel to myofibrils. They lie in between myofibrils. Sarcolemma (outer membrane of the muscle fibre) extends to the interior of fibres at the junction of A and I bands forming T tubules. T tubules are open to the exterior and therefore contain extracellular fluid. At the site where transverse tubule cross the longitudinal tubule there is dilatation called the terminal cisternae and the junction is called the triad. The T tubules cross longitudinal tubules at each A and I band junction. Therefore, in skeletal muscle sarcomere, there are two triads per sarcomere. Due to this, skeletal muscle is the most excitable muscle (Fig. 11.10).

EXCITATION-CONTRACTION COUPLING

What is excitation-contraction coupling?

Excitation-contraction coupling refers to the sequence of events by which an action potential in the plasma membrane of a muscle fibre leads to cross bridge activity by increasing cytosolic calcium concentration.

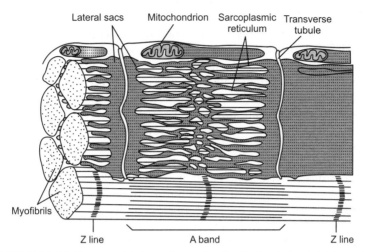

Lateral sacs   Mitochondrion   Sarcoplasmic   Transverse
                                reticulum   tubule

Myofibrils

Z line   A band   Z line

FIGURE 11.10 Transverse tubules and sarcoplasmic reticulum in the skeletal muscle.

What is the mechanism of excitation-contraction coupling in skeletal muscle fibres?

Action potential initiated in the plasma membrane is rapidly conducted on the surface of the muscle fibre and then into the interior of muscle fibre by way of T tubules. This triggers opening of calcium channels in the terminal cisternae. Calcium ions diffuse into the cytosol and get attached to troponin molecule. This results into exposure of active sites on actin molecule. Heads of the myosin molecules get attached to active sites and contraction is initiated.

MUSCLE CONTRACTION

Who put forward the theory of sliding filament hypothesis?

Sliding filament theory was put forward by AI Huxley and HE Huxley in 1954.

What is Fenn effect?

Total energy released by a muscle increases as muscle work increases. This finding is known as Fenn effect. It means that energy released is determined not only by activation process but also by work-load imposed on the muscle.

What is the role of calcium in muscle contraction?

Cytosolic calcium ion concentration determines the number of troponin sites occupied by calcium which in turn determines the number of cross bridges that can bind to actin and exert a force on actin filaments.

Describe the modern theory of muscle contraction.

'Walk-along' theory is the modern theory of muscle contraction, described below.

As soon as actin filament becomes activated by calcium ions, the heads of cross bridges of myosin filament become attached to the active sites of actin filament. There is cyclic attachment and detachment of heads of cross bridges with hydrolysis of ATP which causes movement of actin filaments towards the centre of myosin filament to a small extent with each cross-bridge cycle. Myosin filament has half the cross bridges oriented in one direction from the centre and the remaining half oriented in the opposite direction. Cross-bridge cycles therefore cause the movements of actin filaments on either side towards the centre of myosin filament in each sarcomere thereby causing muscle contraction (reduction in the length of sarcomere).

Single cross-bridge cycle occurs in steps as given below:

Step I. Attachment of head of a cross bridge to active site of actin filament.

Before contraction begins; the heads of cross bridge bind with ATP. The ATPase activity of myosin head immediately causes breaking of ATP to ADP and Pi. Cleavage products remain bound to myosin head. The head of myosin therefore becomes energized. In such a state conformation of head is such that it extends perpendicular towards the actin filament and it gets attached to actin filament. Reaction occurs as follows:

$$A + M.ADP.Pi \xrightarrow{\text{Actin binding}} A.M.A.D.P.Pi \ (A = \text{action}, \ M = \text{myosin})$$

Step II. Power stroke. Bond between head of myosin cross bridge and the active site of actin filament causes a conformational change in the head causing it to tilt towards the arm of the cross bridge. This provides a power stroke for pulling the actin filament towards the centre of myosin filament to a small degree. Energy stored in the head of myosin cross bridge is utilized for power stroke. Reaction occurs as follows:

$$A.M.ADP.Pi \xrightarrow{\text{Bridge movement}} A.M. + ADP + Pi.\uparrow$$

Myosin head still remains attached to active site of actin filament.

Step III. Detachment of head of a cross bridge from active site of actin filament. For cross bridge to repeat the cycle head must get detached. This is caused due to attachment of ATP molecule at the site of release of ADP to the head of a cross bridge. This binding decreases the affinity between myosin head and actin and head of a cross bridge gets detached. The reaction occurs as follows:

$$A.M. + ATP \longrightarrow A + M.ATP$$

Step IV. For next cycle to begin the head of myosin becomes energized. The energized head extends perpendicular towards the action filament and gets attached to the new active site for repeating the cycle. This reaction occurs as follows:

$$M. ATP \xrightarrow{\text{Energized cross bridge}} M. ADP. Pi$$

Thus with each cross-bridge cycle there is movement of actin filament towards the centre of myosin to a small degree (Figs 11.11a and b).

Repeated cross-bridge cycling causes the movement of actin filaments of either side towards the centre of myosin filament of the sarcomere leading to muscle contraction.

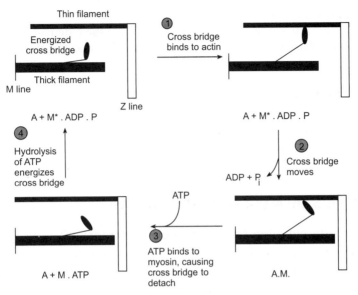

FIGURE 11.11 (a) Cross-bridge cycle.

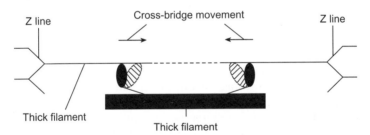

FIGURE 11.11 (b) Power stroke.

What is active state in the muscle? Name factors affecting duration of active state?

The period during which intracellular calcium concentration is above the resting value and cross bridges are cycling is called the active states. The factors affecting active state:

- Intracellular calcium concentration.
- Amount and duration of calcium availability affects intensity and duration of active state.
- Conditions increasing contractile tension affect either the peak or duration of the active state.

What are the functions of ATP in skeletal muscle contraction?

1. Hydrolysis of ATP by myosin energizes the cross bridges providing the energy for force generation.
2. Binding of ATP to myosin dissociates cross bridges bound to actin allowing the bridges to repeat their cycle of activity.

3. Hydrolysis of ATP by Ca^{++}-ATPase in the sarcoplasmic reticulum provides the energy for active transport of calcium back into the cisternae, lowering cytoplasmic calcium, ending the contraction and allowing muscle fibre to relax.

How is normally muscle relaxation caused?

Calcium pump transports Ca^{++} ions present in sarcoplasm during contraction back into the sarcoplasmic reticulum. Removal of calcium from troponin restores blocking action of troponin-tropomyosin complex. Myosin cross-bridge cycles cease and muscle relaxes.

ENERGETICS OF MUSCLE CONTRACTION

How is energy supplied for the muscle contraction?

Energy is supplied in the form of ATP for contraction of skeletal muscle. ATP stored in the muscle initiates the contractile activity but is consumed after a few twitches.

There are three ways in which muscle fibre can form ATP from ADP during contractile activity:

1. *Phosphorylation of ADP by creatine phosphate (CP) (Lohmann reaction)*

$$ADP + CP \xrightarrow{\text{Creatine Kinase}} ATP + C$$

The reaction is rapid and requires only single enzyme. It is reversible and obeys law of mass action. At rest, muscle contains larger quantity of ATP, therefore reaction proceeds from right to left forming creatine phosphate. During muscle contraction, when ATP is utilized, reaction proceeds from left to right forming ATP very rapidly. The amount of CP is limited and therefore amount of ATP formed by this mechanism is only sufficient for contraction of the muscle for a few seconds.

2. *Oxidative phosphorylation of ADP in the mitochondria.* In the mitochondria, there is oxidative phosphorylation of fatty acids and glucose (supplied through blood and also glucose obtained from muscle glycogen). There is requirement of O_2 and nutrient supply for this. For moderate level of exercise with moderate rate of ATP breakdown, most of the energy is obtained by this mechanism. But for intense rapid exercise the rate of ATP synthesized by this mechanism is not able to keep pace with rate of ATP breakdown. Therefore, the next mechanism comes into play (anaerobic glycolysis).

3. *Anaerobic glycolysis.* For exercise level exceeding about 70% of maximal rate of ATP breakdown, ATP is obtained rapidly by anaerobic glycolysis of glucose obtained from muscle glycogen as well as through blood. ATP synthesis by this mechanism occurs at a very fast rate but amount of ATP synthesized per glucose molecule is less (2 ATPs per glucose molecule as compared to 36 ATPs per glucose molecule formed in oxidative phosphorylation). But because the reaction occurs fast and anaerobically, the rate of ATP synthesis can keep pace with the rate of ATP breakdown. Muscle goes in O_2 debt.

During the reaction of anaerobic glycolysis, there is formation of lactic acid. Muscle glycogen is used up. During recovery (after exercise), this glycogen is to be replenished. Lactic acid enters the blood (as blood lactate) and is carried to the liver where it is converted to glucose. This glucose passes to muscle through blood and is converted to muscle glycogen. This is called the Cori's cycle. Thus muscle glycogen is replenished after the exercise. Therefore, greater quantity of O_2 supply is necessary even after the exercise. Amount of excess O_2 utilized during recovery phase is equal to O_2 debt. Longer and more intense the exercise, longer is the time taken to restore glycogen.

What is Lohmann reaction? What is its importance?

Phosphorylation of ADP by creatine phosphate is known as Lohmann reaction. This reaction provides very rapid means of formation of ATP at the onset of contractile activity.

What is efficiency of muscle contraction?

Percentage of energy input that is converted to work is the efficiency of any machine. In case of muscle doing work (e.g. lifting up of load), efficiency is 20% to 25%.

Enumerate the factors affecting muscle efficiency.

- Body size and weight of the person.
- Age.
- Diet and nutritional state.
- Muscular exercise and training.

What is O_2 debt?

After the period of exercise, amount of extra O_2 consumed to remove lactate, replenish ATP, CP and glycogen stores and to replace small amount of O_2 that has been used from myoglobin is called 'O_2 debt'. This amount of extra oxygen consumed is proportionate to the extent to which energy demands during exercise exceeded the capacity for aerobic synthesis of energy stores, i.e. extent to which O_2 debt was incurred, during exercise.

How do you measure O_2 debt?

O_2 debt is measured experimentally by determining O_2 consumption after exercise until a constant basal consumption is reached and then subtracting the basal O_2 consumption from the total O_2 consumed during this period.

MUSCLE TENSION

What is load?

Force exerted by the weight of an object on the muscle is known as load. Thus muscle load and tension are opposing forces.

What is muscle tension?

The force exerted by the contracting muscle on the object is known as muscle tension.

What is isotonic contraction?

Isotonic contraction is the contraction of muscle in which tension remains constant but length of muscle changes.

Muscle consists of contractile elements in parallel with an elastic component (PEC) and in series with another elastic component (SEC). PEC represents the elasticity of structural elements other than the contractile proteins.

Tendon is a series elastic component.

If muscle is suspended vertically from an attachment to a spring, it can be stretched by attaching weights to the lower end. The tension developed in it can be measured. This is a passive tension because here myofibrils act as only passive viscous elements and have very little resistance to stretch. The resistance to stretch mainly resides in series elastic component (SEC) and to some extent in parallel elastic component (PEC).

On stimulation the contractile components convert chemical energy into mechanical work and therefore muscle shortens. The characteristics of PEC and SEC are unchanged during contraction. When muscle shortens, its speed of shortening depends on force that opposes shortening, i.e. the weight of the object to be lifted.

What is isometric contraction?

Isometric contraction is a type of contraction during which length of the muscle remains constant but tension changes.

When two ends of the muscle are fixed and the muscle is not allowed to shorten, then isometric contraction of muscle results on stimulation, e.g. contraction of antigravity muscles to maintain tension in erect posture.

At the onset of such a contraction there is no load opposing the contraction and contractile components (CC) shorten which stretches SEC causing increase in tension which reduces the performance of CC, thereby reducing speed of shortening. The tension which the muscle can develop rises to its maximum, speed of shortening is zero.

Differentiate between isotonic and isometric contraction.

Isotonic contraction	Isometric contraction
1. It is a type of contraction where length of the muscle changes but tension remains constant.	It is a type of contraction in which length of the muscle remains constant but tension changes.
2. Muscle does external work, e.g. lifting of load.	Muscle does not do external work, e.g. contraction of antigravity muscles only for maintaining posture.
3. When muscle is stimulated myofibrils contract and series elastic component (SEC) is stretched initially to cause rise in tension but when tension just exceeds effect of weight, muscle as a whole begins to shorten to cause lifting up of weight and then tension remains constant throughout remaining of shortening and the contraction recorded is due to shortening of contractile component only.	When the muscle is stimulated myofibrils shorten but in doing so stretch the SEC and thus keep length of the muscle constant.

4. Evolution of heat is lesser than that in isometric.
Evolution of heat is more than that in isotonic.

5. Duration is short.
Duration is long.

6. Load determines the velocity of shortening.
Length of sarcomere determines the tension generated.

7. Mechanical efficiency is more.
Mechanical efficiency is less.

Describe the factors determining muscle tension.

1. FACTORS DETERMINING MUSCLE TENSION IN SINGLE MUSCLE FIBRE

- *Frequency of action potential.* Greater the frequency, greater is the tension developed (due to summation).
- *Length of the fibre.* Tension developed is maximum, when length of each sarcomere is 2 to 2.2 microns. At this length the number of active sites exposed for acting with cross bridges is maximum. Decrease or increase in length of sarcomere results into decrease in number of active sites exposed for acting with cross bridges. Tension developed is proportional to the number of cross bridges active at a time, therefore the tension developed is highest at sarcomere length between 2 to 2.2 μ (Fig. 11.12).
- *Diameter of fibre.* Greater the diameter of fibre, greater is the tension developed.
- *Rate of fatigue.* Greater the rate of fatigue, lesser is the tension developed.

2. FACTORS DETERMINING TENSION DEVELOPED IN THE WHOLE MUSCLE

- *Number of active fibres.* Greater the number of fibres contracting, greater is the tension developed. Therefore, as greater and greater number of motor units get recruited, greater is the tension developed.
- *Number of fibres per motor unit.* The number of muscle fibres per motor unit varies with different muscles, e.g. in ocular muscles there are only 10 to 13 fibre per motor unit. In muscles of back there are hundreds of fibres per motor unit. Greater the number of fibres per motor unit, greater rise in tension occurs as more and more number of motor units get recruited.
- *Tension developed by each active fibre.*
- *Number of alpha motor neurons activated.* This depends on impulses coming to alpha motor neurons from higher centres.

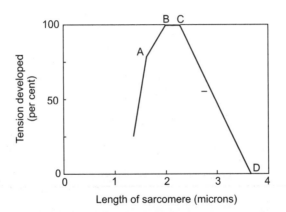

FIGURE 11.12 Length-tension diagram for a single sarcomere.

What is the meaning of the term resting length of muscle or 'L' zero?

The length of the muscle at which the muscle develops the greatest isometric tension is called the 'L' zero length. Normally under-resting state, muscle length is 'L' zero.

TYPES OF SKELETAL MUSCLE FIBRES

Give the classification of skeletal muscle fibres.

For details see Table 11.2.

Table 11.2	Classification of Skeletal Muscle Fibres		
	Type I **(Slow oxidative** **or red fibres)**	**Type II B** **(Fast glycolytic** **or white fibres)**	**Type II A** **(Fast oxidative** **or red fibres)**
1. Diameter	Small	Large	Large
2. Mitochondrial density	High	Low	High
3. Capillary density	High	Low	High
4. Myoglobin content	High	Low	Medium
5. Energy store			
CP stores	Low	High	High
Glycogen store	Low	High	High
Triglyceride store	High	Low	Medium
6. Myosin-ATPase activity	Low	High	High
7. Glycolytic enzyme activity	Low	High	High
8. Oxidative enzyme activity	High	Low	High
9. Ca^{++} pumping ability	Low	High	High
10. Speed of contraction	Low	High	High
11. Speed of relaxation	Low	High	High
12. Force production	Low	High	High
13. Fatigue resistance	High	Low	Low
14. Elasticity	Low	High	High

Give examples of the slow twitch and fast twitch muscle fibres in the body.

Every somatic muscle of the body contains all the three types of skeletal muscle fibres, but fibres of one type are present in majority. Muscles of back and legs contain slow oxidative type (red) of fibres in majority. They can maintain their activity for a long time without getting fatigued.

Muscles of arms contain fast glycolytic fibres in majority. Therefore, these muscles get fatigued very rapidly but large amount of tension can be developed in them in small time.

PROPERTIES OF SKELETAL MUSCLE

Enumerate the properties of skeletal muscle.

- Excitability.
- Contractility.
- Conductivity—can conduct impulse.
- Summation.
- Shows tetanus.
- Shows fatigue.
- Shows absolute and relative refractory period.
- All or none law—obeyed by single motor unit.

What is a motor unit?

Single alpha motor neuron of the spinal cord and group of muscle fibres innervated by it constitute a single motor unit.

What is all or none law? How is it applicable to skeletal muscle?

All or none law is applicable to single motor unit of skeletal muscle. It states that under given physiological conditions, the motor unit gives maximum response (all) or no response (none) to the applied stimulus.

What is simple muscle twitch?

Mechanical response of a muscle to a single stimulus applied to the muscle through nerve is known as simple muscle twitch (in isolated nerve muscle preparation).

What are the causes of latent period in single muscle twitch recorded in isolated nerve muscle preparation?

- Time taken for the impulse to travel from point of stimulation on the nerve to the neuromuscular junction.
- Time taken for the impulse to pass through neuromuscular junctions.
- Time required for different chemical events in the muscle to cause contraction.

- Inertia of the recording lever—Even if muscle contracts because of inertia, lever takes some time to record the contraction. Greater the weight of the lever, greater is the inertia.

What is wave summation or frequency summation?

The increased mechanical response to second stimulus is known as wave summation. If a fibre is repeatedly stimulated by a certain frequency, tetanus is obtained.

TETANUS

What is tetanus?

Tetanus is a sustained state of contraction obtained due to repeated stimulus application at a high rate. It is a type of frequency summation.

What is incomplete tetanus or clonus?

When muscle is repeatedly stimulated at low frequency, there are periods of incomplete relaxation between the summated stimuli. Such a record is called the incomplete tetanus or clonus.

What is critical fusion frequency?

A critical frequency, at which successive contractions are very rapid and fuse leading to sustained state of muscle contraction (tetanus) is called the critical fusion frequency.

What is the mechanism which causes tetanus?

A single action potential releases enough calcium to saturate troponin and all myosin binding sites on thin filament that are initially available. As soon as calcium is released from sarcoplasmic reticulum, it begins to pump back in the sarcoplasmic reticulum and thus calcium concentration in the cytosol begins to fall causing more and more active sites of actin filament to be blocked and become unavailable for cross bridges. Therefore, tension developed in a single twitch is limited.

During tetanic contraction, successive action potential causes release of calcium from sarcoplasmic reticulum before all calcium from previous action potential is pumped back. This results in maintaining high concentration of calcium in the sarcoplasm preventing decline in available binding sites for cross bridges. This allows tension to rise greatly.

FATIGUE

What is muscle fatigue?

The failure of a muscle fibre to maintain a tension as a result of previous contractile activity is known as muscle fatigue.

What is the seat of fatigue in isolated nerve-muscle preparation?

In isolated nerve-muscle preparation, the failure of response after repeatedly stimulating the muscle through its motor nerve is called fatigue. The seat of fatigue is the neuromuscular junction. Repeated stimulation of muscle itself leads to actual muscle fatigue and is due to depletion of muscle glycogen.

What is the seat of fatigue in intact animal?

Seat of fatigue in intact animal is synapses of central nervous system.

What is the mechanism by which fatigue occurs?

Failure of muscle to maintain tension as a result of previous contractile activity is known as muscle fatigue. If muscle is allowed to rest after the onset of fatigue it recovers its ability to contract.

Onset of fatigue and its recovery depend upon (1) intensity and duration of exercise and (2) type of muscle fibres. Fast glycolytic fibres fatigue fairly early and also recover rapidly from fatigue. Slow oxidative fibres do not fatigue early but they also require longer time of rest (up to 24 hours) for complete recovery.

Causes of fatigue. Depletion of ATP though seems to be a logical cause of fatigue, it is not completely true because ATP concentration in the fatigued muscle is only slightly lower than in the resting muscle. However, fatigue develops when rate of ATP synthesis becomes lesser than rate of ATP breakdown in the exercising muscles.

Mechanisms producing fatigue are different in different types of exercises. In short duration high intensity exercise such as weight lifting, short distance running, the main cause of fatigue is increased acidity in muscle cells which accompanies rise in lactic acid (formed due to anaerobic glycolysis). Increased H^+ ion concentration directly inhibits cross-bridge cycles and therefore force generated by them. The second cause is decrease in release of Ca^{++} ions from sarcoplasmic reticulum.

In long duration low intensity exercise such as marathon race depletion of muscle glycogen is the cause of fatigue.

Psychological fatigue. Failure of cerebral cortex to send excitatory signals to motor neurons causes an individual to stop exercising. The muscles are not fatigued (it is not a true muscle fatigue). Athlete's performance therefore depends not only on physical status of appropriate muscles but psychological fatigue also.

Fatigue in isolated nerve muscle preparation. In experiments, muscle contracts on stimulation of the nerve to the muscle. Repeated stimulation of the nerve causes failure of contraction of muscle, but if muscle is directly stimulated it contracts. Here the site of fatigue is neuromuscular junction. Repeated stimulation of nerve causes exhaustion of acetylcholine at neuromuscular junctions. Therefore, there is failure of transmission of impulse from nerve to muscle. After neuromuscular junctions are fatigued, if muscle is repeatedly stimulated true muscle fatigue occurs due to depletion of glycogen.

What is the importance of fatigue?

Relaxation of muscle requires ATP. Calcium pump in the sarcoplasmic reticulum pumps Ca^{++} ions from sarcoplasm into the sarcoplasmic reticulum leading to lowering of Ca^{++} in the sarcoplasm to the resting level. Ca^{++} pump is an active transport mechanism and therefore requires energy. ATP is also required for detachment of myosin head from active site of actin filament.

If contractile activity were to continue without entering into a state of fatigue, the APT concentration in the muscle would decrease to the point that cross bridges would become linked in a rigour position (as no ATP is available for detachment of myosin head from active site on actin and relaxation). This will be damaging to the muscle.

What is muscle tone?

Muscle tone is a state of partial tetanus of the muscle maintained by asynchronous discharge of impulses in the motor nerve supplying the muscle.

What is the effect of temperature on muscle contraction?

At low temperature, excitability of the muscle is reduced and the force of contraction is reduced. As temperature increases there is increase in the force of muscle contraction. It is maximum at 20° to 25°C. Beyond it, there is decrease in force contraction.

COMMON TERMS USED

Name	Description
Hypertrophy	Increase in total mass of the muscle due to increase in size of the certain muscle fibres is known as hypertrophy. Exercise can produce such hypertrophy.
Atrophy	Reduction of muscle mass due to decrease in diameter of muscle fibres is known as atrophy. It is produced due to cutting of motor nerve to the muscle and is known as denervation atrophy.
Hyperplasia	Increase in number of muscle fibres in the muscle is known as hyperplasia. It rarely occurs along with the hypertrophy.
Muscle cramp	Muscle cramp is the involuntary localized painful tetanic contraction of the muscle. It is relieved by stretching the affected muscle.
Muscular dystrophy	Muscular dystrophy is a genetic degenerative disease that leads to progressive wasting (atrophy) and loss of force generating capacity of the muscle.
Muscle fasciculation	Fasciculation is the abnormality detected in the quiescent muscle. Fasciculation is the contraction of group of muscle cells by an impulse through single axon into a motor unit. It is visible through skin as fine rippled movement in a relaxed muscle.
Fibrillation	Fibrillation is another abnormality detected in the muscle at rest. Fibrillation is contraction of muscle cells which have become completely dissociated from neural control (occurs in muscle cells atrophy as in poliomyelitis).

Name	Description
Rigour mortis	Rigour mortis is rigidity that develops in the muscle after death. It is a state of contraction of muscle due to permanent linkage between action and myosin associated with deficiency of ATP. Rigour mortis disappears 24 to 36 hours after death due to autolysis.
Contracture	Contracture is a prolonged contraction of a muscle in absence of action potential.

EMG

What is electromyography and electromyogram (EMG)?

The process of recording electrical potentials in human skeletal muscles is known as electromyography.

As the part of electric current generated is transmitted to the outer surface of the body, the changes in potentials can be studied by either putting the electrodes on the surface of skin covering the active muscle or inserting needle electrodes directly into the muscle concerned. The potentials are recorded on cathode ray oscilloscope. The record obtained is known as electromyogram (EMG). It is obtained during a state of complete relaxation and also with graded voluntary activity.

- Hardly any spontaneous activity is recorded in skeletal muscle of a normal individual at rest.
- With minimum voluntary activity a few motor units discharge. The resultant activity is the effect of summated action potentials in different motor units. No discrete action potentials are recorded.
- Considerable electrical activity is recorded with strong voluntary contraction because of recruitment of large number of motor units.

Clinical application. There are no EMG waves that are diagnostic for a particular disease entity and it is also not possible to sample every muscle of the body. Therefore, EMG is the extension of clinical neurological examination and by itself cannot be used to arrive at a specific clinical entity.

EMG is useful in diagnosis of disorders affecting lower motor neurons, muscles, nerves and neuromuscular junction.

In diseases of motor neuron, motor nerve, muscles normal pattern of EMG is altered, e.g. in lower motor neuron disease, in attempted contraction of the muscle only few motor units are activated resulting in a condition where action potentials remain discrete in the graph.

Destruction of the nerve causes fine regular contractions of individual fibre (fibrillations). Such contractions are not visible and should not be mixed up with fasciculations which are jerky, visible contractions of group of muscle fibres that occur under-resting state in certain pathological states.

EMG is also useful in nerve conduction studies.

NEUROMUSCULAR JUNCTION

STRUCTURE

How is the muscle normally activated?

Muscle activity is controlled by central nervous system through motor fibres to the muscle. Alpha fibres from alpha motor neurons supply skeletal muscles. Impulse passes from nerve to muscle via neuromuscular junction.

Describe the structure of neuromuscular junction.

Alpha type of nerve fibre supplies the skeletal muscle. When fibre comes near the muscle, it loses its myelin sheath and divides into number of branches. Each branch at its termination is distended to form synaptic knob or button, which forms a neuromuscular junction, at the centre of muscle fibre. At this site muscle membrane invaginates forming synaptic gutter. The space between nerve terminal and muscle membrane is called synaptic cleft which is filled by extracellular fluid with reticular fibres forming matrix.

Muscle membrane at the synapse shows large number of folds called subneural clefts. They increase the surface area. Muscle membrane also contains the receptor sites for acetylcholine (channels whose proteins have receptor site for acetylcholine which acts as a ligand and is responsible for opening of the channels when gets attached to the protein) (Fig. 11.13).

The matrix of subneural clefts contains enzymes cholinesterase which can degrade acetylcholine. Nerve terminal or synaptic knob contains large number of vesicles (about three lacs) containing acetylcholine. Mitochondria are also present in nerve terminal.

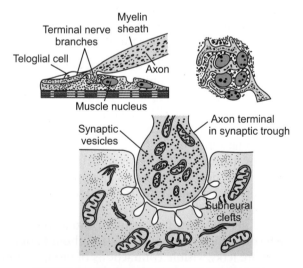

FIGURE 11.13 Structure of neuromuscular junction.

TRANSMISSION OF IMPULSE

Give sequence of the events which causes transmission of impulse through neuromuscular junction.

```
┌─────────────────────────────────────────────────────────────────┐
│ Initiation and propagation of action potential in motor neuron's axon │
└─────────────────────────────────────────────────────────────────┘
                              ↓
┌─────────────────────────────────────────────────────────┐
│   Arrival of impulse at nerve terminal (at synaptic button)   │
└─────────────────────────────────────────────────────────┘
                              ↓
┌───────────────────────────────────────────────────────────────┐
│  Increased permeability of nerve terminal membrane to calcium ions  │
└───────────────────────────────────────────────────────────────┘
                              ↓
┌───────────────────────────────────────────────────────────────────────┐
│ Diffusion of calcium ions from extracellular fluid to the interior of fibre leading to │
│              entry of calcium ions into the terminal               │
└───────────────────────────────────────────────────────────────────────┘
                              ↓
┌───────────────────────────────────────────────────────┐
│   Release of acetylcholine from the nerve terminal     │
└───────────────────────────────────────────────────────┘
                              ↓
┌───────────────────────────────────────────────────────────────────────┐
│ Binding of acetylcholine to the end plate acetylcholine receptors present in the │
│                        muscle membrane                         │
└───────────────────────────────────────────────────────────────────────┘
                              ↓
┌─────────────────────────────────────────────────────────────────┐
│  Opening of acetylcholine gated channels in the end plate membrane  │
└─────────────────────────────────────────────────────────────────┘
                              ↓
┌─────────────────────────────────────────────────────────────────────────┐
│ Entry of mainly $Na^+$ ions and to a lesser extent $Ca^{++}$ ions through these channels │
└─────────────────────────────────────────────────────────────────────────┘
                              ↓
┌─────────────────────────────────────────┐
│   Development of end plate potential     │
└─────────────────────────────────────────┘
                              ↓
┌───────────────────────────────────────────────────────────────────────┐
│ Local end plate potential when reaches a threshold magnitude there is opening to │
│           voltage gated sodium channels at the site              │
└───────────────────────────────────────────────────────────────────────┘
                              ↓
┌───────────────────────────────────────────────────────────────────────┐
│ Initiation of action potential in the muscle fibre by end plate depolarization │
└───────────────────────────────────────────────────────────────────────┘
                              ↓
┌───────────────────────────────────────────────────────────────────┐
│ Propagation of action potential in muscle fibre along the surface and │
│              into the fibre along the 'T' tubules                 │
└───────────────────────────────────────────────────────────────────┘
                              ↓
┌───────────────────────────────────────────────────────────────────────┐
│ Depolarization reaching at triads causing release of calcium into the sarcoplasm │
│         increasing calcium concentration above resting level          │
└───────────────────────────────────────────────────────────────────────┘
                              ↓
┌─────────────────────────────────────────┐
│      Binding of calcium with troponin    │
└─────────────────────────────────────────┘
                              ↓
┌─────────────────────────────────────────┐
│     Initiation of muscle contraction     │
└─────────────────────────────────────────┘
```

DRUGS AFFECTING NEUROMUSCULAR JUNCTION

Name the drugs that block neuromuscular transmission.

Curariform drugs (especially d-Tubocurarine) block the neuromuscular transmission. These drugs compete with acetylcholine for receptor sites of the muscle membrane but cannot increase permeability of the muscle membrane.

Name the acetylcholine-like drugs and their effect.

Methacholine, carbachol, nicotine are acetylcholine-like drugs acting at neuromuscular junction but are not destroyed by cholinesterase. They, therefore, cause prolonged state of spasm in the muscle.

What are anticholinesterases? When are they used?

Drugs like neostigmine, physostigmine, di-isopropyl fluorophosphate act as anti-cholinesterases. They cause increased quantity of acetylcholine accumulation at neuromuscular junction resulting in muscle spasm.

Neostigmine and physostigmine are used for treating the disease known as myasthenia gravis.

MYASTHENIA GRAVIS

What is myasthenia gravis? What is its probable cause?

Myasthenia gravis is a disease of neuromuscular junction. Affected muscles are paralysed because of inability of neuromuscular junction to transmit the signals from nerve to the muscle fibres. Myasthenia gravis is probably an autoimmune disease. There are antibodies produced against proteins of acetylcholine-gated channels. This causes reduction in number of subneural clefts. The magnitude of end plate potential developed is not adequate to stimulate the muscle fibres though release of acetylcholine from nerve terminals is normal.

MUSCLE RIGOUR

What is the nature of contraction of skeletal muscle in the human body?

In the human body, skeletal muscle contractions are tetanic contractions.

What is rigour?

A state of extreme rigidity in a muscle is known as rigour.

What is heat rigour? What is it due to?

Rigour produced by heat (above $50\,^{\circ}C$), e.g. pouring hot saline over the muscle, is known as heat rigour. Heat rigour is due to coagulation of muscle proteins produced by heat, and it is irreversible.

What is rigour mortis? What is it due to? Is it reversible?

State of development of extreme rigidity in the skeletal muscles after death is called rigour mortis. It is due to complete depletion of ATP and phosphocreatine in the muscle. ATP is required to cause separation of cross bridges from actin filaments during relaxation process. Rigour mortis is reversible. When muscle proteins decompose, rigour mortis disappears.

FUNCTIONS OF SKELETAL MUSCLES

State the functions of skeletal muscles in the body.

- To make various body movements by moving the skeletal parts at joints. No muscle in the body acts alone even in simplest movement. A

variety of muscles such as agonists, synergistic, antagonists are involved in each action.
- To maintain joint stability as related to posture.
- A few muscles encircling orifices (anus, lip) act as sphincters.
- Skeletal muscle present in upper one-third of oesophagus helps in swallowing.
- Diaphragm contraction and relaxation causes expansion and contraction of thoracic cavity (respiration).
- Cutaneous muscles, i.e. those having at least one of their attachments to skin, e.g. facial muscles, help in expression of emotions.
- Postural muscles of back and legs support the weight of the body.
- Muscles of arms produce large amounts of tensions rapidly and cause lifting of weights.

COMPARISON OF SKELETAL, CARDIAC AND SMOOTH MUSCLE

Give the comparison of skeletal muscle, cardiac muscle and smooth muscle.

For details see Table 11.3.

Table 11.3	Comparison of Skeletal Muscle, Cardiac Muscle and Smooth Muscle		
	Skeletal muscle	**Cardiac muscle**	**Smooth muscle***
Site	Attached to the skeleton	Attached to the heart	*Single unit*: blood vessels, urinary bladder, gall bladder, gut wall, ureter, bile duct, uterus *Multiunit:* ciliary muscles of the eye, muscles of iris, piloerector muscles in the skin
Composition			
Proteins	Maximum	Less	Less
Glycogen	Less	More	More
ATP and phosphagen	Present	Present	Present

Continued

Table 11.3	Comparison of Skeletal Muscle, Cardiac Muscle and Smooth Muscle—cont'd		
	Skeletal muscle	**Cardiac muscle**	**Smooth muscle***
• Fats	Mainly neutral fats	More phospholipids and cholesterol than others	Mainly neutral salts

Structure of fibre

• Shape of the fibres	Cylindrical	Cylindrical	Spindle shaped
• Nucleus	Single or multiple at periphery	Single, central with many nucleoli	Single
• Contractile proteins and their arrangements	Actin and myosin in the form of filaments arranged regularly	Actin and myosin in the form of filaments arranged regularly	Actin and myosin not arranged regularly
• Striations			
(a) Longitudinal	Present	Present	Present
(b) Cross	Present because actin and myosin filaments arranged regularly	Present because actin and myosin filaments arranged regularly	Not present
(a) Sarcoplasmic reticulum	Very well developed	Well developed but not as much as in skeletal muscles	Moderately developed
(b) T system	Two triads per sarcomere at A-I band junction	One triad per sarcomere at '2' membrane	Not well developed
• Regulating protein	Troponin	Troponin	Calmodulin
• Calcium store and calcium pump in sarcoplasmic reticulum	High	Moderate	Low
• Na$^+$ channels in the membrane	Fast voltage gated Na$^+$ channels present	Fast voltage-gated Na$^+$ channels with slow-voltage gated Na$^+$-Ca^{++} channels	Mainly slow-voltage gated Na$^+$-Ca^{++} channels Very few fast voltage gated Na$^+$ channels

Table 11.3 **Comparison of Skeletal Muscle, Cardiac Muscle and Smooth Muscle—cont'd**

	Skeletal muscle	Cardiac muscle	Smooth muscle*
• Branching of fibres	Not seen	Seen, multiple and in all directions	Not seen
• Connections between fibres	There are no connections—anatomical or physiological	There are no anatomical connections between fibres but they are connected through intercalated discs or gap junctions which have low electrical resistance and are physiological connections between cells (stimulation of one cell causes impulses to be transported to all connected cells)	*Single unit:* like cardiac muscle fibres, are functionally connected through gap junctions *Multiunit:* discrete fibres like skeletal muscles not connected anatomically or physiologically. Each fibre operates entirely independently

Properties

• Autorhythmicity	Not present	Present	Present for some single unit fibres absent in multiunit
• Excitability	High	Moderate. Less as compared to skeletal muscle	Low
• Conductivity	Fast	Slow. Different in different fibres	Slow
• Rate of contraction	Fast	Fast	Slow
• Rate of relaxation	Fast	Fast	Slow
• Refractory period	Short	Long and covers the entire period of contraction	Long
• Tetanus (wave summation)	Possible	Not possible because of long refractory period	Not possible since the process of contractions is long
• Fatigue	Possible	Does not fatigue since long refractory period ensures recovery	Possible but difficult to demonstrate

Continued

Table 11.3	Comparison of Skeletal Muscle, Cardiac Muscle and Smooth Muscle—cont'd		
	Skeletal muscle	**Cardiac muscle**	**Smooth muscle***
• All or none law	Single unit obeys	Obeys as a whole	*Single unit:* obeys as a whole *Multiunit:* by single unit obeys
• Multiple fibre (quantal summation)	Possible	Not possible as it is a functional syncytium	Not possible
• Resting membrane potential	–90 mV	–90 mV	–50 to –60 mV
• Stimulated by	Somatic nerves	Autonomic nerves (a) Sympathetic: excitatory transmitter (norepinephrine) (b) Parasympathetic: inhibitory transmitter (acetylcholine)	Autonomic nerves (a) Sympathetic: inhibitory transmitter (norepinephrine) (b) Parasympathetic: excitatory transmitter (acetylcholine) → Hormones → Local tissue factors causing vasodilatation, e.g. lack of oxygen, excess of carbon dioxide, increased H^+ ions
• Control	Voluntary	Involuntary	Involuntary
• Action potential shape and duration	Spike potential of 1 ms duration	Plateau potential of 0.1 to 0.3 ms duration	*Single unit:* plateau potential of 100 to several 1000 ms. Also spike potential seen of 10 to 50 ms *Multiunit:* spike potential
• Dependence of contraction on extracellular fluid calcium concentration	Not dependent	Partly dependent	Almost totally dependent
• Tonicity	Depends on nerves	Independent of nerves	Independent of nerves
Action of ions			
• Sodium (Na^+)	Excitation	Initiates and maintains heart beat	Probably excitation

Table 11.3	Comparison of Skeletal Muscle, Cardiac Muscle and Smooth Muscle—cont'd		
	Skeletal muscle	Cardiac muscle	Smooth muscle*
• Calcium (Ca^{++})	Present mostly in sarcoplasmic reticulum and stimulates ATPase activity during muscle contractions	Increases strength of contraction and duration of systole	Same as in skeletal muscle
• Potassium (K^+)	Decreases excitability and hastens fatigue	Inhibits contraction and produces relaxations	Same as in skeletal muscle
Metabolism			
• Carbohydrates Lactic acid	Lactic acid is oxidized less easily than glucose and often incomplete	Lactic acid is completely and more readily oxidized than glucose	Same as in skeletal muscle
• Blood supply and oxygen consumption	Moderate	High	Less

Type and duration of action potential in smooth muscles

Single unit
Action potential in single unit smooth muscle is of the following types:

- *Spike potentials:* Typical as seen is skeletal muscle. It occurs in most of the types of single unit fibres. Duration of 10 to 50 ms. Such action potentials are initiated by electrical stimulation, hormones, transmitters or spontaneously.
- *Action potential with plateaus:* Onset is that of spike but repolarization is delayed. Duration of hundred to several thousand milliseconds. Plateaus account for prolonged contraction, e.g. ureters.
- *Slow wave potential in single unit:* This can generate spontaneously the action potentials. Some smooth muscles are self-excitatory and associated with slow wave basic rhythm of membrane potential (e.g. visceral smooth muscle). Cause of slow wave rhythm is not known but probably due to waxing and waning of the pumping of Na^+ outward. Membrane potential becomes more negative when Na^+ is pumped rapidly and less negative when pump is less active. Another suggestion is that conductance of ion channels increases and decreases rhythmically. Slow waves themselves cannot cause muscle contraction but can elicit action potential. When membrane potential rises up to –35 mV (threshold for exciting action potential in smooth muscle), action potential develops and spreads over the muscle.

Multiunit
Depolarization of multiunit: Normally multiunit smooth muscle contracts mainly in response to nerve stimuli like skeletal muscle. The nerve endings release acetylcholine in some multiunit and norepinephrine in others. In both, the transmitter causes depolarization. Even sometimes without action potential, multiunit fibres may have local depolarization called functional potential caused by neurotransmitter and this local potential spreads electrotonically to cause muscle contractions.

SMOOTH MUSCLE

What are the types of smooth muscle?

There are two types of smooth muscle as follows:

1. *Multiunit smooth muscle.* Each fibre in a muscle can contract independently. Its contraction is mainly controlled through nervous signals. It rarely exhibits spontaneous contractions. Functionally it is similar to skeletal muscle, e.g. ciliary muscle of the eye, muscle of iris.

2. *Single unit smooth muscle.* Mass of hundreds of muscle fibres contracts simultaneously as a single unit. It is a type of syncytial muscle. Functionally it is similar to cardiac muscle, e.g. visceral smooth muscle, walls of different viscera (blood vessels, bile ducts, etc.).

What is the source of energy of the smooth muscle?

Fatty acids, acetoacetic acid and to a lesser extent glucose are the sources of energy for smooth muscle.

What is the sequence of events in contraction and relaxation of visceral smooth muscle?

Sequence of events in contraction and relaxation of visceral smooth muscle are:

- Binding of acetylcholine to muscarinic receptors.
- Increased influx of Ca^{++} into the cell.
- Activation of calmodium-dependent myosin light chain kinase.
- Phosphorylation of myosin.
- Binding of myosin to actin and increase in myosin ATPase activity.
- Contraction of the muscle.
- Dephosphorylation of myosin by various phosphatases.
- Relaxation or sustained contraction due to latch bridge mechanism.

What is plasticity of smooth muscle?

Smooth muscle exerts variable tension at any given length. This characteristic is known as plasticity.

If a piece of smooth muscle is stretched, it first exerts increased tension. However, if muscle is held at greater length after stretching, tension gradually decreases. It is consequently impossible to correlate length and develop tension accurately and no resting length can be assigned. Thus smooth muscle becomes more like viscous mass than a rigidity structured tissue and this property is referred as plasticity of smooth muscle.

CHAPTER 12

Cardiovascular System

INTRODUCTION

Enumerate the functions of cardiovascular system.

1. Distribution of metabolites and oxygen to all the body cells.
2. Collection of waste products and CO_2 from different body cells and carry them to excretory organs.
3. Thermoregulation—Carrying of heat from active metabolic sites (where heat is generated) to body surface where it is dissipated. Blood flow through skin varies to enhance or decrease the heat loss to the environment.
4. Distribution of hormones to the target tissues.

Heart which is a muscle pump provides the driving force causing flow of blood for the system whereas arteries are the distributing channels. Veins act as reservoirs and also collect and return the blood back to the heart.

Between arteries and veins, there are capillaries which actually supply blood to tissue cells. They act as exchange vessels because they are thin walled.

Name various chambers of the heart.

Heart is divided into left and right heart. Each half is further divided into two parts—atrium and ventricle. Thus, there are four chambers of the heart: left and right auricles (atria) and left and right ventricles. Right side of the heart collects the deoxygenated blood from tissues and pumps it to the lungs for oxygenation, whereas left heart collects the oxygenated blood from lungs and pumps the oxygenated blood to different tissues. Thus, heart actually has two pumps—right and left.

How are the different chambers of the heart separated?

Left chambers of the heart are separated from the right chambers by a continuous partition. The atrial portion of this partition is known as interatrial septum while ventricular part is known as interventricular septum.

The right atrioventricular opening is guarded by a tricuspid valve so named because it has three cusps, viz. anterior, posterior and medial. Left atrioventricular opening is guarded by a bicuspid valve (mitral) which has two cusps, viz. anterior and posterior.

What are semilunar valves?

From left ventricle arises the aorta which carries blood to the tissues and from right ventricle arises the pulmonary artery (trunk) which carries deoxygenated blood to the lungs. The openings between aorta, pulmonary artery and respective ventricles are guarded by semilunar valves, having three cusps.

What is the function of valves in the heart?

Valves allow unidirectional flow of blood. Atrioventricular valves open towards the ventricles and close towards the atria. They allow blood to flow from atria to ventricles but when ventricles contract, they are closed and thus prevent back flow of blood from ventricles to atria.

Semilunar valves open away from ventricles and close towards the ventricles. These valves open when ventricles contract allowing the blood to flow from ventricles to aorta and pulmonary trunk. They close when ventricles relax thus preventing back flow of blood from aorta or pulmonary trunk into the ventricles.

Describe the course of systemic circulation.

Systemic or greater circulation is responsible for pumping oxygenated blood to different tissues and collecting deoxygenated blood from tissues back to the heart. In this circulation, blood is pumped by the left ventricle to all the tissues (except the lungs) and is returned back to the right atrium. Vessels carrying blood away from heart are termed arteries and those carrying blood from tissues to heart are called veins.

In systemic circuit, blood leaves left ventricle via a single large artery, the aorta. The systemic arteries branch from aorta dividing into progressively smaller branches. The smallest arteries form arterioles which branch into very small, thin walled capillaries only lined by single layer of endothelial cells. Through these, exchange of materials between blood, tissues and cells occurs. Capillaries unite to form thicker vessels called venules (arterioles, capillaries and venules are collectively known as microcirculation).

Venules in systemic circulation unite to form larger vessels called veins. The veins from various peripheral organs unite to form two large veins: inferior vena cava which collects blood from lower portions of the body and superior vena cava collecting blood from the upper half of the body. Through these two veins, blood returns to the right atrium.

Describe the course of pulmonary circulation.

Pulmonary circulation is responsible for pumping the deoxygenated blood to the lungs and collecting oxygenated blood from lungs back to the heart as follows:

Blood leaves the right ventricle via a single large artery, the pulmonary trunk which divides into two pulmonary arteries, one supplying each lung. In the lungs, the arteries continue to branch ultimately forming capillaries that unite into the venules and veins. The blood leaves the lungs via pulmonary veins which empty into the left atrium.

Describe the path of blood through entire cardiovascular system.

Path of blood

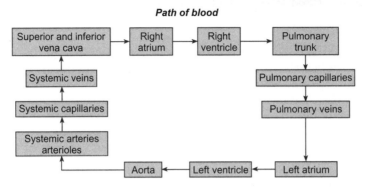

CARDIAC MUSCLE

Describe in short the structure of cardiac muscle.

Cardiac muscle (myocardium) consists of the separate cardiac muscle cells (striated) that are electrically connected to one another by tight junctions. These connections are low resistance pathways and are called intercalated disc. Though there is no anatomical connection between different cardiac muscle fibres from functional point of view, action potential passes from one cardiac muscle cell to the other through gap junctions and cardiac muscle acts as a syncytium of many cardiac muscle cells, i.e. excitation of one cardiac cell causes the action potential to spread to all the other cells. Heart is composed of two separate syncytium—the atrial syncytium (walls of two atria) and ventricular syncytium (walls of two ventricles). Action potential is conducted from atrial syncytium to ventricular syncytium by way of specialized conducting system. Normally there is one functional electrical connection between atria and the ventricles. This is AV node and its extension 'bundle of His'. Because atria and ventricles are two separate syncytium, atria contract a short time ahead of ventricular contraction (Fig. 12.1).

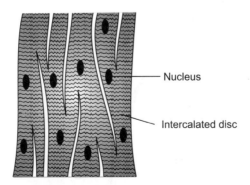

FIGURE 12.1 The syncytial nature of cardiac muscle.

INITIATION AND CONDUCTION OF CARDIAC IMPULSE

What is autorhythmicity?

Cardiac fibres especially, specialized conducting systems have the property of self-excitation because of which they can cause initiation of rhythmic impulses which in turn can cause automatic rhythmic contractions. This property is called autorhythmicity. Sinus node normally initiates the rhythmic impulse and controls the rate of beating of the heart. Thus it is called pacemaker of the heart.

Describe the specialized excitatory conductive system of the heart.

There is a specialized excitatory system which generates rhythmic impulses to cause rhythmic contraction of the heart and special conductive system which conducts these impulses throughout the heart.

EXCITATORY AND CONDUCTIVE SYSTEM (FIG. 12.2)

1. *SA node (sinoatrial node).* It is located near the junction of superior vena cava and the right atrium. It acts as a pacemaker because the rate of impulse generation is highest.

2. *Interatrial tract (Bachman's bundle).* It is a band of specialized muscle fibres that run from sinoatrial node to left atrium. It causes simultaneous depolarization of both the atria, since the velocity of conduction of impulse in this tract is faster than rest of the atrial muscles.

3. *Internodal tracts.* Three pairs of specialized cells connect sinoatrial node to atrioventricular node. They are anterior, middle and posterior. Through them impulses from sinoatrial node reach atrioventricular node to initiate ventricular contraction. These are specialized conducting fibres mixed in the atrial muscle.

4. *AV node (atrioventricular node).* It is located just beneath the endocardium on the right side of the interatrial septum, near the tricuspid valve. Normally it is the only path through which ventricles are activated.

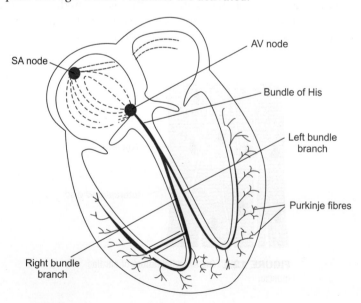

FIGURE 12.2 Special excitatory and conductive system of the heart.

5. *Bundle of His.* It is the continuation of AV node and is located beneath the endocardium on the right side of the interventricular septum. It divides into two branches known as right and left bundle branches. These proceed on each side of the interventricular septum to their respective ventricles.

6. *Purkinje fibres.* These fibres arise from both the bundle branches and branch out extensively just beneath the endocardium of both the ventricles.

Why does sinus node act as a pacemaker of the heart?

Other parts of the conductive system are also capable of generating their rhythm but still SA node acts as a pacemaker because rate of impulse generation by SA node is highest.

Explain the mechanism responsible for sinus nodal rhythmicity.

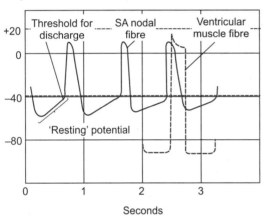

FIGURE 12.3 Rhythmic discharge of an SA nodal fibre.

Sinoatrial nodal fibres have a resting membrane potential which is not steady. It manifests a slow depolarization. This is because of leakage of the resting membrane for sodium. This causes slow diffusion of sodium ions into the SA nodal fibres under-resting condition. The potential therefore, slowly rises from -55 mV due to entry of sodium ions. When potential rises to a threshold level, i.e. -40 mV, the slow voltage-gated sodium-calcium channels open and action potential is initiated. Entry of sodium and calcium through the opened channels causes a rapid depolarization (i.e. action potential). Then at the end of depolarization, potassium channels open and Na^+-Ca^{++} channels close. This causes potassium ions to diffuse out of the fibres resulting into rapid repolarization to -55 to -60 mV. Again because of leakage of membrane to sodium ions, there is slow diffusion of sodium ions causing slow depolarization. When potential reaches a threshold (-40 mV), another action potential is initiated because of opening of slow voltage-gated sodium-calcium channels. Thus, there is initiation of impulses (action potentials) at regular intervals of time (autorhythmicity) (Fig. 12.3).

Describe the impulse conduction from SA node to Purkinje system.

Action potential is initiated in the SA nodal fibres. Ends of SA nodal fibres are fused with surrounding atrial muscle fibres. Therefore, action potential originated in SA node travels outward in these fibres. This way impulse spreads over the atria. Conduction is more rapid in several small bundles of atrial fibres called interatrial tract or band. Conduction through these fibres causes simultaneous depolarization of both the atria. The rate of conduction in these fibres is 1 m/sec.

There are three pairs of internodal tracts (anterior, middle, posterior) through which impulse passes from SA node to AV node fibres.

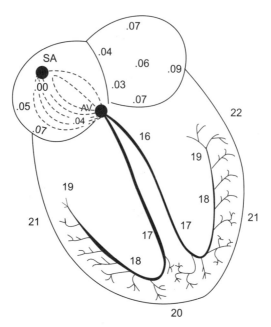

FIGURE 12.4 Transmission of the cardiac impulse through the heart showing the time of appearance (in fraction of a second) of the impulse in different parts of the heart.

Impulse reaches AV node within 0.03 sec after its origin in SA node. At AV node, there is a delay of 0.09 second and further delay in 'bundle of His', for 0.04 second (total delay is 0.13 second) (Fig. 12.4).

CAUSES OF AV NODAL DELAY

- Fibres connecting internodal tract and AV node are called transitional fibres. These are very small fibres conducting the impulse at a very slow rate, i.e. 0.02 to 0.05 m/sec.
- Velocity of impulse conduction in AV nodal fibres is also slow, i.e. 0.05 m/sec.
- Resting membrane potentials of transitional fibres and AV nodal fibres are much less negative than rest of the cardiac muscle fibres.
- There are very few gap junctions connecting successive fibres in the pathway.

Bundle of His conducts impulse from AV node to its left and right branches. Except in certain abnormal states, fibres of AV bundle conduct the impulse from atria to ventricle and not in the reverse direction. This allows forward conduction of impulse. Atrial muscle is separated from ventricular muscle by a continuous fibrous barrier which acts as a barrier to passage of impulse through any other route from atria to ventricles except through AV bundle.

AV bundle passes downward in ventricular septum for 5 to 15 mm and then divides into left and right bundle branches. Through these branches, impulse passes to two ventricles. Branches divide into Purkinje fibres which become continuous with cardiac muscle fibres.

The time taken for impulse to travel from bundle branches to Purkinje fibres is 0.03 second. Through Purkinje fibres, impulse is spread rapidly to ventricular muscle fibres. The velocity of transmission of impulse in ventricular muscle fibres is 0.3 to 0.5 m/sec. It first spreads over the endocardial surface and then the cardiac muscle fibres which are arranged in double spirals. Therefore, impulse does not necessarily travel outwards (towards the surface) but it angulates towards the surface along the directions of spirals. Therefore, transmission from endocardial surface to epicardial surface takes about 0.03 second. Thus total time for transmission in normal heart from initial bundle branches to ventricles is 0.06 second.

Total time required for conduction from SA node to endocardial surface is 0.22 second.

What is the importance of AV nodal delay?

Atria and ventricles are excited at different times and also contract at different times because of AV nodal delay.

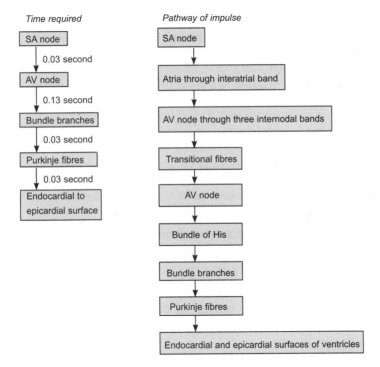

What is the resting membrane potential of normal cardiac muscle?

Resting membrane potential of normal cardiac muscle is from −85 to –95 mV.

Describe the action potential of the cardiac muscle.

Record of action potential in the ventricular muscle shows that there is an initial spike, i.e. rising of resting membrane potential from −85 to −90 mV to a slightly positive value (up to +20 mV) **(Phase-0)**. The positive portion is called overshoot potential. There is a short phase of repolarization **(Phase-1)** due to inactivation of sodium channels. Then membrane remains depolarized for 0.2 second in atrial and 0.3 second in ventricular muscle fibres. This sustained depolarization is seen as plateau **(Phase-2)**. This is due to calcium influx through opening of slow calcium channels. After plateau, due to net efflux of potassium ions, there is abrupt repolarization

(Phase-3). After repolarization is complete, the potential comes back to resting level (Phase-4) (Fig. 12.5).

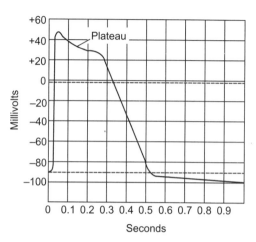

FIGURE 12.5 An action potential from Purkinje fibre of the heart showing plateau.

What is the cause of plateau recorded in cardiac muscle action potential?

1. Initial spike of action potential of cardiac muscle is due to opening of fast voltage-gated sodium channels causing diffusion of sodium ions into the fibres. Plateau is due to opening of slow voltage-gated calcium-sodium channels through which calcium and sodium ions continue to diffuse into the fibre. This causes prolonged phase of depolarization, i.e. plateau.

2. At the onset of action potential, permeability of membrane for potassium decreases about fivefold. This greatly decreases potassium outflux during action potential plateau and thereby prevents repolarization. When slow calcium-sodium channels close at the end of 0.2 to 0.3 second, then membrane permeability for potassium rapidly increases causing rapid outflux of potassium. This results in returning of membrane potential to resting level.

What is the velocity of conduction of impulse in the cardiac muscle?

Velocity of conduction of impulse (action potential) in both atrial and ventricular muscle fibres is about 0.3 to 0.5 m/sec.

How much is the refractory period of cardiac muscle?

Absolute refractory period of atrial muscle is 0.15 second and relative refractory period is 0.03 second. Ventricles have absolute refractory period much longer from 0.25 to 0.30 second and relative refractory period for additional 0.05 second.

Explain the phenomenon of excitation-contraction coupling in the cardiac muscle.

Sarcoplasmic reticulum in the cardiac muscle is less well developed than in skeletal muscle. It is present as a network of tubules surrounding the myofibrils. It has dilated terminals (cisternae) which are located next to the external cell membrane and T tubules. Sarcoplasmic reticulum and cisternae contain high concentration of ionic calcium.

T tubules are continuations of cell membrane and they conduct action potential to the interior of the cell. They invaginate to the interior of the cell at the 'Z' line of sarcomere. Therefore, there is only one T tubule present per sarcomere.

When action potential passes over the cardiac muscle membrane, it passes to the interior of the muscle cells through T tubules.

Action potential acts on the membranes of longitudinal sarcoplasmic tubules to cause instantaneous release of calcium. Calcium ions diffuse into the myofibrils and catalyze chemical reactions that promote sliding of actin and myosin filaments which in turn produce muscle contraction. In addition, in cardiac muscle (as against that in skeletal muscle) extra calcium ions diffuse into the sarcoplasm from 'T' tubules without which contraction strength would be considerably reduced.

'T' tubules of cardiac muscle contain mucopolysaccharides, which are negatively charged and bind an abundant store of calcium ions. 'T' tubules open directly to the exterior and therefore calcium ions in them directly come from extracellular fluid. These calcium ions diffuse into the sarcoplasm when action potential propagates along the 'T' tubules. Because of this, strength of cardiac muscle contraction depends to a great extent on calcium concentration in extracellular fluid; whereas skeletal muscle contraction is hardly affected by calcium concentration in ECF.

What is the duration of contraction in cardiac muscle?

Duration of contraction for atrial muscle is 0.1 sec and for ventricular muscle is 0.3 second.

What is ectopic pacemaker?

When pacemaker is other than SA node it is called ectopic pacemaker, e.g. AV node or Punkinje fibres may act as pacemakers. Ectopic pacemaker causes abnormal sequence of contraction of different parts of the heart.

APPLIED ASPECT

What are the causes of shift of pacemaker?

Causes of shift of pacemaker from SA node to other sites are:

- Rate of discharge in other parts of the heart becomes higher than that of SA node.
- Blockage of transmission of impulse from SA node to AV node.

What is Stokes–Adams syndrome?

When there is AV block, atria continue to beat at the normal rhythm (i.e. of SA node) while new pacemaker develops in Purkinje system of ventricles with a rate of 15 to 40/min. But after a sudden block, Purkinje system does not begin its rhythm immediately. It takes about 15 to 30 seconds. During this time, ventricles fail to contract. Thus the person faints because of lack of blood flow to the brain. This delayed pick-up of heart beat is called Stokes-Adams syndrome. If this period too long, death may occur.

NERVOUS CONTROL OF HEART RHYTHM

Explain the role of autonomic nervous system in controlling heart rhythm.

Heart is supplied by parasympathetic and sympathetic nerves. Parasympathetic supply passes through vagus nerve. Sympathetic supply comes from 1 to 5 thoracic segments of spinal cord. Preganglionic fibres relay in superior, middle and inferior cervical ganglia. Postganglionic nerves supply the heart. Vagi nerves mainly innervate sinus and AV nodes, to a lesser extent the muscle of two atria and even to a lesser extent the ventricular muscle. Sympathetic nerves are distributed to all parts of the heart, especially to ventricular muscles as well as to other areas.

EFFECT OF PARASYMPATHETIC STIMULATION

Parasympathetic stimulation causes release of acetylcholine at vagal nerve endings. It causes: (a) decrease in the heart rate by decreasing the rate of sinus rhythm, (b) decreased excitation of AV node, AV junctional fibres, atrial musculature, thus reducing the rate of transmission of impulse into ventricles. Strong stimulation may completely block the transmission and ventricles may stop beating for 4 to 10 seconds. If it happens, Purkinje system initiates the rhythm causing ventricular contraction at a rate of 15 to 40/min. This phenomenon is called vagal escape.

Mechanism of action. Acetylcholine released at the nerve endings increases the permeability of the fibre membrane for potassium ions. This causes rapid diffusion of potassium to the exterior of the fibre causing hyperpolarization, decreasing excitability of the tissue.

EFFECT OF SYMPATHETIC STIMULATION

Sympathetic stimulation increases the rate of sinus rhythm, rate of conduction of impulse as well as increased excitability in all the portions of the heart. Force of contraction of atria and ventricles increases greatly.

Mechanism of action. Stimulation of sympathetic nerves causes release of norepinephrine at the nerve endings. Probably this increases permeability of cardiac muscle fibre to sodium and calcium. In AV node increased sodium permeability makes it easier for action potential to excite the surrounding portion, decreasing rate of conduction time from atria to ventricles. Increased permeability for calcium increases the contractile strength of the heart.

What is vagal tone?

Right vagus nerve innervates the SA node and liberates acetylcholine from its endings. Normally, vagal activity hyperpolarizes SA node fibres by increasing permeability of SA nodal fibres for potassium. This hyperpolarization slows the firing rate of SA node from its automatic rate of 90 to 120 beats/min to the actual heart rate of about 72 beats/min. This normal vagal activity is called vagal tone.

CARDIAC CYCLE

What is cardiac cycle?

The period of beginning of one heart beat to the beginning of the next is called cardiac cycle.

What is normocardia?

Normal resting heart rate of 60 to 100 beats/min is called normocardia.

What is tachycardia?

Heart rate more than 100 beats/min is termed tachycardia.

What is bradycardia?

Heart rate below 60 beats/min is termed bradycardia. It is commonly seen in well-trained athletes.

Name various cardiac cycle events.

Cardiac cycle includes both electrical (ECG) and mechanical events. Electrical events precede and initiate the corresponding mechanical events.

Name the different mechanical events occurring during cardiac cycle.

Main events in cardiac cycle are: (a) atrial contraction (systole) and atrial relaxation (diastole), (b) ventricular contraction (systole) and (c) ventricular relaxation (diastole).
   The total period of one cycle is 0.8 second.
   Atrial systole is 0.1 second and atrial diastole is 0.7 second.
   Ventricular systole is 0.3 second and ventricular diastole is 0.5 second.
Other events are as follows:

- Atrial systole (0.1 second).
- Ventricular systole consisting of:
   (i) Isovolumic (isometric) contraction (0.05 second).
   (ii) Rapid ejection (0.11 second).
   (iii) Reduced ejection (0.14 second).
- Ventricular diastole consisting of:
   (i) Protodiastole (0.04 second).
   (ii) Isovolumic (isometric) relaxation (0.06 second).
   (iii) Rapid passive filling (0.11 second).
   (iv) Reduced filling (diastasis) (0.19 second).
   (v) Second rapid filling (atrial systole) (0.1 second).

Describe the various events in the cardiac cycle.

   1. *Atrial systole (contraction).* During the period of ventricular relaxation, blood flows from atria to ventricles. About 75% of the blood flows to ventricles before atria contract. Both atria contract almost simultaneously and pump the remaining 25% of blood into the respective ventricles (therefore even if atria fail to function it is unlikely to be noticed unless a person exercises). The contraction of atria increases, the pressure inside the atria to 4 to 6 mmHg in the right atrium and about 7 to 8 mmHg in the left atrium. The pressure rise in right atrium is reflected into the veins and this wave is recorded as 'a' wave (recorded from jugular vein with the help of a transducer).
   Then there is a period of atrial diastole for rest of the cardiac cycle (0.7 second) during which various ventricular events occur in sequence as follows:
   2. *Ventricular systole (contraction).* At the termination of atrial contraction, the pressure of blood in the ventricles rises (normally less than 12 mmHg). Rising ventricular pressure now exceeds the atrial pressure.

This causes closure of AV valves which is a major component responsible for generating first heart sound. Then there are following phases of ventricular systole:

- *Isovolumic or isometric contraction.* At the beginning of this phase AV valves are closed but semilunar valves are not yet opened. Thus ventricular chambers are sealed from both atria and the arteries. The ventricle starts contracting but volume of blood inside both the ventricles remains the same hence this phase is called isovolumic phase of contraction. This phase lasts for about 0.05 second. During this phase ventricles contract as a closed chamber and pressure inside the ventricles rises rapidly to a high value. When pressure in the left ventricle is slightly above 80 mmHg and right ventricular pressure slightly above 8 mmHg, then the ventricular pressures push the semilunar valves open. This causes ejection of blood from ventricles to the respective arteries in next phases.
- *Rapid ejection phase.* As soon as the semilunar valves open, blood is rapidly ejected. About two-third of the stroke volume is ejected in this rapid ejection phase. The duration of this phase is about 0.11 second. Pressure inside the left ventricle rises to 120 mmHg during this phase. The end of rapid ejection phase occurs at about the peak of ventricular and atrial systolic pressure. The right ventricular ejection begins before that of left and continues even after left ventricular ejection is complete. As both the ventricles almost eject same volume of blood, the velocity of right ventricular ejection is less than that of the left ventricle.
- *Reduced ejection phase.* During later two-third of systole rate of ejection declines. During this phase of reduced ejection, rest one-third stroke volume is ejected. This phase lasts for about 0.14 second. During the period of slow ejection ventricular pressure falls to a value slightly lower than that in aorta but still blood continues to empty into aorta because blood flowing out has built up momentum. As this momentum decreases, kinetic energy of momentum is converted to pressure in the aorta. This causes aortic pressure to rise slightly above that of the ventricle.

3. ***Ventricular diastole or relaxation.*** It occurs in following phases:
   - *Protodiastole*—At the end of ventricular systole, ventricles start relaxing allowing rapid fall in the intraventricular pressures. This is the period of protodiastole which lasts for 0.04 seconds. At the end of this phase, elevated pressure in distended arteries (aorta and pulmonary artery) immediately pushes the blood back towards the ventricles which snaps the aortic and pulmonary semilunar valves closed. This is the major component in generating second sound (closure of semilunar valves). It also causes dicrotic notch in the down slope of aortic pressure called incisura. Incisura indicates end of systole and the onset of diastole.
   - *Isovolumic or isometric relaxation*—The ventricles continue to relax as closed chambers as semilunar valves are closed and AV valves are not yet open. This causes rapid fall of pressure inside the ventricles (from 80 mmHg to about 2 to 3 mmHg in the left ventricle). This phase lasts for 0.06 seconds. Because the ventricular volume remains constant, this phase is called isovolumic phase. When ventricular pressures fall below the atrial pressures the AV valves open.

- *Rapid filling phase*—During ventricular systole because AV valves are closed, large amount of blood accumulates in atria because veins continue to empty the blood into them and this causes increase in pressure inside atria. High atrial pressure causes the blood to flow rapidly into the ventricles. Then pressure in both the chambers fall as ventricular relaxation continues.
- *Reduced filling phase or diastasis*—After the rapid filling phase, pressures in atria and ventricles rise slowly as blood continues to return to the heart. This decreases the rate of blood flow from atria to ventricles causing slow filling of ventricles called diastasis.

During rapid filling and diastasis phase about 75% of blood passes from atria to ventricles. Then the next cycle begins with atrial contraction.

What is stroke volume?

Volume of blood that is ejected by each ventricle with each beat is stroke volume. It is 70 ml.

What is ventricular end diastolic volume?

Ventricular end diastolic volume is the volume of blood in the ventricle just prior to the onset of ventricular contraction. Normally left ventricular end diastolic volume is 110 to 120 ml. It is markedly reduced if the heart rate increases. When heart rate increases periods of systole and diastole become shorter. Decreased period of diastole decreases the filling of ventricle and therefore the end-diastolic volume.

What is ventricular end systolic volume?

Volume of blood remaining in the ventricle at the end of ejection is called end systolic volume. It is normally 40 to 50 ml.

What is ejection fraction?

The fraction of end-diastolic volume that is ejected is called the ejection fraction. Normally it is about 60%.

Describe the pressure changes in atria during cardiac cycle.

Atrial pressure curves show three major pressure elevations which are called 'a', 'c' and 'v' waves.

1. The 'a' wave is caused by atrial contraction. Ordinarily, right atrial pressure rises about 4 to 6 mmHg and left atrial pressure rises about 7 to 8 mmHg during this atrial contraction. Wave appears during atrial systole.
2. The 'c' wave occurs when the ventricles begin to contract. It is partly caused by slight back flow of blood into atria at the onset of ventricular contraction but mainly caused due to bulging of AV valves towards the atria because of increasing pressure in the ventricles. This wave therefore appears in the phase of isovolumic contraction of the ventricles.
3. The 'v' wave occurs towards the end of ventricular contraction. It results from slow build-up of pressure in atria due to collection of blood from veins while AV valves are closed during ventricular contraction. This wave

occurs therefore during isometric relaxation phase of ventricle. After this phase AV valves open, allowing rapid flow of blood into the ventricles causing 'v' wave to disappear (Fig. 12.6).

Describe the pressure changes in the left ventricle during cardiac cycle.

Before atrial systole, the pressure inside the left ventricle is almost zero; when left atrium contracts and forces blood into the left ventricle, pressure rises to about 7 mmHg.

At the end of atrial systole, AV valve closes and semilunar valve is not yet open. Ventricle contracts as a closed chamber (isometric contraction) and therefore pressure inside the ventricle rapidly rises from 7 to 80 mmHg.

At the end of isometric contraction, semilunar valve opens and ventricle starts contracting isotonically. This causes pressure to rise to a peak level of 120 mmHg during rapid ejection phase. Then there is reduced ejection phase in which because of decreased volume of blood in the ventricle pressure decreases slightly to 100 mmHg. Then semilunar valve (aortic valve) is closed and ventricular diastole starts.

During isovolumic relaxation phase, ventricle relaxes as a closed chamber and therefore there is a great pressure fall in the left ventricle from 100 mmHg to about 2 to 3 mmHg. Then AV valve opens and ventricular filling begins.

During rapid filling and diastasis though the ventricle is getting filled and volume of blood is increasing because of relaxation of ventricle, pressure in the ventricle drops to almost zero (Fig. 12.6).

Describe the volume changes in the ventricles.

During ventricular diastole, filling of ventricles increases the volume of blood in ventricle, to about 110 to 120 ml which is called end diastolic volume. During ventricular

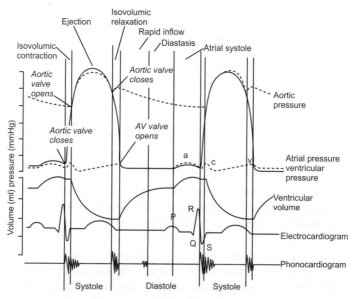

FIGURE 12.6 Events of cardiac cycle showing changes in atrial pressure, left ventricular pressure, ventricular volume, aortic pressure, ECG and phonocardiogram.

contraction, blood flows rapidly out in phase of rapid ejection and comparatively slowly in slow ejection phase leading to fall in volume to 40 to 50 ml (70 ml blood is pumped out). Thus end systolic blood volume is 40 to 50 ml (Fig. 12.6).

What is the function of papillary muscles?

Papillary muscles are attached to the veins of AV valves by the chordae tendineae. Papillary muscles contract when ventricular walls contract and pull veins of the valves towards the ventricle to prevent the excessive bulging of valves towards the atria during ventricular contraction.

Describe aortic pressure changes during cardiac cycle.

Pressure in the aorta varies between 80 and 120 mmHg during cardiac cycle. During the period of rapid ventricular ejection, the pressure in the aorta is slightly less than that of the ventricle. The peak aortic pressure is arterial systolic pressure and occurs at the end of rapid ejection. It is 120 mmHg. Then pressure slightly falls during reduced ejection phase. At the end of reduced ejection phase aortic pressure becomes slightly more than that in the ventricles. This causes closure of semilunar valves, but also causes backward flow of blood. After the aortic valve has closed, pressure in the aorta falls slowly throughout the diastole because blood stored in distended elastic arteries continues to flow to the periphery. Before the ventricles contract again, aortic pressure falls to 80 mmHg (diastolic pressure). The incisura during the down slope of the aortic pressure indicates the end of ventricular systole (Fig. 12.6).

Describe pressure changes in the pulmonary artery during cardiac cycle.

Pressure curve in the pulmonary artery is similar to that of aorta but pressures are low (about one-sixth of that in aorta). Pulmonary artery systolic pressure averages 15 to 18 mmHg and its pressure during diastole is 8 to 10 mmHg.

What is work output of heart?

Work output of the heart can be expressed as stroke work output or minute work output. Stroke work output of the heart is the amount of energy that the heart converts to work during each heartbeat. Minute work output is the total amount of energy that is converted to work in a period of one minute.

∴ Minute work output = Stroke work output × Heart rate.

How does heart muscle derive energy for work?

The energy for work of the heart is derived from oxidative metabolism mainly of fatty acids and to a lesser extent of other nutrients. Therefore, rate of O_2 consumption by the heart is excellent measure of the chemical energy liberated while heart performs the work.

How much is mechanical efficiency of the heart muscle?

Ratio of work output to total chemical energy expenditures (amount of energy converted to work) is called efficiency of heart. Maximum efficiency of normal heart is 20 to 25%. In heart failure, it may reduce to 5–10%.

Describe regulation of pumping of heart.

Pumping of heart is regulated by two mechanisms: intrinsic cardiac regulation, and control by autonomic nervous system.

1. *Intrinsic regulation.* Heart adapts to changes in blood volume it receives. Rate of blood flowing into the heart through veins each minute is known as venous return. Greater the venous return, greater is the pumping ability to pump excess incoming blood into the arteries. This intrinsic ability to adapt to changing volume is called 'Frank-Starling' mechanism of heart. This is because the force of contraction of heart is proportional to initial length of muscle fibre (Frank-Starling law). When there is increased venous return, there is stretch on the cardiac muscle wall which increases the initial length of muscle fibres which in turn increases the force of contraction. Stretch of muscle also increases the heart rate.

2. *Control by autonomic nervous system.*
   (a) Sympathetic stimulation increases the heart rate and also the force of contraction of heart. Thus, volume of blood pumped by heart increases. Also the ejection pressure increases. Sympathetic stimulation can increase cardiac output as much as two to threefold.
   Inhibition of sympathetic system has opposite effects. Under normal conditions, there is a continuous slow rate of discharge through sympathetic fibres to the heart which maintains pumping 30% above that with no sympathetic stimulation. Therefore, when sympathetic activity is inhibited, both heart rate and force of ventricular contraction decrease.
   (b) Parasympathetic (vagal) stimulation decreases the heart rate and force of contraction. The effect on the force is not much because vagal fibres are mainly distributed to the atria and not much to the ventricles. Decrease in strength of heart contraction is only 20 to 30%. Very strong stimulation of vagi can actually stop the heart beat for few seconds but then heart escapes (vagal escape) action of vagus and starts beating but at a lower rate (20 to 30 beats/min).

What are the effects of ions on heart function?
EFFECT OF POTASSIUM IONS

- Excess potassium concentration in extracellular fluid causes heart to become extremely dilated.
- There is blockage of conduction of impulses from atria to ventricle through AV bundle. This is partially caused due to decreased resting membrane potential in cardiac muscles. As membrane potential decreases intensity of action potential also decreases.

EFFECT OF CALCIUM IONS

Excess calcium ions in the extracellular fluid increase force of contraction of heart and heart can go into spastic spasm. Conversely decreased calcium ions cause cardiac flaccidity. Effect of calcium ions is directly on the contracting process.

What is the effect of temperature on heart?

Increase in temperature causes increased permeability of heart resulting into acceleration of self-excitation process. Contractile strength of heart is often enhanced temporarily with moderate increase in temperature. But prolonged elevation of temperature exhausts the metabolic system and causes weakness.

HEART SOUNDS

Give an account of the heart sounds.

Closure of the valves of the heart is associated with audible sounds. Normally the heart sounds are heard with a stethoscope; these are described as first and second heart sounds. Occasionally, the third heart sound which is very weak is heard. But the fourth heart sound is not heard by stethoscope because it has very low frequency. It can only be recorded in phonocardiogram (Fig. 12.7).

Heart sounds are not directly heard over the valves themselves but they are better heard over four auscultatory areas.

- *Mitral area.* This area lies over the apex beat (normally in the fifth left intercostal space three and half inches lateral to the midsternal line).
- *Tricuspid area.* This lies at the lower end of sternum.
- *Aortic area.* This area lies in the right second intercostal space near the lateral border of the sternum.
- *Pulmonary area.* This area lies in the left second intercostal space near the lateral border of the sternum.

Both the heart sounds, first and second are heard in all four auscultatory areas, but at mitral and tricuspid areas first heart sound is better heard because sound caused by A-V valves are transmitted to the chest wall through the respective ventricles. Second heart sound is better heard over the aortic and pulmonary areas because sounds caused by closure of semilunar valves are transmitted to the aorta and pulmonary artery.

1. **First heart sound.** This sound is produced due to closure of A-V valves. Slapping together of valve, leaflets set up vibrations causing vibrations of the adjacent blood, walls of the heart and major vessels around the heart. Contraction of ventricles causes valves to bulge against atria until chordae tendineae abruptly stop the back bulging. The elastic tautness of the valves (tricuspid and mitral valves) then cause back surging blood to bounce forward again into each respective ventricle. This sets blood, ventricular walls and valves into vibration. It causes vibrating turbulence in the blood. Vibrations travel to surrounding tissues and to the chest wall where sound can be heard with the help of the stethoscope. It is like a word LUBB. It is better heard over mitral and tricuspid areas. The duration of the first sound is 0.14 second, and is low pitched.

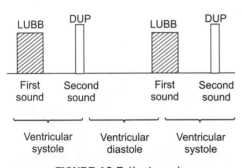

FIGURE 12.7 Heart sounds.

SIGNIFICANCE:

- It indicates the onset of clinical systole of the ventricles.
- The duration and intensity of the first sound indicates the condition of myocardium. If

myocardium is weak, first heart sound is short and low pitched. It is prominent when there is hypertrophy of myocardium.
- Normal first sound also indicates that A-V valves are properly closing (there is no incompetence).

2. *Second heart sound.* The second heart sound is due to closure of semilunar valves. It is of higher frequency than the first sound because of (i) tautness of the semilunar valves in comparison with A-V valves, and (ii) greater elastic coefficient of the arteries (which provide the principal vibrating chambers) in comparison with the much looser ventricular chambers (which are vibrating chambers for the first heart sound).

Thus second heart sound is of higher frequency (high pitched), sharp and of short duration (0.11 sec). It is like a word DUP. The intensity of the sound depends on blood pressure. Sometimes two valves aortic and pulmonary do not close simultaneously during inspiration. This causes splitting of second sound during inspiration.

SIGNIFICANCE:
- It indicates end of systole and beginning of diastole of the ventricles.
- Clear second sound indicates that the semilunar valves are closing properly, i.e. there is no incompetence.
- When the interval between first and second sound is shorter, it indicates clinical systole. When the interval between second heart sound and the next first heart sound is longer, it indicates clinical diastole of the heart.

3. *Third heart sound.* Occasionally a very weak rumbling third heart sound is heard at the middle third of the diastole. It does not appear until middle third of diastole because in early part of the diastole the heart is not filled with blood sufficiently to create even small amount of elastic tension in the ventricles. The frequency of this sound is low and sometimes so low that it cannot be heard, yet it can be recorded in the phonocardiogram. Its duration is 0.04 second. It can be identified by its relation with the second sound and it coincides with descending limb of 'v' wave of jugular venous pulse.

4. *Fourth heart sound.* It is also called atrial sound and is caused by inrushing of blood into the ventricle when atria contract which initiates vibrations similar to those of the third heart sound. It has a very low frequency, i.e. below 20 cycles/sec. Therefore, it can never be heard with the help of stethoscope but it can only be recorded by phonocardiogram. It coincides with 'a' wave of jugular venous pulse.

What is phonocardiogram?

It is a specially designed microphone to detect low frequency. It is applied to the precordium. Heart sounds are amplified and recorded by a high speed recording apparatus (oscillograph). The recording is called a phonocardiogram. Machine is also connected with a mirror arrangement which reflects a beam of light on a moving photographic plate. Sounds thus can be graphically recorded.

ELECTROCARDIOGRAM

What is an electrocardiogram?

Record of the electrical changes during the cardiac cycle is known as electrocardiogram.

Name the machine used for recording ECG.

Electrocardiograph is the machine used to record ECG.

Describe the method of recording ECG.

Action potentials generated in the muscle cells of heart can be recorded by placing recording electrodes on the surface of the skin.

The electrodes are connected to the machine (electrocardiograph). The tracings are usually made at a standard recording speed of 25 mm/sec and amplification (1 mV = 1 cm deflection). These tracings are made over the standard ECG paper. This paper is divided into small squares. Each small square on horizontal axis represents 0.04 sec and on vertical axis represents 0.1 mV.

Most modern electrocardiograph has a direct pen writing recorder that writes electrocardiogram with a pen directly on a moving sheet of paper. Pen is often a thin tube connected at one end to an inkwell; and its recording end is connected to a electromagnet system capable of moving the pen back and forth at high speed. As the paper moves forward, the pen records the electrocardiogram. In other recorder instead of ink pen, special paper is used. The paper turns black on exposure to heat. The stylus (recording pen) is made hot by electrical current flowing through its tip. Another type of paper turns black when electric current flows from the tip of the stylus.

What is a lead?

Lead is the connection between two points on the body surface and the electrocardiograph. Hence a lead consists of:

1. Electrodes (metal plates) which are applied on the surface of the body.
2. The lead wires which connect the electrodes to electrocardiograph. To reduce the electrical resistance between electrode and the surface of the body, jelly is used.

What are bipolar leads?

Bipolar leads mean the ECG is recorded from two specific electrodes placed on the body.

Name the different bipolar limb leads used.

Different bipolar limb leads used for recording ECG are:

- Lead I
- Lead II
- Lead III

Describe the bipolar limb leads.

Three leads are formed by measuring the potential differences between any two of the limb electrodes. The leads are selected by a switch on standard ECG machine.

Lead I. For recording ECG in lead I, negative terminal of the electrocardiograph is connected to the right arm and positive terminal to the left arm. When right arm is negative with respect to left arm, the positive wave is recorded.

Lead II. For recording ECG in lead II, negative terminal of the electrocardiograph is connected to the right arm and positive terminal to the left leg. When right arm is negative with respect to left leg, the positive wave is recorded by electrocardiogram.

Lead III. For recording ECG in lead III, negative terminal of the electrocardiograph is connected to the left arm and the positive terminal to the left leg. If left arm is negative with respect to left leg, ECG records the positive wave.

What is Einthoven's triangle?

Einthoven's triangle is the diagrammatic way of illustrating that the two arms and left leg form apices of triangle surrounding the heart. It is the equilateral triangle with the right and left shoulders and left leg as the three apices. The right leg serves as a ground connector. All four electrodes must be attached to the extremities.

What is Einthoven's law?

Einthoven's law states that if electrical potentials of any two of the bipolar limb electrocardiographic leads are known at any given instant, the third one can be determined mathematically by simply summing the first two (but positive and negative signs of different leads must be observed while making the summation) (Fig. 12.8).

What are unipolar leads? Describe unipolar chest leads.

If the three limb leads are connected to a common terminal through electrical resistance the combined voltage from the three leads will be zero, theoretically. This common terminal can be attached to the negative pole of a galvanometer (indifferent electrode) and a fourth or exploring electrode can be attached to the positive pole. The galvanometer can still only read the potential difference between two points but because the common electrode is at zero volts, other electrode (exploring) will provide the actual or absolute voltage at the body surface. This arrangement of connections is termed a unipolar lead. They are used to record, from standardized sites on precordium. There are six such precordial leads called 'V' leads.

The placement of exploring electrode in leads V_1 to V_6 is as follows:
Lead V_1 in the fourth intercostal space, just to the right of the sternum.
Lead V_2 in the fourth intercostal space just to the left of the sternum.
Lead V_4 in the midclavicular line in the fifth left intercostal space.
Lead V_3 halfway between V_2 and V_4.
Lead V_5 in the anterior axillary line at the same level as V_4.
Lead V_6 in the midaxillary line at the same level as V_4 and V_5.

Describe augmented unipolar leads.

There are three unipolar augmented leads: aVR, aVL and aVF. Any of the three limb electrodes can be used to record cardiac potential in comparison to the

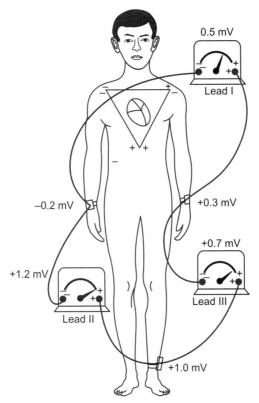

FIGURE 12.8 Conventional arrangement of electrodes for recording the standard electro-cardiographic leads.

common terminal, e.g. voltage recorded in RA (right arm) can be determined by the equation.

RA − (RA + LA + LL) the resulting voltage is small because the potential difference is reduced by the RA potential in common terminal, i.e. (RA + LA + LL).

Disconnecting the RA lead from the common terminal increases the potential difference by 50% and results in augmented limb lead aVR.

aVR is the potential difference between RA and (LA + LL).
aVL is the potential difference between LA and (RA + LL).
aVF is the potential difference between LL and (RA + LA).

In this type of recording two of the limbs are connected through electrical resistances to the negative terminal of the electrocardiograph while the third limb is connected to positive terminal.

The axis of aVR is from −150° to +30°.
The axis of aVL is from −30° to +150°.
The axis of aVF is from +90° to −90°.

Name the different waves and intervals in normal ECG.

Waves and intervals in ECG (Figure 12.9 and Table 12.1)

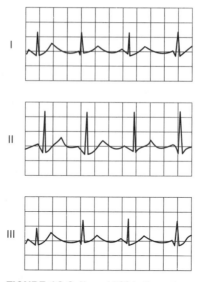

FIGURE 12.9 Normal ECG in three standard leads.

Table 12.1	Normal Waves and Intervals in ECG	
Name	**Description**	**Abnormality**
P wave	It is due to atrial depolarization. It is normally positive (upright) in the standard limb leads and inverted in aVR.	1. 'P' wave is absent in atrial fibrillation. In this condition 'P' waves are replaced by small 'F' waves. 2. 'P' wave is large when there is atrial hypertrophy. It may be also notched. 3. When there is AV nodal rhythm, 'P' wave is inverted.
P-R interval	It is measured from the onset of P wave to the onset of QRS complex. Actually it is PQ interval but Q wave is frequently absent and therefore it is called P-R interval. It is a measure of the AV conduction time and includes the delay through AV node. Its duration normally varies from 0.12 to 0.2 seconds depending upon heart rate.	If P-R interval exceeds 0.2 second, it indicates impaired conduction through AV node. First degree block is produced when PR interval is between 0.2 and 0.3 second. Second degree block is produced when the PR interval is increased to 0.25–0.45 second. When there is complete atrioventricular block, impulses from atria cannot pass to the ventricles. Ventricles start beating at their own rhythm called idioventricular rhythm. ECG shows that there is complete dissociation between P waves and QRS complexes.

Table 12.1	Normal Waves and Intervals in ECG—cont'd	
Name	**Description**	**Abnormality**
QRS complex	It is caused by ventricular depolarization. It is measured from onset of 'Q' to the cessation of 'S' wave. It measures total ventricular depolarization time. Its duration is normally less than 0.08 second. It is a measure of intraventricular conduction time. Voltage of QRS is measured from peak of R wave to the bottom of S wave. It varies between 0.5 and 2 mV (lead III recording lowest and lead II recording the highest voltage).	QRS complex should not exceed 0.1 second. If it is prolonged it indicates bundle branch block. When sum of voltages of QRS complex in three standard leads is greater than 4 mV, it is considered that the patient has a high voltage ECG. The cause of this high voltage in most of the cases is increased muscular mass of the heart (hypertrophy). There may be decreased voltage of ECG due to cardiac myopathies, pericardial effusion (due to short circuiting of electrical potentials generated by heart into pericardial fluid), pulmonary emphysema (due to decreased conduction of electric current through emphysematous lungs). Lungs thus prevent flow of electric current from heart to the surface electrodes. Bizarre QRS pattern is obtained when: • Cardiac muscle is destroyed in various areas and is replaced by scar tissue. • Block in conduction of impulses by Purkinje system will also cause bizarre pattern of QRS complexes. Prominent 'Q' wave indicates old infarction.
Q-T interval	It is measured from beginning of 'Q' wave to the end of 'T' wave. Normally it is 0.35 second. Ventricular contraction usually lasts almost during this interval. It indicates total systolic time of ventricles.	

Continued

Table 12.1	Normal Waves and Intervals in ECG—cont'd	
Name	Description	Abnormality
T wave	It is caused by ventricular repolarization and is normally in the same direction as the QRS complex, since ventricular repolarization follows the path that is opposite to depolarization.	In old age T wave is flattened. Exercise increases its amplitude in healthy hearts. It is inverted when there is ischaemia (sometimes T wave is inverted in lead III without any apparent reason). Abnormalities of 'T' wave in shape, size, duration, direction in leads I and II are of diagnostic importance. These changes indicate myocardial damage associated with cardiac hypoxia (ischaemia). When there is ischaemia of the cardiac muscle, ischaemic portion of the heart takes a longer time for depolarization.
R-R interval	It is the time interval during successive QRS complexes. If it is 1 second, heart rate is 60 beats/min. Normally it is 0.83 second and therefore heart rate is 60/0.83 = 72 beats/min (Fig. 12.9).	
P-P interval	P-P interval is the interval between two successive P waves. Equal P-P intervals indicate rhythmic depolarization of the atria.	
T-P interval	T-P interval is measured from the end of T wave to the beginning of P wave. It measures the diastolic period of the heart. Variable T-P intervals indicate atrioventricular dissociation	

What is 'J' point? What is its significance?

The exact point at which the wave of depolarization just completes its passage through the heart (occurs at the end of QRS complex), all parts of the ventricles are depolarized so that no current is flowing around the heart (even the current of injury disappears). Therefore, the potential of ECG at this instant is exactly zero voltage. This point is known as 'J' point. A horizontal line drawn through all 'J' points is the zero potential line in ECG from which all potentials caused by current of injury must be measured. The potential of current of injury in each lead is the difference of the level of T-P segment of ECG and zero potential time. Potential of current of injury above the zero line is positive (lead I) and potential of current of injury below the zero line is negative (lead III).

What is ST segment shift?

Portion of ECG between end of QRS complex and the beginning of T wave is called ST segment. J point lies at the very beginning of this segment. Whenever there is current of injury, ST segment and T-P segment are not at the same potential level in the record. Actually T-P segment shifts away from zero potential and not the ST segment that is shifted away from the zero axis. Still mostly TP segment of ECG is considered as reference potential level rather than 'J' point. Therefore, when a current of injury is evident in ECG it is called ST segment shift.

What is mean electrical axis?

During most of the cycle of ventricular depolarization, the direction of electrical potential (negative to positive) is from the base of ventricles toward the apex. This preponderant direction of the potential during depolarization is called mean electrical axis (MEA) of the ventricles or the mean QRS vector. The mean electrical axis of normal ventricles is 59 degrees but it can swing to left about 20 degrees or to the right about 100 degrees.

What is right axis deviation? When does it occur? How is it diagnosed?

When mean axis is deviated to right, i.e. MEA of about 170°, it is called right axis deviated. It is caused by right ventricular hypertrophy or right bundle branch block. This can be diagnosed by observing QRS complex in leads I and III. When there is right axis deviation, S wave is prominent in lead I and R wave is prominent in lead III ($S_1 R_3$ pattern).

What is left axis deviation? When does it occur? How is it diagnosed?

When mean electrical axis is deviated to left, it is called left axis deviation, i.e. mean axis is about $-15°$. This is associated with obesity, left ventricular hypertrophy or left bundle branch block. This can be diagnosed by observing QRS complex in leads I and III. When there is left axis deviation, R wave is prominent in lead I and S wave is prominent in lead III ($R_1 S_3$ pattern).

What is sinus rhythm?

Sinus rhythm is present when SA node is the pacemaker. It is assumed if each P wave is followed by a normal QRS complex. P-R and, Q-T intervals are normal and P-R interval is regular.

What is sinus arrhythmia?

In sinus arrhythmia, there is a sinus rhythm except that R-R interval (cardiac rate) varies with respiration. Heart rate normally increases during inspiration and decreases during expiration.

ABNORMALITIES IN RATE AND RHYTHMS*

What is AV nodal rhythm?

When AV node becomes the pacemaker, the rhythm recorded is AV nodal rhythm, i.e. there is ectopic pacing from AV node. It is also called junctional rhythm. It is characterized by inverted 'P' wave and normal QRS complex. The rate is slower than sinus.

What is a premature beat?

Premature beat (premature contraction or ectopic beat) is a contraction of the heart prior to the time that normal contraction would have been expected.

What is premature atrial beat?

When the ectopic focus of the premature beat is located in atrium, atrial premature beat or atrial beat is recorded. The 'P' wave of this beat occurs too soon in the heart cycle. P-R interval is shortened indicating that ectopic origin of the beat is near the AV node.

An interval between premature contraction and next succeeding contraction is slightly prolonged which is called compensatory pause. The reason for this is that the premature contraction originated in the atrium some distance from the sinus node and the impulse had to travel through a considerable amount of atrial muscle before it discharged the sinus node. Therefore, the sinus node discharged very late in premature cycle, and this made the succeeding heart beat also late in appearing. Premature atrial contractions may occur frequently in healthy persons.

What is pulse deficit?

During premature contraction, heart contracts ahead of time. The ventricles are sometimes not filled with blood normally and stroke volume output during the contraction is therefore decreased or sometimes even absent. Therefore, during such a contraction, pulse wave passing to periphery may be so weak that it is not felt at the radial artery. Thus a deficit in the number of pulses felt in the radial pulse in relation to number of contractions in the heart is called pulse deficit.

What is premature ventricular contraction?

When the ectopic focus of the premature beat is located in the Purkinje system or myocardium of the ventricle, ventricular ectopic beat is recorded. Here the QRS complex is usually considerably prolonged and it has a high voltage. T wave has got potential opposite to that of QRS complex.

HAEMODYNAMICS

What is the function of arteries?

Arteries are the vessels which carry blood from heart to the periphery. They transport blood under high pressure to the tissues. For this reason, they have strong vascular walls. Blood flows rapidly in the arteries.

---

*For details refer Vaz M, Kurpad A, Raj T, editors. *Guyton & Hall Textbook of Medical Physiology*. Elsevier: New Delhi, 2013, p. 186.

What are arterioles? What is their function?

Arterioles are small branches of arterial system. They act as control valves through which blood is released into the capillaries. They have strong muscular wall capable of contracting and completely closing and dilating, thereby controlling the blood flowing to the capillaries.

What is the function of capillaries?

Capillaries are thin-walled vessels. Their function is to exchange fluid, nutrients, electrolytes, hormones and other substances between the blood and the interstitial fluid.

What is the function of veins?

Veins are the vessels which carry the blood towards the heart. They are thin-walled and act as major reservoirs of blood. The walls are muscular and therefore veins can contract or expand and reserve small or large volume of blood depending on the needs of the body.

Explain the proportion of blood present in different parts of circulation.

About 84% of the entire blood volume of the body is in the systemic circulation (64% in veins, 13% in arteries, 7% in systemic arterioles and capillaries). Heart contains 7% of blood volume and pulmonary vessels contain 9% of blood volume.

What is the relationship between velocity of blood flow and cross-sectional area of the vessels?

Cross-sectional area of veins is about four times larger than that of arteries. Therefore, there is large storage of blood in venous system as compared to in the arterial system, because velocity of blood flow is inversely proportional to the cross-sectional area.

Which vessels have largest cross-sectional area?

Capillaries have largest cross-sectional area, i.e. 2500 cm^2.

Describe how pressure changes in various portions of circulation.

The pressure in aorta is the highest because blood is pumped by heart continuously in aorta. As blood flows to systemic circulation, pressure falls progressively to approximately zero by the time it reaches the right atrium.

Pressure in aorta varies between 120 and 80 mmHg during systole and diastole of the heart respectively. Average pressure in aorta is about 100 mmHg.

In systemic capillaries pressure drops to 35 mmHg at the arterial ends and about 10 mmHg at the venous end with average functional pressure equal to 17 mmHg.

In pulmonary circulation pressure is much less. In pulmonary artery systolic pressure is 25 mmHg and diastolic pressure is of 8 mmHg. The average pulmonary capillary pressure is about 7 mmHg.

Explain the relationship between pressure, flow and resistance.

Flow of blood through any vessel is determined by two factors:

1. Flow is directly proportional to the pressure difference between the two ends of the vessel.
2. Flow is inversely proportional to the vascular resistance, i.e. impediment to blood flow through the vessel.

$$Q = \frac{\Delta P}{R}$$

Q = Quantity of blood flow
ΔP = Pressure difference at two ends of the vessel
R = Resistance

Name the methods of measuring blood flow.

Blood flow is expressed in ml/sec or L/min. It is measured by:

- Electromagnetic flowmeter.
- Ultrasonic Doppler flowmeter.

What is streamline or laminar flow?

When each layer of blood remains the same distance from the wall while flowing through a long smooth vessel, it is called streamline or laminar flow. When the flow is streamline, blood flows at a steady rate.

What is turbulent flow?

When blood flows crosswise in the vessel as well as along the vessel usually forming whorls in the blood called eddy currents, the flow is said to be turbulent. When eddy currents are present blood flows with much greater resistance than when the flow is streamline because of increased friction of flow caused by eddy currents.

Explain the factors causing tendency for turbulent flow.

The tendency for turbulent flow is directly proportional to the velocity of blood flow, diameter of blood vessel and is inversely proportional to viscosity of the blood divided by its density.

Reynolds' number is a measure of tendency to turbulence to occur. It is calculated as follows:

$$R_e = \frac{V.d}{\dfrac{\eta}{\rho}}$$

V = Velocity of blood flow (cm/sec).
d = Diameter of blood vessel.
η = Viscosity of blood (poises).
ρ = Density.
R_e = Reynolds' number.

When Reynolds' number rises above 200–400, turbulent flow will occur. When it is about 2000, turbulence will occur even in straight smooth vessel. Even in large arteries normally Reynolds' number rises to 200–2000. Therefore, there is always some turbulent flow.

What is resistance to blood flow?

Resistance is the impediment to blood flow.

What is the unit for resistance?

Unit for expressing resistance is the peripheral resistance unit (PRU). If pressure difference between two points in a vessel is 1 mmHg and the blood flow is 1 ml/sec, the resistance is said to be 1 PRU.

Occasionally resistance is expressed in CGS units as dyne sec/cm^5 and is calculated by following formula:

$$R\left(\frac{Dyne}{cm^5}\right) = \frac{1333 \times mmHg}{ml/sec}$$

How much is the total peripheral resistance normally?

At rest, rate of blood flow through circulatory system is 100 ml/sec and the pressure difference from systemic arteries to systemic veins is 100 mmHg. Therefore, total peripheral resistance is 100/100, i.e. 1 PRU. It can increase to 4 PRU when vessels are strongly constricted. It can fall to as low as 0.2 PRU when vessels become greatly dilated.

In pulmonary circulation, the net pressure difference (pulmonary arterial and left atrial pressure) is 14 mmHg whereas rate of blood flow is 100 ml/sec. Therefore, total pulmonary resistance at rest is 0.14 PRU.

What is conductance of flow in a vessel?

Conductance is a blood flow through a vessel for a given pressure difference expressed as ml/sec/mmHg. It is the reciprocal of resistance.

$$Conductance = \frac{1}{Resistance}$$

It changes directly with the diameter of vessel. The relationship is as follows:
$$Conductance \; \alpha \; Diameter$$
Conductance thus increases in proportion to fourth power of the diameter.

What is Poiseuille's law?

Poiseuille's law is the formula which is useful in calculating the rate of blood flow in a vessel. According to it:

$$Q = \frac{\pi \Delta P r^4}{8 \eta l}$$

where, Q = Rate of blood flow.
ΔP = Pressure difference between two ends of the vessel.
r = Radius of the vessle.
η = Viscosity of blood.
l = Length of the vessle.

Thus from the formula it is clear that the diameter of the vessel plays the greatest role in determining the rate of blood flow. This makes it possible for the arterioles, responding with small changes in diameter to nervous or local signals either to turn off completely the blood flow to the tissues or to cause a vast increase in blood flow.

Name the major factors affecting resistance to blood flow.

$$\text{According to Poiseuille's law, } R = \frac{8 \times \eta \times l}{r^4}$$

where, r = radius of vessel, η = viscosity of blood and l = length of the vessel.

How does viscosity of blood affect the blood flow?

According to Poiseuille's law, greater the viscosity, lesser is the blood flow. Viscosity in turn depends upon the haematocrit, i.e. percentage of cells. Greater the haematocrit, greater is the viscosity. Blood flow in very minute tubes exhibits far less viscosity effect because in these tubes red cells instead of moving randomly line up and move through the vessel thus eliminating viscous resistance.

What is the effect of pressure on vascular resistance and tissue blood flow?

Increase in arterial pressure greatly increases the blood flow because of two factors:

- Increase in the force tending to push the blood through the vessel.
- Distension of vessel and decrease in resistance.

What is the importance of vascular distensibility?

All the vessels are distensible. Distensible nature of the arteries allows them to accommodate the pulsatile output of the heart and to average out the pressure pulsation. This provides almost smooth, continuous blood flow through the tissues.

Veins are most distensible vessels; therefore they act as blood reservoirs and store large quantities of blood which can be called into use whenever required.

In pulmonary circulation, veins are similar to those of systemic veins. Pulmonary arteries normally operate under low pressure and have distensibilities about one-half those of veins.

What is the unit of vascular distensibility?

Vascular distensibility is expressed as the fractional increase in volume for each mmHg rise in pressure.

$$\text{Vascular distensibility} = \frac{\text{Increase in volume}}{\text{Increase in pressure} \times \text{Original volume}}$$

What is vascular compliance?

Vascular compliance is the total quantity of blood that can be stored in a given portion of circulation for each mmHg pressure rise.

$$\text{Vascular compliance} = \frac{\text{Increase in volume}}{\text{Increase in pressure}}$$

Compliance of vein is about 24 times that of corresponding artery because it is 8 times as distensible and has a volume 3 times as great. Therefore, compliance is equal to distensibility × volume.

What is the relationship between volume and pressure in arterial system and venous system? What is the effect of sympathetic stimulation?

With mean arterial pressure of 100 mmHg, arterial system (larger and smaller arteries, arterioles) have 750 ml of blood which reduces to 500 ml when pressure falls to zero.

Normally, venous system contains 2500 ml of blood and tremendous changes in the volume are required to change the pressure. Sympathetic stimulation increases the smooth muscle tone of the vessels. This in turn increases the pressure. This causes large volume of blood to shift into the heart.

What is stress relaxation?

When extra volume of blood is suddenly injected into a vessel, at first there will be a large pressure increase but because of stretching of the wall, smooth muscle fibres of the vessel will relax and this will allow pressure to return back towards the normal. This phenomenon is known as stress relaxation.

PULSE

What is pulse?

It is the wave of expansion that passes along the arterial tree from aorta to the peripheral arteries during systole of the heart.

Normally which artery do you choose for feeling the pulse? Why?

Pulse is felt at the radial artery because the artery is superficial and it lies on the bone. On examination of pulse, one notes rate, rhythm, volume, force, tension, equality of both sides, etc.

VENOUS SYSTEM

What is central venous pressure?

Pressure in the right atrium is known as central venous pressure because all the systemic veins open into the right atrium.

Name the factors determining right atrial pressure.

Right atrial pressure depends on balance between ability of atrium to pump the blood into the ventricle and the tendency for blood to flow from the peripheral vessels into right atrium. If right atrium is pumping strongly, the right atrial pressure tends to decrease. Weakness of the atrial wall tends to increase the right atrial pressure. Increase in flow of blood into the right atrium through veins (venous return) increases the right atrial pressure and vice versa.

State the factors increasing the venous return.

1. Increased blood volume.
2. Increased tone in large vessels throughout the body. This increases peripheral venous pressure.
3. Dilatation of arterioles which decreases the peripheral resistance allowing quick flow of blood from arteries to veins.
4. Muscular exercise.

How much is normal right atrial pressure? When does it rise or fall?

Normal right atrial pressure is zero mmHg (i.e. equal to atmospheric pressure). The pressure in the right atrium can rise as high as 20 to 30 mmHg in the following abnormal conditions:

- Heart failure.
- Massive blood transfusion.

Right atrial pressure can decrease to as low as -3 to -5 mmHg due to the following reasons:

- The heart (right atrium) is pumping with vigour.
- Venous return is greatly depressed.

How much is the pressure in the large veins?

Large veins do not offer any resistance when they are distended. But at the entry of thorax most of the large veins are compressed at many points by the surrounding tissues. This impedes the blood flow. Therefore, large veins do offer considerable resistance to blood flow and thus pressure in the peripheral veins is greater than that of the right atrial pressure. It is 4 to 7 mmHg. Venous pressure rises in heart failure.

What is hydrostatic pressure? How much is it in vascular system?

Pressure at the surface of water is equal to the atmospheric pressure, i.e. zero mmHg but the pressure rises by 1 mmHg for each 13.6 mm distance below the surface. This pressure results due to weight of water and therefore is called hydrostatic pressure.

HYDROSTATIC PRESSURE IN VASCULAR SYSTEM

When a person is standing absolutely still

- Hydrostatic pressure in veins between heart and feet is +90 mmHg. Venous pressure at other levels of the body varies between 0 to 90 mmHg.
- Neck veins completely collapse due to atmospheric pressure on the outside of the neck. Therefore, pressure inside them almost remains zero.
- Veins in the skull are in non-collapsible chamber and thus they do not collapse. Therefore, negative hydrostatic pressure (-10 mmHg) exits in dural sinuses of head.

How does hydrostatic factor affect the arterial pressure?

Hydrostatic factor also affects the peripheral pressures in the arteries, e.g. standing person has arterial pressure of 190 mmHg in the feet. Therefore, arterial pressure is stated as pressure at the hydrostatic level of heart.

What is the function of valves in the veins?

The venous pressure in feet is always +90 mmHg in a standing position because of hydrostatic pressure effect. Movement of legs and muscle contractions (muscle pump) squeeze the blood out of veins. The valves are arranged in the veins so that direction of blood can only be towards the heart. This lowers the pressure in the veins. Therefore, in walking adult, venous pressure remains less than 25 mmHg.

What are varicose veins?

The valves in the venous system become incompetent (when there is over-stretching of veins by excess venous pressure as in pregnancy). Stretching of the veins increases their cross-sectional area and valves of the veins no longer remain functional because of which there is failure of muscle pump leading to further increase in size of the veins and destroys the function of valves entirely. Thus large, bulbous protrusions of the veins called varicose veins develop.

How is venous pressure assessed?

Clinically venous pressure is assessed by observing the degree of distension of neck veins. When right atrial pressure is increased up to 10 mmHg, the lower neck veins begin to protrude in sitting position (in normal person in this position neck veins are never distended).

Venous pressure can be measured directly by inserting needle into the vein and connecting it to a pressure recorder. Right atrial pressure can be measured by inserting a catheter through the veins into the right atrium.

What is the function of veins?

Sixty per cent of the circulating blood is present in the venous system. So it serves as a blood reservoir. Especially extensive and compliant areas which act as specific blood reservoirs are liver sinuses, large abdominal veins, venous plexus beneath the skin and spleen.

CAPILLARY SYSTEM

What is the structure of capillary system?

Capillaries are thin-walled vessels which lie between arterioles and venules and supply blood to the tissues. Blood from arterioles passes into metarterioles → capillaries → venules → returns to the general circulation.

Arterioles are highly muscular and can change their diameter. The metarterioles (the terminal arterioles) do not have continuous muscle coat but at the point from where true capillaries originate smooth muscle fibres encircle the metarteriole forming precapillary sphincter. This sphincter can open or close the entrance to the capillaries. Total surface area of tissue capillaries is from 500 to 700 m^2.

Capillary is lined by unicellular layer of endothelial cells which is surrounded by basement membrane on the outside. The diameter of capillary is from 4 to 9 micron barely large enough for the passage of red blood cells, other blood cells squeeze through it. Thin slit lying between two endothelial cells of the capillary wall is called intercellular cleft. Each of this cleft is interrupted periodically by short ridges of protein attachments that hold the endothelial cells together but each ridge in turn is broken after a short distance, so that in between them fluid can percolate through the cleft. Cleft usually has a uniform spacing with a width of approximately 6 to 7 nm. These are termed 'slit pores'. In some tissues, pores in the capillaries have special characteristics. Examples: (a) In the brain, junctions between capillary endothelial cells are tight junctions allowing only small molecules to pass into the brain tissue and therefore act as blood-brain barrier. (b) In the liver, clefts or pores are very wide so that even plasma proteins can pass from the blood into the liver tissues. (c) In kidney number of small oval windows called fenestrae penetrate directly through the middle of endothelial cells in addition to clefts.

Blood flows into the capillaries intermittently, because of phenomenon of vasomotion, i.e. intermittent contraction of metarterioles and precapillary sphincters. This in turn is mainly controlled by concentration of oxygen in the tissues.

What is the function of capillary system?

Function of capillaries is to maintain average rate of blood flow through each tissue. Capillary bed maintains average capillary pressure and average rate of transfer of substances between blood of capillaries and the surrounding interstitial fluid.

Lipid soluble substances can directly diffuse through the cell membranes of the capillary. Water soluble substances cannot pass through lipid membranes of endothelial cells. Such substances pass through the pores.

Capillary dynamics are discussed in chapter on 'Blood'.

What is interstitium? What is present in it?

Spaces between the cells are collectively known as interstitium. It contains fluid known as interstitial fluid and two major types of solid structures—collagen fibres and proteoglycan filaments. Collagen fibres are strong and therefore they provide most of the tensional strength to the tissue. Proteoglycan filaments form fine reticular filaments described as 'brush pile'.

Proteoglycan filaments and fluid entrapped in them has a characteristic of gel and is called tissue gel. Rest of the fluid (which is in very small quantity) forms the free fluid. This amount is very slight (less than 1%). Oedema results when the free fluid in the tissue space increases. Free fluid and gel are continuously interchanging with each other.

State the factors determining fluid movement from blood to interstitial fluid and in opposite direction.

Following factors affect the fluid movement between blood in capillaries and the interstitial fluid:

1. *Capillary pressure.* This tends to force the fluid out through the capillary membrane. At the arterial end of capillary, pressure is from 30 to 40 mmHg and at the venous end of capillary, pressure is from 10 to 15 mmHg and in the middle, pressure is about 25 mmHg.

2. *Interstitial fluid pressure.* This tends to force fluid inward through the capillary membrane. It is about -3 to -5 mmHg.

3. *Plasma colloid osmotic pressure.* This tends to cause inward movement of fluid through the capillary membrane. It is about 28 mmHg.

4. *The interstitial fluid colloid osmotic pressure.* This tends to cause the fluid movement outward through the capillary membrane and it is about 8 mmHg.

All these forces are called Starling's forces.

CONTROL OF BLOOD FLOW

What are the functions of tissue blood flow?

- Delivery of oxygen to the tissues.
- Delivery of other nutrients to the tissues.
- Removal of CO_2 from the tissues.
- Removal of hydrogen ions from the tissues.
- Maintenance of proper concentration of other ions in the tissues.
- Transport of various hormones and other specific substances to the different tissues.

Blood flow to the various tissues is usually regulated at the minimal level that will supply its requirements, neither more, nor less.

Name the local mechanisms controlling blood flow.

Local blood flow control occurs in two different phases:

1. **Acute control** occurs by rapid changes in local constriction of arterioles, metarterioles and precapillary sphincters. This occurs within seconds or minutes.

2. **Long-term control** causes slow change in the flow over a period of days, weeks or even months. This is due to increase or decrease in physical sizes and the number of blood vessels supplying the tissue.

Describe the acute control of local blood flow.

Local blood flow increases with increase in rate of tissue metabolism and vice versa. There are two basic theories for regulation of blood flow:

1. *Vasodilator theory.* Greater the rate of metabolism, lesser is the blood flow and lesser is the availability of oxygen and other nutrients to the tissues. This causes greater release of certain vasodilator substances from the tissues. These substances diffuse to precapillary sphincters, metarterioles and arterioles to cause their dilatation. Different vasodilator substances suggested are adenosine, CO_2, lactic acid, adenosine phosphate compounds, histamine, potassium ions and hydrogen ions. Most of these substances are released in response to oxygen deficiency (especially adenosine and lactic acid). Adenosine plays important role in controlling coronary blood flow. But it is difficult to prove whether sufficient quantities of any single vasodilator substance are formed in the tissues to cause measured increase in blood flow. Probably there is a combined effect of number of vasodilator substances.

2. *O_2 demand theory (nutrient demand theory).* O_2 is required to maintain vascular muscle contraction. In absence of adequate blood flow, there is inadequate supply of oxygen and other nutrients. This causes vasodilatation because of opening of precapillary sphincters and metarterioles.

Normally precapillary sphincters and metarterioles, open and close cyclically (vasomotion). When there is a lack of oxygen, precapillary sphincters cannot contract properly. They open up and remain open for a long time. When O_2 concentration is high, precapillary sphincters and metarterioles close and remain closed until tissue cells consume excess oxygen and oxygen concentration comes back to normal. Similarly, lack of glucose, also has the same effect as lack of O_2 on smooth muscle of precapillary sphincters and metarterioles.

What is reactive hyperaemia?

When blood supply to a tissue is blocked for a few seconds to several hours and then is unblocked, the flow through the tissue usually increases to about five times normal and increased flow continues for few seconds to few hours (depending on how long the flow was blocked). This phenomenon is known as reactive hyperaemia. This is due to metabolic control of local blood flow and explains close relationship between local blood flow regulation and delivery of nutrients to the tissues.

What is active hyperaemia?

When tissues became very active such as during exercise, the rate of blood flow to the tissues increases. This is due to relative lack of nutrients and O_2 leading to local vasodilatation. This is known as active hyperaemia.

What is the effect of arterial blood pressure on blood flow to the tissue?

Blood flow is maintained relatively normal despite of the arterial pressure variation between 70 and 175 mmHg. This is called autoregulation of blood flow. It is explained by two theories:

1. *Metabolic theory.* When arterial blood pressure increases, the excess flow provides too many nutrients to the tissues and it also flushes the vasodilator substances. These two effects cause blood vessels to constrict and flow returns to almost normal despite the increased pressure.

2. *Myogenic theory.* It is observed that sudden stretch on the small blood vessels causes smooth muscles of blood vessel wall to contract. Therefore, when arterial blood pressure increases and stretches the vessel, it causes vascular contraction and reduces the blood flow nearly back to normal. Conversely at low blood pressures, the degree of stretch of the vessel is less, so that smooth muscle of the vessel relaxes and allows increased blood flow.

It is yet doubtful whether myogenic autoregulation is a powerful mechanism.

Explain the long-term mechanism of blood flow regulation.

Long-term mechanism gives far more complete regulation than the acute mechanism. The degree of vascularity of the tissues changes in this mechanism. There is reconstruction of tissue vasculature to meet the needs of the tissue; e.g. arterial pressure falls to 60 mmHg and remains at this level for a long time. The physical structural sizes of the vessels in the tissue increase and also the number of vessels increases.

Probable stimulus for increased or decreased vascularity in many instances is needed for tissue oxygen; e.g. increased vascularity occurs in tissues of many animals which live at high altitude.

Angiogenesis, i.e. growth of new blood vessels occurs mainly in response to angiogenic factors released from: (a) ischaemic tissues, (b) tissues that are growing rapidly and (c) tissues having excessively high metabolic rate.

Many angiogenic factors are small peptides. Three of them are most important. They are endothelial cell growth factor (ECGF), fibroblast growth factor (FGF) and angiotensin. They are released either from the tumours or from other tissues that generally have inadequate blood supply. Deficiency of oxygen and other nutrients leads to formation of these factors. Essentially all the angiogenic factors promote new vessel growth in the same manner. They cause sprouting of new vessels from either venules or capillaries in following steps:

- Dissolution of basement membrane of the endothelial cells.
- Rapid reproduction of endothelial cells.
- Streaming out of new endothelial cells out of the vessel wall in extended cords towards the source of angiogenic factor.
- Continued division of the cells in the cord and their folding in tube.
- Connection of the tube with another tube budding from another donor vessel, forming capillary loop.

What is collateral circulation?

When either an artery or a vein is blocked, a new vascular channel usually develops around the blockage and allows at least partial resupply of blood to the affected tissue. The circulation through these new channels is called collateral circulation.

NERVOUS CONTROL OF BLOOD FLOW

Describe the sympathetic and parasympathetic nerve supply to heart and vessels.

There is autonomic nerve supply to the heart and blood vessels, i.e. sympathetic and parasympathetic supply. The most important system which controls circulation is the sympathetic nervous system.

1. *Sympathetic supply.* All the blood vessels except capillaries, precapillary sphincters and metarterioles are innervated by sympathetic nerves.

Stimulation of sympathetic nerves to small arteries and arterioles causes vasoconstriction and therefore increased peripheral resistance, thus changing rate of blood flow to the tissues. There are very few vasodilator fibres supplying the vessels.

Stimulating sympathetic nerves to large vessels especially veins cause their constriction and therefore blood stored in them is translocated to the heart. This increases the venous return and therefore the cardiac output; thus plays a major role in regulation of cardiovascular function. Stimulation of sympathetic nerves to heart causes increase in the heart rate (positive chronotropic), increase in the force of contraction of the heart (positive inotropic), increased rate of conduction of impulse through the heart (positive dromotropic) and increased excitability (positive bathmotropic).

2. *Parasympathetic supply.* Parasympathetic fibres are carried to the heart through vagus nerve. The effect of parasympathetic stimulation is to decrease the heart rate, force of contraction, rate of conduction of impulse through the heart and decreased excitability (negative chronotropic, inotropic, dromotropic and bathmotropic effects). There is no parasympathetic supply to blood vessels.

BLOOD PRESSURE

What is blood pressure?

Blood pressure is the lateral pressure exerted by flowing blood on the walls of the vessels. Systolic pressure is the maximum pressure during systole and diastolic pressure is the minimum pressure in the arteries during diastole.

Name the methods used for measuring blood pressure.

1. *Palpatory method.* It can only measure the systolic pressure.
2. *Auscultatory method.* It measures systolic as well as diastolic blood pressure.
3. *Oscillometric method.*

How much is normal blood pressure?

Normal systolic pressure in adult is 120 ± 15 mmHg and diastolic pressure varies from 80 ± 10 mmHg.

What is mean arterial pressure?

Mean arterial pressure is the average of all the pressures measured millisecond by millisecond over a period of time. It is determined by adding 60% diastolic and 40% systolic pressure. It is about 100 mmHg.

When mean arterial pressure is chronically above 110 mmHg, person is labelled is hypertensive. Hypertension can be mild, moderate or severe.

What is pulse pressure? What is its significance?

Pulse pressure is the difference between systolic and diastolic pressure. Pulse pressure indicates stroke volume.

VASOMOTOR CENTRE

Describe the vasomotor centre.

Vasomotor centre is situated bilaterally in the reticular substance of medulla and lower third of pons. It transmits impulses through the spinal cord and then through vasoconstrictor fibres to almost all the blood vessels. Following are certain important areas in the centre (Fig. 12.10):

- *Vasoconstrictor area.* It is also called area C-1. It is located bilaterally in the anterolateral portions of upper medulla.

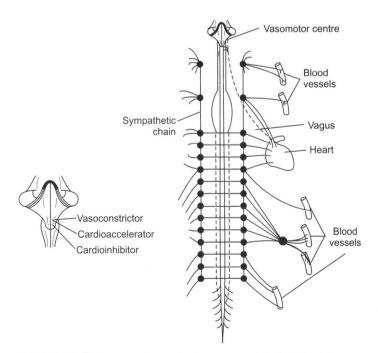

FIGURE 12.10 Anatomy of sympathetic nervous control of the circulation.

- *Vasodilator area.* It is called area A-1. It is located bilaterally in anterolateral portions of lower half of medulla.
- *Sensory area.* It is called area A-2. It is located bilaterally in the tractus solitarius, in the posterolateral portions of the medulla and lower pons. Neurons in this area receive signals from glossopharyngeal and vagus nerves.

What is vasomotor tone?

Vasoconstrictor area of vasomotor centre transmits signals continuously through the sympathetic vasoconstrictor fibres to the blood vessels. These impulses maintain partial state of contraction in the blood vessel which is called vasomotor tone.

How does the vasomotor centre control heart activity?

Lateral portions of vasomotor centre transmit excitatory signals through the sympathetic nerves to the heart. The medial portion of the vasomotor centre which lies near the dorsal motor nucleus of vagus nerve transmits inhibitory impulses to the heart through the vagus nerve.

Thus vasomotor centre can either increase or decrease the heart activity.

Describe the role of higher centres in controlling the vasomotor centre.

Higher centres control the vasomotor centre as follows:

1. *Reticular substance of pons, mesencephalon and diencephalon.* Lateral and superior portions of reticular substance cause excitation of the vasomotor centre. Medial and inferior portions of reticular substance cause inhibition of the vasomotor centre.
2. *Hypothalamus.* Posterolateral portions of hypothalamus cause excitation whereas the anterior part causes mild excitation or inhibition of vasomotor centre.
3. *Cerebral cortex.* Stimulation of motor cortex excites the vasomotor centre because of impulses transmitted to it via hypothalamus. Stimulation of anterior temporal lobe, orbital areas of frontal cortex, anterior part of cingulate gyrus, amygdala and septum can either excite or inhibit the vasomotor centre.

Explain the role of sympathetic vasodilator fibres.

Vasodilator sympathetic fibres mainly supply the skeletal muscles. Anterior hypothalamus mainly controls their activity. It plays role only during muscular exercise causing initial vasodilatation in the vessels of skeletal muscles to cause anticipatory rise in their blood flow.

What is vasovagal syncope?

Fainting occurs when the person has intense emotional disturbances. This is due to intense stimulation of vasodilator fibres to skeletal muscle and at the same time transmission of strong inhibitory signals through the vagus nerve to the heart. There is fall in arterial pressure, decreased blood supply to the brain and person loses consciousness. This effect is known as vasovagal syncope.

Explain the role of nervous system in controlling arterial pressure.

Nervous system is capable of controlling the circulation to cause rapid increase in arterial pressure. This is done by arteriolar constriction, constriction of veins and direct stimulation of the heart. The pressure rises within few seconds. Conversely sudden inhibition of nervous system can cause fall in arterial pressure within 10 to 40 seconds. Thus nervous control of arterial pressure is most rapid.

SHORT-TERM MECHANISMS REGULATING BLOOD PRESSURE

Enumerate the various short-term mechanisms regulating blood arterial pressure.

The various short-term mechanisms regulating blood pressure are:

1. *Neural reflexes:*
   - Baroreceptor reflex.
   - Chemoreceptor reflex.
   - CNS ischaemic response.
   - Atrial reflex.
   - Abdominal compression reflex.
2. *Stress relaxation and reverse stress relaxation.*
3. *Capillary fluid shift mechanism.*

Name the various reflex mechanisms which maintain normal arterial blood pressure.

- Baroreceptor reflex.
- Chemoreceptor reflex.
- Atrial reflex.

Describe the anatomy of baroreceptors.

Baroreceptors or pressoreceptors are stretch receptors and are located in the walls of large systemic arteries. They are extremely abundant in two areas:

- Wall of internal carotid artery slightly above the carotid bifurcation is known as carotid sinus.
- Wall of aortic arch is known as aortic sinus. Baroreceptors are spray-type nerve endings lying in the walls. They are stimulated when stretched.

Impulses from carotid sinus are carried by Hering's nerves to the glossopharyngeal nerve and then to tractus solitarius of medulla. Impulses from aortic sinus are carried through vagus nerve to the tractus solitarius (Fig. 12.11).

Explain the response of baroreceptors to changes in arterial pressure.

Baroreceptors are stimulated on distension of the vessel wall. The carotid sinus represents the most distensible area of the arterial system. Carotid sinus baroreceptors are not stimulated at all when pressure is between 0 and 60 mmHg. They respond progressively more and more rapidly and reach maximum at 180 mmHg pressure.

Baroreceptors respond much more rapidly to changing pressures than to a stationary pressure. The normal operating range of baroreceptor varies from 60 to 180 mmHg. The normal arterial pressure is around 100 mmHg. A slight change in pressure causes strong autonomic reflexes to readjust the pressure.

Thus baroreceptor reflex mechanism functions most effectively in the pressure range where it is most needed.

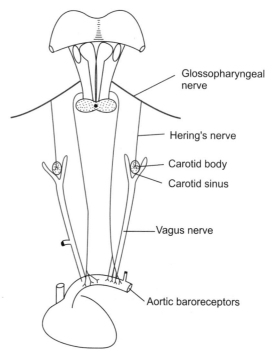

FIGURE 12.11 The baroreceptor system.

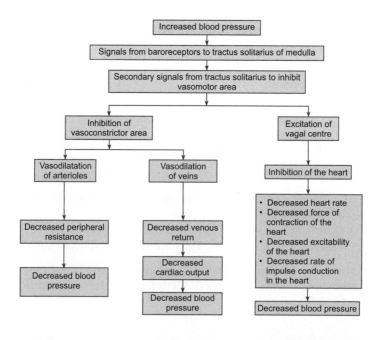

Describe the baroreceptor reflex.

When the blood pressure increases above the normal level, it causes baroreceptor reflex as follows:
Thus the blood pressure returns back to normal.
Exactly opposite sequence of events occurs when blood pressure is lowered.

Explain the buffer function of the baroreceptor reflex.

Baroreceptor system opposes either increase or decrease in arterial pressure and therefore it is called pressure buffer system and the nerves from the baroreceptors are called buffer nerves. This is possible because the baroreceptor system operates within 60 to 180 mmHg pressure.

Baroreceptors therefore relatively maintain constant arterial pressure during various activities or changes in position, e.g. if the person who is lying down suddenly stands, this can cause arterial pressure in the head and upper part of the body to fall and marked reduction can cause unconsciousness. But this is not allowed to occur, because of falling pressure in the baroreceptors. When the person stands, he will elicit baroreceptor reflex resulting into sympathetic discharge minimizing the decrease in pressure in the head and upper part of the body.

Why the baroreceptor system is ineffective in causing long-term regulation of blood pressure?

When there is increase in blood pressure, baroreceptors send impulses but later on rate becomes slower and slower (adaptation).

Describe the role of chemoreceptors in control of blood pressure.

Carotid and aortic bodies contain chemoreceptors which are mainly stimulated by chemical stimuli such as oxygen lack, carbon dioxide excess and hydrogen ion excess. They are profusely supplied with blood and therefore when blood pressure falls below a critical level of 80 mmHg, chemoreceptors are stimulated because of diminished blood flow resulting in diminished O_2 supply and building up of CO_2 and H^+ ions. They send impulse through Hering's nerves (from carotid bodies) and vagi nerves (from aortic bodies) to the vasomotor centre. This elevates arterial pressure. Thus reflex is responsible for bringing arterial pressure back to normal. But this reflex is not very powerful controller of arterial blood pressure. Still it is important as it is stimulated at low pressure and helps in preventing further fall in blood pressure.

Describe atrial reflex.

Atria contain stretch receptors. These are also called low pressure receptors. They play role in minimizing the effect of decreased blood volume on arterial blood pressure. The reflex occurs as follows:

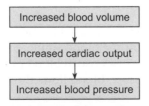

This pressure is brought to normal as follows:

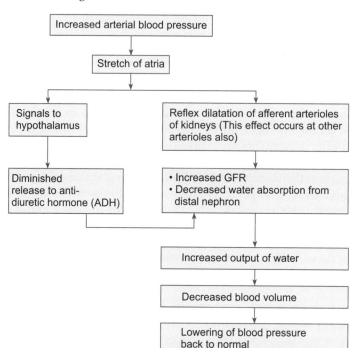

Increase in atrial pressure also causes an increase in the heart rate. This is partly due to direct effect of stretching the sinus node but is mostly due to Bainbridge reflex. Stimulation of stretch receptors in atria → afferent signals through vagus to medulla of brain → efferent signals are transmitted through vagus and sympathetic nerves to increase heart rate and probably also the strength of contraction of heart.

What is CNS ischaemic response?

When blood flow to the vasomotor centre in the brain stem is decreased enough to cause nutritional deficiency (i.e. cerebral ischaemia) the neurons in the vasomotor centre are strongly excited. This is due to accumulation of CO_2 and lactic acid locally near the vasomotor centre. Excitation of vasomotor centre causes strong sympathetic stimulation leading to vasoconstriction leading to increase in blood pressure. Peripheral vessels become totally occluded at certain areas, e.g. kidneys. This most powerful response that activates sympathetic vasoconstrictor system strongly is called CNS ischaemic response. It is initiated when blood pressure falls below 60 mmHg. This acts as an emergency arterial pressure control system. If rise of pressure does not relieve CNS ischaemia, neuronal cells begin to suffer and within 3 to 10 minutes become totally inactive.

What is Cushing reaction?

When CSF pressure rises and becomes equal to arterial pressure, it compresses the arteries in the brain and cuts off the blood supply to the brain. This initiates the CNS ischaemic response. This causes rise in blood pressure. When blood pressure becomes greater than CSF pressure, blood flows through the vessels of brain and ischaemia is relieved. Blood pressure comes to equilibrium at a new level. This effect is called Cushing reaction. It protects the vital centres in the brain.

What is the role of skeletal nerves and muscles in controlling blood pressure?

Though mostly autonomic nervous system controls circulation, the skeletal nerves and muscles play role as follows:

1. *Abdominal compression reflex.* Whenever vasomotor centre is stimulated (e.g. baroreceptor reflex, chemoreceptor reflex) other reticular areas of brain stem are also stimulated. They send simultaneous impulses through skeletal nerves to skeletal muscles of the body especially abdominal muscles. Contraction of abdominal muscles compresses the abdominal venous reservoirs. This causes increased venous return to the heart and therefore increased cardiac output. This overall response is called abdominal compression reflex.

2. *During exercise.* During exercise the skeletal muscles contract and compress the blood vessels. This causes translocation of large quantities of blood from the peripheral vessels into the heart and lungs. This increases the cardiac output.

What is the role of nervous reflexes described above in maintaining the blood pressure?

Nervous reflexes cause rapid, powerful but short-term regulation of the arterial blood pressure. They gradually lose their ability with time because of adaptation of receptors.

What is stress relaxation and reverse stress relaxation?

When blood pressure is high, after some time smooth muscle of blood vessel relaxes leading to vasodilation and fall in blood pressure; this is termed stress relaxation.

When blood volume and pressure is low the vessel constricts over a small volume and pressure inside rises; this is termed reverse stress relaxation.

Explain the role of capillary fluid shift mechanism in regulation of blood pressure.

When arterial blood pressure rises, the pressure at arterial end of capillaries becomes higher than normal. This causes greater fluid to be shifted from capillaries to interstitial fluid. This in turn reduces the total circulating blood volume and venous return and thus reduces the blood pressure.

When arterial blood pressure falls, pressure at arterial end of capillaries and therefore at venous end of capillaries is reduced.

This causes greater absorption of fluid from interstitial space into the capillary. This increases blood volume and therefore the blood pressure.

LONG-TERM MECHANISMS REGULATING BLOOD PRESSURE

What is the basis for long-term regulation of blood pressure?

When there is increase in extracellular fluid volume, it causes rise in blood volume and therefore rise in blood pressure. Rising pressure has a direct effect on kidneys to excrete excess of water (pressure diuresis) and also increase output of sodium (pressure natriuresis). Pressure diuresis and pressure natriuresis bring blood volume back to normal and therefore returning blood pressure back to normal.

Thus pressure diuresis and natriuresis is the fundamental mechanism of long-term regulation of blood pressure. With evolution however multiple refinements have been added to make the fundamental system more exact in its control. Especially important refinement is renin-angiotensin mechanism.

What is the role of salt in renal body fluid mechanism for controlling blood pressure?

Accumulation of salt indirectly increases the extracellular fluid volume because of two reasons:

1. When there is excess salt in the body, there is increased osmolality of body fluids. This increased osmolality stimulates the thirst centre, making person drink large quantities of water to dilute the extracellular fluid. Thus there is increase in extracellular fluid volume.
2. Increased osmolality of body fluids also stimulates hypothalamic posterior pituitary gland system to secrete increased quantities of ADH (antidiuretic hormone). This causes increased reabsorption of fluid from the distal renal tubules. This causes increase in extracellular fluid volume.

What is renin? What is its role in long-term regulation of blood pressure?

Renin is a protein synthesized by juxtaglomerular cells of the kidneys. It is secreted in inactive form called prorenin and is stored in the juxtaglomerular cells. Renin is an enzyme. It acts on the substrate, i.e. plasma globulin or renin substrate or angiotensinogen present in the blood to release angiotensin I. This angiotensin I is converted to angiotensin II by angiotensin converting enzyme present in small vessels mainly in the lungs. Angiotensin II has two principal effects by which it causes elevation of arterial pressure as follows:

- It is a powerful vasoconstrictor. Therefore, causes powerful vasoconstriction of arterioles and to a lesser extent also of veins. Constriction of arterioles increases the peripheral resistance and thus also increases the blood pressure. Mild constriction of veins increases the venous return. This in turn increases the cardiac output. Increased cardiac output increases the blood pressure.
- It directly acts on renal tubules and causes decreased excretion of salt and water. This causes increase in extracellular fluid volume and therefore the blood pressure.
- Angiotensin also increases salt and water retention by kidneys indirectly by stimulating release of aldosterone from the adrenal cortex.

Aldosterone in turn acts on distal renal tubules to cause increased absorption of salt and water.

What is one-kidney Goldblatt hypertension?

When one kidney is removed and a constrictor is placed on the renal artery of the remaining kidney, then within few minutes arterial pressure begins to rise and continues to rise for several days. The hypertension produced in this way is called one kidney Goldblatt hypertension. The early rise in blood pressure is due to renin-angiotensin vasoconstrictor mechanism. The second rise is caused by fluid retention.

What is two-kidney Goldblatt hypertension?

Hypertension that develops when the artery to one kidney is constricted while artery to the other kidney is still normal is called two-kidney Goldblatt hypertension.

What is essential hypertension?

Hypertension of unknown origin is known as essential hypertension. In most of the patients, there is a strong hereditary tendency. It is also called primary hypertension.

What is the importance of renin-angiotensin mechanism?

Despite variable salt intake, long-term level of arterial pressure is maintained normal because of renin-angiotensin system as follows:

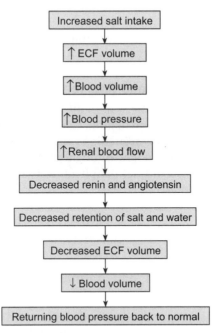

Decrease in salt intake will have exactly opposite effects.

CARDIAC OUTPUT

What is cardiac output? How much is it normally?

Cardiac output is the quantity of blood pumped into the aorta each minute by the heart. It is 5 litres in normal adult person.

What is cardiac index? How much is it normally?

Cardiac index is the cardiac output per square metre of body surface area. It is 3 litres in normal adult person weighing 70 kg.

What is stroke volume?

Stroke volume is the volume of blood pumped by each ventricle per heart beat.

What is venous return?

The quantity of blood flowing from the veins into the right atrium each minute is known as venous return.

What is Frank–Starling's law of the heart?

Frank–Starling's law refers to the relationship between venous return (venous pressure) and cardiac output. An increase in venous return causes greater filling of ventricle during diastole resulting in a greater stretch on the cardiac muscle fibres. This produces a stronger contraction and a greater ejection of blood during systole. Stretch on the SA node also increases the rate of the heart. Stretched right atrium also initiates Bainbridge reflex (passing to vasomotor centre) causing increased heart rate. Thus an increased venous return produces increased cardiac output within physiological limits (Frank–Starling's law). Therefore, venous return is the most important factor controlling cardiac output.

What is the effect of local blood flow regulation on cardiac output?

The venous return to the heart is the sum of all the local blood flows from individual segments of the peripheral circulation. Cardiac output regulation therefore is a sum of all the local blood flow regulations and is therefore determined by all the factors that control local blood flow throughout the body. Cardiac output varies reciprocally to the changes in total peripheral resistance, when arterial blood pressure is maintained normal, i.e.

$$\text{Cardiac output} = \frac{\text{Arterial pressure}}{\text{Total peripheral resistance}}.$$

How much amount of blood can normal heart pump without any excess nervous stimulation?

Normal heart can increase the cardiac output with increased venous return (Frank-Starling law) up to about two and half times its normal. Venous return is limiting factor. So, normal heart without any excess nervous stimulation has the cardiac output up to 13 L/min.

What is hypoeffective heart? Enumerate the factors causing hypoeffective heart.

When the pumping ability of the heart is below the normal, the heart is said to be hypoeffective heart.

Factors causing hypoeffective heart:

- Inhibition of nervous excitation of the heart.
- Valvular heart disease.
- Pathological factors causing abnormal rate and rhythm of the heart beat.
- Increased arterial pressure.
- Congenital heart diseases.
- Myocarditis.
- Cardiac anoxia.
- Myocardial damage or toxicity.

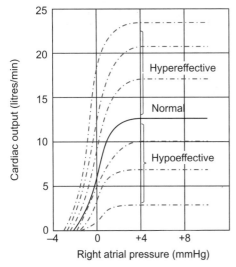

FIGURE 12.12 Cardiac output curves.

What is hypereffective heart? Enumerate the factors causing hypereffective heart.

When the pumping ability of the heart is greater than normal, the heart is said to be hypereffective heart (Fig. 12.12).

Factors causing hypereffective heart:

1. *Nervous stimulation.* When there is sympathetic stimulation of the heart, there is greatly increased heart rate and also increase in the strength of contraction of the heart. Because of these two effects, cardiac output may be increased up to 25 l/min.
2. *Hypertrophy of the heart.* Increase in mass and contractility of cardiac muscle is termed hypertrophy of the heart, e.g. heavy exercise.

When above two effects are combined, cardiac output becomes as much as 30 to 35 L/min.

What is the effect of sympathetic stimulation on cardiac output?

Sympathetic stimulation increases the cardiac output as follows:

1. Increase the strength of contraction of the heart and thus increases cardiac output.
2. Causes peripheral vasoconstriction. Constriction of veins increases the venous return to the heart and thus increases the cardiac output.

Enumerate the methods for measuring cardiac output.*

Cardiac output can be measured by the following methods:

1. *With the help of flowmeter.*
2. *Fick method of measuring output.*

---

*For details refer Vaz M, Kurpad A, Raj T, editors. *Guyton & Hall Textbook of Medical Physiology*. Elsevier: New Delhi, 2013, p. 214.

3. *Indicator dilution method* (Fig. 12.13).
4. *Thermal dilution method.*

SHOCK

What is circulatory shock?

Circulatory shock means generalized inadequacy of blood flow throughout the body to the extent that body tissues get damaged due to too little delivery of oxygen and nutrients.

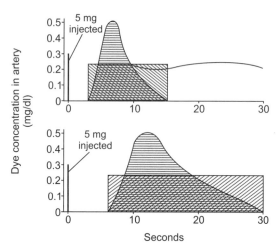

FIGURE 12.13 Dilution method: Dye concentration curves used to calculate two separate cardiac output levels.

Explain the different types of shock and their causes.

1. SHOCK CAUSED BY REDUCED CARDIAC OUTPUT

It is subdivided into:

(a) *Cardiogenic shock,* due to decreased pumping ability of the heart because of cardiac abnormalities, e.g. myocardial infarction, toxic states of heart, severe heart valve dysfunction, heart arrhythmias.

(b) *Shock caused by decreased venous return:*
- *Hypovolumic shock.* There is decrease in blood volume due to any cause, e.g. external or internal haemorrhage (injury, fracture), fluid loss (diarrhoea, vomiting, excess sweating and burns).
- *Decrease in vascular tone,* especially of venous reservoirs as in
  - *Neurogenic shock,* caused by general or spinal anaesthesia, brain damage, emotional fainting.
  - *Anaphylactic shock,* an allergic reaction which causes marked venous and arteriolar dilatation and increased capillary permeability due to release of histamine or histamine like substances.
  - *Obstructive shock,* caused by obstructive blood flow, e.g. tension pneumothorax, pulmonary embolism, cardiac tumour, etc.

2. SHOCK OCCURRING WITHOUT DECREASE IN CARDIAC OUTPUT

It is subdivided into:

(a) *Excessive metabolism of the body* due to which normal cardiac output is inadequate.

(b) *Septic shock.* Abnormal tissue perfusion patterns so that most of the cardiac output is passing through blood vessels besides those that are supplying the local tissues with nutrition. It occurs due to blood borne infection, e.g. peritonitis. Usually there is high fever, vasodilation, high cardiac output and sludging of blood in septic shock.

What are the signs and symptoms of circulatory shock?

- Decreased blood pressure.
- Tachycardia and therefore reduced stroke volume.
- Reduction in velocity of blood flow producing stagnant hypoxia and cyanosis.
- Pale and cold skin due to vasoconstriction.
- Decreased urine output due to reduced renal blood flow and GFR.
- Blood flow to vital organs is affected. Reduced blood flow to brain causes fainting.
- Due to tachycardia there is increase in work of heart but its blood flow is reduced. This leads to excessive production and collection of lactic acid.
- Respiration becomes rapid.
- If patient is conscious, there is intense thirst.
- Agitation, restlessness.

Name the different stages of circulatory shock.

STAGES OF SHOCK

1. *Non-progressive stage* (compensated stages). Normal circulatory compensatory mechanisms eventually cause full recovery without help of outside therapy.
2. *Progressive stage.* Shock becomes steadily worse until death.
3. *Irreversible stage.* Shock progresses to such an extent that all forms of known therapy are inadequate to save person's life.

Explain the different compensatory mechanisms occurring in hypovolumic shock.

In hypovolumic shock there is reduction in blood volume most commonly due to haemorrhage. The degree of shock depends on the amount of blood loss. About 10% of total loss of blood has no effect either on blood pressure or cardiac output. If loss is more, cardiac output is reduced and later on blood pressure decreases.

Circulatory system can recover if degree of loss is not greater than a certain critical amount. Crossing this critical amount causes death as shock itself causes more shock resulting into progressive shock.

If shock is not severe enough to cause its own progression, person recovers. Shock of this lesser degree is non-progressive shock. Circulatory system recovers due to various negative feedback control mechanisms set for maintaining cardiac output and blood pressure. They are termed compensatory mechanisms. These are:

- Rapid or short-term mechanisms.
- Long-term mechanisms.

RAPID COMPENSATORY MECHANISMS

1. *Baroreceptor reflex.* Fall in blood pressure causes lesser degree of stretching of baroreceptors. Discharge from these receptors stimulates vasomotor centre and there is sympathetic stimulation leading to generalized vasoconstriction (sparing

vessels of brain and heart). Vasoconstriction is most marked in skin, kidneys and viscera. This causes shifting of greater amount of blood in circulation. Constriction of veins on account of sympathetic stimulation also causes increased shifting of stored venous blood in circulation leading to increased venous return and cardiac output. In kidneys both afferent and afferent blood vessels constrict but afferent vessels constrict to a greater extent. This leads to reduction in GFR.

2. *Chemoreceptor reflex.* Haemorrhage causes loss of red cells leading to reduced O_2 carrying capacity. The resultant anaemia and stagnant hypoxia as well as acidosis stimulates chemoreceptors which also excite vasomotor centre to cause same effects as those caused by baroreceptor reflex. Fall in blood pressure below 80 mmHg usually initiates chemoreceptor reflex.

3. *CNS ischaemic response.* When blood pressure falls below 50 mmHg this response is initiated. It causes more powerful sympathetic stimulation.

4. *Reverse stress relaxation.* This causes blood vessels to constrict down around the diminished blood volume so that available blood volume is adequately circulated.

5. *Release of epinephrine and norepinephrine.* Haemorrhage is a potent stimulator of secretion of these hormones from adrenal medulla. The increase in blood levels of these hormones contribute relatively little to generalized vasoconstriction. They cause stimulation of reticular formation making patient restless and apprehensive.

6. *Increase in circulating angiotensin II level.* Due to ischaemia there is a secretion of renin from the kidneys which increases level of angiotensin II in blood.

7. **Thirst centre:** This is stimulated which makes person drink more fluid which helps to restore extracellular fluid (ECF).

Increased angiotensin II causes vasoconstriction leading to rise in blood pressure. It also causes increased aldosterone secretion (after about 30 min) which in turn causes increased absorption of salt and water by kidneys which helps in restoring extracellular fluid volume. All these effects help in preventing progression of shock.

8. *Release of excess vasopressin or ADH.* Release of ADH causes retention of water by kidneys and helps in restoring ECF.

9. *Capillary fluid shift mechanism.* Drop in capillary pressure causes fluid from interstitial space to move into the capillaries along most of their course helping to maintain circulatory volume.

From different mechanisms described above, reflexes provide immediate help within 30 seconds of haemorrhage. Angiotensin, vasopressin, reverse stress relaxation require ten minutes to an hour for complete response. Readjustment of blood volume by increased absorption of water from intestine and increased absorption of salt and water from kidneys require 1 to 48 hours. Recovery takes place if shock does not become progressive.

Long-term compensatory mechanisms:

1. *Restoration of plasma volume and proteins.* After a moderate haemorrhage, plasma volume is restored to normal in 12 to 72 hours. There is rapid entry of preformed albumin from extravascular stores. After this initial influx albumin and rest of the plasma protein losses are restored by hepatic synthesis over a period of 3 to 4 days.

2. *Restoration of red cell mass.* There is excess release of erythropoietin which leads to increased rate of erythropoiesis within 10 days. Normal red cells mass is restored in 4 to 8 weeks.

What is progressive shock?

When shock becomes severe enough, structures of circulatory system begin to deteriorate and various types of positive feedback mechanisms develop. These cause vicious cycle of progressively decreasing cardiac output. This is called progressive shock.

What is irreversible shock?

After a shock has progressed to a certain stage, transfusion or any other therapy becomes incapable of saving the life of the person. This is irreversible shock.

What is the treatment for circulatory shock?

The treatment for shock is aimed at correcting the cause and helping physiological compensatory mechanisms.

1. *FLUID REPLACEMENT THERAPY*

- *Blood or plasma transfusion.* If the shock is due to haemorrhage, transfusion of blood is the best therapy. If shock if due to plasma loss, plasma or appropriate electrolytic solution can correct the shock. Plasma substitute such as dextran can be used.
- *Saline.* Less effective.

2. *SYMPATHOMIMETIC DRUGS*

They mimic sympathetic stimulation. They are most useful in neurogenic and anaphylactic shock. They are not useful in haemorrhagic shock.

3. *OTHER THERAPY*

- Head low position.
- Oxygen.
- Glucocorticoids: They are useful because they increase the strength of heart in last stages of shock, by stabilizing lysosomal membranes they prevent release of enzymes of cells and help in metabolism of glucose by the severely damaged cells.

REGULATION OF BLOOD FLOW THROUGH SKELETAL MUSCLE

How is the blood flow through the skeletal muscles regulated?

During the periods of rest, the rate of blood flow to skeletal muscles is 3 to 4 ml/100 g of muscle.

At this time only 20 to 25% of muscle capillaries have flowing blood. During exercise when there are rhythmic contractions of the muscles, all dormant capillaries open up, greatly increasing the surface area and the rate of blood flow to the skeletal muscles. There is rhythmic increase in blood flow between the contractions.

Strong tetanic contraction of the muscle causes compression of blood vessels and even total stoppage of blood supply. Increase in blood supply during activity (exercise) is due to local regulation and also due to nervous control.

Local regulation. Due to exercise, muscles use oxygen very rapidly. This in turn decreases local oxygen concentration leading to vasodilatation. Many vasodilator substances (e.g. adenosine ions, acetylcholine, lactic acid) are also released which cause vasodilatation.

Nervous control. Skeletal muscles are supplied by sympathetic vasoconstrictor fibres and sympathetic vasodilator fibres.

Sympathetic vasoconstrictor nerves. These nerves release noradrenaline on stimulation and cause vasoconstriction and reduced blood flow to muscles. In addition norepinephrine secreted by adrenal medulla also passes into circulating blood to cause vasoconstriction. Adrenaline secreted by adrenal medulla acts on beta receptors of the vessels and causes vasodilatation.

Sympathetic vasodilator fibres. In cat and other lower animals, there are sympathetic vasodilator fibres which secrete acetylcholine at their endings, which in turn causes vasodilatation. Such fibres have not yet been proved in human beings (but adrenaline acting on beta receptors of the vessels causes vasodilatation).

HEART RATE

How much is normal heart rate and how is it regulated?

Normal heart rate varies between 72 and 80 beats/min.

REGULATION OF HEART RATE

Heart rate is adjusted according to the metabolic needs of the body, e.g. it increases during exercise and decreases during sleep so that optimum blood is supplied to the tissues.

Two factors mainly regulate the heart rate as follows:

1. *Local mechanism.* Any factor which affects SA node or junctional tissue affects the rhythmicity and also the heart rate.

2. *Nervous mechanism.* There is cardioinhibitory centre connected with vagus and cardioexcitatory centre connected with sympathetic nerves. Vagus exerts a tonic inhibitory control over the heart which is referred to as vagal tone. In addition vagus is reflexly stimulated through the sinoaortic mechanism. Stimulation of vagus causes decrease in the heart rate, whereas stimulation of sympathetic causes increase in the heart rate.

Cardiac centres, i.e. cardioinhibitory and cardioacceleratory centres are in reciprocal relation, i.e. stimulation of one depresses the other and vice versa. These cardiac centres are influenced either directly or reflexly.

1. Excitement quickens the heart rate and sudden shock lowers the heart rate. These changes are due to impulses coming to centres from the cerebral cortex and the hypothalamus.

2. Heart rate is also influenced reflexly by cardioinhibitory and cardiostimulatory reflexes and reflexes from other parts of the body.

- *Sinoaortic reflex.* When blood pressure rises, baroreceptors are stretched and sensory impulses from them increase the vagal tone, so that heart rate falls.
- *Cardioacceleratory reflexes.* Venous engorgement of the right atrium and the great veins reflexly increases the heart rate. This is known as Bainbridge reflex. Afferent impulses from engorged veins and right atrium pass via afferent nerves to cardiac centre to cause increase in the heart rate. This occurs during muscular exercise (due to increased venous return).
- *Reflexes from other parts of the body.*
  - Hypoxia. Hypoxia stimulates the respiratory centre reflexly through the chemoreceptors. It also stimulates cardiac centre to cause increase in heart rate. Therefore, rapid pulse in heart failure, anaemia, haemorrhage, high altitude, CO poisoning is due to this mechanism.
  - CO_2 excess. It has a direct as well as reflex effect in causing stimulation of the heart rate.
  - Body temperature. Increase in body temperature increases the heart rate by direct action on SA node as well as by stimulating cardioacceleratory centre.
  - Increased intracranial pressure. It directly stimulates the vagus and lowers the rate.
  - Adrenaline. It directly stimulates the heart rate but reflexly inhibits it (adrenaline increases the blood pressure and therefore by sinoaortic reflex mechanism reduces the heart rate).
  - Thyroxine. Thyroxine increases the heart rate by stimulating metabolic rate of SA node, increasing BMR of the body and by stimulating the sympathetic.
  - Exercise. It increases the heart rate by causing increased venous return, Bainbridge reflex, sympathetic stimulation, CO_2 excess, etc.

What is circulation time?

CIRCULATION TIME

Time taken for particle in the blood to flow from one point in circulation to the other is known as circulation time. It measures average linear velocity of blood.

What is plethysmograph?

Plethysmograph is the instrument used to find out total volume of blood flowing through an organ or part.

CARDIAC FAILURE*

What is cardiac failure? What are its causes?

Failure of the heart to pump enough blood to satisfy the needs of the body is called cardiac failure. It may be manifested in two ways:

- Decrease in cardiac output.
- By damming of blood in the veins behind the left or the right heart.

---

*For details refer Vaz M, Kurpad A, Raj T, editors. *Guyton & Hall Textbook of Medical Physiology.* Elsevier: New Delhi, 2013, p. 293.

CAUSES OF HEART FAILURE

- Acute or chronically progressive coronary artery disease.
- Malfunction of heart valves.
- Congenital abnormalities of the heart.
- Severe hypertension.

What are acute and chronic effects of moderate heart failure?

ACUTE EFFECTS

When there is sudden damage to the heart as in myocardial infarction, pumping ability of the heart is immediately depressed. This causes reduction in cardiac output to as low as 2 L/min. It also causes damming of blood in the veins resulting into increased systemic venous pressure so that right atrial pressure rises to 4 mmHg. This low cardiac output still sustains life but is associated with fainting.

When cardiac output becomes low, different circulatory reflexes are activated within 30 seconds, e.g. baroreceptor reflex, chemoreceptor reflex, CNS ischaemic response, reflexes originating in the heart. Due to these reflexes, there is strong sympathetic stimulation within few seconds which causes direct effect on the heart. If musculature of the heart is diffusely damaged but still functional, it strengthens the musculature. Or if the part of the muscle has become non-functional, normal muscle is stimulated and compensates for non-functional muscle. Thus heart becomes a stronger pump. Sympathetic stimulation also causes increased tone in the blood vessels, especially the veins. This results into increased venous return. This, in turn, increases the pumping ability of the heart increasing cardiac output to about 4.2 L/min, adequate to sustain life.

CHRONIC EFFECTS

After the few minutes of acute attack, a prolonged secondary state begins which causes: (a) retention of fluid by the kidneys and (b) progressive recovery of the heart.

- *Retention of fluid by the kidneys.* Decreased cardiac output decreases the urine output and therefore causes retention of fluid and increase in blood volume. When it is moderate, it helps in compensating the diminished pumping ability of the heart. It increases mean systemic filling pressure causing flow of blood towards the heart. Secondly it distends the veins, reduces the venous resistance and increases the flow of blood towards the heart.

  If cardiac pumping ability is greatly reduced (less than 25 to 50% of normal) then blood flow to kidneys is greatly reduced and there is low urinary output. Also there is retention of excess fluid but it has no beneficial effect on circulation as heart is already pumping at its maximal ability. This leads to development of oedema which is detrimental.
- *Progressive recovery of the heart.* Heart gradually recovers because of new collateral blood supply and hypertrophy of undamaged musculature. This is achieved ordinarily within 5 to 7 weeks.

Thus there is compensation for the damage (compensated heart failure) and person has normal resting cardiac output but if he performs heavy exercise, pumping ability of the heart cannot be increased to a desired level and symptoms of acute failure may return, i.e. cardiac reserve is reduced in compensated heart failure.

What is the effect of severe heart damage?

If heart is severely damaged, sympathetic reflexes, fluid retention are not useful in causing weakened heart to pump a normal output. Therefore, cardiac output can never rise enough. Fluid continues to be retained and person develops more and more oedema progressively eventually leading to death. This is called decompensated heart failure. This is treated by: (i) strengthening the heart by giving cardiotonic drugs, and (ii) by administering diuretic drugs.

What is left heart failure? When does it occur?

In large number of patients with acute failure, left sided failure predominates over right sided failure leading to unilateral left sided failure. Very rarely there is unilateral right sided failure. When there is predominant left heart failure, right heart pumps normal quantity of blood to the lungs but blood is not pumped out of lungs into the systemic circulation because of left sided failure. This causes increased volume of blood to be retained in the lungs, increased pulmonary capillary pressure (pulmonary vascular congestion) and pulmonary oedema.

What is high output cardiac failure? When does it occur?

When a person's cardiac output is much higher than normal, and he has signs of heart failure (high right and left atrial pressures, oedema), it is called 'high output failure'. This is due to over beating of heart with increased venous return and not due to decreased pumping ability of the heart.

This is caused due to circulatory abnormality that drastically decreases the total peripheral resistance.

CAUSES

- Arteriovenous fistula.
- Beriberi.
- Thyrotoxicosis.

What is low output cardiac failure?

In many cases of acute heart attacks, there is slow progressive cardiac deterioration and heart becomes incapable of pumping adequate blood flow to keep the body alive. All body tissues suffer and begin to deteriorate, ultimately leading to death, within few hours or few days. This type of circulatory shock is called cardiogenic shock or cardiac shock or power failure syndrome. Patient dies of cardiogenic shock before compensatory processes can return cardiac output to normal.

CORONARY CIRCULATION

Describe the anatomy of coronary blood supply.

The heart receives its nutrient supply through left and right coronary arteries. Only inner 75 to 100 μm of endocardial surface can obtain significant amounts of nutrients from the blood present in heart chambers.

Left coronary artery mainly supplies the anterior and lateral portions of the left ventricle. Right coronary artery mainly supplies most of the right ventricle as well as posterior part of the left ventricle in most of the persons. In about 20% of people, left artery predominates and in 30% both arteries provide nutrients equally. In 50% of people, right coronary artery predominates.

Most of the venous blood from the left ventricles is collected by way of coronary sinus (it is 75% of total coronary flow) and the venous blood from the right ventricle is collected through anterior cardiac veins directly into the right atrium. A small amount of blood is collected through Thebesian veins which directly open into all the chambers of the heart (Fig. 12.14).

How much is the resting coronary blood flow?

Resting coronary blood flow is 225 ml/min or 0.7 or 0.8 ml/g of heart muscle, i.e. 4 to 5% of the total cardiac output.

Describe the phasic changes in coronary blood flow.

During the phases of cardiac cycle there are changes in coronary blood flow. During systole, blood flow in the left ventricle falls to a low value. This is due to compression of intramuscular vessels during systole. During diastole, the blood through coronary capillaries rapidly rises, because there is relaxation of ventricular muscle and therefore there is no longer obstruction to the blood flow.

Blood passing through coronary capillaries of right ventricle also show similar phasic changes. They are far less because force of contraction of the right ventricle is much less (Fig. 12.15).

Describe the arrangement of coronary vessels in different layers of the heart.

On the surface of the cardiac muscle there are large epicardial arteries. From them smaller intramuscular arteries penetrate the muscle. They give rise to nutrient arteries in their way to supply muscle. Immediately beneath the endocardium, there is a plexus of subendocardial arteries. During systole when the left ventricle contracts forcefully, blood flow through subendocardial plexus almost falls to zero. To compensate for this, subendocardial arterial plexus is more extensive than the

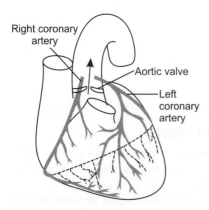

FIGURE 12.14 Coronary circulation.

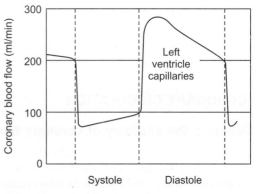

FIGURE 12.15 Phasic flow of blood through the coronary capillaries of left ventricle.

nutrient arteries in the middle and outer layers of the heart. Therefore, during diastole, flow through the subendocardial arteries is considerably greater.

How is the coronary blood flow controlled?

Coronary blood flow is controlled as follows:

1. *Local blood flow regulation.* It is the most important factor which regulates coronary blood flow. Under the resting state, 70% of O_2 is removed by the heart muscles as the blood passes through arteries. Therefore, not much additional oxygen can be provided unless the blood flow increases. Increased oxygen consumption by the heart increases the blood flow proportionately. Yet exact mechanism by which this is done is not certain. Probably decreased oxygen consumption causes release of vasodilator substances such as adenosine (due to increased degradation of adenosine triphosphate) from the muscle cells. This adenosine causes vasodilatation and then reabsorbed back into the cardiac cells to be reused. Hydrogen ions, bradykinin, CO_2, prostaglandins are the other suggested vasodilator substances.

According to other theory, lack of O_2 directly causes vasodilatation because muscles of the vessel wall itself get deficient oxygen. This causes muscle wall relaxation and vasodilatation.

2. *Nervous control.* Autonomic nerves control the blood flow directly as well as indirectly. Normally indirect effects are opposite to direct effect but play important role in control of blood flow.

- *Direct effect.* Distribution of parasympathetic nerve fibres (through vagus) to coronary system is so less that parasympathetic stimulation has very slight direct effect, causing dilatation of coronary arteries.

  Sympathetic nerve fibres extensively innervate the coronary vessels. The transmitters released at their endings are epinephrine and norepinephrine. Norepinephrine acts on alpha receptors and causes vasoconstriction. Epicardial vessels have preponderance of alpha receptors. Epinephrine acts on beta receptors of coronary vessels causing vasodilatation. Intramuscular arteries have preponderance of beta receptors. But overall effect is vasoconstriction of the coronary vessels. Metabolic local factors are more important in controlling blood flow; therefore, they over-ride the effect of nervous stimulation.

- *Indirect effect.* Sympathetic stimulation releases norepinephrine and epinephrine which increase the heart rate, force of contraction of heart and rate of metabolism of heart. Increased metabolism of heart causes relative lack of O_2 supply and sets off the local blood flow regularity mechanisms for dilating the coronary vessels thus increasing the blood flow in proportion to metabolic needs of heart muscle.

  Parasympathetic stimulation releases acetylcholine which causes decrease in heart rate and force of contraction of heart. These effects decrease O_2 consumption of heart and indirectly cause constriction of coronary arteries and decrease in blood flow.

What does cardiac muscle use for its metabolism normally?

Under the resting condition, cardiac muscle uses mainly fatty acids for its energy, rather than carbohydrate. But under anaerobic or ischaemic conditions, glucose is utilized through anaerobic glycolysis.

How is the coronary blood flow measured?

The most common method used for measuring coronary blood flow is nitrous oxide method. This is based on Fick principle. It gives almost accurate value.

PROCEDURE

Person inhales a mixture of 15% nitrous oxide and air for 10 minutes. The amount of nitrous oxide taken in per minute is determined.

During inhalation of the gas several blood samples are taken from an artery and through a catheter introduced into the mouth of coronary sinus (collection of mixed venous blood) at intervals. The nitrous oxide content of each of the blood sample is determined. Arteriovenous difference in nitrous oxide is calculated. Then coronary blood flow is determined by following formula:

$$\text{Coronary blood flow} = \frac{\text{Quantity of nitrous oxide taken up per minute}}{\substack{\text{Difference of nitrous oxide content of arterial} \\ \text{and venous blood}}}$$

Enumerate the factors affecting coronary blood flow.

Factors affecting coronary blood flow are:

1. *Mean aortic pressure.* This is the force for driving blood into the coronary arteries. Rise in mean aortic pressure increases the blood flow and vice versa. But if pressure remains high for a long time, because of increased work load on the heart, heart will go into congestive cardiac failure.

2. *Cardiac output.* Greater the cardiac output, greater is the coronary blood flow.

3. *Metabolic factors.* Increased metabolism of the heart increases O_2 consumption leading to relative hypoxia. This hypoxia causes dilatation of vessels and increase in blood flow (blood flow also increases due to release of adenosine).

4. *Effect of ions.* K+ ions in low concentration cause dilatation of coronary vessels whereas high K+ ion concentration causes constriction of the coronary vessels.

5. *Nervous stimulation.* Already explained.

6. *Hormones.* Thyroid hormone increases coronary blood flow because of increase in metabolism.

Adrenaline and noradrenaline cause increase in blood flow as already explained.

7. *Exercise.* During exercise, coronary blood flow increases because of sympathetic stimulation.

What is ischaemic heart disease?

Ischaemic heart disease is the disease resulting from insufficient coronary blood flow. The most common cause of decreased coronary blood flow is atherosclerosis. Coronary vessel occlusion may occur due to thrombus formation of the atherosclerotic plaque, embolus coming from other areas or coronary vessel spasm due to irritation of smooth muscle.

Describe the collateral circulation in the heart.

In the heart there is almost no communication existing among larger coronary arteries, but many anastomoses do exist among the smaller arteries (20 to 250 μm diameter). They open up within few seconds after the sudden occlusion of larger artery. The blood flowing through them is only one-half that is needed to keep cardiac muscle alive. But collateral blood flow begins to increase and become double by the end of second or third day and reaches to normal by one month. When atherosclerosis causes constriction of coronary arteries slowly over a period of many years, collateral vessels develop at the same time and therefore patient never experiences acute episode of cardiac dysfunction.

What is myocardial infarction?

Immediately after an acute coronary occlusion, the area of muscle that has either zero flow or very little flow that cannot sustain the cardiac muscle function, is said to be infarcted. The overall process is known as myocardial infarction.

Subendocardial muscle normally has difficulty in obtaining adequate blood flow as blood vessels are intensely compressed during systole of the heart. Subendocardial muscle frequently becomes infarcted without any evidence of infarction in the outer portions.

What is angina pectoris?

Development of cardiac pain whenever the load on the heart becomes too great in relation to coronary blood flow is called angina pectoris. Therefore, patient gets pain on exertion. Pain is hot, pressing and constricting type. It is treated by giving vasodilator drugs. Most commonly used vasodilators are nitroglycerin and other nitrate drugs.

What is the surgical treatment for coronary disease?

Following surgical procedures are done for treating coronary disease:

1. *Aortic coronary bypass.* Small vein grafts are anastomosed from the aorta to the side of the more peripheral coronary vessels. Each graft supplies a peripheral coronary artery beyond a block. The vein that is usually used is a long saphenous vein.

2. *Coronary angioplasty.* This is done to open partially blocked coronary vessel (before they become totally occluded) by passing small balloon-tipped catheter under radiographic guidance into the coronary system.

CEREBRAL CIRCULATION

Describe the anatomy of cerebral circulation.

Blood enters the cranium through two internal carotid and two vertebral arteries. Two vertebral arteries combine to form a basilar artery which in turn divides into two posterior cerebral arteries.

Each internal carotid artery divides into middle and anterior cerebral arteries. These six arteries (anterior, middle and posterior cerebral arteries on two sides) intercommunicate with the help of their branches forming circle of Willis. These three vessels supply different parts of brain.

Brain has a very rich blood supply. Grey matter has a greater supply than the white matter. Cerebral arteries are not end arteries. They freely anastomose especially at the circle of Willis. Because of this, blood flows adequately to different parts of brain, especially during the time of emergency. Venous blood drains into large cerebral sinuses (superior sagittal, inferior sagittal, cavernous). All sinuses ultimately form two transverse sinuses which become continuous with the two internal jugular veins.

How is the cerebral blood flow measured?

Cerebral blood flow is measured by nitrous oxide method based on Fick principle.

PROCEDURE

Person inhales 15% nitrous oxide. Blood samples are collected from any peripheral artery and from the jugular vein at frequent intervals, while the subject is inhaling the mixture of nitrous oxide and air. Nitrous oxide content of each sample is determined. Cerebral blood flow per minute is determined from the arteriovenous difference of nitrous oxide and the partition coefficient for N_2O between the blood and the brain.

What is average blood flow to the brain?

Under-resting state, 54 ml of blood is supplied per 100 g of brain tissue per minute or 770 ml/min. Total O_2 consumption by brain is 50 ml/min.

How is the cerebral circulation regulated?

Cerebral blood flow is autoregulated. Various factors help in this autoregulation as follows:

- Arterial CO_2 tension. Increase in CO_2 tension in the arterial blood increases the blood flow by causing dilatation of arterioles (Fig. 12.16).
- Hypoxia. Decreased O_2 supply to the brain also causes vasodilatation. This is due to lack of O_2 supply to smooth muscle of the vessel (causing smooth muscle to relax and cause vasodilatation). Lack of O_2 also causes release of certain vasodilator substances which cause direct effect on the vessel wall causing vasodilatation. The most important of it is adenine.

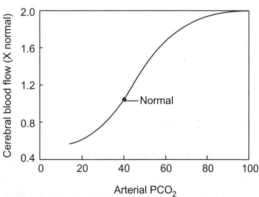

FIGURE 12.16 Relationship between arterial PCO_2 and cerebral blood flow.

Cerebral blood flow depends upon the difference between mean arterial pressure and internal jugular pressure because the difference between these two pressures is the driving force for cerebral circulation. Greater the driving force, greater is the blood flow. Cerebral blood flow is maintained therefore by maintaining general blood pressure through sinoaortic mechanism.

Cerebral blood flow is inversely related to cerebrovascular resistance which in turn depends on:

- Intracranial pressure. It has a negative correlation with blood flow.
- Viscosity of blood. Decreased viscosity increases the blood flow.
- Diameter of cerebral vessels. It is mainly controlled by CO_2, O_2 in blood and neurohormones as described above.

Adrenaline increases the cerebral blood flow.

PULMONARY CIRCULATION—REFER TO RESPIRATORY SYSTEM

CHAPTER 13

Central Nervous System

INTRODUCTION

What are the functions of nervous system?

Nervous system is divided into two main parts:

- Somatic
- Autonomic

Both somatic and autonomic nervous systems have two divisions:

- Sensory division (for collecting information).
- Motor division (for executing the action).

Somatic nervous system collects the information about the changes in the external environment, interprets the meaning of these changes and with the help of skeletal muscles takes appropriate action to neutralize the effect. It also co-ordinates the actions of different skeletal muscles of the body. Thus skeletal muscles are the effector organs of somatic nervous system.

Autonomic nervous system collects the information about the changes that take place in the internal environment, i.e. internal viscera interprets these changes and guides the action and gets the plan executed with the help of smooth muscles, cardiac muscles and secretory epithelium (which are effector organs of ANS).

The higher functions of nervous system include speech, learning and memory.

Name the different parts of the brain.

Different parts of brain are:

1. Forebrain (prosencephalon)
   (a) Telencephalon. Cerebrum with interconnections
   (b) Diencephalon. Thalamus and hypothalamus
2. Midbrain (mesencephalon)
3. Hindbrain (rhombencephalon). pons, medulla and cerebellum.

LEVELS OF CNS FUNCTION

State the levels of central nervous system function.

There are three major levels of central nervous system (CNS) function. They are:

- Spinal cord level.
- Lower brain or subcortical level.
- Higher brain or cortical level.

Give functions subserved at spinal cord level.

Neuronal circuits in the spinal cord can cause:

- Walking movements.
- Withdrawal reflexes for taking the portion of the body away from painful object.
- Reflexes which stiffen the legs to support the body against gravity.
- Reflexes that control local blood vessels, gastrointestinal movements, etc.
- Reflexes that control micturition.

Give functions subserved at lower brain (subcortical) level.

Most of the subconscious activities of the body are controlled in medulla, pons, hypothalamus, thalamus, cerebellum and basal ganglia, e.g.

- Subconscious control of arterial blood pressure and respiration.
- Control of equilibrium.
- Feeding reflexes such as salivation in response to taste of food.
- Expression of emotions like anger, excitement, sexual response, reaction to pain, etc.

What are the functions subserved at higher brain level?

Cortex always functions in association with lower centres of nervous system. Without cerebral cortex functions of lower brain centres are imprecise. Cortex acts a vast storehouse and cortical information is utilized to convert the lower brain function to precise operations.

Cerebral cortex is responsible for thought processes. Here also lower brain centres initiate wakefulness in the cerebral cortex because of which bank of memories can be used for thinking.

TYPES OF CELLS IN NERVOUS SYSTEM

What are different types of cells present in central nervous system?

Central nervous system contains:

1. *Neurons (nerve cells).* There are about 100 billion neurons present in the CNS.
2. *Neuroglial cells.* These are connective tissue cells. They can divide throughout the life but cannot conduct the impulse. They are of the following four types:
    - **Astrocytes.** These are star-shaped cells with many processes and they form skeleton for CNS. They are mainly present in white matter.
      Functions:
      - They provide framework and support the neuronal cells.
      - They form insulation around synapses to prevent spread of impulse.
      - Their processes and footplates on the walls of blood vessels contribute to formation of blood-brain barrier.
      - They store glycogen.
    - **Oligodendrocytes.** They are smaller than astrocytes and have few processes. They form myelin sheath for nerves present within the CNS.

■ **Microglial cells.** They are smaller than oligodendrocytes and mainly do the functions of phagocytosis to clear the cellular debris after injury. They become active when there is damage to the nervous tissue by injury.
■ **Ependymal cells.** They line the ventricles in brain and spinal cord. They are ciliated columner cells. They secrete cerebrospinal fluid.

What is a neuron? What are the various types of neurons?

Neuron or nerve cell is the structural and functional unit of the nervous system. Neuron consists of:

1. Cell body or soma.
2. Protoplasmic processes (nerve fibres). They are of two types:
   ■ *Dendrites.* These are the processes which bring information towards the soma. There may be many dendrites or only a single dendrite.
   ■ *Axon.* It is the process which carries the information away from the cell and is usually single.

According to the site from where dendrites and axon arise, neuron can be classified as follows:

■ *Unipolar neuron* containing only one axon and one dendrite. Axon and dendrite arise from the common stem.
■ *Bipolar neuron* containing one axon and one dendrite. Axon and dendrite arise from opposite poles.
■ *Multipolar neuron* containing one axon and a number of dendrites. Axon and dendrites arise from different sites.

Usually cell surface from which the axon passes shows an elevation which is known as axon hillock.

Describe the structure of a neuron.

Neuron consists of the nerve cell body (soma), the dendrites and the axon (Fig. 13.1).

Soma of the neuron contains usual organelles but centrosome is not functional. It indicates that it is a highly specialized cell and has lost its ability to reproduce. If it is damaged, it is replaced by neuroglial cell. In addition to usual organelles, cytoplasm shows Nissl's granules because of which the cell has spotted appearance. These granules also called tigroid bodies, are collection of RNA. Their number depends on the activity of the neuron. When the nerve fibre is damaged, they get disintegrated (chromatolysis). Cytoplasm also shows thin filamentous structures called neurofibrils which extend from the tip of the dendrite to the tip of the axon.

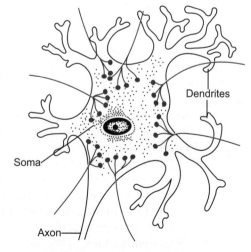

FIGURE 13.1 Structure of a neuron.

Functionally neurons are classified as *afferent neuron* (which collects the information from the peripheral receptors), *efferent neuron* (which sends signals to the effector organs to carry out necessary action) and *internuncial neuron* or *interneuron* (which lies between afferent and efferent neurons).

What is the resting membrane potential of neuronal soma?

Resting membrane potential of neuronal soma is low. Soma of spinal motor neuron has a resting membrane potential of about -65 mV. Lower voltage allows positive and negative control of degree of excitability of a neuron.

NERVE–FIBRES CLASSIFICATION

Refer to question one in chapter 'Nerve and Muscle'.

Synapse
DEFINITION

How are neurons connected to each other?

There is no anatomical connection or continuity between different neurons. They are connected only functionally. These connections are achieved by synapses. So synapse is the functional junction between two neurons.

TYPES

What are the different types of synapses?

Synapses can be of different types depending upon how the connections are established, e.g. axodendritic, axosomatic, axoaxonic.

Most of the synapses occur between axon of one neuron and dendrite or soma of the other neuron.

Synapses can also be classified on the basis of process of transmission of impulses as electrical synapses and chemical synapses.

Chemical synapse is the type in which the first neuron secretes a chemical substance called neurotransmitter at synapse, and this transmitter in turn acts on receptor proteins present in the membrane of the next neuron to excite or inhibit the neuron or to modify its sensitivity. Almost all synapses in the central nervous system of human beings are chemical synapses.

Electrical synapses are characterized by direct open fluid channels that conduct electricity from one cell to the next. Most of these consist of small protein tubular structures called gap junctions which allow free movement of ions from interior of one cell to the interior of the next. In such a synapse impulse can be transmitted in both the directions. Such synapses are mainly seen in invertebrates. In human beings they are present in cardiac and smooth muscles.

What is presynaptic neuron?

Neuron which brings the information towards the synapse is known as presynaptic neuron.

What is postsynaptic neuron?

Neuron which carries information away from the synapse is known as postsynaptic neuron.

STRUCTURE

Describe the structure of the synapse.

As the axon of the neuron approaches the synapse, it branches and loses its myelin sheath. Each branch of the axon shows a slight swelling at its end called synaptic knob or synaptic button, which makes synapse with the soma or dendrite of the postsynaptic neuron. The membrane of the synaptic knob is termed presynaptic membrane. There is a small gap between presynaptic membrane and postsynaptic membrane (200 to 300 Å) which is called synaptic cleft. This gap is filled by the extracellular fluid (Fig. 13.2).

Synaptic knob contains mitochondria and synaptic vesicles. Synaptic vesicles contain the neurotransmitter. When this neurotransmitter is released into the synaptic cleft, it causes either excitation or inhibition of the postsynaptic membrane. Mitochondria provide the ATP required for the synthesis of neurotransmitter.

Postsynaptic membrane contains a large number of receptor proteins which protrude outward in the synaptic cleft. Neurotransmitter released in the synaptic cleft binds with these receptor proteins to cause the effect. Receptor proteins are of two types:

1. **Ion channel receptor proteins.** Which line ion channels (Na^+, $K^+.Cl^-$, etc.). Transmitter released in synaptic cleft by reacting with them causes opening of these channels.
2. **Enzymatic type of receptor proteins.** When neurotransmitter released in the synaptic cleft reacts with them the following effects are caused:
   - Activation of cellular gene for manufacture of additional receptor protein channels in the membrane.
   - Activation of protein kinase which decreases the number of receptor protein channels in the membrane.

Thus there is alteration in the reactivity of the neuron to the transmitter. Such effects are called synaptic modulator effects.

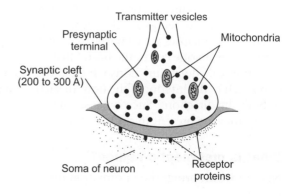

FIGURE 13.2 Physiologic anatomy of synapse.

SYNAPTIC TRANSMISSION

Describe the process of synaptic transmission.

The following events occur in sequential order during synaptic transmission:

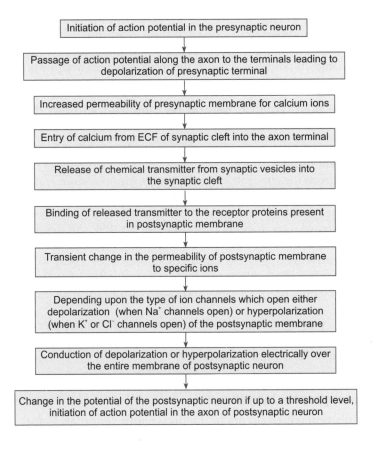

EPSP

What is excitatory postsynaptic potential (EPSP)? How is it produced?

At the synapse when the neurotransmitter released is excitatory transmitter, it acts on the postsynaptic membrane and increases its permeability for sodium ions. This allows a large number of sodium ions to diffuse to the interior of the postsynaptic membrane. This in turn raises the membrane potential in the positive direction (depolarization). This increase in voltage is termed excitatory postsynaptic potential. If the potential rise is high enough, it will elicit action potential in the axon of the postsynaptic neuron. Usually, discharge of a single presynaptic terminal cannot increase the potential to the threshold level, instead simultaneous discharge of many terminals at the same time or in rapid succession is required.

IPSP

What is inhibitory postsynaptic potential (IPSP)? How is it produced?

Transmitter released at the synaptic cleft is an inhibitory transmitter. It causes opening of either K^+ channels or Cl^- channels in the postsynaptic membrane, leading to diffusion of large numbers of K^+ ions from the neuron to the extracellular fluid or large numbers of Cl^- ions to diffuse to the interior of the neuron. This causes postsynaptic membrane potential to become more negative (hyperpolarization). This change in potential is called the inhibitory postsynaptic potential.

How can the postsynaptic neuron be inhibited without development of IPSP?

There is a short circuiting mechanism which causes the inhibition of neuron without development of IPSP.

In some neurons the concentration differences for potassium and chloride ions are such that the Nernst potential of these ions are equal to the resting membrane potential of the neuron. Therefore, even if either K^+ or Cl^- channels open, there is no net transfer of ions in either direction and no IPSP can develop. But when the neuron is excited through other synapse causing inflow of Na^+ ions (because K^+ or Cl^- channels are open), the rapid flux of these ions would nullify the EPSP produced. So far less EPSP will be produced. Greater influx of sodium is therefore required to overcome K^+ or Cl^- flux and cause excitation (may be 5 to 20 times the normal).

This tendency of K^+ or Cl^- ions to maintain membrane potential to resting level (when channels are wide open) masks the effect of sodium current flow by excitatory synapse, thus causing inhibition.

What is presynaptic inhibition?

Type of inhibition which occurs in the presynaptic terminals before the signal even reaches the synapse is known as presynaptic inhibition. This type of inhibition occurs because of axoaxonic synapse. The presynaptic inhibition is caused as follows:

There are three neurons N_1, N_2, and N_3. Neuron N_2 makes a synaptic connection with N_3 to cause its excitation. Axon or axon collateral of neuron N_1 synapses with axon of the neuron N_2. On stimulation of N_1 neuron at this axoaxonic synapse, there is release of inhibitory transmitter which increases the permeability of membrane of axon of N_2 neuron for Cl^- ions. When action potential travels along this axon terminal, magnitude of change in potential produced becomes less (because of entry of negatively charged Cl^- ions). Lesser amount of calcium enters into the terminal because of lesser number of calcium channels which open in this membrane (at synapse between N_2 and N_3). This causes decreased amount of excitatory transmitter to be released at the synapse (excitatory synapse between neuron N_2 and N_3). Thus the size of EPSP produced is less. Here, excitability of postsynaptic neuron is not diminished. Therefore, by presynaptic inhibition, a particular excitatory input can be inhibited without affecting the ability of other excitatory synapses to fire the cell.

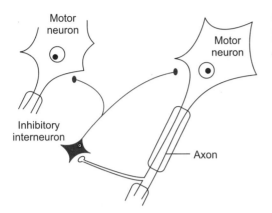

FIGURE 13.3 Renshaw cell or negative feedback inhibition of a spinal motor neuron via an inhibitory interneuron.

Enumerate the types of inhibition in CNS.

The types of inhibition in CNS are:

1. *Postsynaptic inhibition*, i.e. inhibition of postsynaptic neuron. It may be:
   - Direct by development of IPSP or
   - Indirect-postsynaptic neuron can be refractory to excitation because it has just fired and is in its refractory period.
   - Short circuiting mechanism which causes inhibition without development of IPSP as stated above.

2. *Presynaptic inhibition*. Described above.

3. *Renshaw cell inhibition*. This is negative feedback or feed backward inhibition. Impulse generated in motor neuron activates inhibitory interneuron (Renshaw cell) to secrete inhibitory mediator which inhibits motor neuron (Fig. 13.3).

4. *Feed forward inhibition*. This type of inhibition is seen in cerebellum, e.g. stimulation of basket cell produces IPSP in Purkinje cell. However, basket cell and Purkinje cell are excited by the same excitatory input. This arrangement is termed feed forward inhibition; it limits the duration of excitation produced by any given afferent volley.

What are the factors affecting synaptic transmission?

1. General factors. pH, hypoxia, drugs, diseases, etc.
2. Presynaptic factors
3. Postsynaptic factors

PROPERTIES OF SYNAPSE

Name and explain the different properties of synapse.

1. *One way conduction property of synapse.*

Transmission of impulse always occurs from presynaptic membrane to postsynaptic membrane and never in the opposite direction. So the synapse acts like a valve and therefore impulse transmission is unidirectional. This is also called law of dynamic polarity.

2. *Synaptic delay and its causes.*

Some time is required for the passage of impulse from presynaptic membrane to postsynaptic membrane. This is called synaptic delay. Normally, synaptic delay is for 0.5 ms.

CAUSES OF SYNAPTIC DELAY

- Time taken for the release of transmitter.

- Time taken for the diffusion of transmitter through synaptic cleft to post-synaptic membrane.
- Time taken for action of neurotransmitter to bind with receptors on the postsynaptic membrane and to cause the opening of ion channels.
- Time taken for diffusion of ions causing changes in resting membrane potential (development of EPSP or IPSP).

3. *Summation property of synapse.*

Excitation of a single presynaptic terminal on the surface of the neuron will almost never excite (or inhibit) the neuron as sufficient transmitter substance is not released to raise EPSP to a threshold level. So, postsynaptic neuron is stimulated by simultaneous stimulation of large number of presynaptic terminals on it or large number of impulses arising in rapid succession at a single synapse. Thus there are two types of summations, viz. temporal and spatial.

Temporal summation. It occurs due to a large number of impulses coming one after the other at a synapse. At each synapse postsynaptic potential lasts for 15 milliseconds. Therefore, if the terminal is stimulated at a rapid rate, the second stimulus reaches the synapse before the effect of first is over. This causes release of more and more transmitter substance which in turn causes the postsynaptic potential to rise up to a threshold for firing.

Spatial summation. When the postsynaptic neuron receives impulses from a large number of presynaptic terminals simultaneously, effect of all is added up and enough transmitter substance is released to cause change of potential to a threshold level.

Both types of summations occur simultaneously in the neuronal pool.

4. *Convergence property of synapse.*

When large number of presynaptic neurons have synaptic connections on a single postsynaptic neuron, some presynaptic terminals may release excitatory transmitter and others may release inhibitory transmitter. Sum total of these excitatory and inhibitory impulses will decide whether postsynaptic neuron will be inhibited or stimulated. Information coming from large number of neurons is thus integrated to decide the onward effect. This phenomenon is known as convergence (Fig. 13.4).

5. *Divergence property of synapse.*

One presynaptic neuron may have synaptic connections with a large number of postsynaptic neurons because of the large number of branches of its axon. Thus a

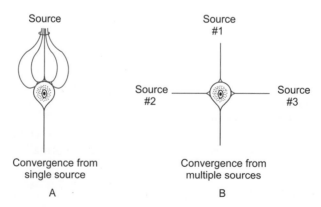

FIGURE 13.4 Phenomenon of 'convergence' on a single neuron.

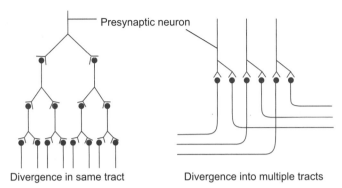

FIGURE 13.5 Phenomenon of 'divergence'.

single impulse is converted to a number of impulses going to a number of post-synaptic neurons. This causes magnification and therefore helps in amplification. This phenomenon is known as divergence (Fig. 13.5).

6. *Occlusion property of synapse.*

Response of simultaneous stimulation of two presynaptic neurons is less than sum total of the response obtained when they are separately stimulated, e.g. stimulation of the presynaptic neuron (A), say, stimulates five postsynaptic neurons and stimulation of neuron (B) also stimulates five postsynaptic neurons, then the total number of postsynaptic neurons stimulated by the stimulation of A and B neurons separately is equal to ten. But if A and B neurons are stimulated simultaneously, number of postsynaptic neurons stimulated is less than ten. This is because some of the postsynaptic neurons are common to both.

7. *Subliminal fringe property of synapse.*

When response obtained by the simultaneous stimulation of two presynaptic neurons is greater than the sum total of response obtained when they are separately stimulated, it is called subliminal fringe. This is exactly opposite to occlusion. Suppose stimulation of neuron A causes stimulation of five postsynaptic neurons, and stimulation of neuron B also causes stimulation of five postsynaptic neurons, then sum of neurons stimulated is ten. But when neuron A and B are stimulated simultaneously, number of postsynaptic neurons stimulated is more than ten.

8. *Facilitation of synapse.*

When presynaptic axon is stimulated with several consecutive individual stimuli, each stimulus may evoke a larger postsynaptic potential than that evoked by previous stimulus. This phenomenon is known as facilitation. This is due to each succeeding stimulus causing greater release of the transmitter but the mechanism by which it occurs is not known. In facilitation, therefore, normally subliminal stimulus from a presynaptic neuron 'primes' the postsynaptic neuron so that another subliminal stimulus can evoke a discharge from the postganglionic neuron. Here the first stimulus is supposed to facilitate.

9. *Property of after discharge of synapse.*

Single instantaneous input results in sustained output signals (i.e. a series of repetitive discharges). This is known as after discharge. Input signal lasts only for one millisecond but output signal lasts for many milliseconds.

10. *Fatigue property of synapse.*

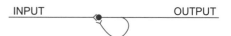

INPUT   OUTPUT

FIGURE 13.6 Reverberating circuit.

Repeated stimulation of synapse causes lesser response either due to exhaustion of transmitter substance or accumulation of waste products or due to refractoriness of postsynaptic membrane to the transmitter substance. Fatigue is a temporary phenomenon. Therefore, fatigue and recovery from fatigue constitute an important short-term mechanism for modulating sensitivities of different neuronal circuits.

11. *Reverberation.*

Passage of impulse from a presynaptic neuron and again back to the presynaptic neuron to cause a continuous stimulation of presynaptic neuron is known as reverberation. The nervous system is a network of fibres and in this network it is possible that a branch of axon of a neuron may establish connection again with its own dendron. This causes reverberation of impulse through the same circuit again and again. This is prevented to some extent by fatigue (Fig. 13.6).

12. *Post-tetanic potentiation.*

A postsynaptic neuron is stimulated with a single stimulus, then with a volley of stimuli (say 100/sec) for two seconds and then again with a single stimulus. This second stimulus evokes a larger postsynaptic response than the first single stimulus. This is called post-tetanic potentiation.

NEUROTRANSMITTERS

Name the different neurotransmitters.

There are about 40 different neurotransmitters and they are classified as:

1. *Small molecule rapidly acting transmitters* which cause acute response:
   - Acetylcholine
   - Amines
     - Norepinephrine
     - Epinephrine
     - Dopamine
     - Serotonin
   - Amino acids
     - Gamma-aminobutyric acid (GABA)
     - Glycine
     - Glutamate
     - Aspartate
2. *Slowly acting neuropeptide transmitters* having prolonged effect:
   - Neuroactive peptides releasing hormones from hypothalamus, e.g. TRH, LH releasing hormone, somatostatin.
   - Pituitary peptides, e.g. ACTH, beta endorphins, vasopressin, oxytocin.
   - Peptides acting on gut and brain, e.g. leucine-enkephalin, methionine-enkephalin, substance P, cholecystokinin, VIP (vasoactive intestinal polypeptide), neurotensin, insulin, glucagon.
   - Neuropeptides from other tissues, e.g. angiotensin II, bradykinin, carnosine, bombesin. Neurons containing neurotransmitter are named accordingly, e.g. cholinergic neurons, adrenergic neurons, dopaminergic neurons, etc.

IMPORTANT NEUROTRANSMITTERS

Where is acetylcholine liberated?

Acetylcholine is released by many neurons in the nervous system. It is specifically released by large pyramidal cells, many neurons of basal ganglia, motor neurons innervating skeletal muscles, preganglionic neurons in autonomic nervous system, postganglionic neurons of parasympathetic nervous system, and some postganglionic neurons of sympathetic nervous system. In most instances acetylcholine is excitatory. At very few places (vagus supplying heart) acetylcholine acts as an inhibitory transmitter.

Where is norepinephrine secreted?

Norepinephrine is secreted by many neurons in the brain stem and hypothalamus.

- Norepinephrine is secreted by area locus ceruleus in pons which determines mood of the mind (arousal and dreaming). This area of pons sends nerve fibres to widespread areas of brain.
- Norepinephrine is also secreted at postganglionic sympathetic nerve endings.
- Tegmentum gives noradrenergic fibres to various parts of the brain.
- Hypothalamus.

Norepinephrine is mainly excitatory, only a few places it is inhibitory.

Where is gamma-aminobutyric acid (GABA) liberated?

Gamma-aminobutyric acid is the most common transmitter in the brain. It is inhibitory and in about one-third of synapses of brain, it is the transmitter. Deficient level of GABA in corpus striatum occurs in patients with Huntington's chorea (uncontrolled movements that characterize this disease are mainly due to diminished effectiveness of GABA).

Where is glutamate released?

Glutamate is released by presynaptic terminals in many sensory pathways as well as areas of cortex. It probably always causes excitation.

Where is dopamine released?

Dopamine is a neurotransmitter released in substantia nigra, ventral tegmentum and corpus striatum. It is mainly inhibitory. In paralytic agitans, there is deficiency of dopamine in nigrostriate pathways. Dopamine is also a neurotransmitter in the hypothalamus. Several drugs used as tranquillizers reduce dopamine content in the brain neurons.

Where is substance P released?

P substance is released by pain fibre terminals of spinal cord, basal ganglia and hypothalamus. It causes excitation.

Where is enkephalin secreted?

Enkephalin is secreted by nerve terminals in spinal cord, basal ganglia, brain stem, thalamus and hypothalamus. It is excitatory to systems that inhibit transmission of pain.

Where is serotonin secreted?

Serotonin is secreted by nuclei of median raphe of brain stem projecting to dorsal horns of spinal cord and hypothalamus. It acts as an inhibitory transmitter for pain pathway of the spinal cord. It is believed to control mood and also cause sleep. Serotonergic neurons are also involved in the regulation of temperature. Inhibition of serotonergic neurons is associated with hallucinations. The drug LSD (lysergic acid diethylamide) used by addicts inhibits serotonergic neurons and produces various hallucinations.

SENSORY SYSTEM

INTRODUCTION

What is sensory system or sensory division of CNS?

Sensory division of nervous system collects the information about external and internal environment and conveys it to the brain.

Sensation is conscious perception of sensory information. It occurs when information reaches the sensory area of the cerebral cortex.

Sensory system therefore consists of:

1. *Sensory receptors.* Receptors are specialized cells present at the end of the afferent nerve.
2. *Afferent neurons.* Information from receptors travels through afferent nerve to sensory area of cerebral cortex through multiple neurons which is termed the sensory pathway.
3. *Sensory cortex.* This is the area of the cortex which receives sensory information.

CLASSIFICATION OF SENSATIONS

How are the sensations classified?

Sensations are broadly classified as general and special:

1. General sensations:
   - Somatic—Superficial and deep
   - Visceral
2. Special sensations:
   - Vision
   - Audition
   - Gustatory
   - Olfactory
   - Equilibrium

RECEPTORS

DEFINITION

What are receptors?

Receptors are non-neuronal specialized cells present at the afferent nerve endings. They are capable of transforming stimulus energy into electrical energy which results into transmission of nerve impulses along the afferent nerve fibres.

CLASSIFICATION

How are receptors classified?

Receptors are classified on the basis of different criteria as follows:

1. *Classification based on the source of stimulus:*
   - *Exteroceptors.* Receptors which receive stimuli from immediate external surrounding, e.g. cutaneous receptors for pain, touch, heat, cold, etc.
   - *Enteroceptors.* Receptors which receive stimuli within the body, e.g. chemoreceptors, baroreceptors.
   - *Telereceptors.* Receptors which receive stimulus coming from the distance, e.g. visual receptors, cochlear receptors.
   - *Proprioceptors.* Receptors detecting changes in muscle length, tension and movements of joints.

2. *Classification based on the type of stimulus energy:*

Stimulus energy	Receptors
• Mechanical	Mechanoreceptor in: • Skin and deep tissue • Joints • Muscle and tendon stretch receptors • Hair cells of cochlea • Hair cells of vestibular apparatus • Baroreceptors of carotid and aortic sinus
• Photic (light)	Photoreceptors of retina (rods and cones)
• Thermal	Cold and warm receptors which detect environmental temperatures
• Chemical	• Chemoreceptors for taste and smell • Aortic and carotid body receptors for detecting level of arterial PO_2, PCO_2 and H^+ ions • Chemoreceptors on the surface of medulla for detecting level of blood PCO_2 • Osmoreceptors in supraoptic nuclei of hypothalamus • Chemoreceptors in hypothalamus detecting levels of blood glucose, fatty acids, amino acids
• Extremes of mechanical, thermal and chemical energy	Nociceptors (detecting pain)

3. *Classification based on type of sensation*, e.g. touch, cold, heat, pain, light, smell, taste, etc.
4. *Classification based on rate of adaptation of receptors:*
   - *Slowly adapting receptors* (tonic or static receptors), which fire action potentials continuously during stimulus application.
   - *Rapidly adapting receptors* (phasic or dynamic receptors), which fire action potentials at a decreasing rate during stimulus application.
5. *Clinical classification of receptors:*
   - Superficial receptors, present in skin and mucous membrane.
   - Deep receptors, present in the muscles, tendons, joints and subcutaneous tissue.
   - Visceral receptors, present in visceral organs.

PROPERTIES

Describe the properties of receptors.

1. *Specificity of response.* Each receptor is easily stimulated (has lowest threshold) by only one type of sensation. Other sensations are almost ineffective in stimulating the receptor, e.g. rods and cones are easily stimulated by light but same light fails to stimulate Pacinian corpuscle.

2. *Generation of receptor potential on stimulation.* Whenever stimulus excites the receptor, it changes the potential across the membrane of the receptor. This change in the potential is called receptor potential. When the receptor potential rises above the threshold for eliciting action potential in the nerve fibre, action potential is generated in the nerve fibre attached to the receptor. Greater the magnitude of receptor potential, greater is the rate of discharge of action potentials in the nerve fibre.

Amplitude of the receptor potential rapidly increases at first with the strength of stimulus but progressively less rapidly with higher stimulus strength. Receptor potential amplitude depends therefore on strength of stimulus. It also depends on the velocity of stimulus application. Amplitude of receptor potential rises with the rate of change of stimulus application (it also applies to the removal of stimulus, e.g. off-response). Another way of varying receptor potential is by adding two or more stimuli together (summation).

Thus magnitude of the receptor potential can vary with stimulus intensity, rate of change of stimulus application, summation and adaptation.

3. *Adaptation.* When a continuous sensory stimulus is applied, the receptors respond at a very high impulse rate at first, then at a progressively lower rate until finally many of them no longer respond at all. All the sensory receptors adapt either partially or completely to their stimuli. Some sensory receptors adapt rapidly to 'extinction' within fraction of a second, e.g. Pacinian corpuscle. Rapidly adapting or phasic receptors react strongly while a change is actually taking place. So they detect the rate at which the change takes place in the stimulus and they have predictive function (change can be predicted ahead of time). Slowly adapting receptors (tonic receptors) continue to transmit impulses to CNS as long as stimulus is present. Therefore, they keep the brain constantly apprised of the status of the body and its relation to its surrounding.

Adaptation is the individual property of the receptor, e.g. rods and cones adapt by changing their chemical composition, mechanoreceptors (Pacinian corpuscle) adapt due to redistribution of fluid. The most obvious function of adaptation is to decrease the amount of sensory information reaching the brain.

4. *Intensity discrimination.* There are two ways for transmitting intensity of stimulus to CNS:

By varying the frequency of action potentials generated by stimulus in the given receptor. Relationship between the stimulus intensity and interpreted intensity is given by the following laws:

- *Weber-Fechner law.* According to this law:

Interpreted intensity = Logarithm of stimulus strength $\times$ constant.

- *Power law.* According to this law:

Interpreted signal strength = $K\,(\text{stimulus} - K_1)_y$

K and K_1 are constants and 'Y' is the power to which stimulus strength is raised.

5. *Projection.* When any part of the sensory path is stimulated, conscious sensation referred to the location of the receptor is produced. This is called law of projection. It helps in judging stimulus quality. This is due to specificity of nerve fibres transmitting only one modality of sensation called 'labelled line' principle. Labelled line mechanism is the mechanism in which stimulus is encoded by the particular neural pathway.

State the differences between receptor potential and action potential.

Receptor potential	Action potential
• Receptor potential is a graded response, i.e. amplitude of receptor potential increases with increasing velocity of stimulus application and increasing strength of stimulus.	Action potential obeys all or none law. Once the stimulus strength is great enough to bring the membrane potential to a threshold level, further increase in stimulus strength does not cause any change in the amplitude. Cannot be added together.
• Can be added together, if second stimulus arrives before the receptor potential developed due to first stimulus is over.	
• Has no refractory period.	
• Mostly it is local and cannot be propagated.	Has a refractory period of about 1 ms. It can be propagated without loss in the amplitude along the nerve fibre. Duration is small (approximately 1 to 2 ms).
• Duration is greater (approximately 5 to 10 ms).	

RECEPTOR POTENTIAL

Describe the mechanism by which receptor potential develops.

Different receptors are excited by different ways as follows:

- Mechanical deformation of the receptor which stretches the receptor and opens the ion channels.
- Application of a chemical to a membrane which also opens the ion channels.
- Change in temperature of the membrane which changes the permeability of the membrane.
- Effect of light (in case of photoreceptors) changes the membrane permeability.

At all instances, the cause of basic change in the membrane potential is a change in receptor membrane permeability, which allows the ions to diffuse more or less readily through the membrane and thereby change the transmembrane potential of the receptor.

What is sensory unit?

A single afferent neuron with its all receptor endings is termed as a sensory unit.

What is receptive field?

A portion of body when stimulated, leads to activity in a particular afferent neuron and is termed receptive field of that neuron. Fields of neighbouring afferent neurons overlap. Degree of overlap varies in different body parts.

CUTANEOUS SENSATIONS

Enumerate the cutaneous sensations. Which type of sensory fibres encodes these sensations?

Touch, vibration, pressure, cold, heat, pain, etc. are the various cutaneous sensations.

About one million nerve fibres innervate the skin. Most are unmyelinated fibres responsible for crude sensations. There are a few large myelinated sensory fibres (group II) which encode sensory quality of touch, vibration and pressure, and a few fibres (group III or A delta and group IV or group C) which carry sensation of temperature and pain.

Name the tactile receptors.

Cutaneous tactile receptors are:

1. *Free nerve endings.* These are present everywhere in the skin and in many other tissues. They detect touch and pressure.

2. *Meissner's corpuscles.* These are encapsulated receptors supplied by A-beta type of myelinated nerve fibres. They are present in non-hairy parts of skin and are abundant at fingertips, lips, etc. They adapt within fraction of a second. They are sensitive to movement of light objects over the surface of the skin. They also detect low frequency vibration.

3. *Merkel's discs.* These receptors are always grouped together in a single receptor organ called 'Iggo dome receptors'. The entire group of receptors present in it are innervated by large single myelinated fibre. They are present in areas where Meissner's corpuscles are present. They are slowly adapting receptors. They along with Meissner's corpuscles play an important role in localizing touch sensations and also in determining the texture of what is felt.

4. *Hair end organs.* Each hair and its basal nerve fibre forms hair end organ. It is stimulated by slight movement of the hair. These receptors mainly detect the movement of objects on the surface of the body.

5. *Ruffini's end organs.* They are present in deeper layers of skin and also in the deeper tissues. They are multibranched encapsulated endings. They adapt very little and therefore continuously signal the state of deformation of the skin and

deeper tissues. They are present in joint capsule where they detect degree of joint rotation.

   6. *Pacinian corpuscles.* They are present immediately beneath the skin, deep in fascial tissues. They adapt very quickly, so they are stimulated only by very rapid movements of the tissues. They detect the tissue vibration or other extremely rapid changes in mechanical state of the tissue.

SENSORY PATHWAY

There are two types of sensory pathways:

   1. *Specific ascending pathways.* Pathway carries only one specific modality of sensation to specific areas in cortex.
   2. *Non-specific ascending pathways.* Pathway carries several sensory modalities. Pathway is responsible for arousal and alertness as it projects from reticular formation to entire cortex.

ASCENDING TRACTS

Name the pathways of transmission of different sensations.

   - *Dorsal column-medial lemniscal pathway* carrying sensations of fine touch, vibration and proprioception.
   - *Anterolateral pathway* carrying sensation of crude touch, pain, heat and cold, tickle, itch, etc.

Describe the dorsal column-medial lemniscal pathway.

All specialized receptors, Meissner's corpuscles, Iggodome receptors, pacinian corpuscles, hair receptors and Ruffini's endings transmit signals through A-beta type of nerve fibres having velocity of transmission from 30 to 70 m/s.

   Free nerve endings transmit the sensations mainly via A-delta type of nerve fibres which conduct impulses at a velocity of 5 to 30 m/s. Some tactile free nerve endings transmit signals through 'C' type of unmyelinated nerve fibres which conduct impulses at a velocity of 2 m/s (these mainly carry the sensation of tickle).

   All these fibres enter the spinal cord via dorsal roots of spinal nerves (Fig. 13.7). After entering the spinal cord, large myelinated nerve fibres from specialized receptors pass medially into lateral margin of the dorsal white columns. On entering, each fibre divides into two branches. Medial branch runs upwards in the dorsal column pathway to the brain. Lateral branch enters the dorsal horn and divide many times synapsing with neurons of intermediate and anterior portions of the grey matter of the spinal cord and do following functions:

   - A few of them form spinocervical tract that joins dorsal column system in the neck or medulla.
   - A few are responsible for local spinal cord reflexes.
   - The remaining form spinocerebellar tracts.

   As stated earlier, majority of A-beta fibres ascend in dorsal column (tract of gracilis and cuneatus or Goll's and Burdach's). These fibres relay in nucleus gracilis and cuneatus in the medulla which acts as a second order neuron. Then fibres cross to the opposite side as arcuate fibres and ascend in brain stem as medial lemnisci. Additional fibres coming from main sensory nucleus also join medial lemnisci (these fibres carry sensation from head region).

Fibres of medial lemnisci terminate in ventral postero-lateral nucleus of thalamus whereas fibres from the trigeminal nerve terminate in the ventral posteromedial nuclei of thalamus. These two nuclei of thalamus are named as ventrobasal complex.

From the ventrobasal complex, third order nerve fibres project to the postcentral gyrus of the cerebral cortex which is somatic sensory area 'I'. A few fibres project to the lowermost lateral portion of each parietal lobe called somatic sensory area 'II'.

In the dorsal column system described above there is distinct spatial orientation of the nerve fibres, e.g.

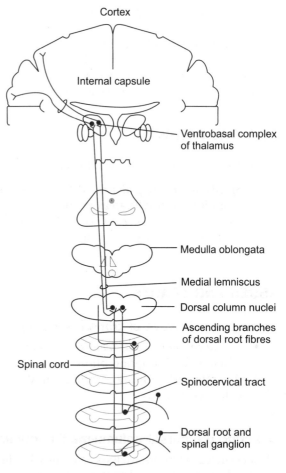

FIGURE 13.7 Dorsal column and spinocervical pathways.

- In the dorsal column, fibres coming from lower parts of the body are in the centre while those coming from progressively higher segmental level form successive layers laterally.
- In the thalamus, tail end of the body is represented most laterally; head and face most medially.
- Fibres end at somatic sensory area I which lies behind the central sulcus located in Brodmann's areas 3, 1, 2. Each side of cortex receives sensory information from the opposite side of the body. Head is represented in most lateral portion and lower part is represented medially. Some areas of the body are represented as large areas on somatic sensory cortex, e.g. lips, face, thumb, whereas entire trunk and lower part is represented by a relatively smaller area.

Somatic sensory area II of the cortex lies posterior and inferior to the lateral end of somatic sensory area I. Degree of localization is poor in this area. Face is represented anteriorly and the legs posteriorly. This area receives signals from both sides of the body from somatic sensory area I and also from sensory areas of the brain receiving auditory and visual signals.

Somatic association areas 5, 7 located behind the somatic sensory area I and above sensory area II receive signals from somatic sensory area I, ventrobasal nuclei of thalamus, visual and auditory cortex. They are responsible for deciphering the meaning of sensory information.

The Pacinian corpuscles are also responsible for detecting vibrations up to 700 cycles/second. Lower vibration frequencies below 100 cycles/second are detected by Meissner's corpuscles.

In addition to fine touch, dorsal column system also carries sensory fibres coming from receptors responsible for position or proprioceptive senses. These carry information about static position as well as rate of movement sense (called kinaesthesia or dynamic proprioception). Both these senses are assessed by knowing the degrees of angulation of all the joints and their rates of change. Multiple receptors help in detecting degree of angulation of joint, e.g. muscle spindles, Pacinian corpuscles, Ruffini's endings and Golgi tendon organs. Pacinian corpuscles and muscle spindles mainly detect rapid rate of change and therefore the rate of movement.

What are the main functions of dorsal column-medial lemniscal system?

1. Carries sensations of fine touch, vibration and proprioception to the cortex.
2. There is a spatial organization in the pathway, i.e. from specific skin areas impulses are transmitted to specific areas of cortex. This helps in tactile localization and two point discrimination. Lateral inhibition, i.e. prevention of lateral spread of excitatory signals in the dorsal column system increases the degree of contrast.
3. Helps in detecting rapidly changing peripheral condition, i.e. vibration sense.
4. Helps in determining the intensity of stimulus over a wide range.
5. Helps in proprioception in detecting the position of different parts of the body under static condition as well as rate of change of movement of different parts during body movements.
6. Helps in perceiving two points discrimination, i.e. capability to distinguish between two points of stimulation. This is mainly possible because of lateral inhibition.

Describe the effects of damage to the dorsal column pathway.

Dorsal column pathway carries sensations of fine touch, tactile discrimination, vibrating sense, joint and position sense. If this pathway is damaged, it is difficult for the person to detect the position without the help of visual apparatus, in erect position. If this person is asked to stand and close the eyes, body cannot maintain balance properly and tends to fall in one direction (Romberg's sign). This condition is known as sensory ataxia (i.e. imbalance due to damage to the sensory pathway). In this, person is able to stand properly only with eyes open. In addition, there is loss of fine touch, tactile discrimination and vibration sense on the affected side.

Describe the anterolateral pathway for transmission of sensory impulses to the cortex.

Impulses of pain, temperature, crude touch, itch and tickle, pressure pass through sensory nerves to dorsal root ganglion and through dorsal root enter the spinal cord. Fibres cross in the anterior commissure of the spinal cord to the opposite side anterior and lateral white columns in which they run upward to the brain.

Anterior division is called anterior spinothalamic tract and lateral division is called lateral spinothalamic tract (Fig. 13.8). Anterior spinothalamic tract mainly carries sensations of crude touch, tickle, itch, etc. whereas lateral spinothalamic tract carries the sensations of pain and temperature. In addition there are spinoreticular (to the reticular system of the brain stem) and spinotectal (to the tectum) pathways.

The anterolateral pathway terminates in two areas:

- Throughout the reticular nuclei of brain stem.
- Ventrobasal complex and intralaminar nuclei of thalamus. Generally, tactile signals and temperature signals terminate in ventrobasal complex. From here the tactile signals go to the somatic sensory areas of the cortex along with the fibres of dorsal column.

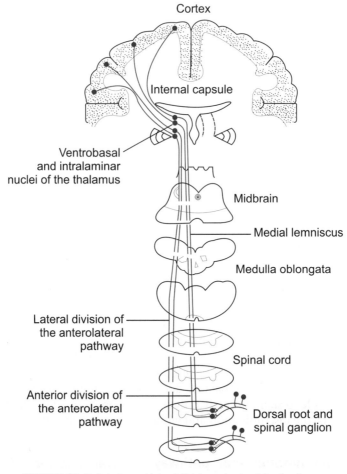

FIGURE 13.8 Anterior and lateral divisions of anterolateral pathways.

Pain signals only partly project to ventrobasal complex of thalamus. Instead most of them enter the reticular nuclei of the brain stem and then to intralaminar nuclei of thalamus.

What are the characteristics of transmission in anterolateral pathway?

1. The velocity of transmission is about one-third as compared to that of dorsal column system (8 to 40 m/sec).
2. Spatial organization in the pathway is poor. Therefore, the degree of localization of sensation is poor.
3. Gradation of intensities judged is far less accurate as compared to those of dorsal column system.
4. Ability to transmit repetitive signals is poor.

Thus anterolateral system is a cruder type of transmission than dorsal column system.

Write the differences between dorsal column and anterolateral pathways.

Dorsal column pathway	Anterolateral pathway
1. Carries sensations of fine touch, vibration and proprioception.	Carries sensations of crude touch, pain and temperature.
2. Velocity of transmission of impulse is high.	Velocity of transmission of impulse is one-third to that of dorsal column pathway.
3. There is spatial organization in the pathway and therefore has good degree of localization and two point discrimination for tactile sensation.	Poor special organization and therefore degree of localization is poor. 500
4. Detects intensity of stimulation over a wide range.	
5. Impulses go to ventrobasal complex of thalamus and then to sensory areas of cortex.	Gradation of intensities judged is less accurate. Pathway mainly terminates in reticular nuclei of brain-stem or ventrobasal complex of thalamus. Only crude touch signals go to sensory areas of cortex from ventrobasal complex of thalamus.
6. Helps in tactile localization, two point discrimination. Helps in detecting positions of different parts of the body.	Helps in detecting crude touch, pain and temperature.

Other Ascending Tracts

Name	Path	Function
Anterior spinocere-bellar tract (lateral white column)	From proprioceptors to anterior lobe of cerebellum	Subconscious kinaesthetic sensations are carried from same as well as opposite side to anterior lobe of cerebellum
Posterior spinocere-bellar tract (lateral white column)	From proprioceptors to anterior lobe of cerebellum	Subconscious kinaesthetic sensations are carried from same side to anterior lobe of cerebellum
Spinotectal tract (lateral white column)	Tract ends in superior colliculi	Concerned with spinovisual reflexes
Spinoreticular tract (anterolateral white column)	From intermediolateral nucleus to reticular formation	Part of ascending reticular system, responsible for consciousness and awareness
Spino-olivary tract (anterolateral white column)	It terminates in olivary nucleus of medulla and then passes to cerebellum	Proprioception
Spinovestibular tract (lateral white column)	It terminates in lateral vestibular nucleus	Proprioception

PHYSIOLOGY OF PAIN

How is the sensation of pain aroused?

Pain sensation is ordinarily aroused by stimuli that damage and risk destruction of the innervated tissue.

What is the purpose of pain?

Pain sensation is different from other sensations because its function is not to inform the quality of stimulus but to indicate that the stimulus is physically damaging. Therefore, though sensation of pain is unpleasant, it is useful. It makes one aware of a harmful agent in close contact with the body and the body gives preferential treatment to this information. It causes the individual to react to remove the pain stimulus to prevent damage to the tissue. Thus pain sensation has a protective function. Pain receptors are non-adaptable receptors, therefore they keep the person apprised of damaging stimulus as long as it persists.

What are the receptors for pain? What are the stimuli which affect them?

Receptors for pain in the skin and other tissues are free nerve endings. These endings are stimulated by excessive mechanical stretch, extremes of heat and cold or specific chemicals. The receptors are therefore, classified as mechanical, thermal or chemical pain receptors.

Some chemicals exciting chemical type of pain receptors are bradykinin, serotonin, histamine, potassium ions, ATP, ADP, acids, acetylcholine, etc. Receptors for pain are termed nociceptors.

Name the viscera which is insensitive to pain.

Parenchyma of liver and alveoli of lungs are insensitive to pain. But liver capsule, bronchi, parietal pleura are very sensitive to pain.

How is pain sensation classified?

Pain sensation is classified as follows:

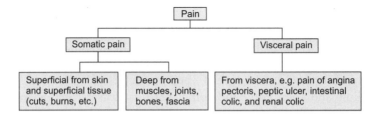

What is slow and fast pain?

Slow pain is the pain which begins after a second or more, after the application of stimulus, but it slowly increases and also lasts for a longer time. It leads to prolonged unbearable suffering. It is burning, throbbing type of pain. It is carried by 'C' type of nerve fibres which are unmyelinated nerve fibres. Pathway for slow pain is more diffuse so slow pain is poorly localized, dull burning sensation. Collaterals from slow pain fibres go to reticular activating system producing emotional perception, i.e. intense unpleasantness. Slow pain produces nausea, vomiting, lowering of blood pressure, generalized reduction in the skeletal muscle tone. Slow pain can arise from both the skin and almost in any deep tissue or organ.

Fast pain is the pain which appears within 0.1 millisecond after the application of stimulus. It is carried by A-delta nerve fibres. These fibres have a small receptive field and there is a topographic representation in the cortex. It is a sharp, pricking acute pain, e.g. pain which occurs when skin is cut with knife. Fast pain is well localized. Usually it is not felt in deeper tissues of the body. It elicits withdrawal reflex and sympathetic response, i.e. increased blood pressure, tachycardia, mobilization of body energy supply.

Describe the mechanism by which the pain is caused.

1. Damaged tissue releases certain chemicals (bradykinin, serotonin, histamine, K^+ ions, ATP, ADP, etc.), of which bradykinin is the most powerful in causing tissue damage pain. These chemicals stimulate chemical pain receptors and cause pain. But they also reduce the threshold for excitation for mechanosensitive and thermosensitive receptors.

2. *Ischaemia*. Blockage of the blood flow to the tissues causes severe pain. Pain is caused due to accumulation of lactic acid in tissues due to anaerobic mechanisms during ischaemia. Other agents such as bradykinin, proteolytic enzymes may also be released.

3. *Muscle spasm.* It causes pain due to direct stimulation of mechanosensitive receptors as well as indirect effect due to spasm of blood vessels.

What are the different reactions to pain?

1. *Emotional.* Pain is accompanied by unpleasantness. Long standing pain causes irritation, frustration, depression, etc.

2. *Muscular.* There occurs a skeletal muscle spasm in the affected region, e.g. spasm of muscles around fractured area. This has a beneficial effect as it causes immobilization of the part and the part gets rest automatically.

3. *Reflex response.* Fast pain sensation is associated with somatic reflex, e.g. pin prick to the sole of foot causing withdrawal of foot.

How is the sensation of pain transmitted to the brain?

Pain sensation has a dual pathway, one for the fast pain and other for the slow pain.

Pathway for the fast pain. Free nerve endings act as receptors and the fast pain impulses are carried by A-delta type of fibres at a velocity of 6 to 30 m/s to dorsal root ganglion and then enter the spinal cord as dorsal root of spinal nerve (formed by axons of cells of dorsal root ganglion) (Fig. 13.9).

On entering the spinal cord, the fibres ascend or descend for one or two segments in the tract of Lissauer lying immediately posterior to the dorsal horn. The fibres terminate on the neurons of the dorsal horn (Lamina I). These neurons give rise to fibres which immediately cross to the opposite side of the cord through anterior commissure and then pass upwards to the brain in the anterolateral columns as neospinothalamic tract.

A few fibres from neospinothalamic tract terminate in reticular areas of the brain stem, but most of them pass upwards and terminate in ventrobasal complex of thalamus along with dorsal column pathway. A few fibres terminate in posterior nuclear group of the thalamus. From thalamus, fibres pass to the basal areas of brain and to the somatic sensory cortex (Fig. 13.10).

When tactile receptors are also stimulated along with fast pain fibres, localization of fast pain is exact. If only pain receptors are stimulated, localization is very poor.

Pathway for slow pain. The impulses of slow pain sensation are mainly carried by group 'C' unmyelinated fibres with few A-delta fibres. The fibres carry impulses to posterior root ganglion and then the axons of cells of dorsal root ganglion form

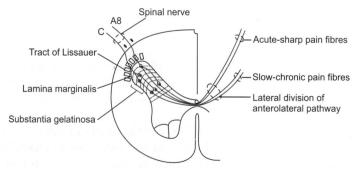

FIGURE 13.9 Transmission of 'acute sharp' and 'slow chronic' pain signals through the spinal cord.

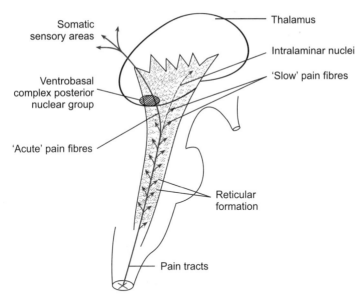

FIGURE 13.10 Transmission of pain signals into the hind brain thalamus and cortex.

the dorsal root which enters the spinal cord and terminate on Lamina II and III of the dorsal horn. Lamina II and III together is known as substantia gelatinosa. From here fibres go to lamina V of the dorsal horn. Last neurons in series give rise to long axons which join the fibres of fast pain upward to the brain in anterolateral column as paleospinothalamic pathway.

Fibres in this pathway terminate very widely in the brain stem in one of the three areas: (a) reticular nuclei of medulla, pons, mesencephalon, (b) tectal area (c) periqueductal grey region.

This lower region is responsible for appreciation of pain. From reticular areas impulses are transmitted to intralaminar nuclei of thalamus, into certain portions of hypothalamus and adjacent areas of basal brain. Localization of pain transmitted in this pathway is very poor.

What is referred pain?

Pain originating in visceral organ is referred to sites on the skin. These sites are innervated by the nerves arising from the same spinal segment as the nerve innervating the visceral organ. Since skin is topographically mapped, and the viscera are not, the pain is identified as originating on the skin and not within the viscera. Referred pain occurs because:

- Sympathetic afferent nerves from the viscus and the somatic afferent nerves from the same dermatome converge on to common neuron of the next order.
- Afferent sympathetic nerve bringing pain sensation from the viscus terminates on second order neuron, but at the same time via collaterals on another second order neuron which is a somatic neuron of the corresponding dermatome.

(Because of this anatomic relationship, diagnosis of visceral diseases is based on location of referred pain, e.g. ischaemic heart pain is referred to the chest and inside of the left arm.)

What are the causes of visceral pain?*

Stimulus must excite diffuse area of the viscus to cause visceral pain. The causes of such diffuse pain are:

1. *Inflammation.* (For detail see chapter on 'Blood'.)
2. *Ischaemia.* Pain is due to acidic metabolic end products or tissue degenerative products (bradykinin, proteolytic enzymes, etc.).
3. *Chemical stimuli.* Damaging substances may leak from the GI tract into the peritoneal cavity, e.g. gastric acid leaking through perforated gastric or duodenal ulcer.
4. *Spasm of hollow viscus.* Pain is caused due to mechanical stimulation of pain endings and ischaemia.
5. *Overdistension of hollow viscus.* Overstretching causes collapse of blood vessels that encircle the viscus.
6. *Parietal pain.* When the disease affects the viscus, it spreads to the parietal wall of the viscus (parietal peritoneum, pleura, etc). These parietal walls are innervated by non-visceral spinal nerves. This causes pain in the area overlying the viscus and is frequently sharp. True visceral pain is carried by autonomic nerves and is referred to areas of the body often far from the painful organ (localization depends on the site of viscus in embryonic life).

Parietal sensation is carried directly into local spinal nerves and therefore is directly felt over the viscus.

What is the effect of complete removal of somatic sensory area on perception of pain?

Complete removal of somatic sensory area of the cortex does not destroy one's ability to perceive pain. This means that lower centres like thalamus, reticular formation are responsible for causing conscious perception of pain.

Describe the pain control system of the brain and the spinal cord.

There is analgesic or pain control system of brain. Major components of this system are:

1. Periaqueductal grey area of the mesencephalon and upper pons surrounding the aqueduct of Sylvius. Neurons in this area send their signals to raphe magnus nucleus.
2. The raphe magnus nucleus is thin midline nucleus located in lower pons and upper medulla. From here, the signals are transmitted through dorsolateral columns to the spinal cord.
3. Pain inhibitory complex located in dorsal horns of spinal cord. Here pain is blocked before it is relayed on to the brain.
4. Periventricular nucleus of hypothalamus and medial forebrain bundle also suppress pain.

In this analgesic system several transmitter substances are involved especially, enkephalin and serotonin.

*For details refer Vaz M, Kurpad A, Raj T, editors. *Guyton & Hall Textbook of Medical Physiology*. Elsevier: New Delhi, 2013, p. 703.

Many fibres from periventricular area and periaqueductal grey area release enkephalin. Fibres terminating in the spinal cord and originating in raphe magnus nucleus cause release of serotonin. This serotonin acts on local cord neurons that secrete enkephalin.

Enkephalin causes presynaptic inhibition of both incoming type C and A-delta fibres, where they synapse in the dorsal horn. This is done by blocking calcium channels in the membranes of nerve terminals. Thus analgesic systems block the pain signals at the initial entry point to the spinal cord. It can block many local cord reflexes that result from pain signal, e.g. withdrawal reflex.

REFLEXES

What is a reflex?

Reflex is the mechanism by which sensory impulse is automatically converted into a motor effect through the involvement of CNS.

Describe the reflex arc.

Pathway for any reflex action is known as reflex arc. It consists of:

- *Afferent limb.* It consists of receptor and afferent or sensory nerve.
- *Efferent limb.* It consists of efferent or motor nerve and effector organ.
- *Centre.* This is the part of CNS where afferent limb ends and either synapses directly with efferent motor neuron or establishes connection with the efferent neuron via internuncial or intercalated neurons.

Classification

Give the classification of reflexes.

Reflexes are classified in different ways:

1. CLINICAL CLASSIFICATION

- *Superficial reflexes.* These are the reflexes which are initiated by stimulating appropriate receptors of skin or mucous membrane. They are usually multisynaptic usually involving moving away from afferent stimulus, e.g. plantar response, abdominal and cremasteric reflexes, corneal and conjunctival reflexes.
- *Deep reflexes.* These are elicited on stroking the tendon. They are basically stretch reflexes and are also called tendon reflexes, e.g. knee jerk, ankle jerk, etc.
- *Visceral reflexes.* These are the reflexes where at least one part of the reflex arc is formed by autonomic nerve, e.g. pupillary reflex, carotid sinus reflex.
- *Pathological reflexes.* These are the reflexes which are not found normally and their presence indicates pathological condition within the body, e.g. Babinski's sign.

2. ANATOMICAL CLASSIFICATION OF REFLEXES

- *Segmental reflexes.* In these, end of afferent neuron and the beginning of efferent neuron are in the same segment of the spinal cord.

- *Intersegmental reflexes*. In these reflexes, end of afferent neuron and the beginning of efferent neuron are in the spinal cord but in different segments.
- *Suprasegmental reflexes*. The centre for such reflex lies above the spinal cord.

3. PHYSIOLOGICAL CLASSIFICATION OF REFLEXES

- *Flexor reflexes*. They are produced when nociceptive (pain) stimulus is applied. Such stimuli cause flexion of the joint, e.g. thorn prick to the sole, causes flexion of knee, hip joints. These reflexes are protective in nature.
- *Extensor reflexes*. Stretch reflexes are extensor reflexes which are the basis of tone and posture.

4. DEPENDING UPON INBORN OR ACQUIRED REFLEXES

- *Unconditioned reflexes*. They are inborn reflexes, i.e. they are present since birth.
- *Conditioned reflexes*. These are the reflexes which develop after birth. Their appearance depends on previous experience.

STUDY OF REFLEXES

How are reflexes studied?

Spinal preparation. Most of the reflexes are studied in spinal animal, i.e. animal where the spinal cord is transected at cervical region and respiration is maintained by respiratory pump. So properties of such reflexes studied are mainly the properties of spinal reflexes.

If spinal cord is transected in the thoracic region, diaphragmatic breathing continues, and artificial respiration is not required.

Decerebrate preparation. Reflexes can also be studied in such a preparation. In this, transection is taken in the brain stem between superior and inferior colliculi.

What is spinal animal?

Spinal animal is the one in whom spinal cord is transected in the neck so that most of the cord still remains functional. This experimental preparation is made to study spinal cord function.

What is decerebrate animal?

Decerebrate animal is the one in whom brain stem is transected in the lower part of the mesencephalon. This experimental preparation is used to study the spinal cord function.

PROPERTIES OF REFLEX ACTION

Explain the properties of reflex action.

Different properties of reflex action are:

1. **Adequate stimulus.** Stimulus for the reflex is usually precise and is called adequate stimulus, e.g. scratch reflex in a dog is initiated only by multiple linear touch stimuli. If multiple touch stimuli are widely separated, reflex is not initiated.

2. **Delay.** There is some interval between application of stimulus and starting of the response which is called delay. It is mainly due to delay at synapses and partly due to time required for passage of impulse along the nerves. It is therefore minimum in monosynaptic reflex.

3. **Spatial and temporal summation.** *Temporal summation.* Application of subminimal (subthreshold) stimulus does not elicit response. But if second subminimal stimulus is applied sufficiently quickly (taking care of refractory period of the nerve), response does occur though individual stimulus is subthreshold. Therefore, two or more subthreshold stimuli applied in succession evoke response because of summation of two EPSPs.

Spatial summation. Two subthreshold stimuli when applied simultaneously at different but closely situated spots can evoke response though each individual stimulus is subthreshold.

4. **Occlusion.** Stimulation of two neighbouring nerves simultaneously evokes lesser response than sum total of the responses obtained when each afferent nerve is separately stimulated, e.g. there are two afferent nerves A and B. Stimulation of A with strong electric shock causes development of tension (T_1) in the muscle. Stimulation of the nerve B with a strong electric shock causes development of tension (T_2) in the muscle.

When both A and B are simultaneously stimulated with strong stimulus, tension developed is lesser than '$T_1 + T_2$'. Nerves A and B stimulate some common neurons, therefore their simultaneous stimulation excites lesser number of neurons than the sum total of neurons stimulated when they are separately stimulated.

5. **Subliminal fringe.** When A and B nerves are stimulated simultaneously with weak shock, the tension developed in the muscle is more than sum total of the tensions developed when A and B nerves are separately stimulated with weak shocks. This can be explained as follows:

Each afferent nerve on entering the spinal cord stimulates two groups of neurons. One group is stimulated adequately and second group subminimally. Each weak stimulus therefore produces action potential in the nerves of group one neurons. The neurons belonging to second group are also excited but only subminimally (so this group is common). When both A and B are simultaneously stimulated, the action potential also develops in second group of neurons and therefore response obtained is greater.

6. **Irradiation.** When the sensory stimulus is too strong, impulse spreads to too many neighbouring neurons in the centre and produces a wider response. It is due to the transmission of impulse through a large number of collaterals of afferents and their interneurons.

7. **Final common path.** Efferent pathway of the reflex arc is formed by motor neurons that supply the extrafusal muscle fibres. All neuronal influences affecting muscular contraction ultimately funnel through the motor neurons, therefore they are called common final paths. Numerous inputs converge on them. On an average about 10,000 synapses are present on the motor neuron. All these converge and determine the activity in the final common path.

8. **Facilitation.** If a reflex is elicited repeatedly at proper intervals the response becomes progressively higher for the first few occasions, i.e. each subsequent stimulus exerts a better effect than the previous one. This is due to facilitation occurring at the synapse.

9. **Inhibition.** Impulses through sensory fibres from protagonist muscles inhibit the action of antagonist muscles, e.g. when flexor muscles of the joint are stimulated extensor muscles are inhibited. Such a reciprocal inhibitory effect is due to inhibitory activity exerted by interneurons.

10. **After discharge.** Continuation of response even after stimulus is over is called after discharge. This is due to discharge from the centre even after stoppage of stimulation, i.e. motor neurons are stimulated through multiple internuncial pathways. Some of them take a longer time to reach motor neurons. Therefore, even after cessation of stimulation impulses travel to motor neurons for a certain period of time. This causes after discharge.

11. **Fatigue.** If a particular reflex is elicited repeatedly at frequent intervals, response becomes progressively feebler and then disappears all together. This is called fatigue. The first site of fatigue is synapse, then the motor endings and lastly the muscle.

12. **Fractionation.** When a stimulus is directly applied to the motor nerve of a muscle, the amount of contraction becomes much higher than when the muscle is stimulated reflexly through a sensory nerve. This is due to the phenomenon of occlusion of the motor neurons when sensory nerve is stimulated. Because of occlusion, the number of motor neurons stimulated is lesser.

13. **Habituation and sensitization.** When a non-injurious stimulus is applied repeatedly, intensity of response becomes lesser, declines and even ceases. This phenomenon is known as habituation.

On the other hand, when the injurious stimulus is repeatedly applied there is intensification of response. This is known as sensitization.

IMPORTANT REFLEXES

STRETCH REFLEX

What is stretch reflex?

Stretching of the skeletal muscle with intact nerve supply causes the muscle to contract. This is known as stretch reflex.

What is a muscle spindle?

Muscle spindles are the stretch receptors embedded with the skeletal muscle. Each skeletal muscle contains muscle spindles. The number is variable. Small muscles of hands and antigravity muscles have more number of muscle spindles.

Describe the structure of muscle spindle.

Muscle spindle is a spindle-shaped receptor. Its tapering ends are attached to the endomysium of the muscle.

Each muscle spindle is made up of 3 to 10 muscle fibres called intrafusal muscle fibres. They lie parallel to the extrafusal muscle fibres of the muscles. These intrafusal fibres do not contain actin and myosin filaments in their central portion, so it is a non-contractile portion (equatorial zone). This portion is the sensory portion of the intrafusal fibres. Depending upon the arrangement of nuclei in this portion, the intrafusal fibre is called either nuclear bag fibre or nuclear chain fibre. Portions on either side are called striated poles (as they have actin and myosin filaments). Each spindle contains 1 to 3 nuclear bag fibres. In these fibres nuclei are congregated into an expanded bag in the central portion. The diameter of the fibre is about double to that of chain fibre.

Each spindle contains about 3 to 9 nuclear chain fibres. They have nuclei aligned in a chain throughout the receptor area.

Nerve supply of the spindle. Central non-contractile portion of each intrafusal fibre is the receptor portion. Sensory fibres supply this area (Fig. 13.11). There are two types of sensory fibres:

- Group Ia fibres which supply nuclear bag as well as nuclear chain fibres. They have a diameter of about 17 microns and carry impulses at a rate of 70 to 120 m/s. These fibres spirally wind round the receptor portion of the fibres and therefore are also known as annulospiral or primary sensory endings.
- Type II fibres having diameter of about 8 microns innervate the receptor portion of mainly nuclear chain fibres on one side of primary endings. They are also known as secondary or flower spray endings.

Motor supply. There are two different types of gamma motor fibres which supply the striated poles of the intrafusal fibres. Gamma-D (gamma-dynamic) fibres supply the striated poles of nuclear bag fibres. Second type of gamma fibres are gamma-static or gamma-S fibres which supply the striated poles of nuclear chain fibres.

Gamma-D fibres control the dynamic response. When they are stimulated, dynamic response of the muscle spindle is greatly increased. Whereas when gamma-S fibres are excited, static response of the muscle spindle is tremendously increased.

When are the muscle spindles stimulated?

Muscle spindles are the stretch receptors and the intrafusal fibres in them lie parallel to the extrafusal fibres of the muscle. Muscle spindles are stimulated when the central (non-contractile) portion of the intrafusal fibre is stretched. Therefore, muscle spindles are stimulated when:

- The entire muscle is stretched.
- Gamma motor fibres are stimulated.

When muscle spindles are stimulated, they cause reflex contraction of the muscle.

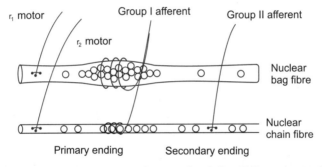

FIGURE 13.11 Central portion of the muscle spindle with its sensory supply.

What is the dynamic stretch reflex?

When length of the spindle receptor increases suddenly, primary endings are stimulated powerfully. They transmit strong signals to the spinal cord and it causes instantaneous, very strong reflex contraction of the same muscle from which signals are originated. This is called dynamic stretch reflex, the function of which is to oppose sudden changes in length, e.g. knee jerk, ankle jerk. Dynamic stretch reflex is over within a fraction of a second. Primary endings (annulospiral endings) are stimulated actively when there is a rapid rate of change in length, i.e. they are stimulated only when the length is actually increasing. As soon as the length stops increasing, their rate of impulse discharge returns back to normal. Conversely when spindle receptors shorten, the discharge through primary endings momentarily decreases. Thus primary endings respond only to rate of change of length of the receptor. Once the length stops increasing or decreasing, their rate of discharge returns back to the background level.

Describe the static stretch reflex.

When the muscle is stretched slowly and kept stretched, signals are continuously sent through both primary and secondary nerve endings. This in turn, causes reflex contraction of the muscle. This is called static response. This static reflex therefore causes muscle contraction as long as the muscle is maintained of excessive length. The muscle contraction thus opposes the force that is causing the excess length, e.g. when the person is standing, gravity causes continuous stretch on the antigravity muscle making them remain in a contracted state as long as gravity is causing the stretch.

What is negative stretch reflex?

When the muscle is suddenly shortened, negative signals from the muscle spindles cause reflex inhibition of the muscle. There is a dynamic as well as a static reflex causing such muscle inhibition. This is called negative stretch reflex.

Describe the reflex arc for stretch or myotatic reflex.

When the muscle is stretched, stretch receptors (muscle spindles) are stretched and therefore stimulated. From stretch receptors afferent impulses run in group Ia and group II fibres, and they directly synapse with the alpha motor neurons without interposition of any neurons. Efferents from alpha motor neurons carry impulses to the extrafusal fibres of the muscle from which the afferent impulses are originated and cause its contraction (Fig. 13.12).

Explain the role of gamma efferents.

Normally, there is alpha-gamma coactivation during the voluntary movements for its proper execution, e.g. when motor control system issues a command to lift a weight, alpha and gamma are coactivated.

- As extrafusal fibre shortens, the intrafusal muscle fibres also shorten.
- If these two types of muscle fibres shorten at the same rate, central region of the intrafusal fibre is neither stretched nor compressed, thus keeping the

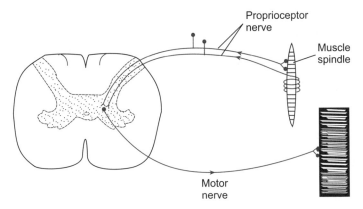

FIGURE 13.12 Neuronal circuit of the stretch reflex.

rate of discharge constant. This indicates that the motor command is being carried out properly.

- If the weight to be lifted is underestimated by CNS, the motor command system does not activate a sufficient number of alpha motor neurons to lift the weight. Thus extrafusal fibres do not shorten to a sufficient degree. However, intrafusal fibres do shorten, the central portion of intrafusal fibre is stretched. This increases the firing rate from muscle spindle fibres, which indicates that motor command is not being carried out. The CNS uses this information to readjust its command. Even before CNS does this adjustment, information provided by group Ia fibres increases the activity of alpha motor neurons (through stretch reflex) and increases the force of muscle contraction to meet the unexpectedly high weight.

When alpha motor neurons are stimulated, simultaneously gamma motor neurons are also stimulated. This alpha-gamma coactivation serves important function as follows:

(a) When gamma efferents are stimulated, the muscle spindle sensitivity is increased. During voluntary movements, fibres of muscle spindle inform the motor control system about the changes in muscle length and provide alpha motor neuron with a source of excitatory input in addition to that coming from higher centres. Following a motor command, when muscle contraction occurs, there is a reduction in firing from the muscle spindle (as there is a shortening of extrafusal fibres, central region of intrafusal fibre is compressed and the firing rate through group Ia fibres is reduced). This unloading is prevented by activity of gamma afferents. Simultaneous stimulation of them shortens the intrafusal fibres simultaneously with shortening of extrafusal fibres. Thus central regions of intrafusal fibres remain stretched during muscle contraction and unloading does not occur. This allows CNS to determine whether its motor commands are carried out properly or not.

(b) *Gamma loop.* CNS is capable of initiating movements directly by stimulating gamma efferents using a pathway called gamma loop as follows:

- Increase in gamma motor activity causes intrafusal fibres to contract and this in turn causes stretching of the receptor portion of intrafusal fibres resulting in an increased discharge through group Ia fibres. These initiate stretch reflex and cause increased activity of the alpha motor neurons thereby increasing the force of contraction of the muscle.

- Though gamma loop is capable of initiating the movements, it normally does not do so. It is usually activated only during alpha-gamma coactivation during all movements and it contributes to excitability and the firing rate of alpha motor activity.

Functions of Stretch Reflex

What are the functions of stretch reflex?

1. *Tone maintenance.* Tone is defined as the resistance offered to active or passive stretch or it can be also defined as sustained partial state of contraction of the muscle under resting condition. This precisely is the action of myotatic reflex. In the brain stem there are two areas—facilitatory area in the pons and inhibitory area in the lower part of medulla. These areas send the impulses to gamma motor neurons. Facilitatory area is intrinsically active, so it continues to discharge facilitatory impulses causing constant activation of gamma motor neurons. This causes stretching of the muscle spindle fibres resulting in reflex and slight contraction of the muscle under resting state (tone). Inhibitory centre in the medulla becomes active only if it receives impulses from the cerebellum or cerebral cortex.

2. *Maintenance of posture.* Static component of myotatic reflex (prominent in medial extensor muscles and antigravity muscles) is the fundamental postural mechanism, e.g. when a person is standing upright, gravity tends to stretch the quadriceps muscle. This stretching elicits stretch reflex resulting in sustained contraction of quadriceps as long as stretch is there. This maintains the extension around the knee joint and the upright posture.

3. *Control of voluntary movements.* Stretch reflex is used by the motor command system to help in the performance of a movement. During activity generated by the motor command system, group Ia fibres from the muscle spindle inform the motor control system about the changes in muscle length and provide the alpha motor neuron with a source of excitatory input in addition to that coming from the higher centres.

Applied Aspect

What is hypotonia? When does it occur?

Decreased tone in the muscle is known as hypotonia. Sometimes there is atonia, i.e. loss of tone. This results mainly due to loss of supraspinal impulses to muscle spindles through gamma motor fibres. Therefore, it occurs when there is transaction of the spinal cord.

What is hypertonia? When does it occur?

Lesion which removes major inhibitory influence on gamma motor neuron increases the sensitivity of the muscle spindles. Myotatic reflex therefore is abnormally active leading to hypertonia or spasticity. This occurs when the animal is made decerebrate by taking a cut between superior and inferior colliculi. This is because impulses coming from cerebellum to the inhibitory medullary area are cut off and therefore the facilitatory area continues to discharge through gamma efferents causing increase in tone of the muscle.

What is clonus?

Oscillation of muscle jerks under appropriate condition is called clonus. Especially, it is demonstrated at ankle jerk oscillation (ankle clonus). If foot is dorsiflexed suddenly and pressure is maintained to keep the foot dorsiflexed, ankle clonus occurs. Clonus occurs when the stretch reflex is highly sensitized by facilitatory impulses from the brain, e.g. in decerebrate animal. If clonus occurs it indicates that the degree of facilitation is high.

GOLGI TENDON REFLEX

What are Golgi tendon organs? What is Golgi tendon reflex?

Golgi tendon organs are the encapsulated sensory receptors through which a small bundle of muscle tendon fibres pass immediately beyond their point of fusion with muscle fibres. Ten to fifteen muscle fibres are usually connected in series with each Golgi tendon organ.

Golgi tendon organs are less numerous than muscle spindles. The Golgi tendon organ is stimulated when the tension is produced in a group of muscle fibres to which the organ is connected. Golgi tendon organs detect the muscle tension (degree of tension in each small segment of the muscle) whereas muscle spindles detect the length of the muscle. When muscle tension increases, signals from Golgi tendon organs are transmitted through group Ib fibres to local areas of the spinal cord. These signals excite the inhibitory interneurons which in turn inhibit alpha motor neurons to inhibit the muscle from which the impulses have originated. Thus stimulation of Golgi tendon organ causes reflex inhibition (relaxation) of the muscle. This is called Golgi tendon reflex. It is also of two types—dynamic and static.

What are the functions of Golgi tendon reflex?

1. Golgi tendon reflex (also called lengthening reaction) is a protective reflex in which the strong and potentially damaging muscle force reflexly causes muscle inhibition. Muscle therefore lengthens instead of trying to maintain the force and risking damage.
2. Plays role in regulating tension during normal muscle activity.

WITHDRAWAL REFLEX

Describe the withdrawal reflex.

If a painful stimulus is applied to any part of the body, the part is withdrawn from the site of painful stimulus. This is the withdrawal reflex. For this several reflex pathways in the spinal cord act together to co-ordinate the activity of all the muscles necessary to produce a smooth movement:

Receptors for the reflex. Receptors for withdrawal reflex are nociceptors located on the free nerve endings, i.e. A delta and C group of nerve fibres.

Upon entering the spinal cord, the pain fibres synapse on many interneurons. Some of these also convey information to CNS. Others form several reflex pathways to cause smooth withdrawal as follows:

1. *Major efferent pathway.* It travels through several interneurons to alpha motor neuron innervating the muscles used to withdraw the limb. So the pathway is multisynaptic. Interneurons form several pathways of different lengths to alpha motor neurons as follows:
   - There are several reverberating circuits which cause after discharge.
   - Under most circumstances minimal number of muscles required to withdraw are activated. This is called a local sign. This depends upon the intensity of painful stimulus. Greater the intensity of painful stimulus, more is the number of muscles activated for withdrawal.
   - *Irradiation.* If the painful stimulus is very strong there is irradiation of impulse to many alpha motor neurons. Thus more number of muscles are activated.
2. *Inhibitory pathways.* Interneurons within the spinal cord terminate on alpha motor neurons supplying antagonist muscles. This is an inhibitory pathway. Therefore, when the limb is withdrawn by flexion movement, extensor muscles are inhibited, so that they do not impede the withdrawal. This type of neuronal organization causing activation of one group of alpha motor neurons and inhibiting its antagonist alpha motor neurons is known as reciprocal inhibition.
3. Interneurons form pathways which cross the spinal cord to innervate extensor motor neurons of the contralateral (opposite) side to cause crossed extensor reflex.

DIFFERENCE IN MONO AND POLYSYNAPTIC REFLEX

Differentiate between monosynaptic reflex and polysynaptic (multisynaptic) reflex.

Monosynaptic reflex	Polysynaptic reflex
• One synapse is present between afferent and efferent neuron.	Many synapses are present between afferent and efferent neuron.
• Example is stretch reflex.	Example is withdrawal reflex.
• Does not show phenomenon of after discharge.	Shows phenomenon of after discharge.
• Latency of response is short.	Latency of response is long.

SPINAL CORD

Describe the structure of spinal cord.

Spinal cord is a cylindrical tube located in the upper two-thirds of the vertebral canal. It extends from the upper border of the atlas to the lower border of L1 vertebra in the adult.

Structure (Fig. 13.13a): The spinal cord shows:

1. The central canal lined by ependymal cells. The terminal part of the central canal is slightly dilated to form the terminal ventricle.
2. The grey matter is arranged like letter 'H' around the central canal and has anterior (ventral) grey columns, posterior (dorsal) grey columns. The lateral grey columns are present in thoracic and first lumbar spinal segments (the columns are called horns in TS). The dorsal columns receive sensory fibres; the axons of ventral column neurons (anterior horn cells) give origin to motor fibres. The neurons of lateral columns give origin to preganglionic sympathetic fibres.
3. The white matter lies outside the grey matter and arranged as anterior, lateral and posterior columns. These columns contain ascending (sensory), descending (motor) nerve tracts (Fig. 13.13b).

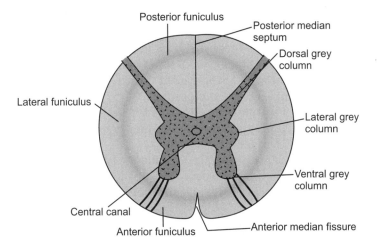

FIGURE 13.13 (a) Internal structure of spinal cord.

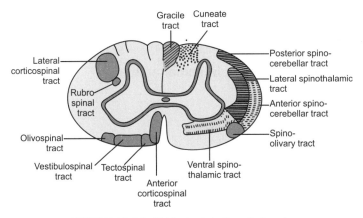

FIGURE 13.13 (b) The tracts in the spinal cord.

Give the organization of grey matter of the spinal cord.

Grey matter of the spinal cord is arranged in the form of 'H'. It shows mainly two anterior and two posterior horns.

What are the types of neurons present in the grey matter of the spinal cord?

The grey matter in the spinal cord contains different neurons as follows:

1. *Sensory relay neurons.* They are located in posterior horn. Sensory signals enter the cord through sensory (posterior) roots. After entering the cord every sensory signal divides into two separate destinations.
   - One branch of the sensory nerve terminates in the grey matter of the cord to elicit local cord reflexes and other effects.
   - Second branch transmit signals to higher levels in the nervous system.
2. *Anterior motor neurons.* They are located in the anterior horns of the grey matter. These neurons are larger than most of the other neurons. There are two types of motor neurons:
   - *Alpha motor neurons.* These are larger, i.e. about 9 to 20 μm in diameter. They give rise to A alpha type of fibres which innervate skeletal muscle fibres. Stimulation of a single neuron excites several muscle fibres and collectively form a single motor unit.
   - *Gamma motor neurons.* They are smaller, i.e. about 5 μm in diameter. They transmit impulses through A gamma type of fibres which innervate intrafusal fibres of the muscle spindles.
3. *Interneurons.* They are present in the anterior horns, posterior horns, and intermedial areas between the two. They are more numerous. Their connections are responsible for integrative functions of the spinal cord.

What is Bell–Magendie's law?

In spinal cord dorsal roots are sensory and ventral (anterior) roots are motor, this is termed Bell–Magendie's law.

SPINAL REFLEXES

Name the different reflexes in spinal animal.

- Stretch reflex.
- Golgi tendon reflex.
- Flexor withdrawal reflex.
- Crossed extensor reflex.
- Postural and locomotive reflexes of the cord.
  - Positive supporting reaction.
  - Cord righting reflexes.
  - Stepping and walking including galloping reflex.
- Scratch reflex.
- Autonomic cord reflexes including mass reflex.

What is spinal shock?

When spinal cord is transected essentially all the cord functions immediately become depressed. This is called spinal shock. Normal activity of the cord neurons depends on tonic discharge from higher centres to a great extent. When spinal cord is transected, this discharge is cut off (particularly discharge transmitted through reticulospinal, vestibulospinal and corticospinal tracts). Because of this there occurs a spinal shock. Following are the features of spinal shock:

1. Arterial blood pressure falls immediately to a low level (up to 40 mmHg) due to blockage of sympathetic activity. In human beings pressure returns to normal within a few days.
2. All skeletal muscle reflexes integrated in spinal cord are totally blocked in the initial stage. In human beings reflexes return within two weeks to several months. The first reflexes to return are the stretch reflexes, flexor reflexes, postural antigravity reflexes and stepping reflexes.
3. Sacral reflexes for control of bladder and colon evacuation are completely suppressed for the first few weeks. They eventually return. The duration of the spinal shock depends on encephalization, i.e. dependence of lower centres on higher centres. In lower animals spinal shock lasts for a shorter period of time. In human beings it lasts for a few weeks to a few months. After this, the spinal neurons gradually regain the excitability. Recovery is sometimes excessive with resultant hyperexcitability of some or all cord functions.

What is mass reflex?

In a spinal animal or human being the spinal cord sometimes suddenly becomes excessively active causing massive discharge of large portions of the cord. The usual stimulus that causes mass reflex is a strong nociceptive stimulus to the skin or excessive filling of a viscus. The effects are:

- Major portion of the body goes into a strong flexor spasm.
- Colon and bladder are likely to evacuate.
- Arterial pressure rises up to 200 mmHg.
- Profuse sweating over large areas of the body.

Precise neuronal mechanism of the mass reflex is not known. Probably it is due to activation of great masses of reverberating circuits in the spinal cord that excite large area of the cord at once.

MOTOR SYSTEM

INTRODUCTION

What is motor system or motor division of CNS?

Different parts of the nervous system which plan, co-ordinate and execute voluntary movements are termed as the motor system (somatic motor system).

The somatic motor system is organized at three levels—higher, middle and lower.

- Higher level: It involves activities of areas of cerebral cortex.

- Middle level: It consists of subcortical structures such as basal ganglia, cerebellum and brain stem nuclei.
- Lower level: It consists of motor nuclei of cranial nerves in the brain stem and alpha motor neurons present in the anterior horns of spinal cord which form the final common pathway for execution of motor movement.

Where is the motor cortex? How is it divided?

Anterior to the central sulcus, occupying posterior third of the frontal lobe is motor cortex. Motor cortex is divided into three separate subareas each of which has a topographical representation of all the muscle groups of the body. These subareas are:

1. *Primary motor cortex.* It lies in the first convolution of the frontal lobes anterior to the central sulcus. Laterally it begins in the sylvian fissure. This area is called area 4 in Brodmann's classification. Body is represented upside down in this area. Important group of muscles (hand muscles, muscles of speech) are represented by larger areas, whereas trunk areas have lesser degree of representation.

2. *Premotor area.* This lies immediately anterior to the primary cortex. It is frequently called area 6. It is responsible for more complex patterns of co-ordinated muscle activity.

3. *Supplementary motor area.* It lies superior and anterior to the premotor area. In this area also there is a topographic representation of the body (leg area lies posteriorly and face area anteriorly). Stimulation of these areas cause bilateral movements. It helps in finer motor control of hands and feet by premotor and primary motor areas.

What is Broca's area?

Premotor area lying immediately anterior to the primary motor cortex and immediately above the Sylvian fissure is called Broca's area for speech. This area makes it possible for a person to speak whole words. This area is closely associated with respiratory function. So, respiratory activation of vocal cords occurs simultaneously with the movements of mouth and tongue during speech.

DESCENDING TRACTS

PYRAMIDAL (CORTICOSPINAL TRACT)

Describe the corticospinal tract.

Motor signals are transmitted directly from the cortex to spinal cord through corticospinal tract (pyramidal tract) (Fig. 13.14).

Corticospinal tract fibres originate from:

- Primary motor cortex (30%).
- Premotor area and supplementary area (30%).
- Somatic sensory areas (40%).

After leaving the cortex, this tract passes through the posterior limb of the internal capsule and then downwards through the brain stem, forming pyramids in the medulla (hence the name is pyramidal tract). Majority of fibres cross to the

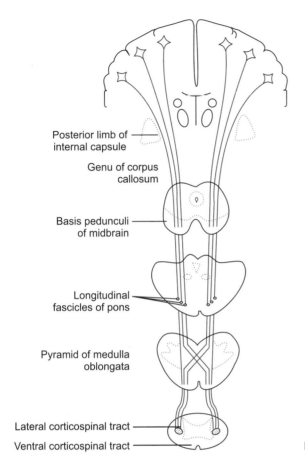

Posterior limb of
internal capsule

Genu of corpus
callosum

Basis pedunculi
of midbrain

Longitudinal
fascicles of pons

Pyramid of medulla
oblongata

Lateral corticospinal tract

Ventral corticospinal tract

FIGURE 13.14 The pyramidal tract.

opposite side and descend in the lateral corticospinal tracts of the spinal cord. These fibres terminate principally on interneurons in the intermediate regions of grey matter of the spinal cord, a few relay on sensory relay neuron in the dorsal horn and some directly on anterior motor neurons.

A few fibres do not cross to the opposite side in the medulla but pass down the cord in the ventral corticospinal tract. But many of these fibres cross to the opposite side in the spinal cord in the neck or upper thoracic region. These fibres are concerned with bilateral control of postural movements by supplementary motor area. The fibres of the corticospinal tract which originate from the giant pyramidal cells (of Betz) present in primary motor cortex are large myelinated nerve fibres with diameter of 16 microns, transmitting impulses at a rate of 70 m/s. The number of Betz cells and therefore the fibres is 34,000 which constitute 3% of the fibres of the corticospinal tract; the total number of fibres present in corticospinal tract is more than 1,000,000. Other 97% of the fibres in the tract are of smaller diameter (less than 4 μ).

These pyramidal tract fibres also send collaterals to other areas of motor control systems thus communicating motor command to the basal ganglia, cerebellum and the brain stem.

The cortical cells that synapse directly on cranial nerves controlling facial muscles perform the same function as pyramidal tract neurons and thus considered a part of the pyramidal system.

What are the functions of pyramidal or corticospinal tract?

Corticospinal tract is the tract through which motor cortex can send impulses to the muscles to initiate the movements. The fibres are mainly distributed in the distal muscle groups. Thus pyramidal tract is responsible for controlling muscles that make precision movements.

These muscles include muscles that move the fingers and hands and the muscles that produce speech.

What is the effect of lesion of the pyramidal tract?

Pure pyramidal tract lesion is very rare. It is usually a lesion of both the pyramidal and extrapyramidal system. Pure pyramidal tract lesion can only be produced in experimental animals. It causes relatively very small motor deficits. Major deficit resulting is weakness and loss of precision in the muscles controlling fine movements of the fingers. Gross movements are not affected. The sign of pyramidal tract lesion is the Babinski's sign (a destruction of the foot region of the area pyramidalis), i.e. on application of the firm tactile stimulation to the lateral sole of the foot, great toe extends upwards and other toes fan outward. Normal response is plantar flexion. Reason is that the corticospinal tract is a major controller of muscle activity for performance of voluntary, purposeful activity. Therefore, when it is damaged and only non-corticospinal system is functional, stimuli to the bottom of the feet cause a typical protective withdrawal reflex. But when the corticospinal system is also fully functional, it suppresses the protective reflex and instead excites higher order of motor function, causing downward bending of toes and foot in response to sensory stimuli from the bottom of the feet, a response which helps us to walk.

EXTRAPYRAMIDAL TRACTS

What is extrapyramidal system?

The term extrapyramidal system is widely used to denote all those portions of the brain and brain stem that contribute to motor control that are not the part of the corticospinal pyramidal system. It includes pathways through basal ganglia, reticular formation of brain stem, vestibular nuclei and also red nuclei. So this system includes various extrapyramidal tracts (Fig. 13.15):

- Rubrospinal tract.
- Lateral vestibulospinal tract.
- Pontine reticulospinal tract.
- Medial vestibulospinal tract.
- Tectospinal tract.
- Interstitiospinal spinal tract.
- Medullary reticulospinal tract.

Except rubrospinal, the remaining tracts form medial system pathways.

Describe the rubrospinal tract. What is its function?

Red nucleus receives many direct fibres from the primary motor complex through the corticospinal tract as well as branching fibres from corticospinal tract. These

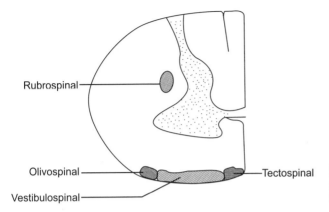

Rubrospinal

Olivospinal ——— Tectospinal

Vestibulospinal ———

FIGURE 13.15 Cross-section of spinal cord showing descending tracts on the left.

fibres synapse in the lower part of the red nucleus. This is called magnocellular nucleus and it contains large neurons similar to Betz cells. These large neurons give rise to the rubrospinal tract which crosses to opposite side in the lower brain stem and follows a course similar to that of corticospinal tract in the lateral column of the spinal cord. Fibres terminate mainly on interneuron along with the corticospinal fibres. Red nucleus also has connection to the cerebellum.

Function. Red nucleus functions in close association with corticospinal tract and together forms lateral motor system of the cord. Red nucleus also has a somatographic representation of all muscles of the body. Along with corticospinal tract, it is responsible for controlling muscles that make precision movements. It is more important in animals. In human beings red nucleus is relatively small.

Describe the reticulospinal tracts.

Throughout the midbrain, pons and medulla, there are scattered group of neurons and nerve fibres collectively known as reticular formation. From these areas two reticulospinal tracts arise: pontine reticulospinal tract and medullary reticulospinal tract.

- *Pontine reticulospinal tract.* Neurons of the pons send axons which are mainly uncrossed down to the spinal cord forming pontine reticulospinal tract present in anterior white column of the spinal cord. Fibres terminate on more ventromedial grey matter throughout the rostrocaudal extent of spinal cord. Fibres cross to opposite side before termination and terminate on contralateral grey matter. This tract is excitatory to motor neurons of proximal extensor muscles (primarily through interneurons).
- *Medullary reticulospinal tract.* From medulla, neurons in reticular formation send their axons to the spinal cord to form medullary reticulospinal tract which lies in the lateral white column of the spinal cord. Fibres descend in both ipsilateral and contralateral side and terminate in the spinal cord grey matter with a wider and more lateral distribution than pontine reticulospinal tract. This tract inhibits proximal limb motor neurons in part through direct connection on motor neuron (on gamma and alpha motor neurons).

Pontine and medullary reticular nuclei mostly function antagonistic to each other. Pontine nuclei are excitatory to antigravity muscles and medullary nuclei are inhibitory to these muscles. Pontine tract excites the motor neurons which excite muscles that support the body against gravity. Pontine nuclei have high degree of spontaneous excitability. In addition, they receive excitatory signals from vestibular nuclei and deep nuclei of cerebellum.

Medullary reticular nuclei transmit inhibitory signals to antigravity muscles. They receive signals from corticospinal tract, rubrospinal tract, etc. They activate medullary inhibitory system to counterbalance excitatory signals from pontine reticular system. When the brain wishes for excitation by pontine system to cause standing, signals from cerebrum, red nucleus and cerebellum disinhibit medullary system.

At other times excitation of medullary reticular system can inhibit antigravity muscles in certain portions of the body to allow those portions to perform motor functions which would be impossible if antigravity muscles opposed the necessary movements.

Describe the vestibulospinal tracts.

There are two vestibulospinal tracts:

1. *Lateral vestibulospinal tract.* Fibres of this tract arise from lateral vestibular or Deiters' nucleus. Tract descends without crossing in anterior white column and terminates ventromedially in spinal grey matter. The terminal distribution is to the extensor motor neurons which innervate proximal postural muscles.

Vestibular nucleus receives afferents from vestibular apparatus mainly from utricles. This pathway is principally concerned with the adjustment of postural muscles to linear accelatory displacements of the body. Lateral vestibulospinal tract mainly facilitates activity of extensor muscles and inhibits the activity of flexor muscles in association with the maintenance of the balance.

2. *Medial vestibulospinal tract.* The fibres of this tract arise from the inferior part of the vestibular nucleus. This part of the vestibular nucleus receives signals from the vestibular apparatus mainly from the semicircular canals. Functionally ventral vestibulospinal tract is the down connection of medial longitudinal bundle (MLB). The tract provides a reflex pathway for movements of head, neck and eyes in response to visual and auditory stimuli.

Describe the tectospinal tract.

Fibres of the tectospinal tract arise from superior colliculi. In contrast to other tracts of extrapyramidal system, the fibres cross the midline in the lower part of tegmentum of the brain forming dorsal tegmental decussation. Then the tract descends through pons and medulla into the anterior white column of the spinal cord. Fibres terminate in upper cervical levels by synapsing on the anterior horn cells through internuncial neurons located in lamina V and VIII of the spinal grey matter. This tract mediates visually guided head movements.

Describe the olivospinal tract.

Olivospinal tract originates from the inferior olivary nucleus. It descends and terminates on anterior horn cells of the spinal cord. Exact connections are unknown. Inferior olivary nucleus receives afferent fibres from cerebral cortex, corpus striatum, red nucleus and spinal cord. It influences muscle activity.

Describe the interstitialspinal tract.

Fibres of interstitialspinal tract arise from interstitial nucleus of Cajal in rostral midbrain. It descends without crossing and travels in anterior column. It terminates on ventromedial spinal grey matter throughout rostrocaudal extent of the spinal cord. This tract helps to mediate the rotation of head and body about the longitudinal axis.

DIFFERENCE BETWEEN LATERAL AND MEDIAL MOTOR SYSTEM

Enumerate the differences between lateral and medial motor system.

Lateral motor system	Medial motor system
• Corticospinal and rubrospinal tracts form this system. The fibres of these tracts mainly originate from cortex and red nucleus.	Except cortico and rubrospinal rest of the motor tracts form this system. Fibres of these tracts primarily originate in the brain stem.
• Fibres are distributed to motor neurons which supply distal muscle groups.	Fibres are distributed to motor neurons which supply proximal muscle groups.
• The main function of this system is to control fractionate movements of the extremities.	The main function of this system is to control posture equilibrium and progression.

DIFFERENCE BETWEEN PYRAMIDAL AND EXTRAPYRAMIDAL SYSTEM

Enumerate the differences between pyramidal and extrapyramidal system.

Pyramidal system	Extrapyramidal system
• Newer in evolution.	Older in evolution.
• Myelination begins at birth and is completed by second to third year after birth.	Myelination begins by 4th month of intrauterine life.
• Onset of function starts after complete myelination.	Onset of function, i.e. gross movements starts before birth.
• Origin is from cortical areas 4, 6, 8, 3a, 3b, 1, 2, 5 and 7.	Origin is diffuse from cortical areas other than those for pyramidal tract and from subcortical areas.
• Relays directly on alpha motor neuron.	Relay is multisynaptic.
• Controls skillful voluntary movements of distal limbs.	Controls gross, synergic, stereotype automatic movements of proximal joints of limbs.
• Control is contralateral. Upper limbs are controlled better than lower limbs.	Control is bilateral. Control of lower limbs is better than that of upper limbs and is mainly for postural adjustments.

What is paralysis?

Paralysis is complete loss of functions and strengths of muscle group or a limb.

Name	Part of body paralysed
Monoplegia	Paralysis of one limb
Diplegia	Paralysis of either both upper limbs or both lower limbs
Hemiplegia	Paralysis of upper and lower limbs of one side of the body
Paraplegia	Paralysis of lower half of the body (both lower limbs)

What are upper motor and lower motor neurons?

Upper motor neurons. Neurons in cerebral cortex, basal ganglia, brain stem nuclei and cerebellum.

Lower motor neurons. Motor neurons in spinal cord innervating muscles, motor neurons of cranial nerves in brain stems.

Lesions in upper and lower motor neurons cause upper and lower motor neuron paralysis respectively.

Effect	Upper Motor Neuron Paralysis	Lower Motor Neuron Paralysis
1. Muscle Tone	Hypertonia leading to spastic type of paralysis	Hypotonia leading to flaccid type of paralysis
2. Superficial Reflexes	Lost	Lost
3. Planter Reflex	Abnormal – Babinski's sign obtained	Lost
4. Deep Reflexes	Exaggerated	Lost
5. Clonus	Present	Absent
6. Wasting of Muscles	Slight	Present
7. Reaction of Degeneration	Not Present	Present
8. Fasciculations and Twitching	Absent	Present
9. Muscles affected	Group of muscles	Individual muscle is affected

TRANSECTION OF SPINAL CORD

What is complete transection of spinal cord? What are its effects?

Complete division of spinal cord is termed complete transection of spinal cord. It commonly occurs due to automobile accidents or gunshot injury.

EFFECTS

Effects depend upon the site of injury. Complete transection in cervical region can be fatal, because of cutting of connections between respiratory centre and respiratory muscles leading to paralysis of respiratory muscles.

Effects of complete transection of spinal cord are described in following three stages:

- Stage of spinal shock.

- Stage of reflex activity.
- Stage of reflex failure.

 1. *Stage of spinal shock.* It is developed immediately and after injury. Cause of spinal shock is not known but perhaps it is related to cessation of tonic neuronal discharge from upper brain stem or supraspinal pathways. Higher the animal, more profound and longer lasting is the spinal shock. This is probably due to encephalization, i.e. greater dependence of spinal cord on higher centres. In cat spinal shock lasts for few minutes in monkeys it lasts for few days and in human beings it lasts for about three weeks.

 There are following effects:

 (a) *Motor.* Below the level of section the muscles are paralyzed. Because of loss of tone muscles are atonic or flaccid. If muscles of all the four limbs are paralyzed it is termed quadriplegia. If muscles of both the lower limbs are paralyzed it is termed paraplegia. Depending upon the site of lesion there can be quadriplegia or paraplegia.

 (b) All tendon jerks are lost (areflexia).

Sensory. All sensations below the level are lost.

Vasomotor. Since sympathetic vasoconstrictor fibres leave the spinal cord between first thoracic and second lumbar segments, the transection of cord below second lumbar segment causes very little effect on blood pressure—sharp fall in BP (about 40 mmHg) when the transection is at first thoracic segment. Due to loss of sympathetic tonic discharge there is arteriolar dilatation leading to fall in BP. Absence of movements further retards the circulation and also the venous returns. Skin becomes cyanotic and liable to bed sores because of lack of nutrient supply.

Visceral. Mainly bladder and bowels are affected. Detrusor muscle of urinary bladder is paralyzed. Sphincter is also paralyzed but regains tone early leading to retention of urine. Bowels become hypotonic resulting in constipation.

 2. *Stage of reflex activity.* If the patient survives the stage of spinal shock, stage of reflex activity follows. At first functional activities of smooth muscles return and urinary bladder becomes 'automatic'. Then sympathetic tone of blood vessels returns and blood pressure is restored to normal.

 Later on tone of skeletal muscle returns. Tone of flexor muscles returns first therefore flexors become less hypotonic than extensors leading to a 'paraplegia in flexion' (both lower limbs are in state of flexion).

 Reflex activity begins to return after a few weeks. The flexor reflexes return first but to elicit flexor reflex a painful stimulus is required. The first reflex which usually appears is Babinski's reflex (Babinski's sign is positive). After a variable time extensor reflexes also return. In some cases, mass reflex can be elicited by scratching the skin over the lower limbs. It causes spasm of flexors muscles of both the limbs, evacuation of bladder and profuse sweating.

 3. *Stage of reflex failure.* Though the reflex movements return, the muscles below the level of injury have less power and less resistance. Usually general condition of the patient starts deteriorating and general infection and toxaemia become common. Due to this the failure of reflex function develops. Reflexes become more difficult to elicit. Mass reflex is abolished. The muscles become extremely flaccid and undergo wasting.

What is incomplete transection of spinal cord? What are its effects?

In incomplete transection there is a partial lesion involving both sides of the spinal cord. Spinal cord is gravely injured but does not suffer from complete division.

Complete transection	Incomplete transection
• Tone returns in flexor muscles first.	Tone returns in extensor muscles first because some descending fibres (e.g. vestibulospinal and reticulospinal tracts) may escape injury. Both these tracts mainly reinforce activity of extensor motor neurons.
• 'Paraplegia in flexion' results because of comparatively higher tone in flexor than in extensor muscles.	'Paraplegia in extension' results because of comparatively higher tone in extensor than in flexor muscles.
• Flexor reflexes return first.	Extensor reflexes (stretch reflexes) return first.
• Mass reflex can be elicited.	Mass reflex is not elicited because the controlling effect of brain stem persists through motor fibres (vestibulospinal and reticulospinal) which have escaped injury.

What is the effect of hemisection of the spinal cord?

When there is a partial transection and damage caused only to half of the spinal cord, typical motor and sensory changes develop after recovery from the spinal shock (Brown-Séquard syndrome). Various changes in Brown-Séquard's syndrome are described as at the level of section, below the level of section and above the level of section.

1. CHANGES AT THE LEVEL OF SECTION

- *Sensory changes.* All the sensations are lost on the corresponding segment on the same side except for the region of overlap due to damage to the posterior nerve roots.
- *Motor changes.* There is lower motor neuron type of paralysis because of damage to the anterior nerve roots. There is a loss of muscle tone, reflexes, and muscle power.

2. CHANGES BELOW THE LEVEL OF SECTION

- *Motor changes.* There is upper motor neuron type of paralysis on the same side, i.e. there is increased muscle tone, exaggerated reflexes, reaction of degeneration is absent and Babinski's sign is obtained. There are no motor changes on the opposite side.
- *Sensory changes.* There is dissociated sensory loss. On the side of damage, vibration, position, joint and fine touch sensations are lost (due to damage to the tract of Goll and Burdach's). Crude touch, temperature and pain persist.

On the opposite side pain, temperature and crude touch sensations are lost. They are lost one to two segments below the level of section. The loss of these sensations is due to damage to anterior and lateral spinothalamic tracts.

3. CHANGES ABOVE THE LEVEL OF SECTION

For one or two segments above the level of section on the same side there is a band of hyperaesthesia, i.e. increased cutaneous sensations. This is due to irritation of neighbouring posterior nerve roots above the level of section. Due to similar irritation of the anterior nerve roots, there is twitching of muscles in upper one or two segments on the same side.

BRAIN STEM

Describe the anatomy of brain stem?

The brain stem consists of the midbrain, pons and medulla oblongata.
Midbrain: It is a short segment connecting the cerebrum with pons.

1. The cerebral aqueduct forms the cavity of midbrain.
2. The part of the midbrain behind the aqueduct, tectum consists of four small swellings called colliculi.
   - The superior colliculi form centre for visual reflexes.
   - The inferior colliculi are concerned with auditory reflexes.
3. The part ventral to the cerebral aqueduct has red nucleus substantia nigra (a black band containing pigmented neurons) and crus cerebri containing descending fibres.
4. Midbrain contains nuclei of III, IV and V cranial nerves.

Pons (means bridge): It joins the midbrain to the medulla oblongata.

1. The ventral aspect of the pons has pontine sulcus with basilar artery.
2. The transverse pontine fibres can be seen on the surface, which are part of the connection between cortex and cerebellum.
3. The pons contains nuclei for V, VI, VII and VIII cranial nerves.

Medulla oblongata: It joins the pons to the spinal cord. It is about 2.5 cm in length and ends at foramen magnum.

1. The lower half of the medulla has central canal while the upper half forms the floor of IV ventricle.
2. The ventral surface has anterior median fissure. On either side of the fissure, are two elevations – pyramid medially and olive laterally. The pyramids are formed by corticospinal fibres which cross (pyramidal decussation) in the lower medulla. The olives are formed by olivary nuclei.
3. From the ventral aspect emerge IX, X, XI, XIIth cranial nerves.
4. In the lower part, axons from gracile and cuneate nuclei cross (sensory decussation) to form medial lemniscus.
5. The medulla contains nuclei of 9–12th cranial nerves.
6. It has many vital centres (cardiac, respiratory, vasomotor centres and reflex centres for vomiting, coughing, deglutition, sneezing).

What are the functions of brain stem?

Brain stem includes medulla, pons and mesencephalon (Fig. 13.16). It contains motor and sensory nuclei that perform motor and sensory functions for face and head region in the same way as the anterior and posterior grey horns of the spinal cord perform. It provides special control functions of:

- Respiration.
- Cardiovascular system.
- Gastrointestinal system.
- Many stereotyped movements of the body.
- Sleep and wakefulness.
- Equilibrium.
- Eye movements.

Whole body movements and equilibrium control occur as follows through reticular formation and vestibular nuclei.

Reticular formation is the relay station for all descending motor commands except those traveling directly to spinal cord through medullary pyramids. It mainly receives motor commands to the proximal and axial muscles of the body and is involved in performance of all the motor activities except fine movements performed by the distal muscles of fingers and hands. The reticular formation is also responsible for maintaining normal postural tone. Neurons within the pontine reticular formation send axons to spinal cord through medial reticulospinal tract. These signals are excitatory to the alpha and gamma motor neurons innervating extensor antigravity muscles. These neurons are prevented from firing too rapidly by inhibitory input derived from the cerebral and cerebellar components of the motor control system. The amount of inhibition is increased to reduce the postural tone and is decreased to enhance postural tone.

Vestibular nuclei are responsible for maintaining tone in antigravity muscles and for co-ordinating the adjustments made by limbs and eyes in response to changes in body position.

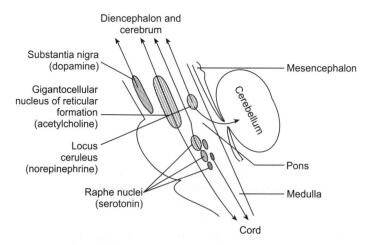

FIGURE 13.16 Centres in the brain stem.

MUSCLE TONE

What is muscle tone? How is it tested?

The resistance of muscle to passive stretch is known as muscle tone. Muscle tone is also described as partial state of tetanus of the muscle in resting state. It is usually tested by moving the relaxed limb of the subject.

How is muscle tone maintained?

Muscle tone is a state of partial tetanus of the muscle, maintained by an asynchronous discharge of impulses in motor nerve supplying muscle.

Tone is mainly maintained reflexly by monosynaptic stretch reflex (spinal). Both afferent and efferent limbs of reflex are composed of large myelinated nerve fibres (12 to 20 microns diameter). Afferent impulses from muscle spindles excite alpha motor neurons which send efferent impulses to the muscle concerned for causing muscle contraction. Though the reflex arc is spinal, supraspinal nervous pathways modify the reflex in intact animal (Chart 13.1).

Supraspinal control. Activity of gamma and alpha motor neurons is modified by both extrapyramidal and pyramidal fibres which terminate on them (directly or through interneurons). Mainly extrapyramidal system is responsible for maintaining tone. It consists of basal ganglia, motor nuclei of reticular formation of brain stem, vestibular nuclei and descending fibres conveying impulses to spinal cord. From cerebral cortex (area 6) also some fibres descend and merge with the extrapyramidal nuclei.

In the brain stem there are bulboreticular facilitatory areas in the pons which discharge facilitatory impulses to spinal motor neurons. These areas in turn receive facilitatory impulses from vestibular nuclei, facilitatory portions of cerebral cortex, cerebellum and basal ganglia. All these impulses keep facilitatory areas constantly active. These areas therefore send continuous impulses to spinal motor neurons.

In medulla, there are bulboreticular inhibitory areas having no intrinsic activity of their own. These areas receive impulses from cerebellum, cerebrum and in turn inhibits bulboreticular facilitatory areas to some extent. But without support from cerebrum or cerebellum these areas cannot inhibit the activity of facilitatory areas.

Normal muscle tone is due to continuous excitatory impulses sent by bulboreticular facilitatory areas to spinal motor neurons (alpha and gamma).

Cerebellum is the site of alpha-gamma linkage. In presence of the cerebellum therefore the muscle tone is maintained through alpha (non-myotatic) and gamma (myotatic) activity. But in the absence of cerebellum, muscle tone is maintained by alpha activity (non-myotatic) only. This can be demonstrated by classical and ischaemic decerebrate rigidity.

When the brain stem is transected at intercollicular level, the rigidity that is produced is termed decerebrate rigidity (classical) leading to increased muscle tone. Section causes total loss of communication between cerebral hemispheres and brain stem (hence the name decerebration). Brain stem therefore no longer receives impulses from cerebral cortex and basal ganglia. As a result, medullary

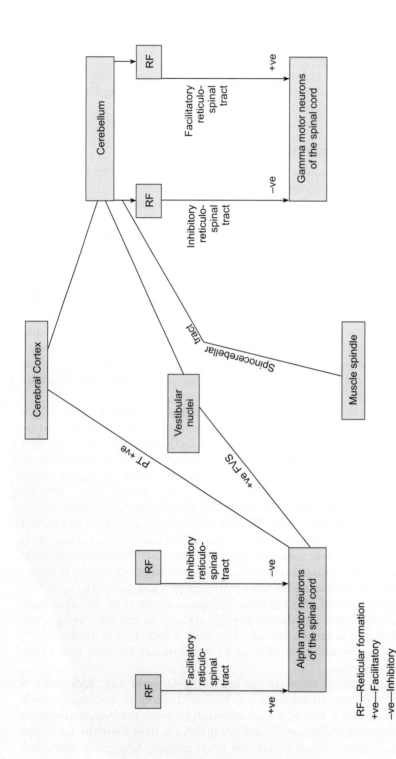

RF—Reticular formation
+ve—Facilitatory
−ve—Inhibitory
FVS—Facilitatory vestibulospinaltract
PT—Pyramidal tract

Chart 13.1 Control of muscle tone. RF—Reticular formation, +ve—Facilitatory, −ve—Inhibitory, FVS—Facilitatory vestibulospinal tract, PT—Pyramidal tract.

inhibitory areas having no intrinsic activity become greatly non-functional (not totally non-functional as they receive impulses from cerebellum). Bulboreticular facilitatory areas therefore become unopposed and continue to discharge excessive facilitatory impulses resulting in increased tone (rigidity). This rigidity is lost by deafferentation (cutting of afferents from muscle). This proves that rigidity is due to increased activity of gamma motor neurons. Rigidity is due therefore to exaggerated stretch reflex.

When common carotid artery and basilar arteries are ligated the similar rigidity is obtained which is termed ischaemic decerebrate rigidity. This rigidity is not lost by deafferentiation. It indicates that hypertonia is induced due to excessive drive of alpha motor neurons.

ABNORMALITIES

What is hypertonia?

Abnormally high muscle tone is known as hypertonia. It is usually found when there are disorders of the descending pathways that result in an imbalance in the facilitatory and inhibitory inputs exerted by them on motor neurons and interneurons. The term spasticity or rigidity is used for the hypertonic muscles.

What is hypotonia?

Hypotonia is a condition of abnormally low muscle tone. It occurs due to cerebellar disease, disorders of alpha motor neurons, neuromuscular junctions and muscles. The term 'flaccid' is used for the hypotonic muscle.

What is classical decerebrate rigidity?

The section of the neural axis in midcollicular region (between superior and inferior colliculi) results in classical decerebrate rigidity. This is due to the removal of cerebral inhibitory inputs to the reticular formation (cerebellar inputs are still retained).

Without these inhibitory inputs pontine reticular formation fires uncontrollably (facilitation takes upper hand) and therefore if such animal is placed over its feet, animal is able to maintain upright posture because of increased tone in the antigravity muscles. Position of the animal is abnormal. Animal stands with hyperextended limbs which act as pillars. Neck and tail are raised and arched. There is also arching of the back. Rigidity is mainly due to increased activity of gamma motor neurons (through gamma loop the activity of alpha motor neurons is increased).

What is ischaemic decerebrate rigidity?

Rigidity like classical decerebrate rigidity can also be produced by tying or occluding blood vessels to the brain (basilar arteries and internal carotid arteries). The rigidity that is produced is called an ischaemic decerebrate rigidity and it is due to increased activity of the alpha motor neurons.

POSTURE AND EQUILIBRIUM

What is posture?

The term posture signifies an unconscious adjustment of tone in different muscles so as to maintain balance during rest as well as during movements.

What is equilibrium?

Equilibrium is to maintain the line of gravity constant at rest and during movement by adjusting the tone in different muscles.

How is equilibrium maintained?

The various parts of neural system play a role in maintaining equilibrium:

1. *Role of vestibular apparatus.* Macula and saccule help in the maintenance of equilibrium under static conditions. They also detect linear acceleration.

Semicircular canals detect angular acceleration and help in maintaining equilibrium during dynamic phase. They also have a predictive function. When the person is in dynamic state, they predict ahead of time that the person is likely to fall off-balance and help nervous system to do adjustments to prevent a fall.

2. *Role of cerebellum.* Impulses from semicircular canals go to flocculonodular lobes of cerebellum. Severe injury to either of these therefore causes loss of equilibrium during rapid changes in direction of motion but does not disturb equilibrium under static conditions.

Impulses from macula and saccule go to uvula of cerebellum. They help in maintaining equilibrium under static condition.

3. *Role of brain stem.* There are four pairs of vestibular nuclei in brain stem:

(a) *Superior vestibular nuclei.* They receive signals from semicircular canals and in turn send signals to medial longitudinal fasciculus to cause corrective movements of eyes, as well as signals through medial vestibular tract to cause appropriate movements of the neck and head.

(b) *Medial vestibular nuclei.* They receive signals from semicircular canals and in turn send signals to medial longitudinal fasciculus to cause corrective movements of eyes, and through vestibulospinal tract to cause appropriate movements of neck and head.

(c) *Lateral vestibular nuclei.* They receive signals from utricle and saccule and in turn send signals through lateral vestibulospinal tract to spinal cord for controlling body movements.

(d) *Inferior vestibular nuclei.* They receive signals from semicircular canals and utricle and in turn send signals to cerebellum and reticular formation of brain stem.

4. *Other factors concerned with equilibrium.*

(a) *Neck proprioceptors.* Vestibular apparatus detects information about orientation of head and movements of head. Information on orientation of head with respect of body is transmitted by neck and body proprioceptors to vestibular and reticular nuclei of brain stem and cerebellum.

(b) *Neck reflexes.* Vestibular and neck reflexes must function oppositely to maintain equilibrium of the entire body. If vestibular apparatus is destroyed, then bending of head causes muscular reflexes called neck reflexes occurring especially in the forelimbs.

(c) *Body exteroceptors and proprioceptors.* Information from other parts of the body besides neck is also important for maintaining equilibrium, e.g. pressure from foot pad informing whether weight is more forward or backward on the feet.

(d) *Visual receptors.* After complete destruction of vestibular apparatus and loss of proprioceptive information a person can still use visual mechanism effectively to maintain balance. But in such a case, if the eyes are closed or the person is moving rapidly, balance is lost.

What is the basic postural reflex?

- The skeleton of the body comprises long bones and multijointed vertebral column held together by ligaments and covered with muscles and is ill-suited to stand against the forces of gravity as the tall human being has to maintain erect posture over a small base. This is true not only for holding the body in erect position but also fixation of body parts over adjoining body segments. Head is also held in erect position while awake, but it cannot be held erect during sleep in sitting position because the centres of gravity of different parts of the body do not lie perpendicular to the articular points of support. The centre of gravity of head passes in front of the centre of gravity of atlanto-occipital joint. Thus head has got always a tendency to roll forwards. To hold the head in erect position cervico-occipital muscles are to be maintained in a state of constant tension. Similar problem is encountered in maintaining the equilibrium of the body in erect position.

- Basic reflex responsible for maintenance of posture is stretch reflex. Pull of gravity initiates this reflex in the antigravity muscle keeping them in contracted state for maintaining the erect body posture. In man, flexors of upper extremity and extensors of lower extremity are the main antigravity muscles. Retractors of neck, the elevators of jaw, supraspinatus, the extensors of back, rectal muscles of abdominal wall, extensors of knee and ankle are the muscles which exhibit the greatest degree of tone. When these muscles completely relax (as in an unconscious person) the body collapses.

Thus postural reflexes help to maintain the body in upright and balanced position. They also provide adjustments necessary to maintain a stable posture during voluntary activity. These postural reflexes include: (i) static reflexes involving sustained contraction of the muscles and (ii) phasic reflexes which maintain a stable postural background for voluntary activity. Both these types of postural reflexes are integrated at various levels in the central nervous system from the spinal cord to cerebral cortex and are affected largely by extrapyramidal pathways. A major factor in postural control is variation in the threshold of spinal stretch reflex caused in turn by changes in the excitability of motor neurons (Fig. 13.17).

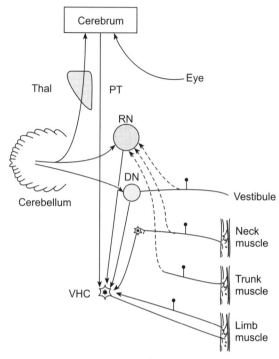

FIGURE 13.17 Regulation of posture. DN = Deiters' nucleus, VHC = ventral horn cell, PT = pyramidal tract, RN = red nucleus.

Describe in short the various postural reflexes.

Reflex	Stimulus	Response	Receptor	Integration
• Stretch reflex	Stretch	Contraction of muscle	Muscle spindles	Spinal cord
• Positive supporting reaction	Sole of palm	Foot extended to support the body	Proprioceptors in distal flexors	Spinal cord
• Negative supporting reaction	Stretch	Release of positive	Proprioceptors in extensors	Spinal cord
• Tonic labyrinthine reflexes	Gravity	Extensor rigidity	Otolith organ	Medulla
• Tonic neck reflexes	(i) Head turned to side (ii) Head turned up (iii) Head turned up down	Extension of limbs on side to which head is turned; Hind legs flexed; Fore legs flexed	Neck proprioceptors	Medulla

Cont'd

Reflex	Stimulus	Response	Receptor	Integration
• Labyrinthine righting reflexes	Gravity	Head is kept erect	Otolith organ	Midbrain
• Neck righting reflexes	Stretch of neck muscles	Righting of thorax, shoulder and pelvis	Muscle spindles	Midbrain
• Body righting reflex on the acting on head	Pressure on the side of the body	Righting of head even when head held sideways	Exteroceptors	Midbrain
• Body righting reflex on the acting on body	Pressure on the side of the body	Righting of body even when head held sideways	Exteroceptors	Midbrain
• Optical righting reflex	Visual cues	Righting of head	Eyes	Visual cortex
• Placing reaction	Various visual, exteroceptive proprioceptive cues	Foot placed on supporting surface in position to support the body	Various receptors	Cerebral cortex
• Hopping reaction	Lateral displacement while standing	Hopping, maintaining limbs in position to support the body	Muscle spindles	Cerebral cortex

DECORTICATE PREPARATION

What is decorticate preparation?

When whole cerebral cortex is removed but the basal ganglia and the brain stem are left intact, the preparation is known as decorticate animal.

HYPOTHALAMUS

STRUCTURE

Describe the structure of hypothalamus.

Hypothalamus is a diffuse nuclear mass which is separated from thalamus by hypothalamic sulcus. It forms the anteroinferior wall of the third ventricle. Nuclear masses of hypothalamus are grouped as follows (Fig. 13.18):

(a) Preoptic area (medial and lateral preoptic nuclei).

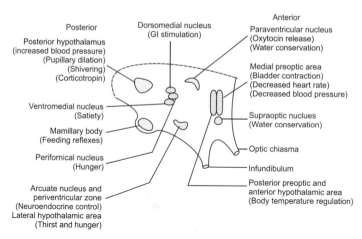

Posterior

Dorsomedial nucleus
(GI stimulation)

Anterior

Posterior hypothalamus
(increased blood pressure)
(Pupillary dilation)
(Shivering)
(Corticotropin)

Paraventricular nucleus
(Oxytocin release)
(Water conservation)

Medial preoptic area
(Bladder contraction)
(Decreased heart rate)
(Decreased blood pressure)

Ventromedial nucleus
(Satiety)

Mamillary body
(Feeding reflexes)

Supraoptic nuclues
(Water conservation)

Perifornical nucleus
(Hunger)

Optic chiasma

Infundibulum

Arcuate nucleus and
periventricular zone
(Neuroendocrine control)
Lateral hypothalamic area
(Thirst and hunger)

Posterior preoptic and
anterior hypothalamic area
(Body temperature regulation)

FIGURE 13.18 Control centres of hypothalamus.

(b) Supraoptic area (supraoptic, suprachiasmatic, paraventricular and anterior nuclei).
(c) Tuberal area (ventromedial, dorsomedial, arcuate, lateral and posterior nuclei).
(d) Mamillary area (medial and lateral mamillary, pre and supramamillary nuclei).

CONNECTIONS

Describe the connections of hypothalamus.

AFFERENTS

1. From other parts of limbic system:
   - Pyriform cortex and amygdaloid nuclei send impulses to ventral pathway to medial forebrain bundle.
   - From amygdaloid nucleus to stria terminalis.
   - From hippocampus and postcommissural fornix to mamillary body. Other hippocampal fibres are carried to medial forebrain bundle which relays in septal nuclei.
   - From restricted region of hippocampus, the medial hypothalamic tract runs to the arcuate nucleus. This pathway and stria terminalis are the only two major afferent pathways running directly to medial hypothalamus. Other afferent fibres take indirect route via medial forebrain bundle and lateral hypothalamus to reach medial hypothalamus.
   - Cingulate gyrus establishes connections with the hypothalamus through its projection to the hippocampus.
2. From midbrain tegmentum there is massive projection to mamillary nuclei and the medial forebrain bundle. Through this route the sensory pathways from the viscera project to hypothalamus (since they do not establish direct connections with it).
3. The frontal cortex and the dorsomedial nucleus of thalamus may send fibres to medial forebrain bundle.

Thus hypothalamus receives information from viscera (about activities of different systems) and limbic cortex. In addition it has got its own receptor systems like glucoreceptors, osmoreceptors, thermoreceptors to detect the composition of body fluids and temperature of the body. In addition, it has many ill-defined connections with reticular formation, basal ganglia and cortex.

EFFERENTS

- Hypothalamus sends fibres to the amygdaloid nuclei and then after relaying, to the pyriform cortex, both in the ventral pathway from lateral hypothalamus and the stria terminalis from the ventromedial nucleus.
- Fibres in the medial forebrain bundle run from hypothalamus to septal nuclei, relay there and then pass to hippocampus.
- Mamillothalamic tract: Fibres from medial mamillary nucleus pass to anterior thalamic nucleus and then to the cingulate gyrus.
- Descending fibres mainly from lateral hypothalamus pass to the reticular formation of tegmentum, to the motor nuclei of bulb and then to the spinal cord, thereby contributing to extrapyramidal facilitatory pathway. These fibres also establish connections to brain stem autonomic nuclei and the lateral horn cells of the thoracolumbar segments and thus control sympathetic outflow. These fibres also establish connection with cranial and sacral parasympathetic outflow.
- From supraoptic and paraventricular nuclei hypothalamo-hypophyseal tract originates and runs to the posterior pituitary.

FUNCTIONS

Describe the functions of hypothalamus.

Though hypothalamus represents only 1% of the brain mass, it has many functions. The functions are classified as: (1) Vegetative and endocrine functions and (2) Behavioural functions.

1. VEGETATIVE AND ENDOCRINE FUNCTIONS

(a) *Regulation of body temperature.* Anterior hypothalamus especially preoptic area is responsible for temperature regulation. Increase in the temperature of blood flowing through this area increases the activity of temperature sensitive neurons whereas decrease in temperature decreases their activity. Anterior nucleus of hypothalamus mainly controls heat loss mechanisms while the posterior hypothalamus controls heat gain mechanisms. Hypothalamus adjusts heat loss and heat gain which helps to maintain body temperature at $37°C$.

(b) *Regulation of water balance.* When the water content of the body is reduced, osmolality of body fluid increases. This is detected by osmoreceptors present mainly in supraoptic nucleus of hypothalamus. The hypothalamus regulates body water in two ways:

- Thirst: There is stimulation of thirst centre located in the lateral hypothalamus. This causes intense desire for water. Animal drinks large quantities of water.

- ADH hormone: Neurons in the supraoptic nucleus are stimulated. They in turn send impulses to posterior pituitary gland to secrete hormone ADH. This hormone reaches kidney tubules through blood and causes increased absorption of water from the collecting ducts of the kidneys. Thus water loss is decreased. When body has excess water exactly opposite events occurs.

(c) *Gastrointestinal and feeding regulation.* In the lateral hypothalamic area, there is the hunger centre. When this is stimulated, it creates a sensation of hunger. In the ventromedial nucleus of hypothalamus, there is satiety centre. When this is stimulated it gives feeling of satisfaction (if animal is eating food it suddenly stops eating). The balanced activity of these two centres is responsible for our normal food intake, which is also guided by conditioning from the cortex.

(d) *Cardiovascular regulation.* Stimulation of posterior and lateral hypothalamus increases the arterial pressure and heart rate. Stimulation of preoptic area decreases both the arterial blood pressure and the heart rate. These effects are transmitted mainly through the cardiovascular control centres in reticular regions of medulla and pons.

(e) *Regulation of uterine contractility and regulation of milk ejection from the breast.* Stimulation of paraventricular nucleus of hypothalamus causes its cells to secrete the hormone, oxytocin. Oxytocin increases the contractility of uterus. It also contracts myoepithelial cells that surround the alveoli of breast and causes milk ejection. At the end of pregnancy, especially large quantities of oxytocin are secreted. Oxytocin helps to promote labour contractions. When the baby suckles the breast, signals from nipple to hypothalamus cause reflex oxytocin release which causes expulsion of milk through the nipple.

(f) *Control of anterior pituitary.* Hypothalamus is connected to anterior pituitary through hypothalamo-hypophyseal portal tract. Neuronal cells present in paraventricular area, arcuate nucleus, and ventromedial nucleus, secrete some releasing and inhibitory hormones. From here these hormones reach median eminence and from there through hypothalamo-hypophyseal tract they reach anterior pituitary and affect release of anterior pituitary hormones as already discussed in the chapter on 'Endocrinology'.

Hypothalamus does the following functions through the releasing hormones:

- Controls the metabolism by controlling thyroid gland.
- Through its influence over adrenal cortex, controls the metabolism of different food stuffs and maintains electrolyte balance.
- Keeps the gonads inhibited. Only when the physical growth is complete this inhibition is removed so that gonads start functioning and gametes are produced (propagation of species). Gonadal hormones acting on the brain bring about physiological changes for mating of male and female.
- Controls the formation of milk by the breasts by controlling prolactin secretion.

2. BEHAVIOURAL FUNCTIONS

(a) Stimulation of lateral hypothalamus not only causes thirst and eating but increases the general level of activity of the animal, sometimes leading to rage or fighting. Stimulation of ventromedial nucleus causes the opposite effect.

(b) Sexual drive is stimulated especially by stimulation of most anterior and posterior portion of hypothalamus.

(c) Hypothalamus along with the limbic structures is concerned with affective nature of sensory impulses, i.e. whether sensations are pleasant or unpleasant.

These affective qualities are also called reward and punishment. Reward centres are located along the course of medial forebrain bundle, especially in lateral and ventromedial nucleus of hypothalamus. Punishment centres are located in the grey area, surrounding the aqueduct of Sylvius, periventricular zones of hypothalamus and thalamus. Almost everything that we do is related in some way to reward and punishment. If we do something that is rewarding, we continue to do it. If we do something that is punishing we cease to do it. Therefore, reward and punishment centres constitute one of the most important of all the controllers of our bodily activities, our drives, our aversions, our motivations.

Sensory experience that is causing neither reward nor punishment is remembered hardly at all, the animal becomes habituated to such sensory experience and then ignores it. But when the sensory experience causes either reward or punishment, the cortical response becomes progressively more and more intense. Thus reward and punishment centres help in selecting the information that we learn.

Strong stimulation of punishment centres causes development of rage. Normally, it is kept in check by counterbalancing activity of ventromedial nuclei of hypothalamus, hippocampus, amygdala and anterior portion of limbic cortex. Stimulation of punishment area in the preoptic region causes anxiety and fear. When reward centres are stimulated there is placidity and tameness.

LIMBIC SYSTEM

Name the structures included in the limbic system.

Hypothalamus, septum, paraolfactory area, epithalamus, anterior nucleus of thalamus, portions of basal ganglia, hippocampus and amygdala are the subcortical centres (Fig. 13.19a). Surrounding these subcortical limbic centres is the limbic cortex composed of ring of cerebral cortex beginning in the orbitofrontal area on the ventral surface of frontal lobe, extending upward in subcallosal gyrus, extending over the top of corpus callosum onto the medial aspect of cerebral hemisphere in the cingulate gyrus, and passing behind the corpus callosum and downward onto the ventromedial surface of temporal lobe to parahippocampal gyrus and uncus. This ring of limbic cortex functions as a two way communication and association linkage between neocortex and lower limbic structures.

Many of the behavioural functions of limbic system are mediated through reticular nuclei and their associated nuclei in the brain stem. Important route of communication between limbic system and brain stem is medial forebrain bundle and second route of communication is short pathways among reticular formation of brain stem thalamus and hypothalamus and other areas of basal brain (Fig. 13.19b).

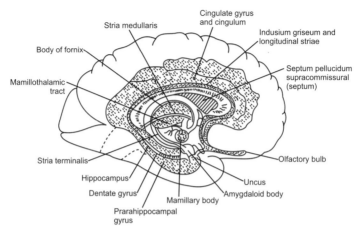

FIGURE 13.19 **(a)** Anatomy of the limbic system illustrated by the shaded areas of the figure.

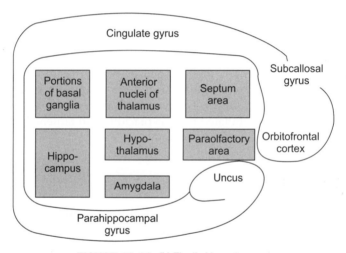

FIGURE 13.19 **(b)** The limbic system.

Describe the functions of important areas of limbic system.

1. *Hypothalamus.* Behavioural functions of hypothalamus are already discussed above.

2. *Amygdala.* In lower animals amygdala is concerned with association of olfactory stimuli with stimuli from other parts of brain. In human beings, basolateral nuclei of amygdala are very well developed and they play an important role in behavioural activities not generally associated with olfactory stimuli.

Amygdala receives neuronal signals from all portions of limbic cortex as well as from neocortex and therefore is called the 'window' through which the limbic system sees the place of the person in the world. Amygdala in turn transmits signals back to the same cortical areas, hippocampus, septum, thalamus and hypothalamus.

Stimulation of amygdala causes the following effects through hypothalamus:
- Increase or decrease in blood pressure (heart rate).
- Increase or decrease in gastrointestinal secretion and motility.
- Defaecation, micturition.
- Pupillary dilatation (rarely constriction).
- Piloerection.
- Secretion of anterior pituitary hormones.

In addition, amygdala stimulation causes the following effects:
- Tonic movements as raising of head or bending of the body.
- Clonic rhythmic movements.
- Circling movements.
- Movements associated with olfaction and eating (chewing, swallowing, etc.).
- Reactions of reward or punishment.
- Erection, copulatory movements, ovulation, uterine activity, premature labour.

Thus amygdala is a behavioural awareness area, that operates at a subconscious level. It projects into limbic system, the present status of a person in relation to both surroundings and thoughts. This information helps to decide the pattern of a person's behavioural response so that it is appropriate for each occasion.

3. *Hippocampus.* It has many indirect connections to many portions of cerebral cortex. Therefore, like amygdala, it is an additional channel through which incoming signals can lead to appropriate behavioural pattern such as rage, passivity, excess sex drive, etc.

Very weak electrical stimuli to hippocampus can cause local epileptic seizures that persist for many seconds. One of the reasons of hippocampal hyperexcitability is that it is a different type of cortex having only three nerve cell layers instead of six found elsewhere in the cortex. Hippocampus is also responsible for consolidation of long-term memories of verbal and symbolic type.

4. *Limbic cortex.* Limbic cortex acts as association area for control of behaviour. Anterior temporal cortex causes gustatory and olfactory associations.

In parahippocampal gyri, there is complex auditory association, and also complex thought association derived from Wernicke's area of the posterior temporal lobe. In the posterior cingulate cortex there are sensory motor associations.

RETICULAR FORMATION

What is reticular formation? Give afferent and efferent connections of reticular formation.

Reticular formation is a diffuse mass of neurons and nerve fibres forming meshwork of reticulum in the central part of brain stem, i.e. medulla, pons and tegmentum.

CONNECTIONS OF RETICULAR FORMATION

AFFERENTS

- Olfactory pathway.
- Optic pathway.
- Auditory pathway.
- Spinal and trigeminal pathway carrying touch sensation.
- Pathways for pain, temperature, vibration and kinaesthetic sensations.
- Cerebral cortex.
- Cerebellum.
- Basal ganglia (caudate nucleus).
- Thalamus.

EFFERENTS

- Cerebral cortex.
- Thalamus.
- Hypothalamus.
- Subthalamus.
- Substantia nigra.
- Red nucleus.
- Cerebellum.
- Spinal cord.

Functionally reticular formation is divided into two systems:

- Ascending reticular activating system (ARAS).
- Descending reticular system.

What is ascending reticular activating system? What are its functions?

Ascending reticular activating system (ARAS) extends from lower pons to thalamus and throughout its course it receives afferent collaterals from auditory, visceral, sensory somatic pathways. It relays efferent impulses to cerebral cortex through midline, intralaminar and reticular nuclei of thalamus. These impulses travel slowly in multisynaptic pathway but are conducted to widespread areas of cerebral cortex (as against impulses which quickly ascend through specific sensory pathways to specific primary sensory area of the cerebral cortex; Fig. 13.20).

FUNCTIONS OF ARAS

(i) Impulses from ARAS pass to widespread areas of cortex. These keep the cortex active and cause desynchronized activity as shown in EEG during wakeful state. These non-specific impulses are therefore responsible for arousal phenomenon, alertness, maintenance of attention and awakefulness. Any type of sensory impulses (somatic or visceral) thus activates ARAS producing arousal phenomenon.

Sympathetic stimulation causing release of epinephrine and norepinephrine produces EEG arousal and behavioural alteration by reducing threshold of reticular neurons in the brain stem.

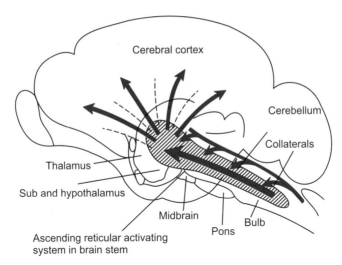

Ascending reticular activating system in brain stem

FIGURE 13.20 Ascending reticular activating system

Cerebral cortex in turn also activates ARAS by sending impulses from certain areas. Thus intracortical events can cause arousal.

- ARAS causes emotional reaction.
- ARAS is helpful in learning and the development of conditioned reflex.

What is descending reticular system? What are its functions?

Descending reticular system is divided into two pathways:

- Descending inhibitory reticular pathway.
- Descending facilitatory reticular pathway.

Descending inhibitory reticular pathway. Stimulation of ventromedial part of medullary reticular formation causes inhibition of movements induced either reflexly or by cortical stimulation. This part of bulbar inhibitory reticular formation is under the influence of inhibitory area of cortex and the caudate nucleus. Bulbar area in turn projects to spinal neurons by reticulospinal pathway (mainly extensor muscles are inhibited).

Anterior and paramedian lobes of cerebellum serve to reinforce the inhibitory influence of these bulbar neurons on spinal neurons.

Descending inhibitory reticular system also inhibits various autonomic functions.

FUNCTIONS

1. *Somatomotor activity.* By inhibiting spinal motor neurons descending inhibitory reticular pathway is responsible for:
    - Smoothness and accuracy of voluntary movements.
    - Regulation of reflex movements.
    - Regulation of muscle tone and maintenance of posture.
2. *Control of vegetative functions.* It causes inhibition of various autonomic functions, e.g. blood pressure, respiration, gastrointestinal functions, temperature, etc.

THALAMUS

STRUCTURE

Describe the structure of thalamus.

Refer Figure 13.21.

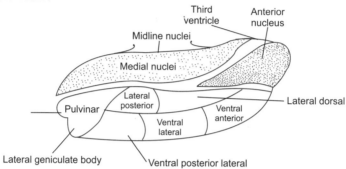

FIGURE 13.21 Thalamic nuclei.

CONNECTIONS

Describe the connections of thalamus.

Functionally thalamus is considered to have extrinsic nuclei, and intrinsic nuclei.

1. *Extrinsic nuclei.* These are cortical relay nuclei. They receive afferent fibres from extrathalamic sources. Axons of these nuclear cells are distributed to primary cortical areas—pre and post central cortices, visual and auditory cortical areas. Different extrinsic nuclei are as follows:

(a) *Posteroventral nucleus.* This receives medial lemniscus and trigeminal lemniscus. The medial lemniscus carries afferent fibres from the gracile and cuneate nuclei and afferent fibres from ventral and dorsal spinothalamic tracts. Hence impulses from touch, pressure, joint, temperature and pain receptors synapse in these nuclei, with the exception of pain, they are relayed to postcentral cortex.

The trigeminal lemniscus carries the same type of afferents from face together with taste fibres.

Muscle afferents from limb which have relayed in 'Z' nucleus (interpolated between head end of gracile and the descending vestibular nuclei) yield fibres which synapse in posteroventral nucleus and then are relayed to area '3a' of the cortex.

In the posteroventral nucleus fibres from the face lie most medially and fibres from legs lie most laterally. Thus there is a topographic arrangement of fibres.

(b) *Lateroventral nucleus.* This receives dentatothalamic fibres from cerebellum carrying proprioceptive information. Nuclear cells of these nuclei projects to precentral motor cortex—area 4 and 6.

(c) *Anterior nucleus.* It receives mammillothalamic tract which carries impulses relayed in mamillary bodies from the hippocampus. The anterior nucleus sends impulses to the cingulate gyrus.

(d) *Medial geniculate bodies.* They receive topically organized projections from auditory fibres from cochlear nuclei and inferior colliculi. They relay in turn to auditory areas of cortex.

(e) *Lateral geniculate bodies.* They receive from primary visual neurons and relay information to the calcarine cortex.

2. **Intrinsic nuclei.** These nuclei receive fibres mainly from the other structures in the thalamus. They are formed of midline, intralaminar, dorsomedial and dorsolateral nuclei and pulvinar. Pulvinar is most developed in primates.

Dorsomedial and intralaminar nuclei have generous connection with the frontal lobes and hypothalamus. Midline and intralaminar nuclei project also to the neostriatum. Pulvinar projects to inferior parietal lobes. The dorsomedial nuclei receive fibres from or project to the precuneate gyrus.

The reticular nucleus which lies between internal capsule and external medullary lamina receives fibres from all the intralaminar nuclei, which in turn are the sites of synapse of afferent tracts from the ascending reticular formation. The impulses from here are relayed to the cortex. These are termed non-specific because the reticulothalamic path exerts great effect on electrical activity of widespread areas of the cortex.

FUNCTIONS

Describe the functions of thalamus.

Functionally thalamus represents the first co-ordinating centre where sensory, motor, autonomic information can be co-ordinated to produce co-ordinate activity. In lower animals, it acts as the highest sensory centre for co-ordination as cerebral cortex is not well developed. In such animals hypothalamus acts as highest autonomic centre and basal ganglia act as highest motor centre. But in man, there is less number of neurons in the thalamus available for interpretation.

FUNCTIONS OF THALAMUS IN MAN

1. Thalamus is the major relay station where all the specific impulses relay before finally terminating in the cerebral cortex. It acts as a crude centre for sense perception.
2. Majority of non-specific ascending impulses from reticular activating system are relayed to thalamus before proceeding to cortex. These fibres when active cause wakefulness, alertness and consciousness.
3. Because of intimate connections between thalamus and frontal cortex and hypothalamus, thalamus is involved in subjective feeling of various emotions. Thus it acts as a part of limbic system.
4. It acts as a relay station for dentatothalamic tract which relays in thalamus and then passes to the cortex. This provides necessary information for skeletal motor activities.

APPLIED ASPECT

What is thalamic syndrome?

Thrombosis of local artery supplying posteroventral nucleus leads to thalamic syndrome. In thalamic syndrome, there is profound muscular weakness, decreased muscle tone, ataxia, loss of discriminative aspects of sensation (loss of sensation of light touch, tactile localization and discrimination) and loss of appreciation of small movements of the joints. All the symptoms and signs occur on the opposite side of the body. In addition to this, there may be altered emotional effects.

BASAL GANGLIA

STRUCTURE

Describe the anatomy of basal ganglia.

Basal ganglia are the group of neurons at the base of cerebral cortex. Basal ganglia include:

- Corpus striatum.
- Subthalamic nucleus.
- Substantia nigra.

The corpus striatum is located lateral to the thalamus. It consists of caudate nucleus (phylogenetically more recent), putamen and globus pallidus (phylogenetically older). Putamen and globus pallidus together form a bean-shaped lenticular nucleus. Caudate nucleus has a tail and head. Between caudate nucleus and putamen lies the anterior limb of internal capsule.

Subthalamus and substantia nigra are located inferior and posterior to the thalamus.

CONNECTIONS

Describe the connections of basal ganglia.

Basal ganglia receive information from all parts of cerebral cortex and project back to motor cortex via ventrolateral and ventroanterior thalamus (Fig. 13.22). Basal ganglia therefore exert influence on voluntary motor performance because of close association with the corticospinal system.

Basal ganglia also send efferents to portions where extrapyramidal tracts originate. They therefore also control non-voluntary motor functions such as maintenance of tone, posture and equilibrium.

Thus basal ganglia control voluntary and non-voluntary motor functions.

AFFERENT CONNECTIONS

(a) *Corticostriate* (from cerebral cortex to putamen). Fibres from pre-motor, supplementary motor cortex and primary somatosensory area pass to putamen (Fig. 13.22).

From all the four lobes of cortex but especially from association areas of cerebral cortex to caudate nucleus (Fig. 13.22).

(b) *Thalamostriate fibres.* Fibres from intralaminar, medial and ventral anterior nuclei of thalamus pass to caudate nucleus and putamen.

(c) *Nigrostriate fibres.* From dorsomedial part of substantia nigra fibres pass to caudate nucleus and putamen. These are dopaminergic fibres. They are distributed in a topically ordered manner (Fig. 13.23).

(d) From median raphe nucleus (pons) of brain stem fibres pass to putamen and caudate nucleus.

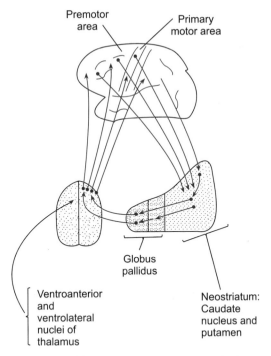

FIGURE 13.22 Feedback circuit from the cerebral cortex to the basal ganglia.

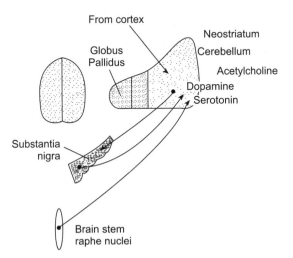

FIGURE 13.23 Interrelationship between neostriatum and substantia nigra and raphe nuclei in the brain stem.

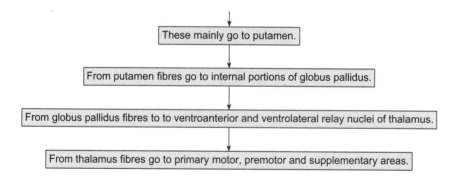

These mainly go to putamen.

| From putamen fibres go to internal portions of globus pallidus. |

| From globus pallidus fibres to to ventroanterior and ventrolateral relay nuclei of thalamus. |

| From thalamus fibres go to primary motor, premotor and supplementary areas. |

EFFERENT CONNECTIONS

From caudate nucleus and putamen fibres go to globus pallidus from where all efferent fibres arise. Efferents arise in the form of two tracts: (a) striothalamic or ansa fascicularis and (b) striosubthalamic or ansa lenticularis.

(a) *Striothalamic fibres.* They arise from internal segment of globus pallidus and go to ventroanterior and ventrolateral nuclei of thalamus from where they pass to motor cortex.

(b) *Striosubthalamic fibres.* They arise from globus pallidus and go to red nucleus, subthalamic body nuclei of reticular formation and substantia nigra.

NEURONAL CIRCUITS (Fig. 13.24)

1. *Putamen circuit.* The fibres mainly originate from premotor and supplementary motors areas of the motor cortex and primary somatosensory areas of sensory cortex.

This circuit is mainly responsible for executing learned patterns of movements, e.g. writing of letters of alphabets.

In association with primary putamen circuit there are three following circuits:

(a) From putamen → external globus pallidus → subthalamus → relay nuclei of thalamus → motor cortex.

(b) From putamen → internal globus pallidus → substantia nigra → relay nuclei of thalamus → motor cortex.

(c) From external globus pallidus → subthalamus → external globus pallidus.

Abnormalities of function of putamen circuit leads to athetosis, hemiballismus and chorea.

2. *Caudate circuit* (Fig. 13.25). From different association areas of cerebral cortex fibres pass to caudate nucleus.

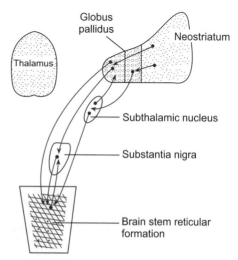

FIGURE 13.24 An older pathway involving basal ganglia.

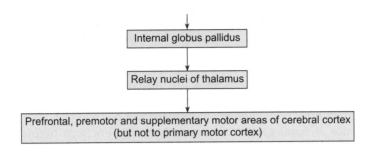

Thus returning signals only pass to accessory motor regions that are responsible for sequential pattern of movements. Caudate nucleus plays role in cognitive control of motor activity (thinking process of brain) by controlling timing and scaling of movements.

CONNECTIONS OF SUBSTANTIA NIGRA

Substantia nigra is a crescentic mass containing melanin.

Afferent connections. It receives fibres from:

- Precentral gyrus of cerebrum.
- Caudate nucleus.
- Subthalamic nucleus.

Efferent connections. (i) Globus pallidus and (ii) red nucleus.

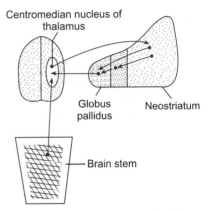

FIGURE 13.25 Pathway for transmission of signals from the basal ganglia to the brain stem reticular formation.

CONNECTIONS OF SUBTHALAMIC NUCLEUS

Subthalamic nucleus lies lateral and ventral to red nucleus. It is connected to red nucleus, substantia nigra, globus pallidus. It is a part of extrapyramidal system.

FUNCTIONS

Describe the functions of basal ganglia.

1. VOLUNTARY MOTOR ACTIVITY

In association with the corticospinal system basal ganglia control the complex pattern of voluntary motor activity.

(a) *Cognitive control of motor activity.* Most of the motor actions occur as a consequence of thoughts generated in the mind. This process is known as cognitive control of motor activity. Basal ganglia play a role because caudate nucleus extends into all lobes of cerebrum and it receives large amount of input from the association areas of the cerebral cortex. Association areas are the areas which integrate different types of sensory and motor information into thought patterns. After the signals pass from cerebral cortex to caudate nucleus, they pass to globus pallidus and then through ventroanterior and ventrolateral relay nuclei of thalamus, they return back to prefrontal, premotor and supplementary motor areas of cortex. Due to these connections basal ganglia help in cognitive control of motor activity.

(b) *Change of timing and to scale the intensity of movements.* Two important capabilities of the brain in controlling the movements are:

- To determine how rapidly it is to be performed (timing).
- To control how large the movement will be (scaling).

In absence of basal ganglia timing and scaling functions become very poor. Basal ganglia function is association with the motor cortex. In animals, basal ganglia is the highest motor co-ordination centre. In higher animals it acts as an important co-ordinating centre of extrapyramidal system.

(c) *Semiautomatic movements.* Swinging of arms while walking are carried out subconsciously at the level of basal ganglia. Crude movements of facial expression that accompany emotion are controlled by basal ganglia. Various movements like movements of limbs while swimming, control of clutch, brake while driving though in initial stage require constant attention, they are carried out subconsciously by basal ganglia as they become routine. By subconscious control of ordinary activities, basal ganglia relieve cortex from routine acts so that cortex can be free to plan its action.

Gross body movements are carried out by basal ganglia and only finer movements require assistance of motor cortex. Putamen circuit is responsible for execution of complex patterns of motor activity, e.g. writing of letters of alphabets.

2. CONTROL OF REFLEX MUSCULAR ACTIVITY

Basal ganglia exert inhibitory effect on spinal reflexes and regulate activity of muscles which maintain posture.

3. CONTROL OF MUSCLE TONE

Gamma motor neurons, muscle spindle and therefore the muscle tone are controlled by basal ganglia, especially substantia nigra. In lesion of basal ganglia, muscle tone increases.

EFFECTS OF DAMAGE*

What are the effects of the damage to the basal ganglia?

Depending upon whether facilitatory or inhibitory portion of basal ganglia is damaged, there may recur hypokinetic syndrome and hyperkinetic syndrome.

1. *Hypokinetic syndrome.* Hypokinesia is reduction in body movements, e.g. Parkinson's disease or paralysis agitans. This results from widespread damage of that portion of substantia nigra, pars compacta which sends dopamine-secreting nerve fibres to the caudate nucleus and putamen.

---

*For details refer Vaz M, Kurpad A, Raj T, editors. *Guyton & Hall Textbook of Medical Physiology.* Elsevier: New Delhi, 2013, p. 797.

Cause. Dopamine secreted in caudate nucleus and putamen is inhibitory transmitter. Therefore, destruction of substantia nigra theoretically removes the inhibition and allows these structures to become overactive and cause continuous output of excitatory signals to the corticospinal motor control system.

Disease is characterized by:

- Rigidity of most of the musculature of the body. It is lead pipe type of rigidity (when one tries to bend the limb, the resistance is offered throughout the movement).
- Tremors are involuntary, rhythmic, oscillatory movements. Tremors of Parkinson's occur in all waking hours.
- Akinesia means difficulty in initiating the movement.
- Semiautomatic movements like swinging of arms while walking are lost. Face is expressionless and is described as mask-like face.

Treatment. Drug L-dopa is effective. It is converted to dopamine in the brain and dopamine restores the normal balance between inhibition and excitation.

2. **Hyperkinetic syndrome.** It is of 3 different types: (a) chorea, (b) athetosis and (c) hemiballismus.

(a) *Chorea.* There are involuntary repetitive, short range movements of different groups of muscles. Because they are rapid, short range movements, they are like movements of dance and they are therefore known as St. Vitus' dance. The disease is also known as Huntington's chorea. It is a hereditary disorder due to loss of most of the cell bodies of GABA secreting neurons in the caudate nucleus. The axon terminals of these neurons normally cause inhibition in globus pallidus and substantia nigra. Loss of this inhibition is believed to allow spontaneous outbursts of globus pallidus and substantia nigra activity to cause distortional movements.

(b) *Athetosis.* In this there are slow worm-like movements of longer range mainly seen in upper extremity. This is due to lesion in the globus pallidus.

(c) *Hemiballismus.* In this there are sudden flailing movements of an entire limb. It is due to lesion in the subthalamus.

CEREBELLUM

STRUCTURE

Describe the structure of cerebellum.

Cerebellum is made up of two cerebellar hemispheres connected with each other by vermis (Figs 13.26, 13.27 and 13.29).

Cerebellar hemisphere has grey matter outside and white matter inside. White matter has many nuclear masses called roof nuclei. From medial to lateral side they are (Fig. 13.28):

Nucleus fastigius.
Nucleus globosus.
Nucleus emboliformis.
Nucleus dentatus.

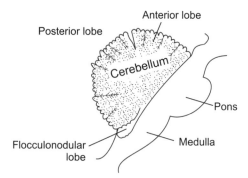

FIGURE 13.26 Anatomical lobes of the cerebellum.

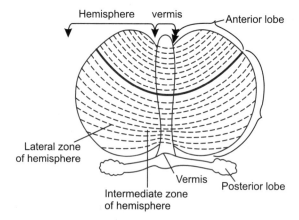

FIGURE 13.27 Functional parts of the cerebellum.

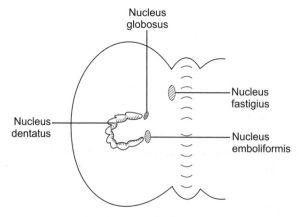

FIGURE 13.28 Cerebellar nuclei.

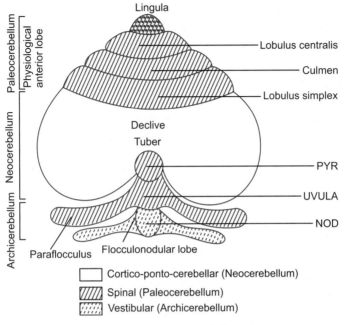

Lingula
Lobulus centralis
Culmen
Lobulus simplex
Declive
Tuber
PYR
UVULA
NOD
Paraflocculus   Flocculonodular lobe

Paleocerebellum
Physiological anterior lobe
Neocerebellum
Archicerebellum

☐ Cortico-ponto-cerebellar (Neocerebellum)
▨ Spinal (Paleocerebellum)
▨ Vestibular (Archicerebellum)

FIGURE 13.29 Primate cerebellar cortex.

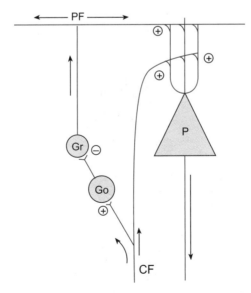

PF
⊕
⊕
⊕
P
Gr ⊖
Go
⊕
CF

FIGURE 13.30 Functional unit of cerebellum. PF = Parallel fibres, P = Purkinje cell, Gr = Granule cell, Go = Golgi cell, CF = Climbing fibre.

Why cerebellum is called silent area?

Cerebellum is called 'silent area' of the brain because electrical excitation of this structure does not cause any sensation and rarely causes motor movement.

CONNECTIONS

Describe the connections of cerebellum.

1. *Afferent connections of cerebellum.* All the afferent fibres of cerebellum except afferents from cerebral cortex, ventral spinocerebellar tract and tectocerebellar tract enter through inferior cerebellar peduncle. Inferior cerebellar peduncle therefore, is the main entrance gate of cerebellum (only fibres which find exit through it are cerebellovestibular fibres) (Fig. 13.31). Fibre groups present in inferior cerebellar peduncle are:

- *Dorsal spinocerebellar tract.* These fibres bring sensory information from muscles, joints (proprioceptors) and the skin. Through this cerebellum receives information about degree and distribution of contraction of muscles, position of limbs and posture.
- *External arcuate fibres.* These fibres carry cutaneous and deep sensations as well as impulses from capsules of the joints.
- *Reticulocerebellar fibres.* Fibres from reticular formation go to cerebellum.
- *Olivocerebellar fibres.* These fibres are from inferior olive. Inferior olive in turn receives fibres from basal ganglia and collaterals of pyramidal tract.
- *Vestibulocerebellar fibres.* These fibres come from vestibular nuclei which in turn receive information from vestibular apparatus.

Afferents passing through middle cerebellar peduncle. Pontine nuclei receive collaterals from the pyramidal tract. They in turn send the fibres to cerebellum—called

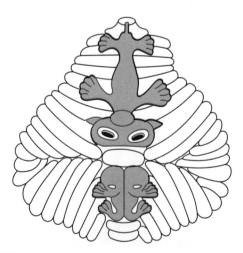

FIGURE 13.31 Sensory projection areas on the cortex of cerebellum (homunculi).

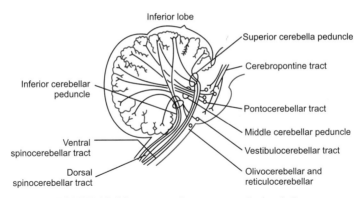

Inferior lobe

Superior cerebella peduncle

Cerebropontine tract

Inferior cerebellar peduncle

Pontocerebellar tract

Middle cerebellar peduncle

Ventral spinocerebellar tract

Vestibulocerebellar tract

Dorsal spinocerebellar tract

Olivocerebellar and reticulocerebellar

FIGURE 13.32 Principal afferent tracts to the cerebellum.

cerebro-pontocerebellar fibres which travel through middle cerebellar peduncle (Fig. 13.32).

Afferents passing through superior cerebellar peduncles. (a) Ventral spinocerebellar tract: These fibres carry impulses from muscles and joints (proprioceptors) and the skin.

(b) Tectocerebellar tract: Visual and auditory information from the cortex enters through these fibres which pass from tectum of the brain to the cerebellum.

All the afferent fibres except the fibres from inferior olive, after entering the cerebellum form connections with the granular cells. These fibres are called mossy fibres. Fibres from inferior olive after entering the cerebellum ascend upward to reach molecular layer. These are called climbing fibres. Axons of granule cells as well as climbing fibres form synapses with the dendrites of Purkinje cells. Impulses from granule cells produce subminimal excitation of Purkinje cells whereas climbing fibres can immediately activate Purkinje cells. Purkinje cells are inhibitory and they send their impulses to roof nuclei. Inhibition may be tonic (if activation is through granular cells) or momentary (if activation of Purkinje cells is through climbing fibres). Collaterals from all the fibres send facilitatory impulses to roof nuclei; impulses from Purkinje cells inhibit them. Roof nuclei in turn send efferents to control the motor activity.

Narrow band in the centre of cerebellum is called vermis. To each side of vermis there is a large, laterally protruding cerebellar hemisphere which is divided into intermediate zone (lateral to vermis) and lateral zone. As shown in Figure 13.31 there is a topographical representation of different parts of the body on vermis and intermediate zones of cerebellum. As shown in the figure there are two such representations on vermis and intermediate zone. In these representations axial portions of the body lie in the vermis parts whereas limbs and facial regions lie in intermediate zone of cerebellum. These topographical representations receive afferent signals from all the respective parts of the body as well as from the corresponding topographical motor areas in the cortex and brain stem. In turn they send motor signals to motor cortex, red nucleus and reticular formation. However, large lateral portions of cerebellar hemispheres do not have topographical representations of the body. These portions receive signals entirely and exclusively from the cerebral cortex and premotor areas of frontal cortex, somatosensory and sensory association areas of parietal cortex. These connections play an important role in planning and coordinating rapid sequential muscular activities of the body.

2. *Efferent connections of cerebellum.* All the efferent fibres except cerebellovestibular travel through superior cerebellar peduncle which is therefore called exit gate of cerebellum.

Efferents passing through superior cerebellar peduncle. (a) Efferent fibres to motor cortex (area 4): They form dentato-rubro-thalamo-cortical path. It is a multisynaptic path, synapsing at least in red nucleus and thalamus. The fibres originate from dentate nucleus which is recent in origin and most well developed in man. There is also cerebello-thalamo-cortical path having same function, i.e. controlling influence over the motor cortex.

(b) Efferents to reticular formation—Anterior horn cells are controlled by the cerebellum through reticulospinal tracts (direct fibres from cerebellum to anterior horn cells do not exist).

Efferent fibres passing through inferior cerebellar peduncle. Through this peduncle cerebellovestibular fibres pass to vestibular nuclei. These efferents control anterior horn cells of the spinal cord through vestibulo-spinal tract.

Control of cerebellum is ipsilateral (Figs 13.33 and 13.34).

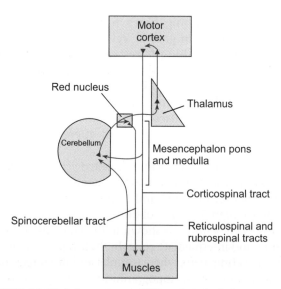

FIGURE 13.33 Pathways for cerebellar control of voluntary movements

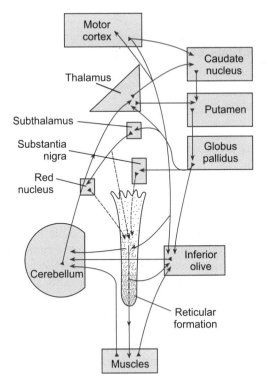

FIGURE 13.34 Pathways for cerebellar error control of voluntary movements.

STRUCTURAL UNIT

Describe the functional unit of cerebellum.

Functional unit of cerebellum is shown in Figure 13.30. There are such 30 million units in cerebellum. The output from functional unit is through deep cerebellar nuclear cells. These deep nuclear cells continuously fire action potentials at resting. Output activity of these cells can be modulated upward or downward.

Deep nuclear cells receive excitatory inputs from climbing and mossy fibres. They receive inhibitory input from Purkinje cells present in cerebellar cortex. Normally balance between these two effects is slightly in favour of excitation.

What is delay line negative feedback signal?

In execution of rapid motor movement, input signals from motor cortex or brain stem initially increase deep nuclear cells excitation. Then few milliseconds later feedback inhibitory signals from Purkinje cell circuit inhibit deep nuclear cells. Thus first there is rapid excitatory signal sent by deep nuclear cells in motor pathway followed within fraction of a millisecond by inhibitory signals. These inhibitory signals help in providing damping, i.e. they prevent muscle movement from overshooting its mark.

FUNCTIONS*

Describe the functions of cerebellum.

Cerebellum is not able to initiate any motor activity but assists the action initiated from any other region of the neural axis. Thus cerebellum controls both voluntary as well as non-voluntary motor activity (tone, posture and equilibrium).

FUNCTIONALLY CEREBELLUM IS DIVIDED INTO:
(a) Vestibulocerebellum.
(b) Spinocerebellum.
(c) Cerebrocerebellum.

FUNCTIONS OF VESTIBULOCEREBELLUM

Vestibulocerebellum mainly consists of flocculonodular lobes and adjacent parts of vermis. It controls equilibrium and postural movements in association with brain stem and spinal cord. It controls balance between agonist and antagonist muscles, muscle contractions of the spine, hips and shoulders during rapid changes in body position.

Most important problem in controlling balance during rapid movement is time required for proprioceptive information to reach the brain from different parts of the body. Even with most rapidly conducting spinocerebellar fibres (120 m per second) the time required is 15–20 milliseconds. Therefore, in rapid movements, it is not possible for return signals from brain to reach peripheral parts of the body at the same time that the movements actually occur.

Vestibulocerebellum calculates in advance the rate and direction of movement from these, Brain can know the progression of movement and do the correction for the next sequential movement within a few milliseconds.

FUNCTIONS OF SPINOCEREBELLUM

Spinocerebellum mainly consists of vermis (of anterior and posterior cerebellum) and intermediate zone on both the sides of vermis.

By feedback control of distal limb movements it does:

(a) Damping for preventing overshoot,
(b) Controlling ballistic movements.

Intermediate zone of cerebellar hemispheres receives signals from:

(a) Motor cortex, red nucleus midbrain giving information of intended sequential plan of movements through cortico-ponto-cerebellar tract.
(b) It also receives signals from periphery (especially from proprioceptors of limbs) informing cerebellum about how actual movement has occurred through dorsal and ventral spinocerebellar tracts.

---

*For details refer Vaz M, Kurpad A, Raj T, editors. *Guyton & Hall Textbook of Medical Physiology.* Elsevier: New Delhi, 2013, p. 784.

Intermediate zone compares actual movements with intended movement and sends corrective signals through interposed nucleus. These corrective signals are sent to cerebral motor areas through thalamus and magnocellular partition of red nucleus. Rubrospinal and corticospinal tracts ultimately innervate anterior horn cells of spinal cord which controls distal parts of limbs. Thus this allows motor system to provide smooth, co-ordinate movements of agonist and antagonist muscles of distal parts of limbs.

Damping function: Almost all movements of the body are pendular. Because of momentum, all pendular movements have a tendency to overshoot, this is detected by cerebrum. If cerebellum is not functional and correction is done to cause reverse movement (in opposite direction) but by momentum arm overshoots again and appropriate corrective signals are again sent. This causes oscillation back and forth across the intended point for several cycles (intention tremor occurring in cerebellar disease). If cerebellum is intact, appropriate subconscious signals stop the movements exactly at the intended point and prevent intention tremor. This is called **damping**.

Control of ballistic movements: The example of ballistic movement is movement of fingers during typing. They are so rapid that it is not possible to receive feedback signals from periphery. Entire movement is preplanned and set into motion to go specific distance and then stop. When cerebellum is damaged automatism of such ballistic movement is lost.

FUNCTIONS OF CEREBROCEREBELLUM

Cerebrocerebellum is mainly formed of lateral zones of cerebellar hemisphere. It is mainly important in planning, deciding the sequence and timing the different complex movements, i.e. for development of 'motor imagery' of movements to be performed. In human beings lateral zones are greatly enlarged. This makes human being plan and perform intricate, sequential patterns of movements.

Lateral zones of cerebellar hemispheres do not have direct input from periphery. It mainly gets information from cerebral cortical premotor area, primary and association somatosensory areas because they are concerned with planning and timing of sequential movements.

PLANNING OF SEQUENCE OF MOVEMENTS

Lateral parts of cerebellar hemisphere communicate with the premotor and sensory portion of the cerebral cortex and there is two way communications between these areas and also the areas of basal ganglia. Plan is transmitted from cerebral cortex to cerebellum and two-way traffic between two areas provides appropriate transition from one movement to the next. Thus movement progresses smoothly.

Timing function: Lateral cerebellar hemisphere also provides appropriate timing for each movement, without which succeeding movements may begin too early or too late.

Cerebellum also plays a role in predicting events, e.g. rates of progression of auditory and visual phenomena. From changing visual scene person can predict how rapidly he can approach an object.

CEREBELLAR DAMAGE*

Describe the features of cerebellar damage.

Common causes of cerebellar damage are: Thrombosis of the artery supplying cerebellum,Tumour or Injury.

When cerebellar lesions involve deeper cerebellar nuclei as well as cerebellar cortex, the following signs and symptoms are developed:

- *Dysmetria.* Because of cerebellar damage, movements ordinarily overshoot their intended mark and then conscious portion of the brain overcompensates in the opposite direction for the succeeding movements. This effect is called dysmetria.
- *Ataxia.* Ataxia is disturbance in voluntary movements.
- *Past pointing.* Due to cerebellar damage the movement goes beyond the intended point. It is a manifestation of dysmetria.
- *Failure of progression.* Control over rapid motor movements is lost. No progression of movement can occur. Person is not able to do rapid movement, e.g. rapid alternate pronation and supination of hand. This is known as dysdiadochokinesis.
- *Dysarthria.* Failure of progression of movements of laryngeal, mouth, respiratory muscles causes jumbled vocalization. This is called dysarthria.
- *Intention tremor.* Involuntary tremors occur during voluntary movements. It is due to failure of overshooting and failure of damping due to absence of cerebellar motor control.
- *Cerebellar nystagmus.* It occurs during damage to flocculonodular lobes. Tremor of eyeballs occurring at rest (when neither person nor the visual scene is moving) is called cerebellar nystagmus.
- *Rebound.* Normally cerebellum offers a feedback support to stretch reflex. Without cerebellar support strong activation of muscles fails to occur allowing over-movement of the limb in unwanted direction. This is known as rebound.
- *Hypotonia.* Damage to dentate and interpositus nucleus leads to hypotonia.

CEREBRAL CORTEX

STRUCTURE

Describe the structure of cerebral cortex.

There are two cerebral hemispheres and they are most massive in human beings. In cerebrum, outside is the grey matter (cortex) and inside the white

---

*For details refer Vaz M, Kurpad A, Raj T, editors. *Guyton & Hall Textbook of Medical Physiology.* Elsevier: New Delhi, 2013, p. 787.

matter. Each cerebral hemisphere is divided into four lobes due to three fissures (sulci):

- Central fissure or fissure of Roland
- Lateral or Sylvian sulcus
- Parieto-occipital sulcus

DIFFERENT LOBES

- *Frontal lobe.* Part of cerebral hemisphere lying in front of the central fissure.
- *Parietal lobe.* Part of cerebral hemisphere lying between central fissure and parieto-occipital sulcus.
- *Occipital lobe.* Part behind the parieto-occipital sulcus.
- *Temporal lobe.* Part below the Sylvian sulcus.

Functionally. Occipital lobe serves the functions of vision. Temporal lobe serves auditory functions. The parietal lobe has cutaneous, deep and gustatory sensory functions whereas frontal lobe has the motor function. The part in front of motor region of the frontal lobe has large number of neurons which participate in the process of interpretation of information. Intelligence and personality depend on the development of this part of frontal lobe which is called prefrontal lobe.

Cerebral cortex is 2-4 mm thick and under microscope is divisible into six different layers as follows:

- *Molecular layer.* Outermost layer is made up mainly of nerve fibres (dendrites and axons of lower layers) and a few nerve cells.
- *External granular layer.*
- *External pyramidal layer.*
- *Internal granular layer.*
- *Internal pyramidal layer.*
- *Polymorphic layer.* It is the innermost layer formed of neurons of different sizes and shapes.

Most incoming specific sensory signals terminate in layer IV. Most of the output signals leave cortex from layer V and VI. Layers I, II and III perform most of the intracortical association functions with a large number of neurons especially in layers II and III making horizontal connections with the adjacent cortical areas.

All these 6 layers are not found everywhere in the cortex. Cerebral cortex is divided into allocortex, mesocortex and neocortex. Only neocortex has 6 layers.

Cerebral cortex is divided into 50 different areas known as Brodmann areas based on histological structural differences (Fig. 13.35).

In the frontal lobe. In front of central fissure there is primary motor area (area 4); anterior to it is the premotor area (area 6); anterior to area 6 is area 8 or frontal eye field. Inferior to it, is area 44 (Broca's area for speech) 45, 46, 47. Anterior to area 6 are areas 8, 9, 10 (most anterior).

In the parietal lobe. Just behind the central fissure, there are somatic sensory Brodmann areas 1, 2, 3, 5, 7 and 40.

In the temporal lobe. In superior temporal gyrus are auditory areas 41, 42. Inferior to areas 41, 42 there are areas 22, 21 and 20.

In the occipital lobe. There are areas 17, 18, 19—primary and association visual areas.

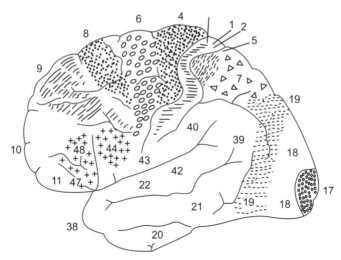

FIGURE 13.35 Different areas on the lateral surface of the human cerebral cortex.

CONTROL OF VOLUNTARY MOVEMENTS

Describe the initiation and control of voluntary movement.

Motor control system is a highly complex system and is a highly integrated network in which all parts work together to produce a movement as follows:

1. Idea of a movement is generated within the cortical association area of the parietal lobe.
2. Idea is transferred to the motor areas of frontal lobe when it is organized into a motor command.
3. The command is sent to the spinal cord for execution of the movement and coordinated movement is produced by modifying the motor command as follows:
   - Basal ganglia provide the motor patterns necessary to maintain the postural support required for motor commands to be carried out properly.
   - The cerebellum receives information from the motor cortex about the nature of intended movement and from the spinal cord about how well it is performed.
   - This information is used to adjust the motor command so that the intended movement is executed smoothly.
   - The brain stem is the major relay station for all motor commands (except those requiring greatest precision which are transformed directly to the spinal cord).

The brain stem is also responsible for maintaining normal body posture during the motor activity.

   - The spinal cord contains the final common pathway through which movement is executed. By selecting the proper motor neurons for a particular task and by reflexly adjusting the amount of motor neuron activity, the spinal cord plays an important role in the co-ordination of motor activity.

FRONTAL LOBE

CONNECTIONS AND FUNCTIONS

Describe the connections and functions of frontal lobe.

Frontal lobe extends from frontal pole to the central sulcus and below it is limited by lateral sulcus. It forms one-third of the cortical surface.

It is subdivided into two main areas—precentral cortex and prefrontal cortex.

1. PRECENTRAL CORTEX

It is the posterior part of frontal lobe and includes lip of central sulcus, precentral gyrus, and posterior part of superior, middle and inferior frontal gyri. Stimulation of different points in this area causes activity of discrete skeletal muscle. It is therefore called the excitomotor area of cortex.

It has following important areas:

(a) *Primary motor area (area 4).* It extends over precentral gyrus and the adjoining anterior wall and lip of central sulcus. It also extends over the medial surface of the hemisphere. This area contains all the six layers of cortex. Special feature of this area is the presence of giant pyramidal cells called Betz cells, in ganglionic layer.

Function. This area is a centre for volition. There is topographic representation of different muscles of the opposite side of the body in this area. Face and mouth regions are represented near Sylvian fissure, arm and head areas in the mid portion, and trunk near the apex of the brain. Leg and foot areas are represented in area which dips into the longitudinal fissure. Thus body is represented upside down (however face is not represented in inverted manner). Degree of representation of different muscles is different. Major part of the area controls muscles of hands and speech.

Electrical stimulation of this area causes discrete isolated movements on the opposite side of the body.

Area 4S. It forms a narrow strip anterior to area 4 and is called the suppressor area. It inhibits movements initiated by area 4.

(b) *Premotor area.* It lies anterior to primary motor area and has areas 6, 8, 44 and 45. It has all the six layers of cortex but no Betz cells unlike that in primary motor cortex.

Area 6. It lies anterior to area 4 and is divided into two parts, upper 6a and lower 6b. Topographical organization of this area is roughly the same as that of primary cortex. Cells from this area contribute fibres to pyramidal tract.

Nerve signals from premotor area cause pattern of movements involving group of muscles to do a particular task. Premotor area sends signals to primary motor area to excite multiple group of muscles, by way of basal ganglia and back through the thalamus to primary motor area.

Area 8. It is termed frontal eye field and lies anterior to area 6. It is concerned with eye movements. It receives afferents from occipital lobe and dorsomedial nucleus of thalamus and sends efferents to nuclei of third fourth and sixth cranial nerves.

Stimulation of this area causes conjugate movements of eyes to opposite side, opening and closing of eyelids, lacrimation and pupillary dilatation.

Area 44 or Broca's area. It lies immediately anterior to primary motor cortex and immediately above the Sylvian fissure. This area (especially in dominant hemisphere) causes activation of vocal cords, simultaneously with movements of mouth and tongue during speech. Damage to this area causes motor aphasia, i.e. inability to speak the word though vocalization is possible.

Area of hand skill. In premotor area anterior to primary motor cortex for hands and fingers, is a region called area for hand skills. When this area is damaged, hand movements become incoordinated and non-purposeful (motor apraxia).

(c) *Supplementary motor area.* It lies immediately anterior and superior to premotor area, mainly in longitudinal fissure. This area also has topographical organization for control of motor functions, with leg area lying most posteriorly and faces area most anteriorly. Stronger electrical stimulation of this area is required to cause muscle contraction as compared to other areas, but these contractions are often bilateral, e.g. bilateral grasping movements of both hands simultaneously. This area in association with premotor area provides attitudinal movements, fixation movements of different segments of the body, and positional movements of head, eyes, etc.

CONNECTIONS OF PRECENTRAL CORTEX

Afferents. (a) Fibres from adjacent regions as follows:
- Somatic sensory area of parietal cortex.
- Adjacent areas of frontal cortex anterior to the motor cortex.
- Subcortical fibres from auditory and visual cortices.

(b) Subcortical fibres passing through corpus callosum connect corresponding areas of cortices in the two sides of brain.

(c) Somatic sensory fibres directly from ventrobasal complex of thalamus bringing cutaneous, tactile, joint and muscle signals.

(d) Tracts from ventrolateral and ventroanterior nuclei of thalamus which inturn receive from cerebellum and basal ganglia. They cause co-ordination between functions of motor cortex, basal ganglia and cerebellum.

(e) Fibres from intralaminar nuclei of thalamus to cause general level of excitability of motor cortex.

Efferents. (a) Corticospinal tract (pyramidal tract) is the most important efferent pathway. 30% of fibres arise from primary motor area, 30% from premotor and supplementary motor area (40% from somatic sensory area).

(b) Large number of fibres from motor cortex or collaterals from pyramidal tract go to deeper regions of cerebrum and brain stem as follows:
- Axons of Betz cells send collaterals to adjacent areas of cortex. These collaterals inhibit adjacent areas (lateral inhibition) and sharpen the boundaries of excitatory signals.
- Large number of fibres goes to caudate nucleus and putamen from where additional pathway goes to brain stem.
- Some fibres go to red nuclei and then to spinal cord through rubrospinal tracts.

- Some fibres go to reticular substance and vestibular nuclei of brain stem. From here fibres pass to spinal cord through reticulospinal and vestibulospinal tracts. They also go to cerebellum through reticulocerebellar and vestibulocerebellar fibres.
- Large number of fibres synapses in pontine nuclei and pass to cerebellum (pontocerebellar fibres).
- Collaterals also go to inferior olivary nucleus and then to cerebellum through olivocerebellar tract.

2. PREFRONTAL CORTEX (ORBITOFRONTAL CORTEX)

It is the part of frontal lobe lying anterior to areas 8 and 44, and is known as prefrontal lobe. It includes orbital gyri, medial frontal gyrus and areas 32. Prefrontal cortex has different Brodmann's areas such as 9, 10, 11, 12, 13, 14, 23, 24, 29 and 32 (Figs 13.36 and 13.37).

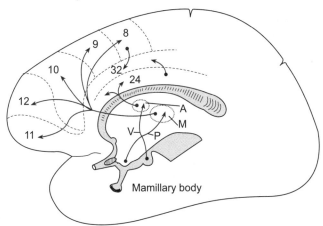

FIGURE 13.36 Afferent connections to prefrontal cortex. A = Anterior nucleus of thalamus, M = Medial (dorsomedial) nucleus of thalamus, V = Mamillothalamic tract, P = Fibres from hypothalamus to 'M'.

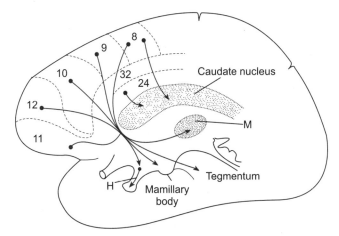

FIGURE 13.37 Efferent connections of prefrontal lobes. H = Tract from pituitary hypothalamus to posterior, M = Medial (dorsomedial) nucleus of thalamus.

CONNECTIONS OF PREFRONTAL CORTEX

Afferents.   (i) Anterior nuclei of thalamus to cingulate gyrus (areas 23, 24, 29, 32).
(ii) Medial dorsal nucleus of thalamus to areas 9, 10, 11, 12.
Efferents.   (i) From areas 9, 10 to ventral and medial dorsal nuclei of thalamus.
(ii) From areas 9, 10 to reticular formation in the tegmentum.
(iii) From area 10 to pontine nuclei.
(iv) From area 24 to caudate nucleus.
(v) From hippocampal region to mamillary body of hypothalamus.

Functions of prefrontal cortex. (a) It is the centre for planned actions—prefrontal association areas in close association with motor cortex plan complex patterns and sequence of motor movement. Through fibres from parieto-occipitotemporal association areas, it receives preanalyzed sensory information which is necessary for planning. Output from prefrontal area to motor cortex passes through caudate nucleus-thalamus circuit. It provides sequential components of motor movements.

(b) It allows the person to concentrate on central theme of thought. It helps in depth and abstractness of thought and thereby in elaboration of thought.

(c) Short-term memories are registered here. Prefrontal cortex can keep track of many bits of information and also has ability to recall this information bit by bit for subsequent thoughts. It is therefore called a seat of intelligence or an organ of mind.

(d) It is a centre for higher functions like learning, emotions, memories and social behaviour. It is responsible for various autonomic changes during emotional condition because of its connections to hypothalamus and brain stem.

It has the following intellectual abilities to:

- Prognosticate.
- Plan the future.
- Delay action in response to incoming sensory signals so that sensory information can be weighed until the best response is obtained.
- Consider the consequences of motor actions before their performance.
- Solve complicated mathematical, legal and philosophical problems.
- Correlate avenues of informations in diagnosis of rare diseases.
- Control one's activity according to the moral laws.

Describe the functions of parietal lobe.

Major areas present in parietal lobe and their functions are:

1. *Primary sensory area (Areas 3, 1 and 2).* This is the highest area of general conscious sensations. It receives from thalamus the fibres conveying impulses from spinothalamic tracts (touch, pain and temperature), lemniscal system (muscle and joint proprioceptors). In the most anterior of postcentral gyrus located deep in Sylvian fissure there is Brodmann area 3a responding to muscle, tendon,

joint, stretch receptors. Many signals from this area spread directly to the motor cortex and help in control of muscle function. Somatic sensory area 1 is responsible for:

- Localizing different sensations in different parts of the body.
- Judging critical degrees of pressure against the body.
- Judging exact weights of objects.
- Judging shapes or forms of object.
- Judging texture of the material.

Appreciation of size, shape, texture and weight of the object is called stereognosis. Lesion in this area leads to disturbances in localizing and discriminating tactile stimulus. It leads to astereognosis, loss of spatial recognition, appreciation of relative intensities of different stimuli.

Inferior part of postcentral gyrus contains centre for taste and general sensations from tongue. Lesion of this part causes loss of taste and general sensations of opposite half of the tongue.

2. *Sensory association area (areas 5 and 7).* This area lies behind the somatic sensory area 1. It receives signals from somatic sensory area 1, ventromedial nuclei of the thalamus, other areas of thalamus, visual and auditory cortex. This area gives the person the ability to recognize complex objects and complex forms by the process of feeling them. Because it receives information from various sensory cortical areas, it gives an idea of the state of the body as a whole, so that the individual develops body image on which he develops motive which is the basis of subsequent action. Damage of these areas produces a sensory deficit called 'amorphosynthesis' in which condition the person neglects about one-half of the body and therefore cannot perform complicated motor acts satisfactorily.

OCCIPITAL LOBE

CONNECTIONS AND FUNCTIONS

Describe the connections and functions of occipital lobe.

Occipital lobe is mostly formed of sensory and association area and has only a slight motor function.
It contains visual cortex having three areas:

- Primary visual cortex (area 17).
- Visual association area (area 18).
- Visual association area or occipital eye field (area 19).

Area 17 is situated at posterior pole and calcarine fissure of occipital lobe. It receives afferents from lateral geniculate body. It functions as a cortical visual centre. It is concerned with perception of visual impulses.

Area 18 lies on the convexity just above area 17. It receives afferents from area 17. It is concerned with the interpretation of visual information. The exact meaning of visual image is interpreted and integrated here, e.g. meaning of written language. Lesion in this area causes inability of a person to interpret the meaning of what is seen or read.

Area 19 is situated just above area 18 and receives afferents from area 17 and pulvinar.

TEMPORAL LOBE

CONNECTIONS AND FUNCTIONS

Describe the connections and functions of temporal lobe.

Temporal lobe mainly has sensory and association areas as follows:

1. *Areas 41 and 42.* These are primary auditory areas situated in anterior transverse gyrus and lateral surface of superior temporal gyrus.

They receive auditory fibres from medial geniculate body and pulvinar of thalamus. The basal turn of cochlea is represented anteriorly and the apical turn posteriorly.

It is a centre for hearing. Here pitch and intensity of the sound are perceived.

2. *Area 22.* It is audiopsychic area or association area situated in superior temporal gyrus. It is responsible for interpreting the meaning of what is heard.

3. *Areas 21 and 20.* They are situated in the middle and the inferior temporal gyri respectively. These are auditory association areas. They receive impulses from primary area and are responsible for analysis, interpretation and integration of auditory impulses.

DOMINANT HEMISPHERE

What is dominant hemisphere?

The general interpretative functions of Wernicke's area and the angular gyrus, and also the functions of speech and motor control areas are usually much more highly developed in one cerebral hemisphere than in the other. This hemisphere is called the 'dominant hemisphere'. In about 95% of the people, left hemisphere is the dominant one. The dominance is primarily for language or verbal symbolism-related intellectual function; the opposite hemisphere is dominant for some other types of intelligence.

What is Wernicke's area? What is its function?

Wernicke's area is the sensory area of the dominant hemisphere for interpretation of language and is closely associated with primary and secondary auditory areas of temporal lobe.

Because of this close association, the first introduction to language is by way of hearing. If this area in the dominant hemisphere is destroyed, the person loses almost all intellectual functions associated with language or verbal symbolism, such as ability to read, ability to perform mathematical operations and even the ability to think through logical problems.

HIGHER FUNCTIONS

SPEECH

What is speech?

Speech is a symbol through which human beings communicate with each other. It is restricted to man alone. Physiologically there are two forms of speech:

- Spoken words.
- Written words.
- There are two aspects to communication: (i) sensory aspect involving ears and eyes and (ii) motor aspect involving vocalization and its control.

Describe the sensory aspect of communication.

Visual and auditory association areas of the cortex are responsible for the ability to understand the written word or spoken word. Sensory, visual, auditory association areas, all meet one another in the posterior part of the superior temporal lobe, where parietal, occipital and temporal lobes come together. This area of confluence of the different sensory interpretation areas is especially highly developed in the dominant hemisphere and plays important role in the brain function called 'intelligence'. It is known as Wernicke's area and is responsible for interpretation of the complicated meanings of different sensory experiences (meanings of what is heard or read). Stimulation of this area causes a highly complex thought, e.g. complicated visual scene seen in childhood, auditory hallucination such as of a musical piece. This means that activation of Wernicke's area can call forth complicated memory patterns involving more than one sensory modality and many of the memory patterns are stored here. Wernicke's area lies near the auditory areas but the angular gyrus lies between visual area and the Wernicke's area. If this is destroyed, the person is able to see the words and even know they are words but is not able to interpret their meanings. This condition is called word blindness. However, the person can still interpret the auditory experience (what is heard) as usual.

When a person hears a particular word, impulses go to primary auditory area and association auditory area. From this, information goes to Wernicke's area which interprets and understands the word, and then sends impulses to Broca's area for speaking the word that is heard. When a person reads a certain word, information first goes to areas 18, 19 (visual areas), then from here to angular gyrus and from here to Wernicke's area for interpretation of word that is read. If this word is to be spoken, impulses go to Broca's area.

Destruction of Wernicke's area, therefore, results into sensory aphasia (aphasia means defective speech). In this condition, the person fails to interpret the complicated meaning of different sensory experiences.

Describe the motor aspect of communication.

Broca's area in the dominant hemisphere is responsible for activation of vocal cords simultaneously with the movements of mouth and tongue during speech and is therefore responsible for motor aspect of speech.

Broca's area is responsible for formation of words by exciting laryngeal respiratory muscles and muscles of mouth simultaneously. Normally, when a person hears or reads the word it goes from auditory or visual cortex respectively to Wernicke's area which decides what is to be expressed aloud, then from Wernicke's area the impulses go to Broca's areas and then to area 4 to cause expression of thought into accepted symbols (spoken/written words). The speech involves: (i) formation in mind the thoughts to be expressed and choice of words to be used and (ii) motor control of vocalization itself.

Formation of thought and choices of words is the function of sensory areas of the brain (Wernicke's area).

Motor control of vocalization is controlled by Broca's area (control of word formation) and then signals from here are transmitted to motor cortex to control speech muscles.

Damage to Broca's area causes motor aphasia. The person is capable of deciding what he wishes to say but he cannot make his vocal system emit words though it is capable of producing noises.

LEARNING

What is learning? Explain the different forms of learning.

Learning is ability to alter behaviour on the basis of experience. There are two forms of learning:

1. *Non-associative learning.* It is learning about a single stimulus. It is of two types:

Habituation. It occurs when a neutral stimulus is repeatedly applied. When the stimulus is applied for the first time it is novel and evokes reaction. This response is called orientation reflex or 'what is it' response. Lesser and lesser response is evoked on repeated stimulation. Eventually the subject totally ignores the stimulus and thus gets habituated to it.

Sensitization. It is opposite to habituation. In this repeated stimulation produces greater and greater response if it is coupled one or more times with an unpleasant or pleasant stimulus. The mother who sleeps through many kinds of noise but wakes promptly when her baby cries is an example.

2. *Associative learning.* It involves learning about relations between two or more stimuli at a time. There are two types of conditioning:

(a) *Classical conditioned reflex.* It was studied by Pavlov. A conditioned reflex is a reflex response to stimulus that previously elicited little or no response, acquired by repeatedly pairing the stimulus with another stimulus that normally does produce the response. In Pavlov's experiment, placing meat in the mouth of dog for causing salivation was used as an unconditioned stimulus (US). A bell was rung just before meat was placed in dog's mouth and this was repeated a number of times. Ringing of bell acted as a conditioned stimulus (CS). After CS and US were paired for sufficient number of times CS produced response, i.e. salivation originally evoked by US. This way a large number of somatic, visceral and other neural changes can be made to occur as conditioned reflexes. Conditioning of visceral response is known as biofeedback.

(b) *Operant conditioning*. It is a form of conditioning in which animal is taught to perform some task (operate on the environment) in order to obtain a reward or to avoid punishment. The US is a pleasant or an unpleasant event and CS is a light or some other signal that alerts the animal to perform the task. Conditioned motor responses that permit an animal to avoid unpleasant event are called conditioned avoidance reflxes, e.g. an animal is taught that by pressing a bar it can prevent an electric shock to the feet. Similar responses also occur in human beings. These are very strong and sometimes can be learned with a single pairing of the CS and the US.

Any process, learned by one cerebral hemisphere is transferred to the other through corpus callosum.

CONDITIONED REFLEX

What is conditioned reflex?

Conditioned reflex is the one which develops after the birth. This is a form of learning. There are different forms of conditioning:

- *Type I*. In this conditioning, stimulus is followed by unconditioned stimulus, e.g. in classical Pavlov's experiment, ringing of bell (conditioning stimulus) is followed by food (unconditioned stimulus).
- *Type II* (Instrumental conditioning). Where subject has control over the stimulus, e.g. if electrode is placed in reward area, animal repeatedly presses the bar. It is conditioned to press the bar whenever it sees it. Here the animal has control over the stimulus.

What is the importance of conditioned reflex?

Conditioned reflexes are important in the processes of learning and behaviour. Some psychiatric disorders are related to conditioned reflex.

Describe the characteristic features of conditioned reflex.

1. For developing a conditioned reflex, animal must be alert and in good health.
2. The conditioned stimulus must begin to operate before the unconditioned stimulus is applied, e.g. bell must begin to sound before any food is put into the mouth. The conditioned stimulus should be allowed to continue to act so as to overlap the unconditioned stimulus, e.g. bell continues to ring while the animal is being fed.
3. Any suitable stimulus, if suitably employed may become a conditioned stimulus.
4. For a conditioned stimulus to retain the new properties, it is essential that it should be followed by unconditioned stimulus, i.e. ringing of bell must be followed by giving food. The process of following up a conditioned stimulus with the basic unconditioned stimulus is termed reinforcement.

5. If after establishing the conditioned reflex, conditioned stimulus is carried out several times without unconditioned stimulus, conditioned reflex no more occurs, e.g. if ringing of bell is carried out several times and is not followed by placing of food, it soon ceases to elicit salivary flow, i.e. conditioned reflex is abolished.

MEMORY

What is memory?

Memory is the ability to recall past events at the conscious or unconscious level. The ability of human brain to store and retrieve memories is perhaps the most important ability:

Memory stores include:

1. Vocabulary.
2. Knowledge of language.
3. All facts which person learns.
4. All people known.
5. All skills which one learns.
6. On playing, e.g. walking, talking, swimming, etc.

Brain stores all this diverse information so that it can be easily assessed and used.

How do you classify memory?

Memory is classified as:

(i) *Short-term memory.* It includes memories that last for seconds or at the most minutes unless they are converted to long-term memories.

(ii) *Intermediate long-term memory.* It lasts for days to weeks but eventually is lost.

(iii) *Long-term memory.* Once stored this type of memory can be recalled up to years or even a life time long.

What is the mechanism of short-term memory?

Short-term memory lasts for a few seconds, e.g. memory up to 7-10 digits telephone numbers. Memory only lasts as long as the person continues to think about the numbers.

Suggested mechanisms of short-term memory:

1. *Continual neuronal activity.* This is due to travelling of signal through a circuit of reverberating neurons.

2. *Presynaptic facilitation or inhibition.* This occurs in the synapses that lie on the presynaptic terminals and not in the subsequent neuron. This causes prolonged facilitation or inhibition for as long as few seconds to a minute.

3. *Synaptic potentiation.* When train of impulses passes along the presynaptic terminal, the amount of calcium ions in presynaptic terminal increases with each impulse. When it becomes greater, there is prolonged release of neurotransmitter at the synapse.

What is the neural mechanism of intermediate long-term memory?

Intermediate long-term memory lasts for many minutes to many weeks. This results from temporary physical or chemical changes or both at the presynaptic terminal.

1. One terminal is from primary input sensory neuron and terminates on the surface of the neuron that is to be stimulated. This is called sensory terminal. The other terminal lies on the sensory terminal and is called facilitator terminal. Changes occur as follows:
   - Stimulation of facilitator neuron at the same time so that the sensory neuron is stimulated. It causes serotonin release at the facilitator synapse on sensory presynaptic terminals.
   - Serotonin acts on the receptors present in the sensory terminal surface and activates adenyl cyclase which causes formation of cyclic AMP.
   - Cyclic AMP activates protein kinase which causes phosphorylation of a protein that is the part of potassium channels. This blocks the channel and the blockage can last for a few minutes to a few weeks.
   - Blockage of potassium channels prolongs the action potential which causes activation of calcium channels. Large quantities of calcium enter the sensory terminal causing greater release of transmitter which greatly facilitates synaptic transmission. Thus when sensory neuron and facilitator neuron are simultaneously stimulated, facilitator neuron causes prolonged change in sensory terminal that produces memory trace.
2. Second suggested mechanism for intermediate long-term memory: Stimuli from two separate sources acting on a single sensory neuron can cause long-term changes in the membrane properties of the entire postsynaptic neuron under appropriate conditions.

What is the mechanism for long-term memory?

Long-term memory is due to actual structural changes at the synapse that enhance or suppress signal conduction. There is no real demarcation between prolonged type of intermediate long-term memory and long-term memory.

Suggested mechanism for long-term memory:

1. There is increase in total area of the vesicular release site in the presynaptic terminal during development of long-term memory traces. Increase in vesicular site starts within hours after initiating the training session.
2. There is also increase in the number of transmitter vesicles in the presynaptic terminal.

In addition, there is also increase in number of terminals themselves, i.e. the number of synapses increases. These effects facilitate transmission of signals which is the basis of learning. It is also possible that there is change in the number of neurons in the used circuits. For short-term memory to be converted into either intermediate long-term or long-term memory it must become consolidated, i.e. memory must in some way initiate the chemical, physical and anatomical changes in the synapses that are responsible for the long-term type of memory. This process requires 5 to 10 minutes for minimum consolidation and an hour or more for maximal consolidation. This occurs due to phenomenon of rehearsal, i.e. rehearsal of the same information again and again.

MEMORIES PLACED INTO LONGER-TERM

Memory storehouses are codified into different classes of information. During this process, similar information is recalled from the memory storage bins and is used to help the process of new information. The new and old are compared for similarities and differences. Thus during the process of consolidation, the new memories are not stored randomly in the brain but are stored in direct association with other memories of the same type.

Hippocampus is one of the important output pathways of reward and punishment areas of limbic system. All these reward and punishment signals together provide the background mood and motivation of the person. Among these is the drive in the brain to remember either pleasant or unpleasant. The hippocampus is one of the important sites for storage of long-term memory.

Wernicke's area which is a major locus of intellectual operations also helps in memory storage. It helps in analysis of memory so that it can be stored in association with similar old memories.

What is retrograde amnesia?

Inability to recall memories from the past is known as retrograde amnesia. Amnesia is much greater for recent events rather than for events of distant past. Memories of distant past are rehearsed so many times that the memory traces are deeply engrained and elements of these memories are stored in the widespread areas of the brain.

What is anterograde amnesia?

Inability of the person to establish new long-term memories of those types of information that are basis of intelligence is called anterograde amnesia. This occurs on removal of hippocampus.

EEG

What is electroencephalogram? How is it recorded?

Recording of electrical potentials from the surface of the brain is known as electroencephalogram. It is recorded by placing electrodes on the outer surface of the head.

Name the different types of waves recorded in EEG.

The intensities of brain waves recorded from the scalp vary from 0 to 200 μV and their frequencies range from 50 or more cycles per second. Much of the time brain waves are irregular and no general pattern is obtained. At other times distinct patterns do appear. Character of the waves depends on the degree of activity of cerebral cortex.

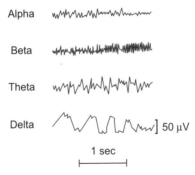

FIGURE 13.38 Different types of normal EEG waves.

Different waves recorded in a normal person are classified as alpha, beta, theta and delta waves (Fig. 13.38).

1. *Alpha waves.* These are rhythmic waves with frequency of 8-13 cycles/s. They are recorded from normal adult person when they are awake in quiet resting state of cerebrum. These waves occur intensely in occipital region, but can be recorded also from parietal and frontal regions.

Voltage of alpha waves is 50 µV. During sleep, alpha waves disappear. They also disappear when person is awake and his attention is directed to some specific type of mental activity. In such condition alpha waves are replaced by asynchronous, higher frequency but lower voltage beta waves. Merely by opening the eyes, alpha waves disappear because visual sensation causes replacement of alpha waves by beta waves. Alpha waves result from spontaneous activity of non-specific thalamocortical system.

2. *Beta waves.* They have frequency of more than 14 cycles/second to 80 cycles/second. They are frequently recorded from the parietal and frontal region during activation of CNS or during tension.

3. *Theta wave.* These waves have a frequency of 4 to 7 cycles/second and are recorded during emotional stress, disappointment and frustration. They are mainly seen in brain disorders.

4. *Delta waves.* They include all the waves in EEG below 3.5 cycles/ second. They occur in deep sleep, in infancy and in serious organic brain damage. They occur strictly in the cortex independent of activities in lower regions of the brain, therefore they occur in sleep when cortex is released from the activating influence of lower centres.

SLEEP

What is sleep? What are the types of sleep?

Sleep is defined as unconsciousness from which the person can be aroused by sensory or other stimuli. There are multiple stages of sleep such as light sleep, deep sleep, etc.

There are two types of sleep:

1. *Slow wave sleep (SWS).* In this type of sleep, brain waves are very slow.

2. *Rapid eye movement or REM sleep.* During this type of sleep, eyes undergo rapid movements despite of the fact that the person is still asleep.

Describe the sleep cycle.

There is an orderly progression of sleep stages and states during a typical sleep period. When an individual falls asleep, the light stage of SWS sleep is entered first. During next hour or so the person passes progressively in deeper stages of sleep until deep sleep is reached. After about 15 minutes of deep sleep, depth of sleep starts decreasing and continues to do so until the person re-enters the light stage of sleep about 90 minutes after the start of the first sleep cycle. At this point, individual passes from SWS to REM sleep. This cycle repeats itself about 5 times during night. After the second cycle, the intervals between periods of REM sleep become shorter and the duration of each of period of REM sleep becomes longer. As morning approaches, an individual spends less time in the deeper stages of SWS and periodically awakens. This sleep cycle is typical of adult.

During infancy, about 16 hours of every day are spent asleep. This decreases to 10 hours during childhood and 7 hours during adulthood. In elderly people sleep becomes 6 hours/day.

Prematurely born infants spend 80% of their time in REM sleep. In full-term infants REM sleep is 50%. Total time of REM sleep is reduced to 1.5 to 2 hours by puberty and remains unchanged thereafter.

Describe slow wave sleep (SWS).

Slow wave sleep is a restful type sleep which a person experiences during first hour of sleep after having been kept awake for many hours. Slow wave sleep progresses in an orderly way from light to deep sleep. Light sleep is characterized by EEG which shows high-amplitude waves of 12 to 15 cycles/second called spindles which periodically interrupt alpha rhythm.

During moderate sleep, the EEG displays slower and larger theta waves. The deepest stage of SWS produces EEG pattern of very slow waves 4 to 7 cycles/second and large waves which are called delta waves. Usually it is dreamless sleep.

SWS is characterized by progressive reduction in consciousness and an increasing resistance to being awakened. Muscle tone is reduced. Heart and respiratory rates are decreased. Body metabolism is lowered (Fig. 13.39).

Describe rapid eye movement (REM) sleep.

This is the state of sleep characterized by rapid eye movements and therefore is known as rapid eye movement sleep. It is also called dream sleep because dreaming occurs during REM sleep. During this state, EEG shows fast waves with high frequency and low amplitude (like waking state) though person is unresponsive to environmental stimuli and thus is asleep. Therefore, it is also called paradoxical sleep or desynchronized sleep. Eyes are not the only organs active during this sleep. The middle ear muscles are active, penile erection occurs, heart

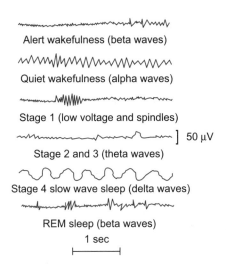

Alert wakefulness (beta waves)

Quiet wakefulness (alpha waves)

Stage 1 (low voltage and spindles)

] 50 μV

Stage 2 and 3 (theta waves)

Stage 4 slow wave sleep (delta waves)

REM sleep (beta waves)

1 sec

FIGURE 13.39 Progressive changes in brain waves during different stages of sleep and wakefulness.

rate and respiration becomes irregular and there are occasional twitches of limb musculature. Muscle tone is tremendously reduced so the frequency and intensity of muscle twitching does not produce injuries or does not make the person awake (Fig. 13.39).

How is the waking state maintained?

Waking state is maintained by signals from reticular activating system to the cortex.

What is the mechanism of sleep?

Mechanism of sleep is not very clear and has been explained by several theories:

1. *Passive theory of sleep.* It was thought earlier that excitatory areas of reticular activating system send signals to cortex and are responsible for waking state. Fatigue of reticular activating system makes it inactive, and causes sleep. This is the passive theory of sleep.

2. *Active theory of sleep.* Some centres located in mid pons actively cause sleep by inhibiting other parts of the brain.

3. *Stimulation of raphe nuclei in the lower half of the pons and in the medulla causes sleep.* Nerve fibres from these nuclei are spread widely in the reticular formation, upward into the thalamus, neocortex, hypothalamus and most of the areas of limbic system. Fibres also run downwards in the spinal cord terminating on posterior horn cells to inhibit incoming pain signals. Most of these endings secrete serotonin which is probably the major neurotransmitter associated with production of sleep. Excitation of raphe nuclei stimulates some areas in nucleus tractus solitarius for promoting sleep through serotonergic system (stimulation of certain areas of tractus solitarius also produces sleep). Stimulation of several regions in the

diencephalon, e.g. suprachiasmatic nucleus of the hypothalamus, diffuse nuclei of thalamus also produces sleep. Discrete lesions of raphe nucleus produces a state of wakefulness.

Other possible transmitters related to sleep are muramyl peptide and non-apeptide which accumulate in blood and CSF when animal is kept awake for several days. When they are injected in the third ventricle, they cause sleep. Therefore, it is possible that prolonged wakefulness causes progressive accumulation of a sleep factor in the brain.

What is the mechanism of REM sleep?

Large acetylcholine secreting neurons in the upper brain stem reticular formation through their extensive fibres activate many portions of brain and are responsible for the development of REM sleep.

CSF

Describe the formation, circulation and absorption of cerebrospinal fluid (CSF).

Formation. Cerebrospinal fluid is mainly formed in the choroid plexuses of lateral and to some extent third ventricles of the brain. It is formed by processes of filtration and secretion (because it is not merely an ultrafiltrate of plasma).

Circulation. CSF formed in lateral ventricle through foramen of Monro enters the third ventricle, then from here it passes through aqueduct of Sylvius to the fourth ventricle.

CSF passes then to the foramina of Luschka and Magendie and occupies the subarachnoid space and is distributed all over the brain. Small amount also enters the central canal of the spinal cord.

Absorption. Arachnoid villi of the sagittal sinus project from arachnoid mater. These villi come in contact with the venous blood of sagittal sinus. Pressure within the sinuses is low, colloid osmotic pressure of venous blood is high whereas that in the CSF is low. All these factors help to transfer CSF into the venous blood.

How is CSF collected?

In some diseases examination of CSF is diagnostic. It is collected by putting needle between 3rd and 4th lumbar spinous processes into the subarachnoid space within the vertebral canal. There is no risk of damaging the spinal cord as it ends at the level of first lumbar vertebra.

What are the functions of CSF?

1. Covers the brain from inside as well as outside and acts as a cushion. If there is any injury to head, because of presence of CSF, the impact

of injury is distributed all over the brain and thus no single area of the brain has to bear high degree of impact. Thus damage to the brain is prevented.

2. If there is brain injury or an inflammation leading to brain oedema, CSF escapes from the subarachnoid space into the venous sinuses and provides some room so that brain is not pressed.

3. Also carries nutrients to the brain.

BLOOD-BRAIN AND BLOOD-CSF BARRIER

What is blood-brain barrier?

Blood-brain barrier is physiological barrier to the movement of many substances from capillary blood into or out of brain. It maintains constancy of environment in and around brain.

Blood-brain barrier is highly permeable to water, CO_2, O_2, liquid soluble substances like alcohol, anaesthetic drugs, etc. It is slightly permeable to electrolytes and totally impermeable to plasma proteins and non-lipid soluble large organic molecules.

What is blood-CSF barrier?

Transfer of materials from blood to cerebrospinal fluid apparently takes place very slowly because their is blood-CSF barrier. This barrier is mainly associated with the endothelia of choroid plexus and also in part with those of meningeal capillaries of pia. Lipid soluble substances very easily pass through this barrier than non-lipid soluble substances.

AUTONOMIC NERVOUS SYSTEM

What is autonomic nervous system?

Autonomic nervous system is the one which controls the visceral functions.

Give general organization of autonomic nervous system.

The centres for autonomic nervous system are located in the spinal cord, brain stem and hypothalamus.

Cerebral cortex, limbic cortex can transmit impulses to these lower centres and can influence autonomic control. Autonomic system also operates through visceral reflexes. The efferent autonomic signals are transmitted to the body through two major subdivision:

- Sympathetic nervous system.
- Parasympathetic nervous system.

Give physiologic anatomy of sympathetic nervous system.

The sympathetic nerves originate in the spinal cord between segments T_1 and L_2 and pass from here first into the sympathetic chain (chains of ganglia lying on the two sides of the spinal column) and then to the tissues and organs. Each sympathetic pathway from spinal cord to the tissue has two neurons. Preganglionic neuron situated in the intermediolateral horn of the spinal cord. Preganglionic fibres pass through anterior roots of spinal nerves to the ganglia of the sympathetic chain. The neurons of sympathetic ganglia act as postganglionic neurons. From here postganglionic sympathetic fibres pass to the different organs (segmental distribution of sympathetic nerves). Preganglionic sympathetic fibres pass without synapsing from intermediolateral horn of the spinal cord, through sympathetic chain, through splanchnic nerves finally to adrenal medullae. They stimulate secretory cells of adrenal medulla (which act as postganglionic neurons) to secrete hormones epinephrine and norepinephrine. Preganglionic sympathetic fibres release acetylcholine whereas postganglionic sympathetic fibres release norepinephrine (Fig. 13.40).

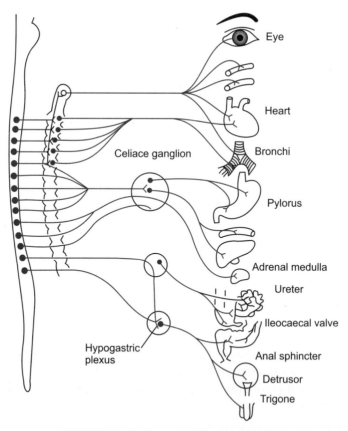

FIGURE 13.40 The sympathetic nervous system.

Give physiologic anatomy of parasympathetic nervous system.

Parasympathetic fibres leave central nervous system through cranial nerves III, VII, IX and X and the second and third sacral spinal nerves (craniosacral outflow). About 75% of fibres pass in vagus nerve.

These fibres are preganglionic fibres. They pass to the organ and synapse in the ganglia which lie near the organ. From the ganglia, postganglionic parasympathetic fibres supply the organ. Pre and postganglionic fibres release acetylcholine at the endings (Fig. 13.41).

Describe the effects of sympathetic stimulation.

Effects of epinephrine and norepinephrine are already described in the chapter on 'Endocrinology'.

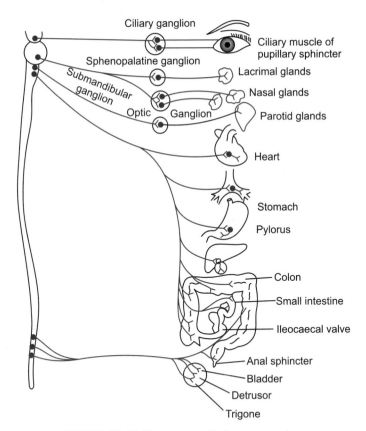

FIGURE 13.41 The parasympathetic nervous system.

Enumerate the effects of parasympathetic stimulation.

Organ	Effect of parasympathetic stimulation
• Eye	
Pupil	Constricted
Ciliary muscles	Contraction (accommodation for near vision)
• Glands	
Nasal	Stimulation of copious secretion containing many enzymes from enzyme-secreting glands
Lacrimal	
Parotid	
Submandibular	
Gastric	
Pancreatic	
Sweat glands	Sweating of palm and hands
Apocrine glands	No effect
• Heart	
Muscle	Slow rate, decreased force of contraction
Coronaries	Dilatation
• Lungs	
Bronchi	Constricted
Blood vessels	Dilated
• Gut	
Lumen	Increased peristalsis and tone
Sphincter	Relaxed
• Liver	Slight glycogen synthesis
• Gall bladder and bile ducts	Contraction
• Kidney	No effect
• Urinary bladder	
Detrusor	Contracted
Trigone	Relaxed
• Penis	Erection

Index